Society, Health and
Population during the
Demographic Transition

Society, Health and Population during the Demographic Transition

Editors: Anders Brändström and Lars-Göran Tedebrand

Almqvist and Wiksell International, Stockholm, Sweden

Report No. 4 from the Demographic Data Base, Umeå university

Proceedings of the international conference "Society, Health, and Population during the Demographic Transition", Umeå university, Sweden, August 18-21, 1986. The conference was financed by The Bank of Sweden Tercentenary Foundation, The Swedish Council of Planning and Coordination of Research, The Swedish Medical Research Council, Umeå Municipality and Umeå university. The printing of this book has been financed by The Swedish Council for Research in the Humanities and Social Sciences.

Cover illustration: Smallpox vaccination in Stockholm. *Ny Illustrerad Tidning 1874*
Compositing work: Anita Bengtsson and Berit Eriksson
© Anders Brändström and Lars-Göran Tedebrand
Distribution: Almqvist & Wiksell International, Stockholm, Sweden
ISBN 91-22-01216-8
Printed by Umeå universitets tryckeri, Humanisthuset, Umeå university, Umeå 1988

Contents

5

Introduction

Lars-Göran Tedebrand

Twenty years ago our knowledge of the decline in western mortality was fairly rudimentary. In England there was little factual material available for groups below the peerage in economic and social status. As far as other countries are concerned, available data for France strongly suggested a lower mortality rate in the second half of the eighteenth century than in the first. Even Swedish data pointed in the same direction.

As a result of the vast expansion of historical population studies during the last decades the main features in the mortality decline have been revealed. In most western countries expectation of life at birth improved during the 19th century. Death rates fell much more heavily among children and teenagers than among adults. However, further studies have revealed interesting national irregularities in the decline of infant and child mortality. Decisive changes in adult mortality did not occur until after 1900. Still we know too little about the details in the epidemiological transition.

The causes of the remarkable decline in crude death rates and the changes in the disease panorama have been under intensive debate during the last 10-15 years. The view that the decline should mainly be attributed to improvements in medical technology has been vigorously challenged by, for instance, Thomas McKeown. According to McKeown long-term changes in mortality rates ought to be explained by advances in material conditions especially nutrition and possibly housing standards.

As is well-known, McKeown in his turn has been challenged in recent years. Historical demographers have argued that the modern rise of population in England, for instance, depended more on a rising birth rate explained by changes in nuptiality and age of marriage than on a falling death rate. The complexity in the nutrition-morbidity/mortality link has been discussed. Other principal explanations as alternatives to nutrition have come into focus: reductions in the virulence of pathogens, acquired immunities, public sanitation etc. The decline in mortality now seems to have been conditioned by a series of complex and often interwoven factors: social, economic, cultural, medical, political, psychological and biological. The real scientific answers to the complexity in the mortality decline and the general improvement in people's health can only be isolated by using a broad interdisciplinary approach.

A variety of materials, methods and theories are used by researchers from different disciplines in many countries when analyzing the determinants behind the changes in morbidity and mortality during the demographic transition. Some of them are reflected in this report volume from the international conference "Society, Health, and Population during the Demographic Transition" held at Umeå University, 18-21 August, 1986. The following sessions were organized: Infant, child and maternal mortality; Causes of death and classification of diseases; Urban disease and mortality; Society and medicine; Health and nutrition and Changes and patterns in rural mortality. All the papers and most of the comments are included in this volume. The comments refer to the original and unrevised versions of the papers.

The organizers and the editors want to express their gratitude towards the funds and the contributors who made the conference possible.

Infant, Child and Maternal Mortality in Western Europe: A Critique

Robert Lee

It is now commonly accepted that there is a clear need to link the analysis and interpretation of population characteristics to their socio-economic context.[1] This is particularly the case in relation to changes over time in infant and child mortality, which have been conditioned by a series of complex mechanisms — social, economic, cultural, psychological and biological.[2] Moreover, in terms of assessing long-term trends in mortality, infant mortality, in particular, remains a central focus for research. Not only could infant deaths selectively account for between 40 and 60 per cent of the total death rate (as Lithell indicates[3]) but in a country such as Sweden, in contrast to Germany and other European states, the secular decline in infant mortality from the late eighteenth century onwards constituted the main component in the overall fall in the death rate.[4] Similarly in Italy, during the period 1863/1865-1953/1955 the combined fall in infant and child deaths (0-5 years) accounted for 63 per cent of the registered decline in the crude death rate.[5] Indeed the traditional model of the demographic transition has often posited a close relationship between improving survival chances of children and the fertility decline,[6] despite the continuing absence of conclusive evidence,[7] and the findings from the Princeton studies that there is little evidence of a general, positive cross-sectional association of marital fertility and mortality in the pre-transitional era,[8] at least at the national aggregate level. This result is confirmed at the regional level in Larsson's analysis of spatial patterns in Swedish nineteenth century demographic change.[9]

The five papers presented in this session, despite methodological differences, provide in their own fashion an important extension to existing knowledge in this field. However, given the time constraints imposed on the discussant, it would be virtually impossible at this juncture to provide a full critique of each separate paper. In order to foster a broader debate, therefore, the following commentary will be structured in such a way as to hopefully stimulate a more general and wide-ranging discussion of some of the central issues raised in this session.

One immediate issue that warrants consideration relates to the level of aggregation and the relative representativeness of the data samples employed in the analysis. Both Margareta Larsson and Oiva Turpeinen base their papers on a regional analysis of demographic data at the rural deanery, or *prosteri,* level, in order to establish changes over time in the spatial pattern of specific variables, specifically infant mortality and fertility. Given that the *prosteri* were essentially administrative units, of a political or ecclesiastical nature, which varied extensively in terms of area and absolute population size, reflecting, perhaps, earlier patterns of land colonization, their suitability for demographic analysis of this kind needs to be carefully examined. It would be useful in this context, particularly in view of the time period covered in Margareta Larsson's paper, to extend the spectrum of potential multivariate relationships and the comparability over time of demographic indices by including available data on employment and occupational structure, population density and migration levels, and the disease panorama. This approach, if feasible, would certainly improve our ability to explain the divergent spatial dynamics of infant mortality and fertility in the period under consideration, and the disparate trends in infant mortality in specific Finnish deaneries. Indeed a more rigorous analysis of the underlying socio-economic structure of the rural deaneries is important, not only because of the apparent existence of different regional demographic regimes in Sweden,[10] but also in view of the general predominance in pre-industrial and industrialising Europe of local demographic peculiarities,[11] "local diversity" across a broad range of demographic variables,[12] and the continuing persistence in nineteenth century Europe of local value systems.[13]

However if the utilisation of regional analysis frequently leads to a reassessment of national models of demographic change, to what extent will this process be replicated at an even lower level of aggregation? The problem of representativeness and comparability, moreover, is also unavoidable in studies based on the family reconstitution of individual parishes and village populations. John Knodel wisely disclaims any pretense at scientific randomness in relation to his sample of 14 German village populations. But given the increasing acceptance by economic and social historians of the need to reconstruct both the problematical term of "peasant" and "community",[14] it is difficult to establish the degree to which Knodel's sample adequately represents the immense diversity in occupational distribution, inheritance systems and land-holding patterns in eighteenth and nineteenth century Germany. The relatively limited number of available family reconstitution studies generally only serves to aggravate the problem, as do unfortunate data deficiencies for Knodel's Bavarian villages for the second half of the eighteenth century.

Similarly, in relation to Margit Rosenberg's fascinating material from Norwegian maternity hospitals, the analysis of changes in birth-weight, breast-feeding, post-partum amenorrhoea and infant mortality over time is complicated by the excessive predominance of unmarried women in the sample, at least until 1887. The *Fødselsstiftelsen* almost certainly had the same function as institutionalised *Gebäranstalten* in Germany: they were a place of last resort, particularly in the earlier decades of the nineteenth century, for unmarried women, frequently dismissed from domestic service or regular employment on account of their illicit pregnancy during the critical third trimester of the pregnancy. They were frequently bereft of effective kinship support, and, to judge from the Munich maternity hospital records, seldom well fed, having travelled extensive distances to seek whatever institutional shelter that might be available. In turn they were obliged to provide the raw material for trainee midwives, were subject to extensive breast-feeding propaganda and, dependent upon their length of hospitalisation, prevented from returning to work immediately after delivery. Given the gradual change over time in the social class composition and marital status of the clients of the *Fødselsstiftelsen,* and the growing acceptability of institutionalised childbirth, great care must be exercised in assessing the significance of changes in recorded birth-weight etc. over any extended period.

A further methodological problem is evident in the case of Margareta Larsson's paper, although, to be fair, she is herself aware of it. In order to assess the changes in the spatial pattern of fertility and infant mortality, calculations are based on mean values for two two-year periods (1805/1806 and 1855/1856 respectively). While this approach may be to some extent acceptable in terms of a fertility analysis, even discounting the importance of regional changes in nuptiality which need to be incorporated in the paper, infant mortality historically was subject to high annual variation[15] and invariably reacted rapidly to short-term economic fluctuations.[16] The explanatory power of the paper would be substantially strengthened if the apparent "uncertainties, arising from temporary disturbances, mainly epidemics"[17] could be analysed in greater detail, with the mean demographic rates for the two two-year periods firmly anchored in a robust historical context by utilising a decennial mean.

There is clearly a general consensus in the papers presented at this session that the pattern and practice of infant feeding exercised a crucial role in determining contemporary levels of infant mortality. The factors affecting the spatial diffusion of different infant feeding practices, however, have still to be explained in a convincing manner. Within this context the recent contributions of Ulla-Britt Lithell have been most salutary in focusing attention on the nature and extent of women's work as a critical factor influencing the viability and extent of breast-feeding. On the basis of this type of approach, infant mortality rates in historical populations can be used as an indicator of "living conditions for women".[18] However, interpretive problems still remain in this area. Lithell's data on infant mortality rates for the decade 1840-1849 reveal a high degree of variation not only between coastal and inland parishes, but also within the two distinct types of parish with analogous employment and economic structures.[19] The evidence for the parish of Vähäkyro is also somewhat contradictory, in that despite the cessation of tar production employing extensive female labour, and a concomitant improvement in women's overall living conditions, "... one of the main agricultural regions in Ostrobothnia showed one of the highest infant mortality rates during the nineteenth century".[20] Perhaps the persistence of relatively high infant mortality rates in this specific parish was primarily a function of emergent agrarian capitalism, linked with the growth of a significant export trade, which, in turn, had important ramifications for the labour function of both married and single women, as was the case in other territories bordering on the Baltic in the early decades of the nineteenth century.[21]

However the growing concern with the organisation of peasant society, specifically in relation to the nature and extent of women's work within both the family home and the local agrarian economy gives rise to a number of further interesting questions.[22] If the work function of women was such a critical variable in determining infant feeding practices, how was it that radically different approaches to infant care could apparently co-exist within relatively small regional areas, as the data on breast-feeding in Sweden for the period 1869-1874 indicate?[23] Moreover there were areas where both artificial and breast-feeding methods existed side by side.[24] Clearly any increased maternal involvement in subsistence-related activity will inevitably mean that less time will be available for child and specifically infant care, and the abandonment or premature curtailment of breast-feeding will lead to reduced immunity for infants. But are we to assume that longer-term fluctuations and trends in infant mortality, such as the particularly high level of infant mortality reported for certain localities in the second half of the seventeenth century[25] were also directly linked to critical changes in the nature of women's work or a significant cyclical shift in the delicate balance of female familial and work responsibilities?

Furthermore, are we to assume that the inter-familial distribution of resources has always in pre-industrial and industrialising Western Europe conformed with an established gender hierarchy, with mothers required to maximise their subsistence-related activities according to seasonal or cyclical need, and consistently obliged to sacrifice their own share of familial resources? Or is it the case, as Medick and Sabean have argued, that the increasing spread of commercial and capitalist relations in the nineteenth century reinforced the existing unequal distribution of social power, above all between men and women, with important consequences for the extension of differential gender-specific health conditions?[26] How can one reconcile this apparently reactive role of women, determined primarily by changing economic conditions of work and employment, with the assertion that women were not powerless in preindustrial families, although the constraints of family membership may well have greatly affected their opportunities for individual autonomy?[27] If women's work in agriculture was traditionally "equally hard",[28] with important demographic consequences, a German proverb from the Bremen region would seem to indicate that this had always tended to be the case: *"Wo die Frau arbeitet nicht, da gibt kein Brodt im Hause".*[29]

It has also been argued that the relatively quick response to official campaigns designed to promulgate breast feeding, at least in certain areas of Sweden in the nineteenth century,[30] is a clear indication of the absence of any significant cultural or economic determinism in the sphere of infant feeding practices. If it was the case, as Lithell has indicated in an earlier publication,[31] that breast-feeding was not practised in Petalax because husbands claimed that it destroyed the beauty of their wives, then clearly educational improvements and pro-breast-feeding campaigns may well have had an important impact on infant feeding practices. However it is salutary to note, in this respect, that J.P. Frank's proposal of compulsory breast-feeding *(Stillzwang)* within his concept of medical police was not taken up by any absolutist state in eighteenth century Germany. Moreover the process of medicalisation in the nineteenth century was not a linear development and other areas of compulsory regulation, such as smallpox inoculation, frequently failed to provide the nascent medical profession with any immediate improvement in their credibility in the eyes of the general population. The state in Hamburg, for example, repeatedly attempted to intervene to reduce infant mortality, specifically by controlling the extent of wet-nursing. But these attempts were largely ineffective, and the last "angel-maker" *(Engelmacherinnen)* was condemned and executed as late as 1904 for murdering infants in her charge.

Indeed if cultural factors affected infant feeding practices and group control determined individual choice,[35] then it is equally relevant to examine available data for any potential differential treatment of daughters,[36] particularly as evidence for a gender-specific distinction in infant and child care has already been presented for nineteenth century Ireland.[37] It is clearly difficult to decide how much of a sex mortality differential was biologically determined and how much was the result of broader environmental factors, as these two sets of factors were inextricably intertwined.[38] However John Knodel's findings are very explicit in this respect, with on balance, equal probabilities of dying for both sexes between exact ages one and five.[39] A similar focus in other studies of village and parish populations would clearly be desirable. However demographers would probably benefit considerably from the incorporation in their analysis of trends in vital rates of historical and ethnographical material, even if documenting changes in peasant tradition and customs "will be difficult enough".[40] Infant feeding practices and childbirth itself were often rooted in specific attitudes toward the life and death of children, which, in turn, frequently reflected the contemporary conditions of peasant life. Childbirth, for example, was seldom allowed to interfere significantly with the work process, illegitimate babies were frequently born in the privy, with the birth experienced primarily as a bowel evacuation. Moreover, according to Schulte,[41] the South German practice of *himmeln lassen* (to let die) can be viewed as an accepted and customary form of postnatal family planning. Unless historical studies of village populations and rural communities can incorporate a broader analysis of ethnographical material, our ability to correctly interpret the complex causal factors affecting trends in key demographic variables, such as infant and child mortality, will invariably be impaired.

The evidence presented on the relationship between socio-economic status and the mortality risks of infants and children, however, remains somewhat inconclusive. Ulla-Britt Lithell's data from Vähäkyro does not reveal any significant difference in the infant mortality rate for farmers and non-farmers,[42] although it is conceded that there may well have been a substantial variation between the expanding group of lodgers and other socio-economic groups in terms of infant mortality rates. John Knodel finds little association between socio-economic status and child mortality risks, and Oiva Turpeinen, in an earlier publication,[43] found no specific links between infant mortality levels and social or economic differences in the Pietarsaari deanery. And yet other authors, utilising family reconstitution data and contemporary statistical material, have found an inverse relationship between economic status and infant mortality levels.[44] In Cartmel, differences in child mortality were greater between social groups than between the sexes, and in Ditfurt the children of *Kossaten* and labourers had a higher life expectancy than the children of farmers *(Ackermänner)*.[45] Indeed according to Imhof the propertyless were in any case forced to rely on breast-feeding because they were simply too poor to buy milk substitutes.[46] Economic necessity, therefore, condemned them to practice breast-feeding and to enjoy, by definition, lower levels of infant mortality. To some extent this hypothesis is borne out in Margit Rosenberg's paper which indicates a substantially longer breast-feeding period among the lowest social strata, at least in the pre-1920 sample.[47] Indeed it has frequently been assumed that in a population with a low standard of living, breast-feeding, ceteris paribus, is likely to be relatively common.[48]

Occupational evidence, in this respect, remains somewhat confusing and contradictory. The apparent absence of any clear association between socio-economic status and the probability of dying before age five in the sample fourteen villages implicitly tends to undermine the assumption that infant feeding practices, child care and relative levels of infant and child mortality were predicated on the living conditions of women. Peasant society, throughout many parts of Western Europe, was already highly stratified by the early eighteenth century, and the so-called "individualization of agriculture",[49] the expansion of freehold peasant ownership in countries such as Sweden,[50] and the broader structural changes associated with the development of agrarian capitalism had aggravated even further existing

14

socio-economic differentials. Moreover, in terms of marriage patterns, peasant society frequently evinced a high level of socio-economic group endogomy.[51] To portray German village life, as a whole, as having been characterised by "pervasive poverty",[52] as a means of explaining the relatively homogeneous levels of mortality across different socio-economic groupings is patently incorrect in the light of the differential responsiveness of specific sections of peasant society in the latter decades of the eighteenth century to macro-economic price stimuli,[53] and the evidence for significant economic stratification in most rural areas from inventory data. But if the practice of infant feeding and general attitudes to child care were not determined by economic criteria, but by tradition and custom (however defined), reinforced, perhaps on a face-to-face basis, through dominant group control, then infant and child mortality rates cannot be used as a useful indicator of general living standards or the gender-specific position of women. Moreover, to complicate the picture even further, Kintner has also argued in relation to German data, that the relationship between infant feeding practices and local customs cannot be analysed statistically.[54]

The utilisation of occupational evidence as a proxy for socio-economic status, is in any case itself problematical. A person's occupation could frequently differ from one register and from one year to another,[55] and socio-economic indices tend to become obsolete over time.[56] Categories such as "farmers" and "non-farmers"[57] appear to be rather crude and impressive, if we are concerned to elucidate the precise relationship between the nature of the family economy, socio-economic status and infant and child mortality. Equally in relation to the sample fourteen German villages reservations must still exist (as I am sure John Knodel well knows), concerning the precise occupational groupings employed in the analysis. What specific criteria are we to employ to distinguish between the different categories of "farmers"? Are those employed within the domestic economy in proto-industrial production to be classified as "proletarian" (itself a rather problematic term within an eighteenth century context), or among the artisans and skilled? To what extent did changes in the relative terms of trade between agricultural and non-agricultural production significantly affect the balance of activity in the "mixed" category? Indeed is there not an implicit risk of creating an a-historical construct by assuming that a farmer in East Friesland, with fertile land and surplus factors of production, specifically manure, enjoyed the same economic standard of living as his impoverished and undercapitalised equivalent in Bavaria? If this is the case, then irrespective of the excellence of the demographic analysis, the relationship between socio-economic status and differential infant and child mortality must remain an open question.

Differentials in socio-economic status, however, also have implications, on a gender-specific basis, for maternal nutritional levels. Although it is true to say that even modern studies are still frequently inadequate in terms of exposing the precise mechanisms by which nutrition is related to death,[58] an adverse or deteriorating maternal nutritional status will affect neonatal mortality levels, specifically through greater prematurity, an increased likelihood of difficult labour and a lower birth weight. Malnutrition and severe poverty, if associated with vitamin deficiencies and rickets, might also lead to contracted pelvises and a higher frequency of stillbirths.[59] Significantly, as in the case of late nineteenth century Montreal,[60] Margit Rosenberg reports a decrease in average birth weight, albeit on a far more modest scale and conditioned, perhaps, by factors that may well have been specific to the disproportionate number of unmarried women in the sample. The explanation tentatively offered for this phenomenon is that "periods of unemployment and reduced wages" for women employed in the textile industry and match factories, not only counterbalanced the "general rise" in economic life,[61] and the fall in the relative price of foodstuffs, but presumably led to a noticeable deterioration in nutritional levels. However no employment or wage data are utilised in the analysis and no attempt is made to explore the potential effect of environmental factors, including overcrowding, population density etc., in a sufficiently rigorous fashion.[62] The problem is further compounded by the amalgamation of material from three separate urban centers, with potentially different environmental structures, into one uniform data set.

On the other hand Oiva Turpeinen's dramatic portrayal of the cataclysmic effects of the 1868 catastrophe in Finland on infant mortality levels, which might have been able to elucidate the relationship between chronic malnutrition and this key demographic variable, fails to realise its full potential. It is impossible to explore the possible existence of a malnutrition threshold because of the failure to incorporate in the analysis adequate data on neonatal mortality trends in the period under consideration. Moreover any analysis of this relationship on the basis of the radically changing regional pattern of infant mortality would be complicated by the possible enforced resumption of breast-feeding in traditionally non-breast-feeding deaneries, as a result of the slaughter of animals and reduced cow milk supplies. However, given data availability, the crisis of 1868 can clearly be utilised as a means of providing a more rigorous assessment of the relationship between nutrition and infant mortality.

Nutritional standards, however, particularly among the working-class depended on a wide range of individual factors. Within an urban context food was only one of many items of expenditure and changes in accommodation expenditure often had immediate short-term ramifications in terms of outgoings on food. The price of basic items such as bread, even in the nineteenth century, fluctuated considerably and any objective analysis of the nutritional content of a typical working-class diet is hampered by the existence of widespread food adulteration.[63] More significantly rapid urbanisation may well have accentuated the severity of the problem of food adulteration, and polluted water mains together with the difficulty of supplying milk to urban centers,[64] may have contributed to widespread milk adulteration. Equally

16

damaging from a nutritional point of view would have been excessive alcohol consumption during pregnancy (and per capita alcohol consumption in Sweden rose dramatically during the nineteenth century),[65] as well as the increasing recourse to patent medicines containing narcotics.[66]

There is clearly a need to examine the relative effect of broader environmental factors on both maternal nutrition and the susceptibility of infants and children to disease and death. This is the case both in relation to the developing urban population centers of nineteenth century Europe, and to rural areas, where the impact of sanitary improvements and new housing developments remained extremely restricted before the beginning of the twentieth century. If infected water and milk accounted for a significant proportion of infant deaths from gastro-intestinal disorders, particularly during the summer months, inadequate housing, poor ventilation and persistent damp directly encouraged bronchitis, pleurisy and pneumonia among infants in autumn and winter.[67] Moreover poor sewage and endemic dirt in densely populated urban areas provided the perfect background for the spread of infectious diseases to which infants inevitably were specifically susceptible. Given the evidence of high urban-rural infant mortality differentials in the nineteenth century,[68] it would be particularly useful if greater attention could be focussed on the complex factors affecting trends in urban infant and child mortality over time. Even within the context of the Finnish crisis of 1868, urban centers, with a more established framework for charitable poor relief, may well have witnessed a disproportionate level of selective immigration from adjacent, or more distant, rural areas, with clear implications for the recorded trends in infant mortality in rural deaneries.

Inevitably it has been impossible to do full justice to the range of results contained in the papers presented at this session, or to pursue a wide range of specific queries. Collectively the five papers under consideration extend our understanding considerably of the complex social, economic and cultural factors affecting historical trends in infant, child and maternal mortality. But it cannot be a coincidence that the respective authors of these papers come from such a wide spectrum of disciplines—demography, history, sociology and informatics. Perhaps it is only on the basis of such a broad interdisciplinary approach that the factors determining levels, trends and differentials in these critical demographic variables will be fully understood.

Notes

1. E.A. Wrigley, 'The Prospects for Population History'. *Journal of Interdisciplinary History,* 12, 2 (1981), p. 115.

2. G. Masuy-Stroobant, 'La Surmortalité infantile des Flandres au cours de la deuxième moitié du XIXe siècle. Mode d'alimentation ou mode de développement?', *Annales de Démographie Historique* (1983), p. 231.

3. U-B. Lithell, 'Child Care—A Mirror of Women's Living Conditions. A community study representing 18th and 19th century Ostrobothnia in Finland', *In this volume.*

4. A. Brändström, *'De Kärlekslösa Mödrarna'. Spädbarnsdödligheten i Sverige under 1800-talet med särskild hänsyn till Nedertorneå.* Umeå (1984), passim, and specifically p. 241.

5. E. Hoffman, *The Sources of Mortality Changes in Italy since Unification* (New York 1981), p. 178.

6. G. Carlsson, 'The Decline of Fertility: Innovation or Adjustment Process', *Population Studies,* vol. 20 (1966), pp. 149-174.

7. R. Gehrmann, 'Einsichten und Konsequenzen aus neueren Forschungen zum generativen Verhalten im demographischen Ancien Régime und in der Transitionsphase', *Zeitschrift für Bevölkerungswissenschaft,* Vol. 5 (1979), p. 475.

8. P.C. Mathiessen and J.C. McCann, 'The Role of Mortality in the European Fertility Transition: Aggregate-Level Relations', S.H. Preston (Ed.), *The Effect of Infant and Child Mortality on Fertility* (New York 1978), p. 15.

9. M. Larsson, 'The Old in the New: Spatial Patterns in the 19th Century Demographic Change', *In this volume,* Ibid. *Fruktsamhetsmönster, produktionsstruktur och sekularisering* (Stockholm 1984).

10. G. Sundbärg, 'Bidrag till Sveriges officiella statistik, serie A: Befolkningsstatistik', *Statistiska Centralbyrån* (Stockholm 1890, 1900).

11. D.S. Smith, 'A Homeostatic Regime: Patterns in West European Family Reconstitution Studies', R.D. Lee (Ed.), *Population Patterns in the Past* (New York 1977), p. 27.

12. J. Knodel, 'Child Mortality and Reproduction Behavior in German Village Populations in the Past. A Micro-Level Analysis of the Replacement Effect', *University of Michigan. Population Studies Center, Research Report,* No. 81-1 (1981).

13. O. Löfgren, 'Arbeitsteilung und Geschlechterrollen in Schweden', *Ethnologia Scandinavica* (1975), pp. 49-72. Ibid. 'Family and Household among Scandinavian Peasants', *Ethnologia Scandinavica* (1974), pp. 17-52.

14. R.J. Evans and W.R. Lee (Eds.), *The German Peasantry. Conflict and Community in Rural Society from the Eighteenth to the Twentieth Centuries* (London 1986), p. x.

15. O. Turpeinen, 'The Percentage of Deaths under One Year of Age of All Deaths in Finland in 1749-1865', *Yearbook of Population Research in Finland* (1984), p. 47.

16. T. Bengtsson and R. Ohlsson, 'Population and Economic Fluctuations in Sweden, 1749-1914', T. Bengtsson, G. Fridlizius and R. Ohlsson (Eds.), *Pre-Industrial Population Change* (Lund 1984), p. 286.

17. Larsson (1984), p. 3.

18. Lithell (1986), p. 22.

19. Ibid.

20. Ibid.

21. W.R. Lee, 'The Impact of Agrarian Change on Women's Work and Child Care in Early Nineteenth-Century Prussia', J.C. Fout (Ed.), *German Women in the Nineteenth Century. A Social History* (New York 1984), pp. 234-255.

22. Ibid, p. 249.

23. G. Broström, A. Brändström and L-Å. Persson., 'The Impact of Breastfeeding Patterns on Infant Mortality in a 19th Century Swedish Parish, *Newsletter No. 1 from the Demographic Data Base* (Umeå 1981), p. 29.

24. Brändström (1984), p. 245.

25. A. Bellettini and A. Samoggia., 'Evolution differentielle et mouvement saisonnier de la mortalité infantile et enfantine dans la Banlieue de Bologne (XVIIᵉ XIXᵉ siècles)', *Annales de Démographie Historique* (1983), pp. 195-207.

26. H. Medick and D.W. Sabean, 'Interest and Emotion in Family and Kinship Studies: a Critique of Social History and Anthropology' H. Medick and D.W. Sabean (Eds.), *Interest and Emotion. Essays on the Study of Family and Kinship* (Cambridge 1984), pp. 14-15.

27. L.A. Tilly, J.W. Scott and M. Cohen., 'Women's Work and European Fertility Patterns', *Journal of Interdisciplinary History,* 6 (1976), pp. 447-476.

28. E.S. Riemer and J.C. Fout (Eds.), *European Women. A Documentary History, 1789-1945* (1983), p. 4.

29. T. Hodgkin, *Travels in the North of Germany.* (London 1820), Vol. 1, p. 266.

30. Broström, Brändström and Persson (1981).

31. U-B. Lithell, 'Breast-feeding Habits and Their Relation to Infant Mortality and Marital Fertility', *Journal of Family History* (1981), p. 183.

32. A.E. Imhof, 'Säuglingssterblichkeit im europäischen Kontext, 17-20. Jahrhundert. Ueberlegungen zu einem Buch von Anders Brändström', *Newsletter no 2 from The Demographic Data Base* (Umeå 1984), p. 7.

33. C. Huerkamp, 'The History of Smallpox Vaccination in Germany: a First Step in the Medicalization of the General Public', *Journal of Contemporary History,* 20 (1985), pp. 617-635.

34. R-J. Evans, *Death in Hamburg. Society and Politics in the Cholera Years 1830-1910* (Oxford, forthcoming), ms. p. 265.

35. Smith (1977).

36. R. Wall, 'Inferring Differential Neglect of Females from Mortality Data', *Annales de Démographie Historique* (1981), pp. 119 130.

37. R.E. Kennedy, *The Irish: Emigration, Marriage and Fertility* (1973), pp. 52-53.

38. R.D. Retheford, *The Changing Sex Differential in Mortality* (1975), p. 15.

39. J. Knodel, 'Two Centuries of Infant, Child and Maternal Mortality in German Village Populations', *Umeå conference paper* (1986).

40. J. Knodel, and C. Wilson., 'The Secular Increase in Fecundity in German Village Populations', *Population Studies,* Vol. 35 (1981), p. 79.

41. R. Schulte, 'Infanticide in Rural Bavaria in the Nineteenth Century' H. Medick and D.W. Sabean (Eds.), *Interest and Emotion. Essays on the Study of Family and Kinship* (Cambridge 1984), p. 91.

42. Lithell (1986).

43. O. Turpeinen, 'Infant Mortality in Finland 1749-1865', *Scandinavian Economic History Review,* XXVII, 1 (1979), pp. 1-23.

44. C. Winberg, *Folkökning och Proletarisering* (Partille 1975).

45. R. Finlay, 'Differential Child Mortality in Pre-industrial England: the Example of Cartmel, Cumbria, 1600-1750', Annales de Démographie Historique (1981), pp. 67-79; P. Stephen, 'Geburtlichkeit und Kindersterblichkeit in einem Dorf im 17. und 18. Jahrhundert', *Aerztliche Jugendkunde,* Bd. 75, Heft 3 (1984), p. 178-189.

46. Imhof (1984) p. 13.

47. M. Rosenberg, 'Birth-Weight, Breast-feeding, Postpartum Amenorrhoea and Infant Mortality in 3 Norwegian Cities during the Late 19th and early 20th Century', *In this volume.*

48. Lithell (1986).

49. O. Osterud, *Agrarian Structure and Peasant Politics in Scandinavia* (Oslo 1978), p. 113.

50. K. Tønnessen, 'Tenancy, Freehold and Enclosure in Scandinavia from the Seventeenth to the Nineteenth Century', *Scandinavian Journal of History,* 6 (1981), pp. 202-203.

51. Smith (1977).

52. Knodel (1986).

53. H. Harnisch, *Kapitalistische Agrarreform und Industrielle Revolution* (Weimar 1984); Ibid, 'Peasants and Markets: The Background to the Agrarian Reforms in Feudal Prussia East of the Elbe, 1760-1807', Evans and Lee (1986), pp. 37-70.

54. H.J. Kintner, 'Trends and Regional Differences in Breast-Feeding in Germany from 1871 to 1937', *Journal of Family History,* Summer (1985), pp. 163-182.

55. Lithell (1982), p. 74.

56. R. Spree, 'Die Entwicklung der differentiellen Säuglingssterblichkeit in Deutschland seit der Mitte des 19. Jahrhunderts', A.E. Imhof (Ed.), *Mensch und Gesundheit in der Geschichte* (Husum 1981), passim.

57. Lithell (1986).

58. S.C. Watkins and E. van de Walle, 'Nutrition, Mortality, and Population Size: Malthus' Court of Last Resort', R.I. Rothberg and T.K. Rabb (Eds.), *Hunger and History. The Impact of Changing Food Production and Consumption Patterns on Society* (Cambridge 1985), p. 16.

59. Evans (forthcoming), p. 244.

60. W.P. Ward and P.C. Ward, 'Infant Birth Weight and Nutrition in Industrializing Montreal', *American Historical Review* (1984), pp. 324-345.

20

61. Rosenberg (1986).

62. A.I. Hermalin and J. Knodel, 'Biological Factors affecting Infant and Child Mortality: An Assessment Based on 18th and 19th Century Reproductive Histories', *Population Studies Center, University of Michigan,* 83-37 (1983), p. 18.

63. Evans (forthcoming), p. 215.

64. B. Duden and U. Ottmueller, *Der suesse Bronnen. Zur Geschichte des Stillens* (Courage 1978), Heft 2.

65. G. Fridlizius, 'Sex Differential Mortality and Socio-Economic Change. Sweden 1750-1910', *In this volume.*

66. Ward and Ward (1984), p. 337.

67. Evans (forthcoming).

68. J. Knodel, 'Town and County in Nineteenth-Century Germany: A Review of Urban-Rural Differentials in Demographic Behavior', *Social Science History,* 1, 3 (1977), pp. 356-382.

Two Centuries of Infant, Child and Maternal Mortality in German Village Populations

John Knodel

Knowledge about mortality for Germany prior to the latter part of the nineteenth century, especially for the population living outside of cities, must be based primarily on information contained in registers of deaths or burials kept by ecclesiastical authorities in local parishes. The development of the family reconstitution technique in historical demography, in connection with procedures to analyze the data it produces in ways that avoid or minimize potential inherent biases, has considerably expanded our ability to document the conditions of mortality under which German villagers lived in the past. While it is difficult to determine adult mortality with any degree of precision from family reconstitution data, relatively precise estimates of infant and child mortality are possible. In addition, estimates of the special situation of maternal mortality can also be derived without great difficulty.

The purpose of the present paper is to explore levels, trends, and differentials in mortality for a sample of 14 German village populations during the eighteenth and nineteenth centuries based on reconstituted family histories contained in village genealogies *(Ortssippenbücher)*, a source unique to Germany. The focus is on infant, child and maternal mortality, although rough estimates of life expectancy at birth are also presented. The villages are located in five different states or regions of Germany: 4 in Baden, 1 in Württemberg, 3 in Bavaria, 4 in Waldeck, and 2 in East Friesland. While the villages cannot be considered a random sample of the rural population of the period, they do cover a moderate range of demographic conditions and represent diversity in occupational distribution, inheritance systems, and religious affiliation. One interesting feature of Germany during the period of study was the sharp regional differences in the prevalence and duration of breastfeeding and this is also reflected in the sample. For example, the villages in Bavaria are located in areas where, at the turn of the nineteenth century at least, most mothers either did not breastfeed their infants at all or did so for a very short time, while in the area of the East Friesland villages, almost all mothers nursed their infants and the average duration of breastfeeding was close to a year.

The data set on which the present study is based has been developed in connection with a broader study of demographic behavior in the past. Thus, except as noted in the discussion of maternal mortality, the analysis is limited to births to couples for whom complete reproductive histories are known, i.e. only couples that could be considered in observation until the death of the first spouse to die. In general, the data appear to be reasonably accurate with the exception of certain fairly readily identifiable periods of incomplete or imprecise registration of infant and child deaths. Data from these periods are excluded from the present study. Because of apparently variable treatment of stillbirths in the parish registers of the different villages, especially between Catholic and Protestant villages, stillbirths are included in the infant mortality rates unless specifically indicated to the contrary. Overall, the data represent more than 9,000 reproductive histories, covering some 48,000 births. The nature and quality of the genealogies, the rules of selection, and the nature of the sample are discussed at some length in a forthcoming monograph.[1]

Trends and levels of infant and child mortality

National-level life tables providing detailed information on age-specific levels of mortality are available for Germany only after 1870. Several German states produced life tables for earlier years although only exceptionally for periods prior to the mid-nineteenth century. These data indicate a steady and substantial decline in the mortality of children above age one, as well as some evidence of decline in infant mortality during the last third of the nineteenth century when the first national-level life tables were compiled.[2] There is little evidence available from official statistics, however, to determine how long these trends had been under way. Given the different implications of alternative sequences in fertility and mortality decline for understanding the demographic transition, and the real possibility that infant and child mortality trends may have differed substantially, information on long term trends prior to the period covered by official statistics takes on added importance.[3]

The probabilities of dying before age one ($_1q_0$), between exact ages one and five ($_4q_1$), and between exact ages five and 15 ($_{10}q_5$) are shown in Figure 1 from the mid-eighteenth century to the early twentieth century for the combined sample as well as regional groupings of villages. While the combined sample is clearly composed of a non-random selection of German villages, results for the end of the nineteenth century correspond reasonably closely to the national levels infant and child mortality indicated by official statistics.[4] At a more local level, both the level and trend of infant mortality indicated for the four Baden villages during the last half of the nineteenth century correspond closely to the official statistics at the district level.[5]

Figure 1. Trends in infant and child mortality.

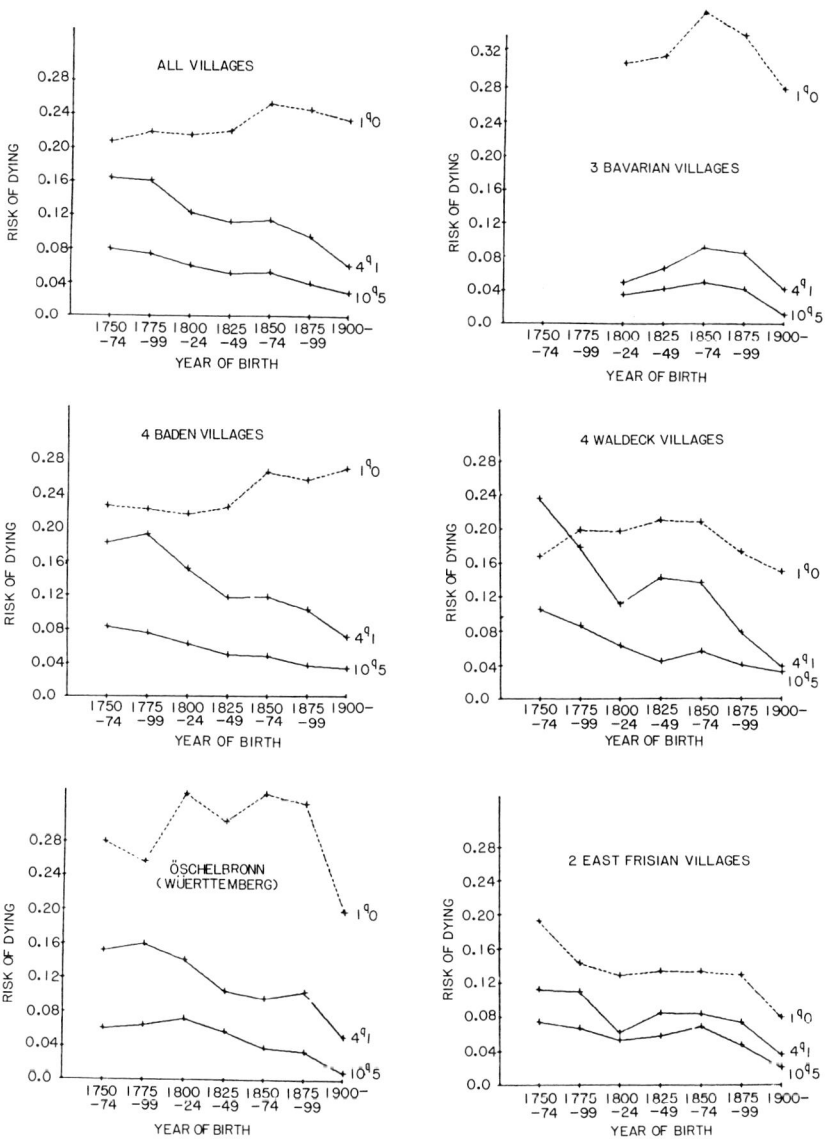

Notes: The calculations of $_1q_o$ include stillbirths.

Probably the most striking feature of the results is the indication that infant and child mortality generally follow divergent paths from the end of the eighteenth to the beginning of the twentieth century. For the sample as a whole, infant mortality reaches its highest level during the third quarter of the nineteenth century and declines only moderately by the start of the twentieth century, while in contrast the probabilities of dying between ages one and five and between ages five and 15 decline almost steadily from the mid-eighteenth century. The pronounced rise in infant mortality during the third quarter of the nineteenth century, largely evident for the sample as a whole, is absent in the Waldeck and East Frisian villages. The modest fall in infant mortality for births from 1900 onward for the combined sample is the result of a slight increase in infant mortality in the Baden villages combined with a sharp drop everywhere else. The general pattern of an earlier decline in child mortality than in infant mortality, however, holds for most of the regional groupings with the main exception being the Bavarian villages for which equivalent indices are shown only from 1800 on because of the lack of exact death dates for many infant and child deaths prior to that time. For the East Frisian villages, the trends in infant and child mortality are somewhat closer to being parallel than elsewhere. Given that infant mortality is at a higher level than child mortality, even parallel declines would reflect greater proportionate reductions in child than in infant mortality.

The tardiness in the decline in infant mortality relative to improvements in mortality at childhood ages above one appears not to be unique to Germany but rather a common feature of the demographic transition in much of Europe.[6] One possible contributing factor to the decline of child mortality, particularly at ages immediately following infancy, was the introduction of smallpox inoculation which became compulsory in a number of German states very early in the nineteenth century.[7]

A realistic assessment of the linkages between changes in mortality and fertility associated with the demographic transition clearly needs to incorporate measures of mortality which go beyond just the first year of life. In the case of Germany, judging from the results for the combined sample of all villages, improvements in child mortality were to some extent cancelled out by rising infant mortality during parts of the eighteenth and nineteenth centuries. The result is that the probability of surviving to age 15 fluctuated within a relatively narrow range until the beginning of the twentieth century.

Substantial differences in the levels of infant and child mortality for the various regional groupings of villages are also apparent. One important determinant of these differences, especially in infant mortality, was undoubtedly the variation in the prevailing infant feeding practices. The highest infant mortality rates are found for the Bavarian villages which are located in areas where breastfeeding was known to be relatively rare during the nineteenth century, while the lowest infant mortality was found for the East Frisian villages where breastfeeding was probably most extensive.

Interestingly, the risk of dying in the first four years following infancy is relatively low in the Bavarian villages perhaps reflecting a selection process in which only the hardier infants survived the high mortality before age one. One possible mechanism accounting for the relatively low early child mortality in the Bavarian villages might be the absence of weanling diarrhea since many children in the Bavarian villages were either not breastfed at all or weaned long before the end of the first year of life. In other villages, where a substantial proportion of children might have been breastfed longer than a year, the increased risk of mortality following weanling might contribute significantly to the early child mortality rate.

As mentioned above, the estimation of adult mortality from family reconstitution data is considerably more problematic than the calculation of infant and child mortality. Without information on mortality risks at all ages, it is not possible to calculate a complete life table and thus not possible to calculate directly an estimate of life expectancy at birth. One alternative is to indirectly estimate life expectancy through the application of model life tables (i.e., generalized hypothetical life tables embodying typical age patterns of mortality risks at different overall levels of mortality). All that is required is to determine which model life table embodies mortality risks in infancy and childhood that match most closely those of the observed population. The life expectancy at birth indicated in that model life table is then taken as the life expectancy corresponding to the observed data. While the procedure is relatively simple, the validity of the results is uncertain and thus can be considered only as rough estimates, especially when they refer to periods or regions other than those on which the construction of the model life tables are based. Indeed, the use of model life tables within historical demography has not been without criticism.[8]

Probably the best known and most widely used model life tables are the regional model life tables developed at Princeton University by Coale and Demeny.[9] They are based on over 300 actual life tables thought to be of reasonable accuracy. Most refer to European populations or populations settled by Europeans overseas and date from the last third of the nineteenth century through the post-World War II period. Four different regional "families" of model life tables were created: The West Tables cover much of Western Europe as well as overseas European settlements and other non-European populations; the East tables cover mainly Central European countries and draw heavily on German life tables; the North and South tables are derived mainly from life tables from Scandinavian and Southern European countries respectively. The East, North, and South groups are separated out because they revealed age patterns with substantial and significant deviations from the world average while the West pattern is in a sense a residual one thought to have most general applicability.

The four regional model life table families differ substantially from one another with respect to the age structure of mortality within infancy and childhood as well as with respect to the relationship of infant and child mortality to adult mortality. Since German life tables including a number from the late nineteenth century were an important component of those determining the East model, we might expect the East model to fit the experience of the sample villages most closely. In actuality, the situation is more complicated both because there were substantial variations regionally within the sample in the age pattern of mortality during the first years of life and because trends in infant and child mortality diverged during the period under observation. The result is that the model life table family which best fits the age pattern of mortality in infancy and childhood differs both over time and across regional clusters of villages.

The values of $_1q_0$, $_4q_1$, and $_5q_5$ as observed in the entire sample over time and in several regional clusters of villages for selected periods are compared in Figure 2 with the equivalent model life table values from each of the four model families. The model life table values for $_4q_1$ and $_5q_5$ are equivalent in the sense that in each case they are associated with a value of $_1q_0$ that is identical to the observed value (after excluding stillbirths).[10] Thus the observed and model values of $_1q_0$ are necessarily the same but the observed and model values at older ages agree only if actual and model age patterns are identical. The comparison is extended only to age 10 rather than to age 15 in order to minimize possible biases that might affect the observed values of older childhood mortality due to the selection of cases to be included in the analysis.[11] The purpose of this comparison is to show how the age patterns of mortality in infancy and childhood varied over time and among regional groupings of villages.

One distinctive feature of the East pattern of mortality, to which Germany is generally assumed to conform, is the relatively low childhood mortality compared to a given level of infant mortality. This same pattern is evident for the combined sample of all villages for the years 1850 onward and the fit between the East model values and the observed values is quite close. This pattern, however, is a result of the declining trend in early childhood mortality during the nineteenth century in the face of persistent, even slightly rising, infant mortality. Thus for the first half of the nineteenth century, the age structure of infant and child mortality differs from that in the second half and, for the combined sample of all villages, no longer resembles the East pattern. Rather it is much closer to that embodied in the West pattern. Moreover, for the eighteenth century, prior to the decline in child mortality, results for the combined sample resemble most closely the North pattern. Thus in the case of the combined sample of villages, the divergent trends in infant and child mortality over the eighteenth and nineteenth centuries resulted in shifts in the age pattern of mortality under age ten sufficient to alter the fit with respect to the model life table family to which the observed experience conformed most closely. Schofield and Wrigley in studying infant and child mortality in England also found that a sufficient change in the age pattern occurred to af-

28

Figure 2. Observed values of $_4q_1$ and $_5q_5$ and corresponding regional model life table values matched on $_1q_0$.

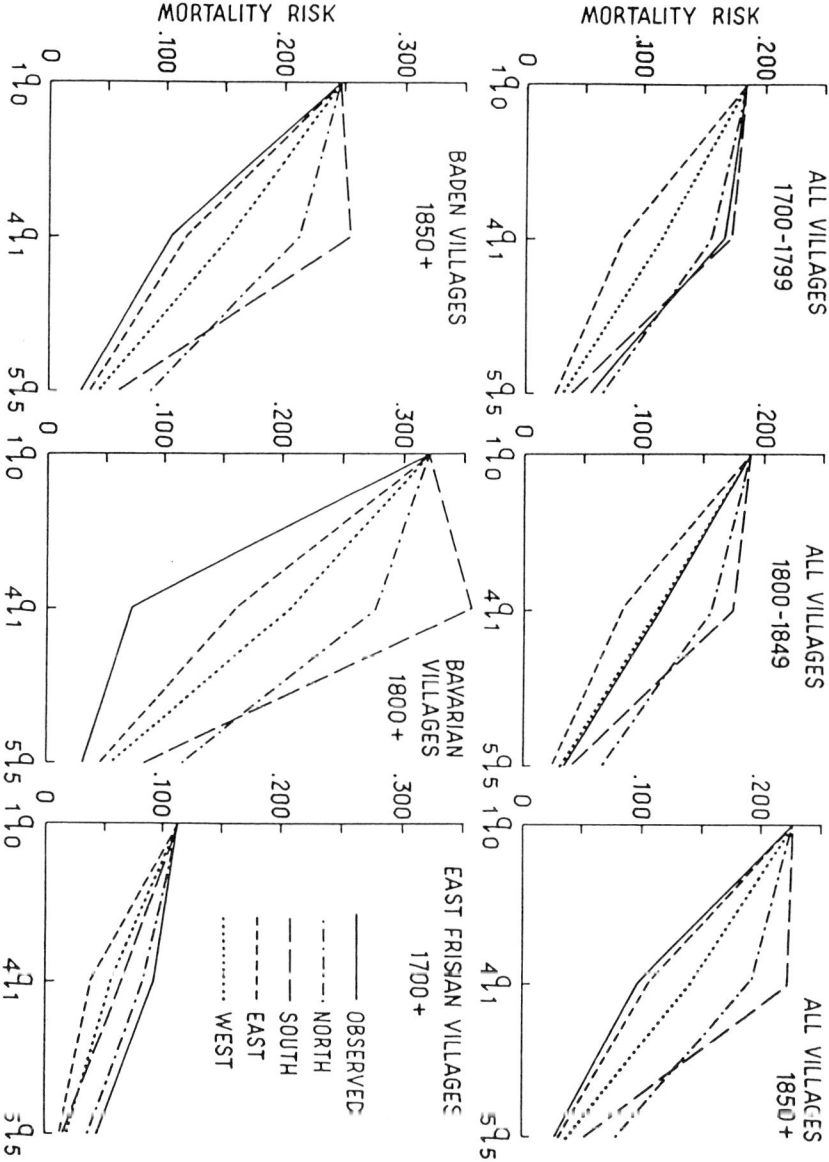

Notes: Values of $_1q_0$ exclude stillbirths.

fect the extent to which the observed data best fit particular model life table families.[12] These results caution against assuming that mortality patterns as observed in the late nineteenth century or during the twentieth century on which the different families of model life tables have been determined, will necessarily apply for earlier periods. In the case of Germany, it appears that as far as mortality under age ten is concerned, the distinctive East pattern only emerged toward the end of the nineteenth century and may not have applied during earlier years.

Also shown in Figure 2 are equivalent comparisons for several regional groupings of villages between the observed age pattern of mortality under age ten and the model life table values corresponding to the observed mortality risk under age one. For the four Baden villages during the period from 1850 onward, the age pattern of mortality appears to most closely fit the East model. Although the degree of conformity is fairly close, the observed drop-off in childhood mortality compared to infant mortality is actually slightly more extreme than embodied in the corresponding East model. A far more pronounced example of this is provided by the Bavarian villages from 1800 onward. While the East pattern comes closest of the four model life table families to that observed in the Bavarian villages, the fit is still poor. Mortality risks between exact ages one and five and between exact ages five and ten as observed are much lower relative to infant mortality risks than embodied even in the East pattern. In both the cases of the Baden and the Bavarian villages, the possible transference of some stillbirths to the early infant death category may contribute to the exaggerated East pattern but, especially in the latter case, could hardly account for all of it. An opposite situation characterizes the East Frisian villages from 1700 onward where childhood mortality is relatively high compared to the observed level of infant mortality. The pattern conforms most closely to the North model with values of $_4q_1$ and $_5q_5$ being even higher relative to $_1q_0$ than implied by the North model.

Quite possibly, differences in the infant feeding practices account at least in part for the different age patterns of infant and child mortality observed for the regional clusters of villages as well as the deviations from the model life table patterns. The Bavarian villages represent the extreme case of little or no breastfeeding and thus the minimal amount of protection from mortality risks during infancy. At the same time there should be an absence of problems associated with weaning later in childhood in these villages. The Frisian villages probably represent the opposite situation or at least a marked contrast in this respect to the Bavarian villages. For Germany as a whole, at least during the latter part of the nineteenth century, the overall East pattern to which it conforms appears to result from a combination of patterns far more extreme than the East such as in the areas of Bavaria and elsewhere, where little breastfeeding occurs, and the opposite pattern in areas such as East Friesland, where breastfeeding was extensive. Thus caution must be used when choosing a model life table family to apply to particular regional groupings of villages given the substantial differences in the age pattern of mortality that characterize them.

In order to estimate life expectancy at birth (e_0) from the Coale Demeny life tables, the corresponding life table from each of the four regional families was determined by matching the observed probability of dying before age ten (excluding stillbirths) with the model life table characterized by that probability.[13] Results are shown in Table 1 for the regional groupings of villages by year of birth of children and for each of the four families of regional life tables. In order to determine which of the four model families fit best with the observed data, the sum of the absolute deviations from the observed values of $_1q_0$, $_4q_1$, and $_5q_5$ and those embodied in the chosen model life tables was calculated. The model for which the sum of the absolute deviations was a minimum was judged to be the best fitting and the life expectancy for that particular model is underlined in the results.

These results should only be considered as rough estimates given the uncertainties about the applicability of model life tables to historical data and particularly the possibility that the model which best fits the age pattern of infant and child mortality may not necessarily be the one that best fits the age structure of mortality over a wider age range. If we are willing to accept that for the combined sample as a whole the appropriate model shifts from North to West to East, a moderate but steady increase in life expectancy of about five years is indicated over the span covered by the present study. If, on the other hand, we were to assume that the East model, or for that matter any of the other three models, was the most appropriate throughout the period, a more modest increase in life expectancy would be indicated as well as, with the exception of the West model, a slight reduction in life expectancy between the first and second halves of the nineteenth century. Regardless of the trend in life expectancy indicated, the results are fairly consistent in indicating that during most of the period under study life expectancy at birth was in the range of 35 to 40 years.

Substantial variation according to the regional grouping of the villages is suggested by the results. If we accept the estimate corresponding to the best fitting model for each time period the following results are indicated: there appears to be little improvement in life expectancy in Oeschelbronn; a worsening of life expectancy in the Bavarian villages; some improvement in the Baden villages between the eighteenth and early nineteenth centuries but not during the nineteenth century; and substantial improvement of almost twelve years of life expectancy in the Waldeck villages and over eight years in the East Frisian villages. In the latter case, however, all the improvement occurred between the eighteenth and early nineteenth centuries and none between the first and second halves of the nineteenth century. Thus while the results cannot be taken as precise estimates of life expectancy at birth, the contrasts between the regional clusters of villages are pronounced enough to suggest strongly that mortality conditions and improvements were substantially better in some than in others.

Table 1. The observed probability of dying before age 10 (excluding stillbirths) and corresponding life expectancy at birth (e_0) according to Coale-Demeny regional model life tables by year of birth and regional clusters of villages.

	Observed $_{10}q_0$	e_0 According to model			
		North	South	East	West
4 Baden Villages					
pre 1800	.404	32.3	*34.0*	34.0	31.1
1800-49	.330	38.4	40.3	40.0	*40.0*
1850+	.345	37.1	39.0	*38.8*	39.6
Öschelbronn (Württemberg)					
pre 1800	.378	34.4	*36.2*	36.1	33.1
1800-49	.384	33.8	35.6	*35.5*	32.6
1850+	.359	35.9	37.8	*37.6*	36.3
3 Bavarian Villages					
1800-49	.357	36.1	38.0	*37.8*	36.8
1850+	.410	31.8	33.5	*33.5*	30.6
4 Waldeck Villages					
pre 1800	.366	*35.3*	37.2	37.0	34.6
1800-49	.294	41.6	*43.6*	43.0	40.3
1850+	.259	45.0	*47.0*	46.1	43.6
2 East Frisian Villages					
pre 1800	.277	*43.1*	45.1	44.5	41.8
1800-49	.190	*51.6*	54.2	52.5	50.4
1850+	.189	*51.7*	54.3	52.6	50.5
All Villages					
pre 1800	.364	*35.5*	37.3	37.2	35.1
1800-49	.311	40.1	42.0	41.6	*38.7*
1850+	.323	39.0	41.0	*40.6*	39.4

Notes: The corresponding regional model life table was determined by matching the observed value of $_{10}q_0$. Values in italics of e_0 are from the regional model judged to best fit the observed values of $_1q_0$, $_4q_1$, and $_5q_{10}$ determined by the minimum sum of the absolute differences between the observed and model life table values.

Occupational and status differentials

The probability of dying before age five is presented in Table 2 according to the occupation of the child's father. As the results show, differentials in child mortality among these broad occupational groups were rather modest and indeed far less pronounced than differences among regional clusters of villages. In the East Frisian villages, where child mortality is generally low, this is the case for all major occupational groupings while in Oeschelbronn and the Bavarian villages, where child mortality is generally high, it is high for all occupational groupings. There is a slight tendency for children with fathers in proletarian occupations to experience risks of dying slightly above average, although this is neither pronounced nor very consistent across regional clusters or over time within clusters. There are also no clear differentials in the trend of infant mortality according to the broad occupational groups or any evidence for any of substantial improvement in infant mortality during the last half of the nineteenth century compared to earlier years.

Table 2. The probability of dying before age 5 ($_5q_0$) by occupational group, year of birth and regional clusters of villages.

			Occupational group		
	Farmers	Prole-tarians	Artisans and Skilled	Mixed, Other, Unknown	Total
4 Baden Villages					
Pre 1800	.364	.411	.367	.378	.376
1800-49	.317	.332	.328	.297	.322
1850+	.320	.369	.337	.333	.337
Total	.328	.361	.339	.331	.340
Öschelbronn (Württemberg)					
Pre 1800	.385	.391	.363	.420	.389
1800-49	.357	.436	.439	.386	.402
1850+	.417	.362	.369	.358	.382
Total	.390	.393	.389	.391	.390
3 Bavarian Villages					
Pre 1800	(.517)	.449	.334	.352	.381
1800-49	(.403)	.350	.371	.316	.351
1850+	.351	.424	.389	.408	.400
Total	.390	.400	.371	.355	.379
4 Waldeck Villages					
Pre 1800	.306	.389	.295	.357	.337
1800-49	.311	.282	.320	.303	.304
1850+	.264	.298	.254	.263	.271
Total	.291	.310	.284	.324	.303
2 East Frisian Villages					
Pre 1800	.258	.267	.335	.272	.274
1800-49	.143	.223	.198	.157	.195
1850+	.183	.189	.230	.177	.189
Total	.209	.230	.267	.208	.226
All Villages					
Pre 1800	.329	.350	.350	.361	.346
1800-49	.300	.320	.332	.295	.309
1850+	.308	.331	.329	.316	.321
Total	.311	.324	.335	.326	.324

Notes: Results in parentheses are based on less than 100 cases.

In brief, the results suggest that socioeconomic position, at least as indicated by occupation, made little difference in terms of the mortality risks experienced by the children in the families. The relatively homogeneous levels of mortality across different socioeconomic groupings within each regional grouping of villages may reflect the pervasive poverty that characterized German villagers in general, even those that were relatively better off. The fact that the major social groupings within the village appear to have shared a more or less common risk of child loss suggests that child mortality was largely determined by exogenous forces beyond their control, at least to the extent their behavior was bound to local regional customs such as infant feeding practices or other infant care practices that could exert important influences on infant and child mortality.

Sex differentials

Sex differentials in infant and child mortality are of particular interest because of their potential to reflect preferential treatment of one sex over the other although interpretation of mortality results in this connection is not without substantial difficulties[14]. In the past, traditional child care practices in parts of Europe probably contributed to infant and child mortality and may have served as a way of limiting family size. Thus in the absence of birth control, selective neglect could potentially serve not only as an effective substitute but also as a way to adjust the sex composition of the family. Even if traditional child care practices were unrelated to such motivations, provided there were strong preferences for children of one sex over the other, those of the preferred sex might receive better treatment, such as receiving more and better food or better quality care, and as a result experience lower mortality rates than children of the less preferred sex.

Without having to make a judgment regarding the motivations behind traditional child care practices, it seems reasonable to argue that if there were strong preferences for one sex over the other, children of the less favored sex would suffer relatively more "neglect", if only in the sense of receiving less or poorer quality food or care. As a result, they would experience higher mortality rates. This apparently is the case today in much of South Asia where there seems to be little doubt that the main factors behind the excessive female mortality at young ages are worse malnutrition and generally preferential treatment of sons.[15] Favored treatment of sons is also thought to account for excess mortality among daughters in nineteenth-century Ireland.[16]

In his recent study of mortality in modern populations, Preston finds females to have a greater mortality advantage in low mortality populations than in high mortality populations.[17] In a substantial number of the latter, females actually experience higher death rates than males. The relationship between sex differentials and mortality level is probably due in part to a positive association between level of mortality and the extent of preferential treatment given males. But there is undoubtedly an important biological aspect to the relationship as well. For example, the importance of relatively sex-neutral infectious diseases increases at higher levels of mortality. Other factors beyond this compositional effect also appear to be at work.[18] There is reason to expect, then, that independent of sex discriminatory practices, females would not experience as great a relative advantage in high mortality situations, such as our German villages, as would be found in low mortality situations, such as in modern day Germany. If innate biological factors alone were operative, however, female children still should experience at least some modest advantage.

Even in high mortality populations where unequal treatment of sons and daughters is known to exist, it is often only after infancy that females experience a clear mortality disadvantage. This is apparent from relatively recent data from Ceylon, Pakistan, and Bangladesh and historically in Ireland.[19] Apparently the innate biological advantage plays a more important role in determining sex differentials during the first year of life than in subsequent childhood years. Boys may be particularly disadvantaged with respect to neonatal mortality, an important component of overall infant mortality.[20] Moreover, mortality differences due to discriminatory feeding might be evident only after a child is weaned, since breast milk has the same content whether being fed to a boy or a girl.

A detailed age breakdown of infant and child mortality is presented in Table 3. Focusing on the results for the villages collectively, there appears to be a pronounced female advantage under age one, followed by a slight advantage between ages one and two and a disadvantage between ages two and five. The combination of a small advantage for girls during the second year of life and a small disadvantage during the next three years results in essentially equal probabilities of dying between exact ages one and five ($_4q_1$) for both sexes. Furthermore, the risk of dying between exact ages five and fifteen ($_{10}q_5$) is also close to equal for males and females. In infancy, girls show the greatest advantage during the first month of life and the least advantage toward the end of the first year. While the decreasing advantage of girls probably reflects in part the increasing importance of the relatively sex-neutral infectious diseases, the lack of any advantage at all after the second year of life and indeed even a small disadvantage between ages two and five suggests the possible existence of discriminatory child care practices favoring sons, although to only a modest extent.

Results for the separate villages or village groups are generally similar. The Bavarian villages appear most exceptional with a substantial female advantage persisting through age five but reversing between five and fifteen when in any event mortality appears to be unusually low.[21] In all villages or village groups, female infant mortality is lower than male although in each of the four Baden villages (Grafenhausen, Herbolzheim, Kappel, and Rust) the female advantage disappears during the later months of infancy. In addition,

Table 3. Infant and early childhood mortality by sex of child and ratio of female to male mortality by village.

| | $_1q_0$ | $_4q_1$ | $_{10}q_5$ | Probability of dying between exact ages | | | | | | |
				0 & 1 month	1 & 3 months	3 & 6 months	6 & 9 months	9 & 12 months	1 & 2 years	2 & 5 years
Grafenhausen										
boys	.266	.120	.057	.126	.064	.050	.035	.023	.056	.068
girls	.240	.126	.049	.113	.050	.041	.036	.024	.058	.072
ratio	0.90	1.05	0.86	0.90	0.79	0.82	1.04	1.03	1.04	1.07
Herbolzheim										
boys	.252	.160	.057	.109	.053	.057	.032	.029	.075	.092
girls	.220	.166	.061	.088	.049	.042	.033	.029	.071	.102
ratio	0.87	1.04	1.07	0.81	0.92	0.75	1.02	1.01	0.95	1.11
Kappel										
boys	.214	.103	.057	.103	.047	.041	.023	.019	.047	.058
girls	.194	.102	.046	.089	.035	.032	.032	.020	.044	.061
ratio	0.91	0.99	0.82	0.86	0.76	0.78	1.44	1.06	0.93	1.04
Rust										
boys	.257	.115	.048	.125	.052	.048	.037	.023	.086	.062
girls	.225	.125	.049	.092	.044	.052	.034	.026	.058	.071
ratio	0.87	1.09	1.00	0.73	0.85	1.08	0.90	1.12	1.04	1.14
Öschelbronn										
boys	.309	.127	.056	.170	0.53	.036	.055	.035	.059	.072
girls	.271	.134	.047	.132	.057	.036	.036	.029	.061	.076
ratio	0.88	1.06	0.84	0.78	1.08	1.34	0.66	0.83	1.03	1.06
3 Bavarian villages										
boys	.359	.082	.035	.176	.092	.085	.042	.022	.037	.047
girls	.270	.059	.043	.125	.058	.068	.034	.017	.034	.026
ratio	0.75	0.72	1.24	0.71	0.62	0.80	0.81	0.78	0.93	0.55
4 Waldeck villages										
boys	.196	.140	.067	.098	.029	.027	.029	.028	.065	.080
girls	.169	.143	.067	.085	.026	.025	.020	.024	.062	.086
ratio	0.86	1.02	1.01	0.86	0.90	0.95	0.69	0.86	0.96	1.07
Middels										
boys	.138	.067	.047	.075	.024	.018	.014	.015	.030	.038
girls	.104	.067	.051	.055	.014	.018	.018	.011	.024	.043
ratio	0.75	1.00	1.09	0.74	0.56	0.55	1.30	0.73	0.81	1.14
Werdum										
boys	.166	.117	.076	.095	.031	.022	.014	.014	.045	.076
girls	.154	.099	.075	.083	.031	.019	.012	.017	.044	.057
ratio	0.93	.084	0.99	0.87	1.01	.087	.085	1.24	0.98	0.75
All villages										
boys	.239	.124	.057	.117	.048	.042	.031	.024	.057	.071
girls	.207	.125	.056	.095	.041	.037	.028	.023	.056	.073
ratio	0.87	1.01	0.98	0.81	0.85	0.89	0.90	0.97	0.97	1.04

Notes: Calculations of $_1q_0$ and the probability of dying between exact ages 0 and 1 month include stillbirths. The ratio of female to male mortality was calculated before rounding mortality rates as shown.

with only the exceptions of the Bavarian villages just noted and Middels, mortality between ages two and five was higher for girls.

In a recent article, Wall has suggested that if there were neglect of female children during the period prior to deliberate family limitation, this should show up more strongly in, or perhaps be entirely limited to, children of higher birth ranks.[22] He argues that the first few children will undoubtedly be wanted, regardless of sex, since families want heirs, even if there is no real property to transmit and that, at least in the European case, when there are no sons, daughters will suffice. He therefore suggests examining sex differentials in infant and child mortality according to birth rank. His own evidence in several English parishes points to excess female mortality in infancy being more common among higher-order births although his findings are not conclusive.

To examine the possibility of such a relationship in the German villages, Table 4 shows the ratio of female to male mortality in infancy and in childhood. There appears to be little systematic relationship between sex differentials in mortality and birth rank and, clearly, no consistent pattern of excess female mortality among higher birth ranks. Based on these findings, it seems reasonably safe to conclude that any neglect of female infants that might have existed was as likely to manifest itself among earlier births as it was among later births.

Maternal mortality

Calculation of adult mortality from family reconstitution data is problematic because of the difficulty of determining with any precision the period during which individuals can be considered under observation and hence at risk of dying for those individuals for whom a death date is unknown. In the special

Table 4. The ratio of female to male mortality in infancy and childhood according to birth rank and regional clusters of villages.

	Birth rank				
	1—2	3—4	5—6	7+	Total
4 Baden villages					
$_1q_0$	.86	.85	.88	.92	.88
$_4q_1$	1.03	1.14	1.09	.90	1.04
$_{10}q_5$	.98	1.07	.92	.86	.97
Öschelbronn					
$_1q_0$	.93	.74	.90	.92	.88
$_4q_1$	.97	1.07	.98	1.17	1.06
$_{10}q_5$	1.05	.79	.64	.80	.84
3 Bavarian villages					
$_1q_0$	.67	.70	.79	.85	.75
$_4q_1$	.65	.97	.85	.49	.72
$_{10}q_5$	1.99	1.97	.51	1.19	1.24
4 Waldeck villages					
$_1q_0$	.88	.85	.94	.80	.87
$_4q_1$	1.12	.82	1.05	1.21	1.02
$_{10}q_5$	.91	.88	1.70	.88	1.02
2 East Frisian villages					
$_1q_0$	.94	.80	.75	.91	.86
$_4q_1$	.82	.96	.81	1.07	.88
$_{10}q_5$	1.04	1.17	.71	1.06	1.01
All villages					
$_1q_0$	.87	.83	.87	.91	.87
$_4q_1$	1.00	1.04	1.02	.97	1.01
$_{10}q_5$	.99	1.04	.96	.90	.98

case of maternal mortality, provided it is defined as the risk of dying during or shortly after confinement and expressed as a rate relative to the number of confinements, this problem is essentially absent. The beginning of the period of risk is clearly defined by the birth of a child and ends, according to different definitions, within a few weeks or months following confinement. Since it is unlikely that many women migrate out of a village shortly after giving birth and, among those few who do, that they died in some other village within the specified period, women for whom no death date is known can be safely assumed to have survived the critical period after confinement.

There are special problems in measuring maternal mortality from reconstituted family histories that are essentially inherent to the parish register sources on which they are typically based.[23] The most important one is the fact that maternal mortality may be associated with miscarriages or stillbirths, events that are at best only poorly recorded in the registers. In such cases, the woman's death does not appear to follow a reproductive event in the reconstituted family history and thus is not classified as maternal mortality. To the extent this occurs, maternal mortality is underestimated.

Unlike the previous analyses, the examination of maternal mortality must be based on only six of the fourteen villages in the sample. The reason for this is that the data set used for the broader study of demographic behavior and on which the previous analyses have been based is restricted to couples for which the death date of at least one spouse is known. Such a restriction will tend to bias estimates of maternal mortality upward since the wife's death date is more likely to be known in cases where the wife died at or shortly following childbirth than in cases where she survived the reproductive age span. For six of the fourteen villages included in this study, however, all couples in the village genealogy were coded and thus are available for the calculation of maternal mortality based on women free from this restriction, thereby avoiding the biases that would otherwise result. Hence the following analysis of maternal mortality is based on all women in the six fully-coded villages rather than the usual restricted sample of women in all 14 villages used in the previous analyses. Consideration is limited to mortality following local confinements (i.e. those occurring in the village) and for which an exact date of confinement is known.

Both in historical and contemporary studies, a variety of definitions of maternal mortality appear to be used in practice. Some studies provide statistics on maternal mortality which are based on causes of death rather than simply on time since confinement. While a definition based on cause of death would be more precise, it is obviously impractical for most historical studies where such information is lacking. It is also impractical for use in many developing countries today where cause-of-death information is incomplete or faulty. Thus a number of other studies simply classify deaths to women within some period following the birth of the last child as constituting a maternal death. This risks misclassifying some deaths occurring shortly after but unrelated to childbirth as maternal mortality and missing others which in fact result from childbirth but which occur past the time span used for determining maternity-related deaths.

Even when the definition is based on the length of time following childbirth, the period chosen is not uniform in all studies and may involve deaths up to three months following confinements. Based on the six fully-coded villages, maternal mortality rates, expressed as maternal deaths per 1000 confinements, are presented in Table 5 according to different durations of periods following confinement. Probably the most common definition involves deaths within the first six weeks following childbirth. This is apparently the definition recommended by the World Health Organization as well as the American College of Obstetrics and Gynecology.[24] The latter also recommends distinguishing between maternal deaths occurring within the first seven days and those occurring later since the first week following confinement is the most dangerous period of time. As indicated by our results, such deaths involve roughly half or more of all maternal mortality during most time periods covered.

Since all couples including those married 1900 were processed in the fully-coded villages, trends through the first half of the twentieth century can be examined. Moreover, since an examination of individual villages did not reveal

Table 5. Maternal deaths per 1000 confinements according to different definitions of maternal death, and percent of deaths in first 42 days following confinement that occur in first 7 days, by year of confinement, combined sample of 6 villages.

Year of confinement	Maternal deaths per 1000 confinements, in first days following confinement				Of deaths in first 42 days % in First 7 Days	Number of confinements
	7 Days	42 Days	60 Days	90 Days		
1700-49	5.4	9.5	10.3	10.8	57	3888
1750-99	4.3	7.6	8.3	9.1	57	6048
1800-24	4.2	7.8	8.2	9.4	55	4257
1825-49	6.9	11.3	11.7	11.7	61	5389
1850-74	5.6	10.8	11.0	12.3	52	5381
1875-99	4.0	9.7	10.2	10.8	42	5476
1900-24	1.9	4.1	4.9	5.1	47	4679
1925-49	0.3	0.9	0.9	0.9	—[a]	1699

Notes: This table is limited to the six fully-coded villages (Kappel, Rust, Öschelbronn, Braunsen, Massenhausen, and Middels). Results are based on local confinements for which an exact date of confinement is given. Women with unknown death dates are assumed to have survived past stated reference periods.

[a] Fewer than 10 deaths in first 42 days.

lower maternal mortality during periods when registration of infant and child deaths was deficient, periods when death registration for infant and child deaths were poor are not excluded. The results suggest that little improvement in maternal mortality occurred prior to the turn of the twentieth century and indeed that conditions during the mid-nineteenth century may have been somewhat worse than during previous periods. It is difficult to know how general the trends based on our sample of six villages are.

One possible explanation for a rise in maternal mortality during the middle of the nineteenth century, if indeed such an increase is genuine, could be in the initial increase in total demand for labor necessitated by agricultural reforms and which is thought to have been met in part by an extended workload for peasant women. Apparently there was generally little period of rest either during pregnancy or immediately after childbirth for women in rural society in Germany at the time.[25] However, in an extensive review of maternal mortality statistics from a variety of sources including a number referring to German populations, Shorter discerns no consistent evidence of an increase in maternal mortality during the mid-nineteenth century.[26] Data he presents for Prussia covering the years 1816 through 1894 indicate fairly steady maternal mortality ranging from 7.6 to 9.5 maternal deaths per 1000 deliveries until the end of the third quarter of the century and then somewhat lower rates than that for the last quarter of the century.

It is noteworthy that the general level of maternal mortality indicated for Prussia was similar to that indicated by our sample of six villages, at least until the end of the nineteenth century. Moreover, national statistics for Germany during the first quarter of the twentieth century as presented by Shorter indicate a maternal mortality rate of between 3.5 and 5.0 maternal deaths per 1000 live births, again reasonably consistent with the rates indicated by the sample of six villages. These comparisons indicate agreement only in terms of the rough order of magnitude, however, due to a lack of strict comparability in definitions of maternal mortality.

The general picture presented by the data from the six villages and confirmed by Shorter's extensive review of maternal mortality in a number of Western countries is that childbearing throughout the eighteenth and nineteenth centuries was associated with a risk of death many times higher than in recent times and that substantial improvement occurred only during the twentieth century. In West Germany by the late 1970s, childbearing carried with it a risk of only about .2—.3 deaths per 1000 births, only a fraction of the levels found in the sample villages during the eighteenth and nineteenth centuries.[27] Given the far lower rate of childbearing today than in the past, a maternal death has become a very rare event. The 1 percent or so chance of death associated with each confinement in the sample villages during the eighteenth and nineteenth centuries, in conjunction with considerably higher fertility at that time, meant that a significant proportion of women ended their lives as the result of reproductive activity. Given the average age at which women started childbearing in combination with the average rate of childbearing, a 1 percent chance of dying at each confinement would lead roughly to a 5 percent cumulative chance of a woman dying due to childbirth before reaching the end of her reproductive span.

Table 6 indicates the maternal mortality rates for the different villages as well as for the marital status of the union, the sex of the child, and the multiple birth status of the confinement for confinements occurring during the eighteenth and nineteenth centuries. For the six villages combined, almost a 1 percent chance of death for the mother within six weeks was associated with each confinement. Some variation is evident across villages, although given the infrequent occurrence of a maternal death, some statistical fluctuation would be expected. Data presented by Shorter for East Friesland, based apparently on a large number of cases, indicate a maternal mortality rate more than twice as high as the rate characterizing the East Frisian village of Middels.[28] In addition, when maternal mortality is calculated based on the restricted sample of women selected for the present study in Werdum, the other East Friesland village in the sample, and compared to the same rates calculated for Middels based on the restricted sample of women, far higher rates are indicated for Werdum. Thus is does not appear that the low rate for Middels is typical for East Friesland generally.[29]

Higher maternal mortality is associated for non-marital unions than for marital unions. Part of this difference is due to confinement order. A substantially higher proportion of confinements associated with non-marital compared to marital unions are first confinements and, as indicated below, maternal mortality associated with first confinements (11.7 deaths per 1000 confinements) is above average. Nevertheless, since non-marital maternal mortality is higher than that associated with all first confinements, this appears to be only part of the explanation. The small number of cases on which the non-marital maternal mortality is based must also be kept in mind. Indeed, the differences between non-marital and marital maternal mortality are not statistically significant at the .05 level even without taking into account differences in confinement order.

Maternal mortality associated with the birth of a boy is higher than that associated with the birth of a girl. Whereas the difference is small and not statistically significant at the .05 level, it is in the expected direction. Given the larger average size of newborn males, an increased risk is expected to be associated with the birth of boys. Far more dangerous are confinements associated with multiple births. Despite the small number of such cases in our sample, the difference in maternal mortality associated with single and multiple births is statistically significant at the .05 level.

Among the most often studied aspects of maternal mortality is its relationship to mother's age and order of confinement.[30] There is general agreement that biological causes at least partly underlie age and confinement order differences in maternal mortality while differences in overall levels of maternal

Table 6. Maternal deaths within six weeks of confinement per 1000 confinements, by village, by marital status of union, by sex of child, and by multiple birth status of confinements, for confinements occurring 1700-1899.

	Maternal deaths per 1000 confinements	Number of confinements
Village		
Kappel	7.4	6487
Rust	10.3	9976
Öschelbronn	11.9	5033
Braunsen	11.0	1722
Massenhausen	10.3	2899
Middels	6.5	4322
All 6 villages	9.5	30439
Marital status of union[a]		
Marital	9.2	28771
Non-marital	13.2	1667
Sex of child[b]		
Boy	9.4	15603
Girl	8.7	14700
Multiple birth status		
Single	9.2	29960
Multiple	25.1	479

Notes: This table is limited to the six fully-coded villages (Kappel, Rust, Öschelbronn, Braunsen, Massenhausen, and Middels). Results are based on local confinements for which an exact date of confinement is given. Women with unknown death dates are assumed to have survived past the end of the six-week reference period.

[a] Premarital confinements to women who later marry the father are included under marital unions; one confinement of a woman in a union of unknown marital status is excluded.

[b] In cases of a multiple birth, the confinement is included under the sex of the first-born child; a small number of confinements for which the sex of the birth is unknown are excluded.

mortality are largely a result of non-biological causes such as socioeconomic levels, cultural practices, and the state of and accessibility to medical technology. To the extent that age at confinement and number of children ever born are associated with socioeconomic status (or the other relevant characteristics), the association between maternal mortality and age of mother and confinement order can also reflect non-biological influences. For example, if women of lower socioeconomic status are more likely than women of higher socioeconomic status to start childbearing earlier and to continue longer, and if they are also disadvantaged with respect to their health and access to health facilities, we would expect maternal mortality at the extreme childbearing ages to be higher than at other ages even in the absence of any biological effects. The same can be said for maternal mortality associated with confinements of higher orders if lower socioeconomic status women are disproportionately represented among those who have above average numbers of births. One advantage of examining the association of maternal mortality with age of mother and confinement order for earlier periods, when deliberate fertility control within marriage was less common, is that the non-biological influences should be less important.

Maternal deaths per 1000 confinements are shown in Figure 3 according to the age of mother at confinement and according to confinement order based on confinements in the eighteenth and nineteenth centuries for the six fully-coded villages combined. The J-shaped relationship between maternal mortality and age which typifies most populations is clearly evident. The extent to which maternal mortality is higher at the later childbearing ages, however, is somewhat less pronounced than is typical in most contemporary populations including those in high mortality developing countries for which reliable data are available. Nortman points out that the age differentials typically widen as the level of mortality is reduced.[31] According to her estimates for high mortality populations (defined as those with more than 1.0 maternal deaths per 1000 confinements), maternal mortality in the age group 40-44 is typically twice as high as that for the unweighted average of all age groups through 40-44. In the results for the six German villages, the same calculation indicates that the 40-44 age group of women experienced maternal mortality rates only about 40 percent higher than the unweighted average up to that age group. Given the fact that the overall level of maternal mortality in the German villages during the eighteenth and nineteenth centuries was about four times as high as the average of Nortman's high mortality populations, the more attenuated relationship with age observed for the German villages may simply represent a more extreme case of less pronounced differentials as the overall level increases across populations. However, it may also reflect less self-selection at higher ages of women in low socioeconomic categories than occurs in more modern populations.

The relationship of maternal mortality with confinement order is less pronounced than the association with maternal age but again a J-shaped curve, although considerably flattened, roughly describes the relationship. Particularly sharp is the drop between maternal mortality rates associated with first and second confinements. While maternal death rates increase generally with rising confinement order, not until confinements of the sixth order and above is the level characterizing first order confinements reached again.

Given the inevitable association between age and confinement order, it is of some interest to examine maternal mortality controlling for both simultaneously. The results of such a comparison are indicated in Table 7.

Figure 3. Maternal mortality within six weeks of confinement by age of mother and confinement order, 1700-1899.

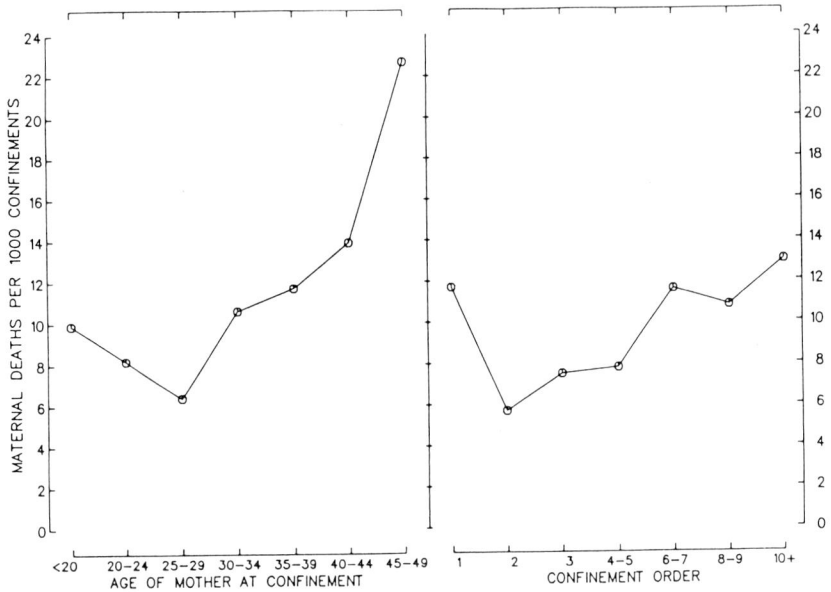

Notes: Results are limited to the six fully-coded villages only and are restricted to local confinements for which an exact confinement date is known and to first marriages of women with no previous union resulting in an illegitimate birth.

Table 7. Maternal deaths within six weeks of confinement per 1000 confinements, by age and confinement order, for confinements occurring 1700—1899.

Age at Confinement	Confinement order		
	1	2—5	6+
Under 20	(11.7)	—	—
20—24	10.5	3.2	—
25—29	8.0	4.9	(6.2)
30—34	(22.0)	8.5	12.3
35—39	(23.3)	10.1	11.0
40—44	—	(18.5)	13.2
45—49	—	—	(20.2)

Notes: This table is limited to the six fully-coded villages (Kappel, Rust, Öschelbron, Braunsen, Massenhausen, and Middels). Results are based on local confinements for which an exact date of confinement is given and are restricted to first marriages to women who had no previous unions resulting in an illegitimate birth. Women with unknown death dates are assumed to have survived past the end of the six-week reference period. Results in parentheses are based on less than 500 confinements.

44

Caution is required in interpreting the results because of the extent of statistical fluctuation that can be expected due to insufficient numbers of cases when examining a phenomenon with a low frequency of occurrence such as maternal mortality. In order to reduce the problem, broad groupings of confinement order have been made after separating out the first confinement order which is of particular interest given the relatively high level of maternal mortality associated with it in the absence of control for age. Even when we examine only confinements of the first order, the general J-shaped curve with age persists. Little confidence, however, can be placed in the results indicating the small difference between maternal mortality associated with ages under 20 which is based on few cases, and the lower levels for women in their twenties. Some limited data for other populations suggest that for women bearing their first child, a monotonic increase in maternal mortality with age rather than a J-shaped relationship holds.[32]

At higher confinement orders, maternal mortality also increases fairly steadily with age, at least judging from the two broad confinement order categories into which confinements after the first have been grouped. For both categories, however, there are insufficient cases of women under age 20 to determine their level of maternal mortality. Also in the group of sixth and higher order confinements there are insufficient numbers of women below age 25 to make this determination. Nevertheless, the results suggest that the higher mortality of women under 20 compared to those in their twenties when confinement order is not controlled is to a large extent an artifact of the concentration of first order confinements at younger ages. The results also reveal that first order confinements consistently have a higher maternal mortality associated with them than higher birth orders even when age is controlled. Indeed, without exception, for the broad confinement order groups shown, the highest maternal mortality is found for women at their first confinement.

Summary and conclusions

One of the most striking findings to emerge from the present study is the divergent path followed by infant and child mortality from the mid-eighteenth to the beginning of the twentieth century. The results show fairly clearly that reductions in child mortality above age 1 preceded improvements in infant mortality. The combination of somewhat worsening infant mortality and improving early child mortality resulted in a situation in which the probability of dying between birth and age 5 showed little consistent trend, fluctuating around a level of 30 percent during most of the eighteenth and nineteenth centuries. The divergent paths of infant and child mortality underscore the difficulty of applying model life tables, which assume a fixed pattern of relations among mortality rates at different ages, to historical populations over long periods of time.

Pronounced regional differences in the levels of infant and child mortality are evident and appear to be related to differences in the prevailing infant feeding practices. In contrast socioeconomic status, at least as indicated by occupation of the father, shows little association with mortality risks experienced by the children. This lack of socio-economic differences emphasizes the probable role of local or regional infant feeding customs, common to all classes, as a key determinant of infant mortality.

Differences in mortality risks during infancy and childhood were evident between the sexes. Females tend to experience lower infant mortality rates but lose their advantage by the early childhood ages. It is difficult to draw any firm conclusions from the mortality data about the extent to which male children were given preferential treatment. If this was the case, the evidence suggests it bore no relationship to birth order as has sometimes been hypothesized.

Maternal deaths are the one aspect of adult mortality that can be investigated easily with family reconstitution data. In German village populations during the eighteenth and nineteenth centuries, there was roughly a 1 percent chance of death for women associated with each confinement. In combination with relatively high fertility, this meant that a woman had approximately a 5 percent cumulative chance of dying due to childbirth before reaching the end of her childbearing span. Thus, not an insignificant proportion of women died as a result of their reproductive efforts.

Notes

1. J. Knodel, *Demographic Behavior in the Past: German Village Populations in the 18th and 19th Centuries* (Forthcoming, Cambridge University Press).

2. J. Knodel, *The Decline of Fertility in Germany, 1871-1939* (Princeton 1974).

3. P. Matthiessen and J. McCann, 'The Role of Mortality in the European Fertility Transition: Aggregate-Level Relations', S. Preston (Ed.), *The Effects of Infant and Child Mortality on Fertility* (New York 1977), pp. 47-68.

4. For the period 1875-1899, our combined sample yields the following values: $_1q_0$ (excluding stillbirths) = .226; $_4q_1$ = .095; and $_{10}q_5$ = .039. This compares to an unweighted average of the three decade estimates at the national level for the period 1871-1900 as follows: $_1q_0$ = .226; $_4q_1$ = .117; and $_{10}q_5$ = .053.

5. The most appropriate comparison appears to be with the district of Ettenheim. Grafenhausen, Kappel, and Rust were all located in the district of Ettenheim during the last half of the nineteenth century. Herbolzheim also belonged to Ettenheim during the mid-part of the period but due to redistricting, was part of two other districts at other times within the 50-year span. Excluding stillbirths, $_1q_0$ in the four Baden villages was .246 during 1850-1874 and .243 during 1875-1899. In comparison, the infant mortality rate (infant deaths per 1000 live births in the district of Ettenheim was as follows: 248 in 1856-1863, 248 in 1864-1869, 244 in 1875-1880, 257 in 1885-1890, and 213 in 1891-1895, *Beitraege zur Statistik der inneren Verwaltung des Grossherzogtums Baden,* No. 46.

6. Matthiessen and McCann (1977).

7. W.R. Lee, 'Germany', W.R. Lee (Ed), *European Demography and Economic Growth* (London 1979), Chapter 4, pp. 144-195; W.R. Lee, 'The Mechanism of Mortality Change in Germany, 1750-1850', *Medizin-historisches Journal*, 15 (1980), pp. 244-268.

8. R.S. Schofield, 'Statistical Problems', *International Population Conference, Liege 1973*, Volume 3, pp. 45-57.

9. A.J. Coale, and P. Demeny, *Regional Model Life Tables and Stable Populations* (Princeton 1966); A.J. Coale and P. Demeny, *Regional Model Life Tables and Stable Populations*, 2nd edition (New York 1983).

10. Since the Coale-Demeny model life tables are given separately for males and females, the l_x values have been combined based on a sex ratio of birth of 105 for the purpose of matching the observed values which are for both sexes combined.

11. Knodel (forthcoming).

12. R.S. Schofield and E.A. Wrigley, 'Infant and Child Mortality in England in the Late Tudor and Early Stuart Periods', C. Webster (Ed.), *Health, Medicine, and Mortality in the Sixteenth Century* (Cambridge 1979), pp. 61-95.

13. Model life table values of $_{10}q_0$ were estimated for the two sexes combined as indicated in the preceding footnote. A simple arithmetic average of male and female life expectancy was used to represent the combined sex life table at any given level.

14. R. Wall, 'Inferring Differential Neglect of Females from Mortality Data', *Annales de démographie historique* (1981), pp. 119-140.

15. R.H. Cassen, *India: Population, Economy, Society* (New York 1978); L.C. Chen, Emdadul Huq, and S. D'Souza, 'Sex Bias in the Family Allocation of Food and Health Care in Rural Bangladesh', *Population and Development Review*, 7 (1981), pp. 55-70; M.A. El Badry, 'Higher Female than Male Mortality in Some Countries of South Asia: A Digest', *Journal of the American Statistical Association*, 64 (1969).

16. R.E. Kennedy, *The Irish Emigration, Marriage, and Fertility* (Berkeley, Ca 1973); E.A. Wrigley, *Population and History* (New York 1969).

17. S.H. Preston, *Mortality Patterns in National Populations* (New York 1976).

18. Preston (1976), p. 153.

19. G. T. Curlin, L.C. Chen, and S.B. Hussain, *Demographic Crisis: The Impact of the Bangladesh Civil War (1971) on Births and Deaths in a Rural Area of Bangladesh* (Dacca 1975); El Badry (1969); Kennedy (1973), pp. 59-60.

20. R. Naeye, L.S. Burt, D.L. Wright, W.A. Blanc, and D. Tatter, 'Neonatal Mortality: The Male Disadvantage', *Pediatrics*, 48 (1971), pp. 902-906.

21. Statistics for all of Bavaria show a similar strong female advantage in infant mortality. For example, from 1835/1836-1868/1869, the infant mortality rate for the entire kingdom averaged 41.2 per 100 live births for males and 35.7 for females. W.R. Lee, *Population Growth, Economic Development and Social Change in Bavaria 1750-1850* (New York 1977), p. 6.

22. Wall (1981).

23. B.M.W. Dobbie, 'An Attempt to Estimate the True Rate of Maternal Mortality, Sixteenth to Eighteenth Centuries', *Medical History*, 26 (1982), pp. 79-90; E.A. Wrigley and R.S. Schofield, 'English Population History from Family Reconstitution: Summary Results 1600-1799', *Population Studies*, 37 (1983), pp. 157-184.

24. A.E. Imhof, 'Unterschiedliche Säuglingssterblickeit in Deutschland, 18. bis 20. Jahrhundert—Warum?', *Zeitschrift für Bevölkerungswissenschaft,* 7 (1981), p. 152; E.C. Hughes, 'Obstetric-Gynecologic Terminology with Section on Neonatal Mortality and Glossary of Congenital Abnormalities', *American College of Obstetrics and Gynecology* (Philadelphia 1972), p. 454.

25. Imhof (1981), pp. 343-382; W.R. Lee, 'Family and Modernization: The Peasant Family and Social Change in Nineteenth Century Germany', R. Evans and W.R. Lee (Eds.), *The German Family* (London 1981), pp. 148-174; D. Sabean, 'Small Peasant Agriculture in Germany at the Beginning of the Nineteenth Century: Changing Work Patterns', *Peasant Studies,* 7, 4 (1978), pp. 218-224.

26. E. Shorter, *The Evolution of Maternal Mortality, Eighteenth to Twentieth Centuries* (Unpublished manuscript).

27. According to the 1979 United Nations Demographic Yearbook, maternal mortality in West Germany was 31.1 per 100,000 live births in 1977 and 23.1 per 100,000 in 1978. Apparently a maternal death is determined by cause of death rather than time since confinement. A.E. Imhof, 'Women, Family and Death: Excess Mortality of Women in Childbearing Age in Four Communities in Nineteenth-Century Germany', Evans and Lee (1981), p. 161 indicates that, based on a definition of deaths within six weeks of pregnancy termination, the maternal mortality rate in West Germany in 1973 was 45.9 per 100,000 births. This compares to a figure of 37.9 for 1973 according to the U.N. Yearbook based on cause of death.

28. Shorter (Unpublished manuscript).

29. Based on the restricted sample of women, the maternal death rate in Werdum per 1000 confinements was 21.4 compared to 8.3 for Middels.

30. L.G. Berry, 'Age and Parity Influences on Maternal Mortality: United States 1919-1969', *Demography,* 14 (1977), pp. 297-310; J.T.P. Bonte and H.P. Verbrugge, 'Maternal Mortality: An Epidemiological Approach', *Acta Obstetricia et Gynecologica Scandinavica,* 46 (1967), pp. 445-474; D. Nortman, 'Parental Age as a Factor in Pregnancy Outcome and Child Development', *Reports on Population-Family Planning,* 16 (New York 1974).

31. Nortman (1974).

32. Nortman (1974).

Birth Weight, Breast-Feeding, Postpartum Amenorrhea and Infant Mortality in Three Norwegian Cities during Late Nineteenth and Early Twentieth Century

Margit Rosenberg

Material and methods

In Norway, records from the earliest maternity hospitals are still preserved. The first maternity hospital was established in Oslo (Christiania) in September 1818. The hospital is still functioning, and the archive containing all birth records from 1818 up until today is intact. The hospital "Fødselsstiftelsen" was founded partly to "render maternity patients from the classes without means, good and inexpensive services".[1] The other main purpose of the hospital was to train midwives.

The records have all been written by the midwives. The information is given in a detailed and systematic way for each woman, but printed forms were not introduced until 1912. The information about each woman and child contained in the records varies somewhat from one period of time to another. The material used in the present study, was primarily collected to study various aspects of breast-feeding. Before 1860 and after 1930 the women in Christiania were not asked about breast-feeding of any previous children, so the time period covered by our investigation is between these years.

In Bergen, the first hospital was established in 1861, on the same lines as the hospital in Christiania. The records from Bergen are included in our material from 1878 up until 1941. In Trondheim, the first maternity hospital, a charitable institution, was started in 1908. The first records contained only sparse information about the parturient women. But in 1934, new forms were introduced, and we have been able to use the records from then and up until 1984. Due to changing standards of records, those included in our material are from different time periods in the three cities. These periods overlap partially and together they cover a period of 120 years. Detailed description of the material is found in Liestøl, Rosenberg and Walløe [2].

In short, the material contains records from multiparous women with information about previously born children. In order to make comparisons between some of the variables, a certain number of primiparous women have also been included. The information about the current delivery which is of interest to us, concerns the sex and birthweight of the child, whether or not the child was born alive, and if it died during the time at the hospital — on which day. The multiparous women have given information about the duration of breast-feeding of any previous children, the corresponding postpartum amenorrhoea, whether the child is still alive at the time of the current birth, and if dead, when and of what cause the child died. Information about the mother is also given: her name and age, where she was born and where she lived, her parity, her age of menarche, her menstrual cycle and the date of the last menstruation. Various social parameters are given, such as her marital status, her husband's occupation if married or her own occupation if unmarried. The year, date and serial number are given for each record. In our material we have included all these items of information. The records also gave detailed information about the pregnancy, the delivery and the childbed, but we have not included this in our material.

The woman's social relations are stated by the marital status variable and the occupation variable. To do this, we classified the occupations in seven different categories; the first four for married women and the last three for those not married. Group 1 contains husbands' occupations of highest status, and group 4 occupations of lowest social status. The three groups for the unmarried women's occupations are organized similarly. The occupation categories and where to place the different occupations have been decided after discussion with historians.

In Norway up until World War II, most of the children were born at home, also in the cities. Our material will therefore not be a representative sample of the population except perhaps for the last decades. The further we go back in time, the more the lower classes are overrepresented. Before 1885, the material consists mainly of women from the working classes, and nearly twice as many unmarried as married women. The women of higher social categories from that period present in our material cannot be regarded as a random sample from the corresponding social classes in town. The social categories will therefore be used simply to pinpoint the differences between social groups. The description will mainly show the secular trend in the working classes.

The sample includes 200-300 records taken at random from 2 to 5 years around every 10th year from each of the three maternity clinics. These are records from multiparous women, as the main object for the total investigation was to study breast-feeding and adjoining relationships. To compare some of the variables, we have added around 80 (50-110) records for every 10 years from primiparous women. We eventually had data from 8015 women. From a pilot study we have record information from another 1137 women, different from those studied in the "new" investigation but with less information on each woman. Thus, for part of the analysis, we have material from the three cities consisting of a total of 9152 individual women.

The information we decided to include, was collected manually and filled in on a special form, one for each record. Afterwards, the data was input to a DEC-10 computer via a similar on-screen form. For processing the collected information we have used the BMDP-program system for statistical analysis.

Results and discussion

There is a long tradition of using growth data to mirror the social conditions in a population. From Norway there are internationally well known investigations on, for instance, height of military conscripts [3], weight and height of schoolchildren [4] and on the age when girls get their first menstrual bleeding, the age of menarche [5]. Birth weight, in particular, may be used as an indication of the condition for women in a society. We know that during the Dutch hunger period in 1944-1945 [6] and the German Siege in Leningrad 1941-43 [7], the birth weights fell due to serious, acute undernourishment. It is more difficult to find out how less severe malnutrition over some length of time influences birth weight.

Fig. 1 gives a picture of the secular trend in birth weight in Norway from 1860 to 1984, separated for unmarried and married women. Due to only a small number of unmarried mothers after about 1930, I have not plotted the birth weights after that year. The dotted line is the regression line from after 1930. There is an overall increasing tendency throughout the period. A multiple regression analysis showed an increase of about 180 g from 1860 to 1960—given the other variables are kept constant. We have, however, found a minor decreasing tendency of about 70 g before 1900. But this decrease is statistically significant only among unmarried women. This is in great contrast to the decline of about 430 g for both married and unmarried women which Ward and Ward have found in their material from Montreal from 1851 to 1905 [8].

In the multiple linear regression analysis with birth weight as the dependent variable, we were, after a set of preliminary analysis on both the whole material and various subgroups, left with six independent variables of significant influence: the year of giving birth, the mother's age of menarche, her marital status (unmarried or married), the sex of the child, parity and a variable which we have called "primiparity". "Primiparity" is the extra gain in birth weight when going from parity 1 to 2. We had to introduce this new variable because of a nonlinear relation between parity and birth weights. The birth weight increases linearly with parity from parity 2 and upwards, but the increase from parity 1 to 2 is much larger. We have a moderate decrease in birth weight with increasing age of menarche, the regression coefficient is 14.39 g per increasing year. The regression coefficient tells us that there is a difference of 67.86 g between unmarried and married mothers, the married having the heaviest babies. Boys are on an average 112.32 g heavier than girls.

Figure 1.

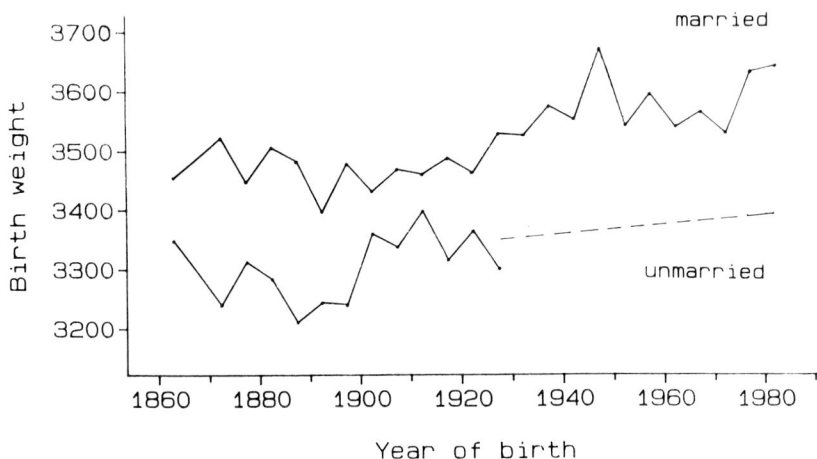

We have tried to split the material in different time periods, but ended up with only two periods, before and after 1900. There are only two variables, the year of birth and the marital status, which have a change over time of any importance. The change occurs at the turn of the century.

In the year of birth variable we have found a decreasing tendency before 1900. But how can this decrease be explained? In Oslo and to some degree in Bergen, during the second half of the last century, there was a change in economic and demographic circumstances due to industrialization. The economic life in Norway had a general rise during the second half of the nineteenth century [9]. The textile industry, however, had problems in the late seventies and eighties as a consequence of the international crisis from 1873 onwards. During these periods there was some unemployment in this industry and the employees were forced to work shorter hours and the wages were reduced by 5-20 % [10]. The textile industry employed mostly women. The match factories constituted another important industry which employed mostly women. The employees in this industry were also paid very low wages. These facts resulted in the first organized strike for better working conditions in Oslo, in 1889 in the match factory and in 1890 in Christiania Canvas factory. The conditions in these two industries may have been partly responsible for the decreasing birth weights for unmarried women before 1900. Unmarried women workers constituted, for instance, 77.4 % of the employees in the textile industry. Considerable migration to the cities with people living in close quarters and thereby poor living conditions, may also have been partly responsible.

Another interesting point concerning the unmarried women is that women working in factories had children with substantially lower birth weights than women working as maidservants or in trade (about 150 g). It is reasonable to believe that the women working in factories probably lived under the worst

52

conditions of all. The maidservants, for instance, were generally provided with housing and food by the family they worked for. Both housing and nutrition for these women would certainly have been worse than for the majority of married women, but the conditions cannot have been so bad as for the factory workers. But in spite of the difference in birth weight which we have found, we know from contemporary sources that the girls themselves preferred to work in factories.

The decline in birth weight among women observed before 1900 coincides with a declining age of menarche [11]. How decreasing birth weight can correspond to simultaneously declining age of menarche may seem unclear, particularly as the living condition factor seems to have opposing effects on these two variables. Liestøl has earlier shown that the age of menarche seems to be more dependent on the conditions for the woman in her early life than on the conditions in later years.[12] In Norway, during the time period in question, there was a general economic rise. This led to better living conditions for the greater part of the population, including most of the children born both in Oslo and elsewhere. In turn, the age of menarche declined. At the same time, the industrialization process caused a deteriorating situation for part of the population. Judging from mortality statistics, unmarried women living in towns were especially seriously affected. Birth weights, which probably are more dependent on conditions during pregnancy, may therefore still have declined marginally.

Fig. 2 illustrates how breast-feeding habits have varied with time during the last 120 years. This curve includes all children born in all the three maternity hospitals. We see that for a period of over 60 years, from 1860 to 1920, breast-feeding habits were quite stable, except for a decline in the number of women breast-feeding for 12 and especially 18 months. The fraction of mothers who breast-fed for the time periods up to and including 3, 6 and 9 months respectively, began to decline about 1920, at first quite modestly, then succeeded by a steeper fall. The bottom point was reached in 1967 with only just over 30 % of the women breast-feeding up to and including 3 months and as few as about 5 % breast-feeding up to and including 9 months. After that, the trend has changed completely and we have experienced a distinct upward tendency. The final points in the curve, after 1980, may indicate that a plateau level was reached about 1980 and that this level of breast-feeding was comparable with the 1940 values.

The materials from the three cities are only partly overlapping. In the overlapping periods, however, the distribution of breast-feeding duration and the trends in breast-feeding are the same for the two cities Oslo and Bergen, and for Bergen and Trondheim, respectively. This indicates fairly congruous curves from the different cities during the whole period 1860-1984. When looking at the unmarried and married mothers separately, we find the same picture as in fig. 2 except for the curves of married mothers lying above the curves of unmarried.

Figure 2.

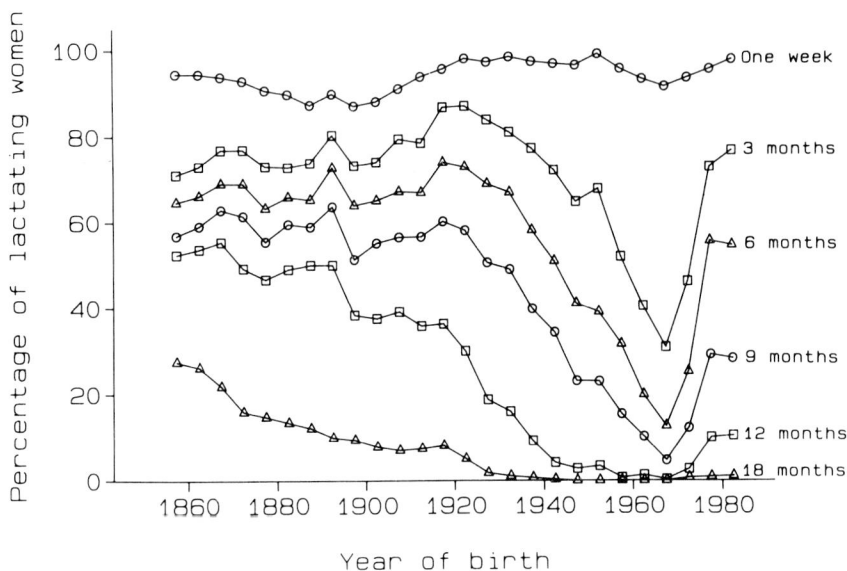

When we analysed the development of breast-feeding in more detail, we looked into three different time periods separately: 1) up to and including 1920, 2) 1921-1967, 3) after 1967, depending on when the important changes have taken place. In this paper I shall concentrate on the first period.

Before 1920 we have seen that the distribution of the lengths of breast-feeding was remarkably stable for a very long time, except for a decline in the number of women breast-feeding for 12 and 18 months. After a preliminary regression analysis, we were left with a quite reduced number of variables which seemed to influence breast-feeding to a greater or smaller extent in this time period. The most important variable is the marital status. Married mothers breast-fed their children considerably longer than the unmarried mothers did. The difference appears to be about three months from the multiple linear regression analysis. A much more modest part does the age of menarche play. Up until 1920 it seems that with increasing age of menarche, the breast-feeding increases with just under one week per year, both for married and unmarried.

Concerning parity, the importance lies in the greater difference in lactation period between the first and the second child. The second child is breast-fed about one month longer than the first child. In the subsequent parities, there is a minimal decreasing tendency. As a control, we have analysed separately the mothers who have had 3 or more children and those with 4 or more children respectively. The results from these analyses were not qualitatively different from what we have found when analysing the total material. As an extra control, we have investigated the breast-feeding pattern of subsequent children of individual mothers. We found the same tendency here as found earlier. The habit of breast-feeding the second child longer than the first one with a following small reduction from the second child to the third, from the third to the fourth etc., seems to be the general pattern.

The year of birth for the child and the mother are strongly correlated. When one of them was taken care of in the regression, the effect of the other nearly disappeared. After a series of analyses of the sudden change in breast-feeding practice in the late sixties, it became clear that the year of birth of the child was the most important variable of the two, at least at that time. This variable has therefore been kept in the regression analysis when assessing the influence of the other variables. The regression coefficient for the mother's age was very small, but indicated a marginal positive association between age and breast-feeding.

The geographical variables do also play a modest part in influencing breast-feeding. Before 1920, after analyses of different combinations of the mother's birthplace and in which town the delivery took place, we were left with the variable born in the countryside as the most important. The regression coefficient indicates that mothers who were born in the Norwegian countryside on an average breast-feed their children about three weeks more than the mothers born in towns or cities.

The occupation variable plays an important part in influencing breast-feeding practice. When studying this variable, we have to separate the mothers into groups of married and unmarried. Referring to married mothers first, we have before 1920 found a substantial longer breast-feeding period among the lowest social strata compared with the highest ones. The difference is about 10 weeks between the extremities in social status (group 1 includes senior officials, academics etc., group 4 comprises manual workers, farm hands etc.). After 1920 the influence of occupation has gone through an interesting development. Analyses have shown that there was a turn in the influence after World War II. Up until that time we have found a difference of about one month in the same direction as before 1920, the lowest social strata giving breast for the longest time. After World War II we have, however, found a corresponding difference but of opposite direction. The women of the highest social status do now breast-feed their children for the longest periods. The difference is at first just under one month, growing to about one and a half month between group 1 and group 4.

Unmarried women constitute a varying proportion of the material during the investigated period. After 1920 they constitute only a very small part. Therefore, no significant influence of the occupation variable on breast-feeding could be expected here. However, neither in the time period before 1920 did we detect any significant influence of the occupation variable among unmarried mothers.

To understand how lactation influences fecundity, we have to study at which time women get their menstruation back after giving birth, the postpartum amenorrhoic period. But, to get the menstruation back after a period of postpartum amenorrhoea may occur in three principally different ways: without lactating at all, after giving up lactation or while still lactating. We have tried to study these three situations separately. To study amenorrhoea in on-going lactation, we have used statistical methods which take into account that the observed period may finish either because lactation is given up or because the menstruation returns. Therefore, we have used the so called survival analysis which allow censored observations. To study the factors influencing amenorrhoea, we have used Cox regression models.

In the analysis of amenorrhoea in on-going lactation, it was revealed that there was a considerable fall in median duration of amenorrhoea around 1900. The duration of amenorrhoea was very stable before 1900, for 50 % of the women their menstruation had returned at 12 months after delivery. Around 1900 the duration of the amenorrhoic period dropped down and was followed by a slight downward tendency. After 1900, 50 % of the women had recommended menstruating at 6 months after delivery.

In the regression analysis, we have used 10 independent variables which could influence the length of amenorrhoea. These variables included the woman's social relations—her marital status, her or her husband's occupation, her birthplace, where she lives etc. It appeared that only three variables were of any importance:

1) in which year the child was born
2) the woman's age of menarche
3) if the woman was primiparous or multiparous

Fig. 3 gives a picture of the effects of the above variables. This figure shows estimated survivor function plots for amenorrhoea in on-going lactation—estimated by the regression analysis. The abscissa is time in months, the ordinate is the fraction of women who still haven't got their menstruation back. In this figure one has to keep the curve in the middle, the reference curved marked A, in mind, and compare the other curves with that one. This curve describes a thought cohort of women who have given birth in 1890, whose age of menarche are 12 and who are multiparous. We see that 50 % of the women have got their menstruation back after about 8 months. The effect of parity is shown in the curve at the bottom, marked B. This curve comprises a thought cohort of women who have given birth for the first time, but otherwise are identical with the women behind the reference curve. Primiparous get their menstruation back a little earlier than multiparous, 50 % is now 5.5 months. The curve at the top, marked C, shows the influence of the age of menarche. This curve represents a thought cohort of women with a late age of menarche, 16 years, but who are otherwise identical to the women in the reference curve.

Figure 3.

```
      .+....+....+....+....+....+....+....+....+....+....+....+....+....+....+....+....+.
 1.0  +**C                                                                            +
      .  *
      .  *C
      .  *CC
      .  B*C
 .90  +   *C                                                                          +
      .  *AC
      .   * C
      .   * CC
      .   *  C
 .80  +   *     C                                                                      +
      .  BAA  CCC
      .  B A    C
      .   B A    CC
      .   BA     CC
 .70  +   B A     CCC                                                                  +
      .   BB A      CC
      .   B AAA     CC
      .    B  AA      CC
      .    B  A        CC
 .60  +    B   A        CCC                                                            +
      .    BB AA          C
      .    BB AAA           C
      .     BB   AA         CCC
      .     B    AA          CCC
 .50  +     B     A           CC                                                       +
      .     BBB   AA           CCCC
      .      BB   AA            CCCCC
      .      B    AA             CCCC
      .      BB    AA             CCCCCCCCC
 .40  +       BB    A                      CC                                          +
      .       BB    A                       CCC
      .       B    AAA                        CCC
      .       BBBB   AA                         CCC
      .         B   AAA                          CC
 .30  +         B    AAA                                                               +
      .         BB    AAA
      .         BBB   AAAAA
      .          BBB    AAAAAA
      .           BBB    AAAAAAAA
 .20  +           BBBB     AAA                                                         +
      .            BBBB      AAAA
      .            BBBBBBBBBBBB   AAA
      .                BBBB     AAA
      .                 BBBB
 .10  +                  BBBBB                                                         +
      .                   BB
      .
      .
      .
 0.0  +                                                                                +
      .+....+....+....+....+....+....+....+....+....+....+....+....+....+....+....+....+.
        2.    6.     10     14     18     22     26     30
      0.    4.    8.     12     16     20     24     28     32
```

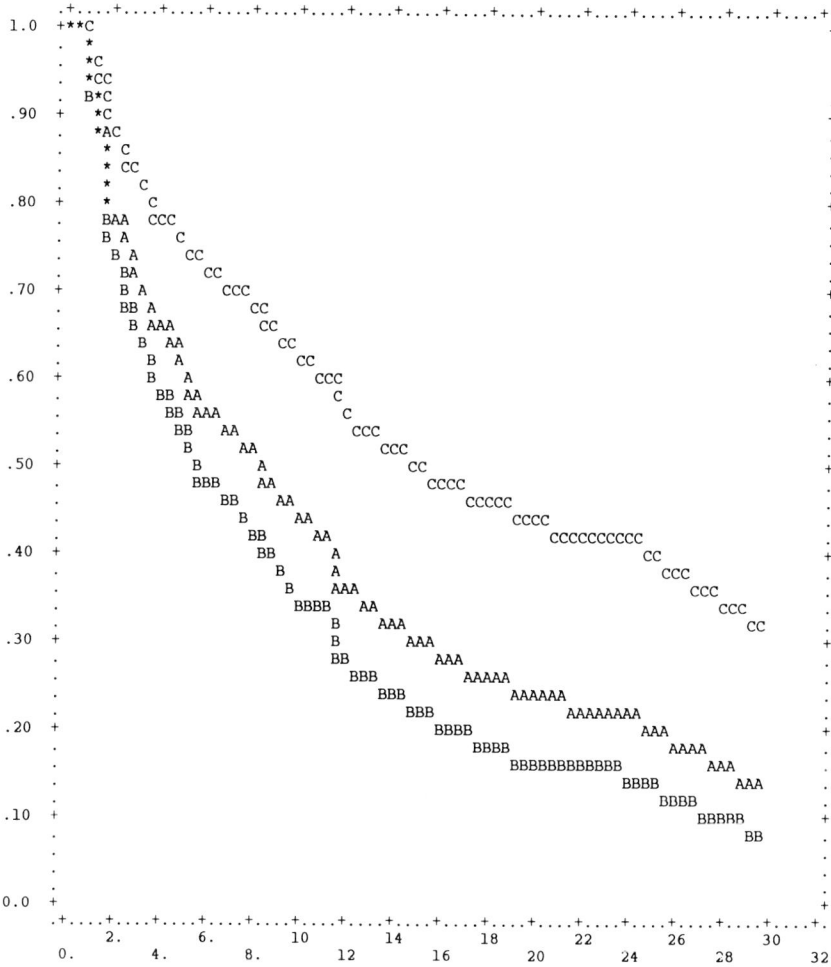

We see that these women have a long period of amenorrhoea, 50 % of the women have recommenced menstruating at about 15 months. Fig. 3 is based on the material from the years up to and including 1900. We have also performed an analysis on the material after 1900. The curves from this analysis are quite similar with the ones in Fig. 3. They show the same tendency and the same relationship between the different variables, except that the effect of the variable age of menarche is somewhat less.

When looking at these curves one might believe that it was improved living conditions, for instance better nutrition, which have caused the substantial decline in postpartum amenorrhoea. In our analysis it seems that neither the marital status nor her or her husband's occupation influence the length of amenorrhoea. These variables, which we have used as indicators of the woman's social situation, do, however, play an important part in other analysis, for instance of birth weight and lactation. Therefore, it does not seem that the woman's own nutrition influences the length of amenorrhoea to any great extent, at least within the variations of nutrition which are found in Oslo and Bergen in the last century. In severe malnutrition the situation may, of course, be different. Our hypothesis is that the decline in the length of postpartum amenorrhoea from 1860 up until today, is caused by a changed feeding pattern and how early, and to what extent supplementary food is introduced.

Concerning infant mortality in the second half of the last century, we have just started out the analyses. The few results presented here will therefore be only preliminary results. During the first year of life, the death rate for the infants who have not been breast-fed was roughly the double of what was the case for those who have been given breast. The death rate for the infants born by unmarried mothers was also roughly the double of those born by married mothers, both when the infants were given breast and when not. Thus, the infants who were absolutely worst off, were the not breast-fed ones born by unmarried mothers. After a year, nearly half of them were dead.

Notes

1. F.G. Faye, 'Om Fødselsstiftelsen i Christiania fra dens begynnelse i Aaret 1818 til Udgangen af 1846', *Norsk Magazin for Laegevidenskaben,* 2 (1847), pp. 321-364.

2. K. Liestøl, M. Rosenberg and L. Walløe, *Breast-Feeding Practice in Norway 1860-1984* (manuscript 1987).

3. V. Kiil, 'Stature and Growth of Norwegian Men During the Past Two Hundred Years', *Skrifter utgitt av Det Norske Videnskaps Akademi i Oslo,* I. Mat.-Naturv. Klasse No 6 (1939); L.G. Udjus, *Anthropological Changes in Norwegian Men in the Twentieth Century* (Oslo 1964).

4. G.H. Brundtland, K. Liestøl and L. Walløe, 'Height, Weight and Menarcheal Age of Oslo Schoolchildren During the Last 60 Years', *Annals of Human Biology,* 7 (1980), pp. 307-322.

5. J.E. Brudevoll, K. Liestøl and L. Walløe, 'Menarcheal Age in Oslo During the Last 140 Years', *Annals of Human Biology,* 6 (1979), pp. 407-416.

6. Z. Stein, M. Susser, G. Saenger and F. Marolla, *Famine and Human Development. The Dutch Hunger Winter of 1944-1945* (Oxford 1975).

7. A.N. Antonov, 'Children Born During the Siege of Leningrad in 1942', *Journal of Pediatrics,* 30 (1947), pp. 250-259.

8. W.P. Ward and P.C. Ward, 'Infant Birth Weight and Nutrition in Industrializing Montreal', *The American Historical Review,* 89 (1984), pp. 324-345.

9. Central Bureau of Statistics of Norway, Nasjonalregnskap 1865-1960 (National Accounts 1865-1960), *Norwegian Official Statistics,* XII (1965), p. 163.

10. H. Torstensson, *Ugifte mødre og barnefedre i Kristiania på 1800-tallet,* Hovedoppgave i historie vår 1985 (Oslo 1985).

11. Brudevoll, Liestøl and Walløe (1979).

12. K. Liestøl, 'Social Conditions and Menarcheal Age: The Importance of Early Years of Life', *Annals of Human Biology,* 9 (1982), pp. 521-537.

Infant Mortality in Finland 1865-1869

Oiva Turpeinen

Introduction

In Finland the general trend of IMR (infant mortality rate) has been in decline since 1750 (Fig. 1). Whereas IMR was 217.6 (infant deaths per thousand live births) in 1751-1800, it was 197.5 in 1801-1850, 164.9 in 1851-1900 and 91.4 in 1901-1950. From 1971 to 1980 the figure was only 9.6.

Figure 1. IMR (Infant mortality rates) in Finland 1751-1975 and in Finnish cities 1811-1975 (log. scale).

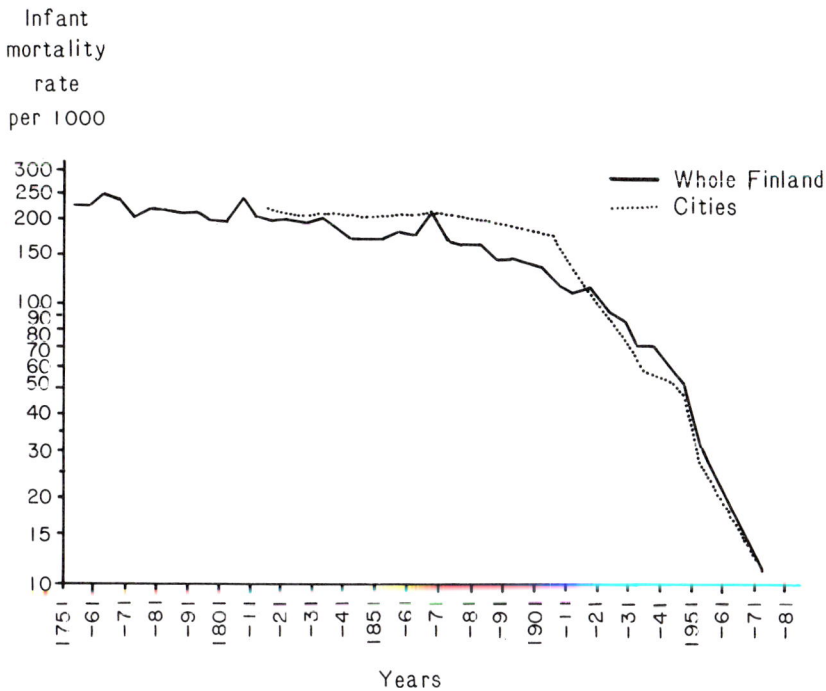

Source: K. Pitkänen, Infant Mortality Decline in a Changing Society, *Yearbook of Population Research in Finland* XXI (1983), p. 48.

The central reason given by many studies for the decline of infant mortality is that breast feeding became a general practice in passing from the 18th to the 19th century.[1]

Although the trend of IMR was downward, there were immense yearly fluctuations until about 1870 (Fig. 2).[2] At times IMR rose to prodigious figures; the highest of all was recorded in 1868, no less than 391.7. The present article will concentrate on this disastrous year, though other critical years — 1865-1867 and 1869 — will also receive some attention, especially with regard to regional differences. My article is based for the most part on a broader study I have made which is completed in manuscript form.

Infant and age-specific mortality

Fig. 3 and Table 1 show how mortality in 1868 grew violently in all age groups.[3]

It should be stressed that the mortality crisis of 1868 was not confined to children and the old: an exceptionally great number of Finns died who were at the best age for work, marriage and fertility. During 1868 in Finland a total of 137,700 died and 43,800 were born. The difference was thus 93,900, at least five per cent of the population.

Table 1. Infant and age-specific mortality in Finland 1865—1869

	1865	1866	1867	1868	1869
IMR	193.7	217.6	223.4	391.7	140.5
1—2	55.3	73.5	69.5	142.2	49.5
3—4	27.7	33.0	36.4	110.4	35.8
0—4	79.7	92.0	94.0	168.6	68.5
5—9	11.8	14.6	15.5	59.9	16.1
10—14	5.1	6.8	6.6	27.0	7.5
15—19	6.1	7.6	7.6	20.8	7.3
20—24	7.9	10.9	11.0	24.5	9.1
25—29	8.3	12.6	13.3	30.0	10.6
30—34	9.5	14.1	15.2	38.5	11.3
35—39	10.8	17.4	20.9	47.1	12.6
40—44	13.5	21.9	27.9	67.3	16.4
45—49	17.6	28.5	35.2	85.3	19.1
50—54	22.6	36.9	47.1	108.8	26.1
55—59	27.0	45.0	59.7	131.5	34.6
60—64	44.4	60.5	82.2	156.4	46.0
65—	103.0	134.7	178.8	268.9	100.4
Mortality rate	25.9	33.6	38.1	77.5	25.2
Crude birth rate	34.2	32.2	32.3	24.6	33.7

Figure 2. Infant mortality rates in Finland 1751-1870.

per thousand

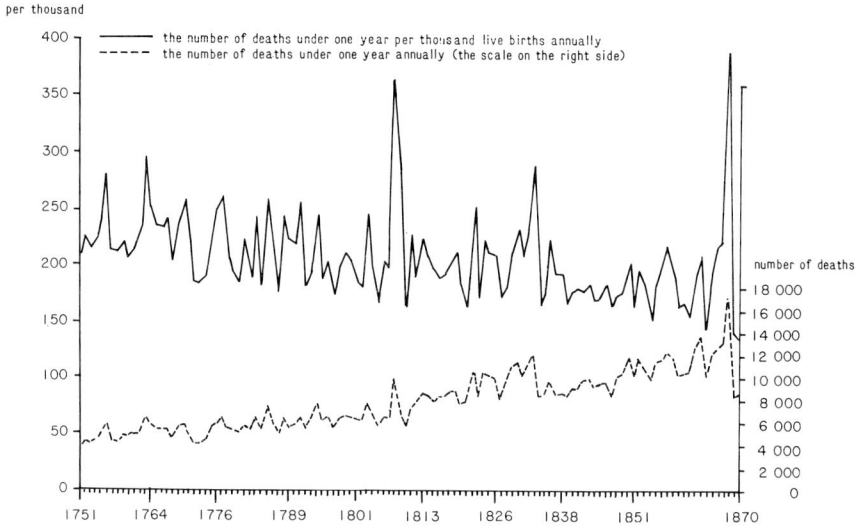

Regional differences in the death rate were enormous in 1868 (Map 1). In some deaneries it rose above 120 per thousand. In central Finland the figure was clearly greatest, but in the south-east, in Åland and in the north it was low. In these areas mortality was less than 40 per thousand.[4]

Regional differences in infant mortality

The extent of regional differences from 1865 to 1869 is indicated by maps 2-6 — see also Appendix Tables 1-2.[5] The maps for 1865 and 1869 are similar. This is no accident. Both maps show in what areas IMR was greater or smaller than what was traditionally normal. In a sense this continuity was broken by the years 1866-1868. The crisis developed and matured in 1866-1867, reaching its height in 1868.

It was in 1868 that IMR assumed exceptionally shocking proportions. In the deanery of Jämsä, for instance, it reached the appalling level of 697.5 per thousand and in the deanery of Lapua 693.2. Regional differences in that year were truly immense, for in Åland the rate was only 160.6 and in the extreme north of Lapland no more than 234.9.

Causes and consequences

In explaining the catastrophe of 1868 two background factors must be stressed: unusual poverty caused by crop failures, and infectious diseases which were rampant at the same time.

63

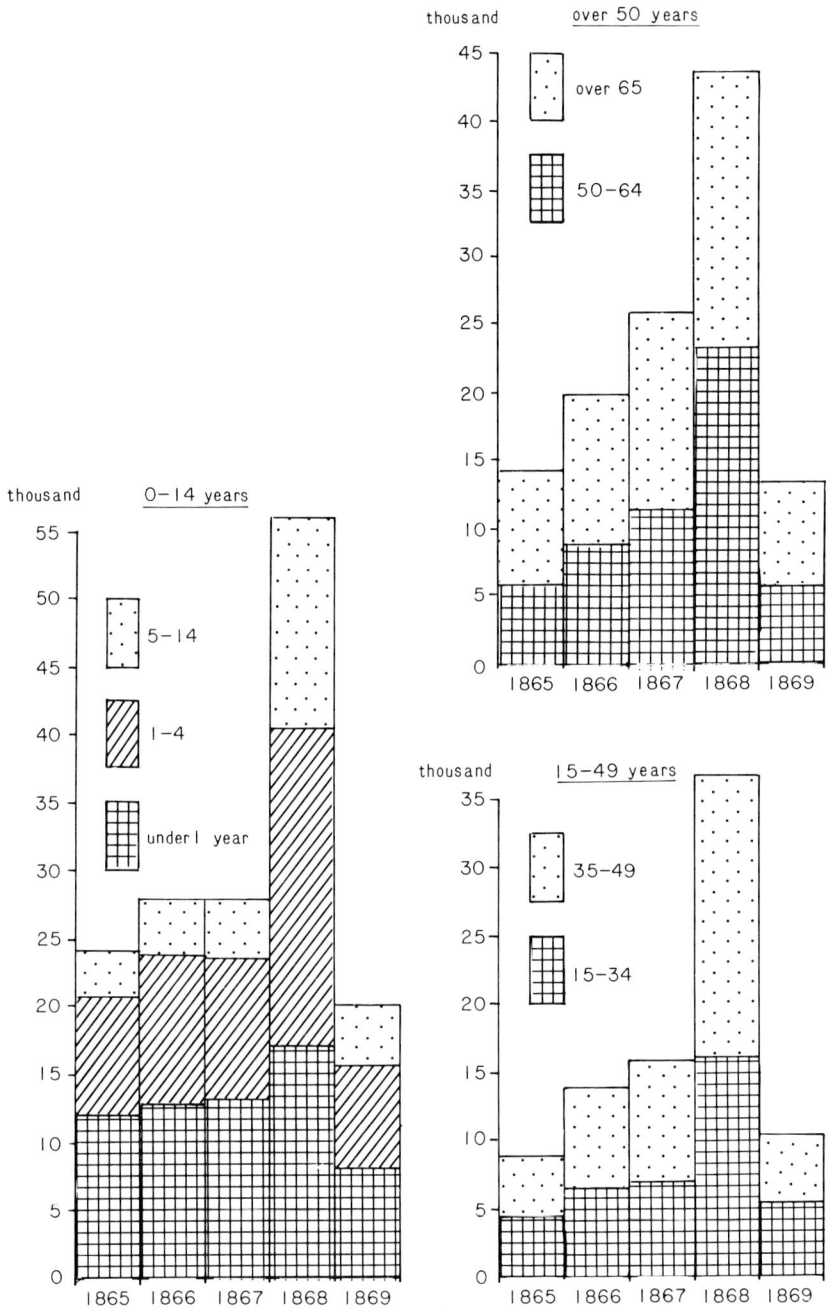

Figure 3. The number of deaths by age groups in Finland 1865-1869.

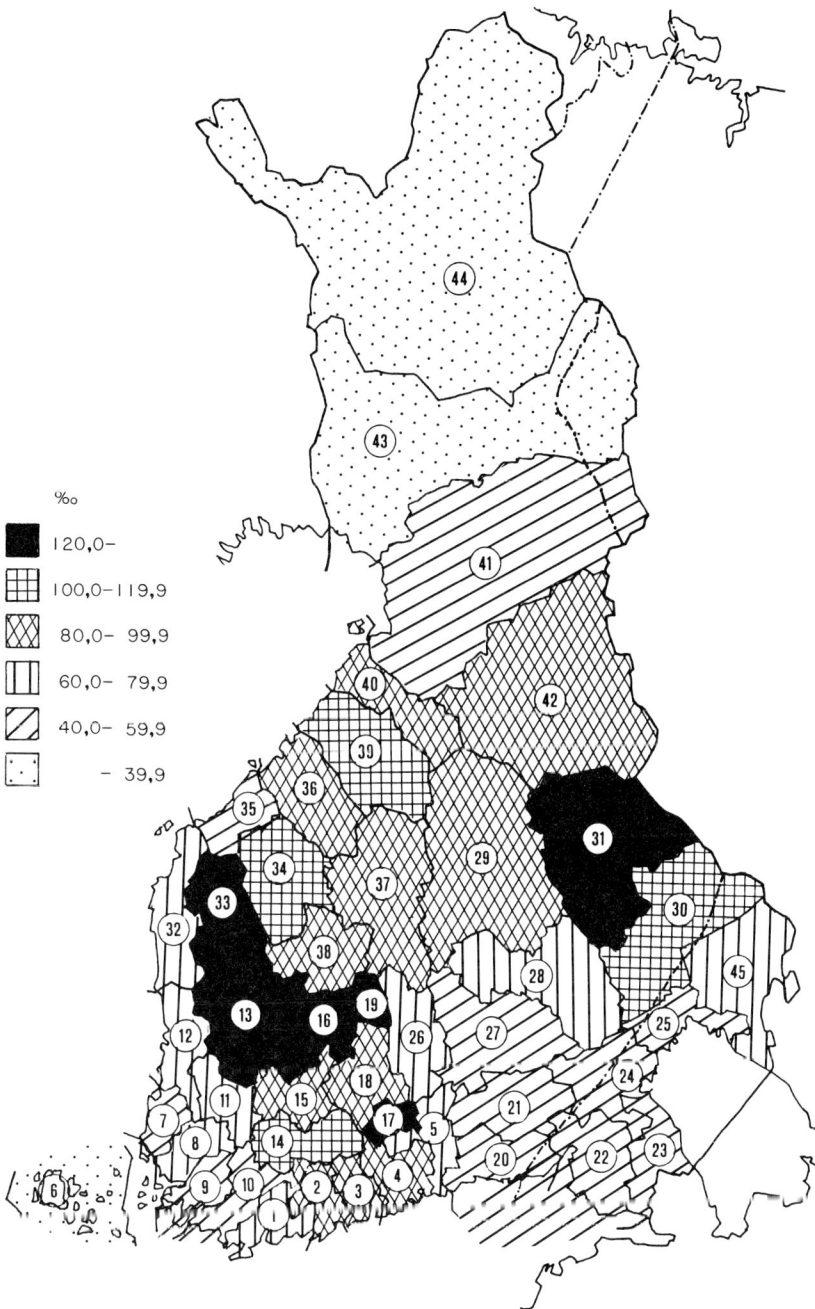

Map 1. Crude death rate in Finland 1868

‰

■	120,0-
⊞	100,0-119,9
⊠	80,0- 99,9
▥	60,0- 79,9
▨	40,0- 59,9
⬚	- 39,9

Map 2. Infant mortality in Finland 1865

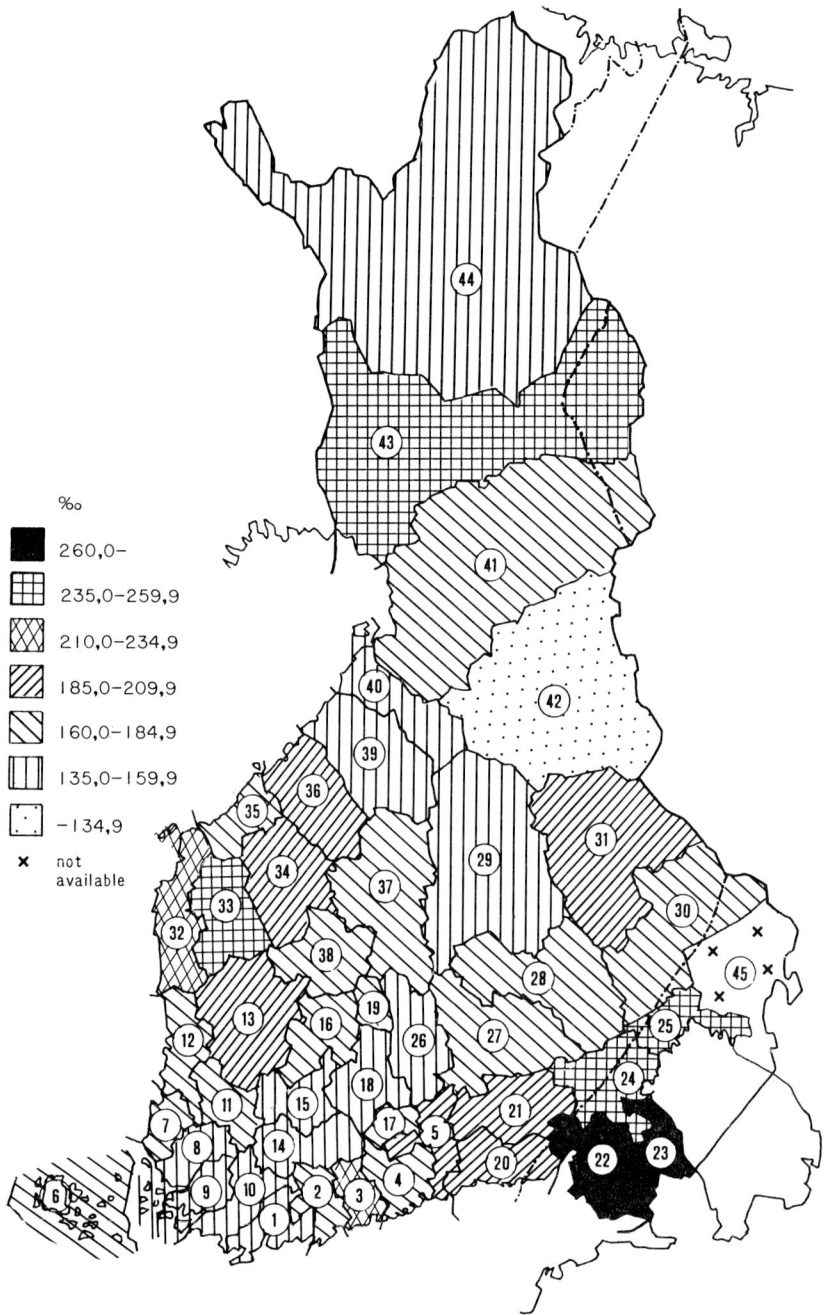

‰

- ■ 260,0-
- 235,0-259,9
- 210,0-234,9
- 185,0-209,9
- 160,0-184,9
- 135,0-159,9
- -134,9
- × not available

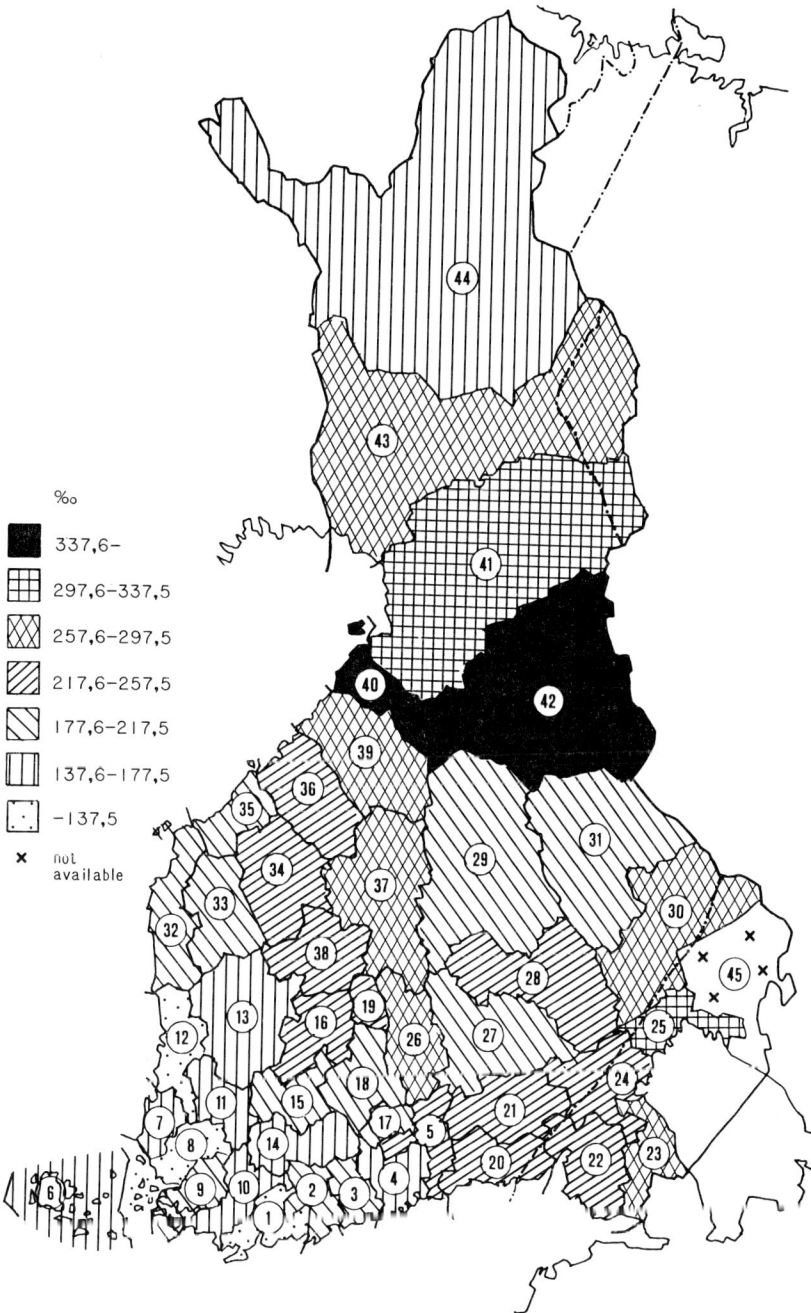

Map 3. Infant mortality in Finland 1866

‰

- ██ 337,6—
- ⊞ 297,6—337,5
- ▨ 257,6—297,5
- ▨ 217,6—257,5
- ▨ 177,6—217,5
- ▥ 137,6—177,5
- ⬚ —137,5
- ✕ not available

Map 4. Infant mortality in Finland 1867

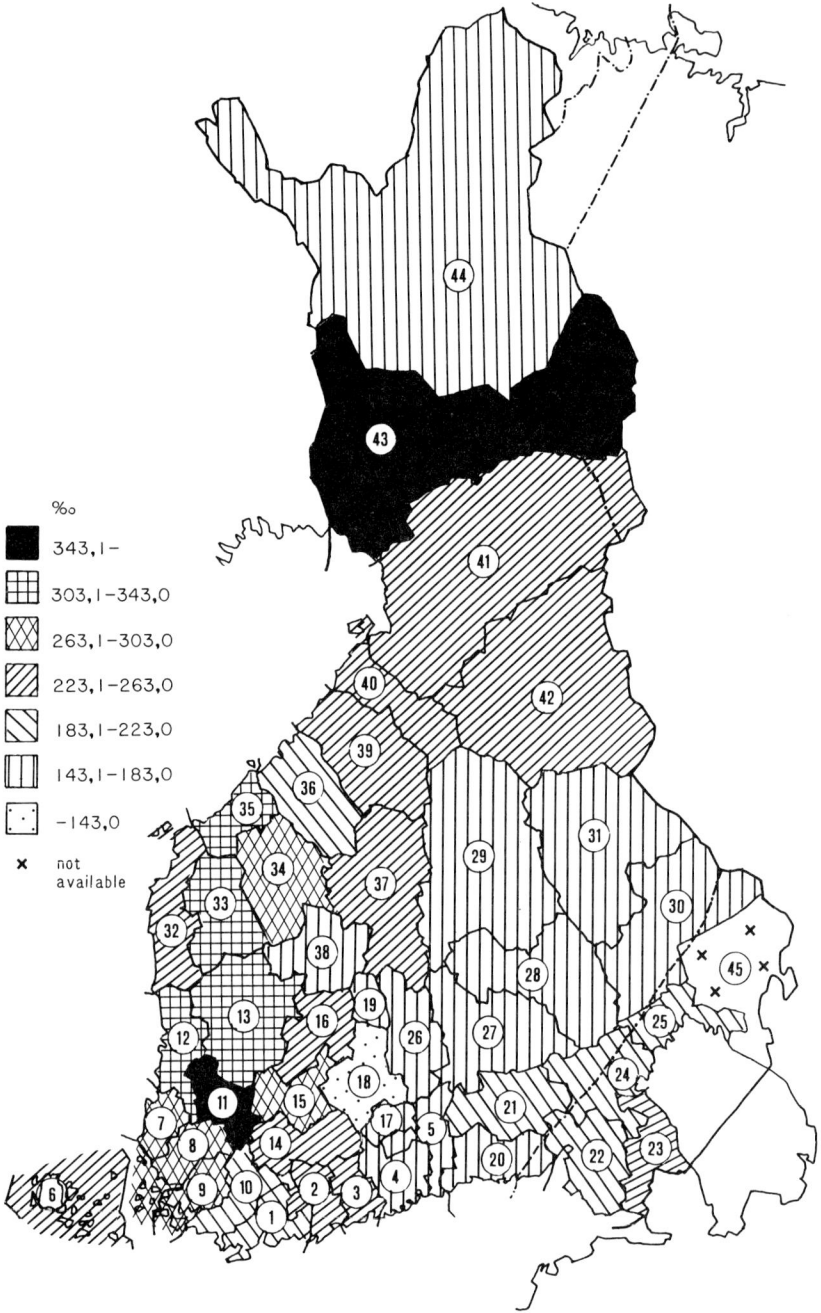

‰

- ■ 343,1–
- ⊞ 303,1–343,0
- ▨ 263,1–303,0
- ▨ 223,1–263,0
- ◪ 183,1–223,0
- ▥ 143,1–183,0
- ⬚ –143,0
- × not available

Map 5. Infant mortality in Finland 1868

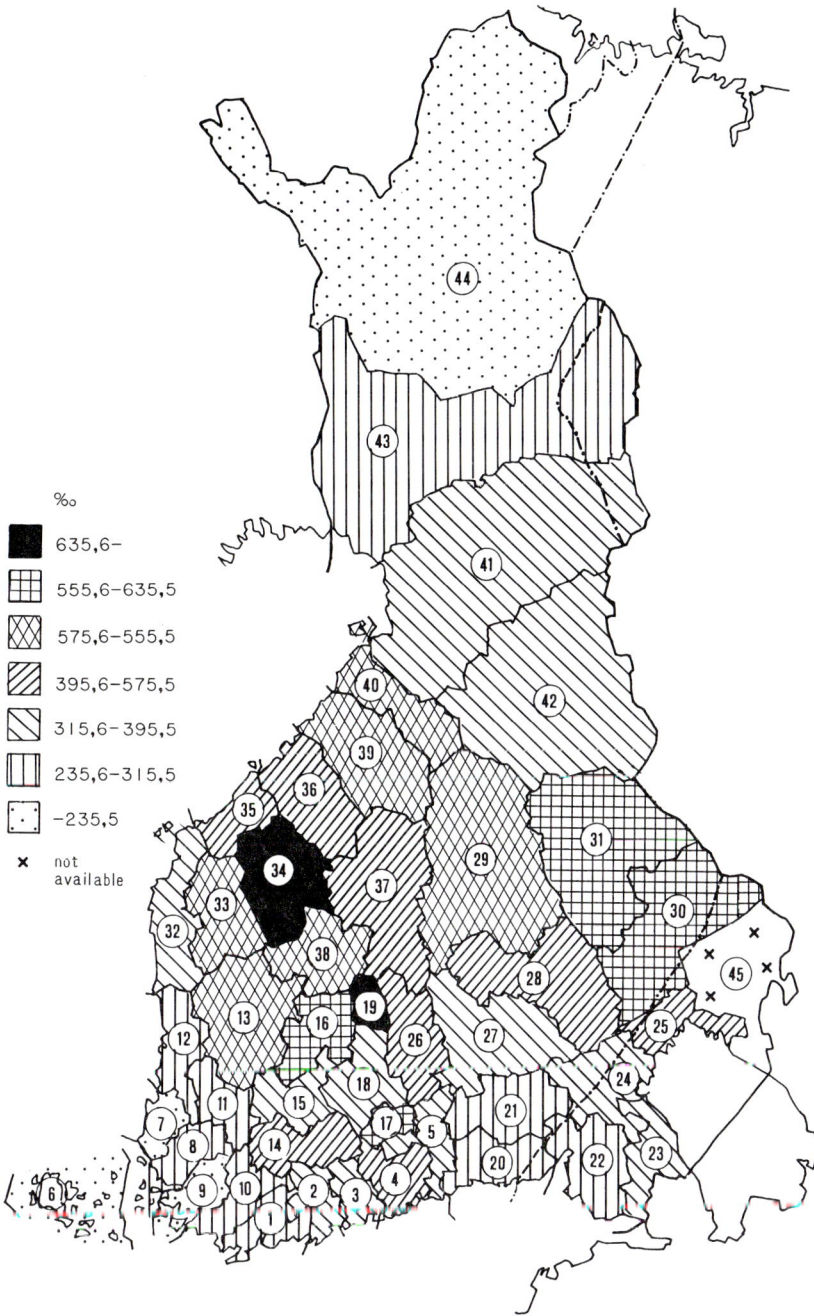

‰

- ■ 635,6–
- ⊞ 555,6–635,5
- ▨ 575,6–555,5
- ▨ 395,6–575,5
- ◩ 315,6–395,5
- ▥ 235,6–315,5
- ⸬ –235,5
- ✕ not available

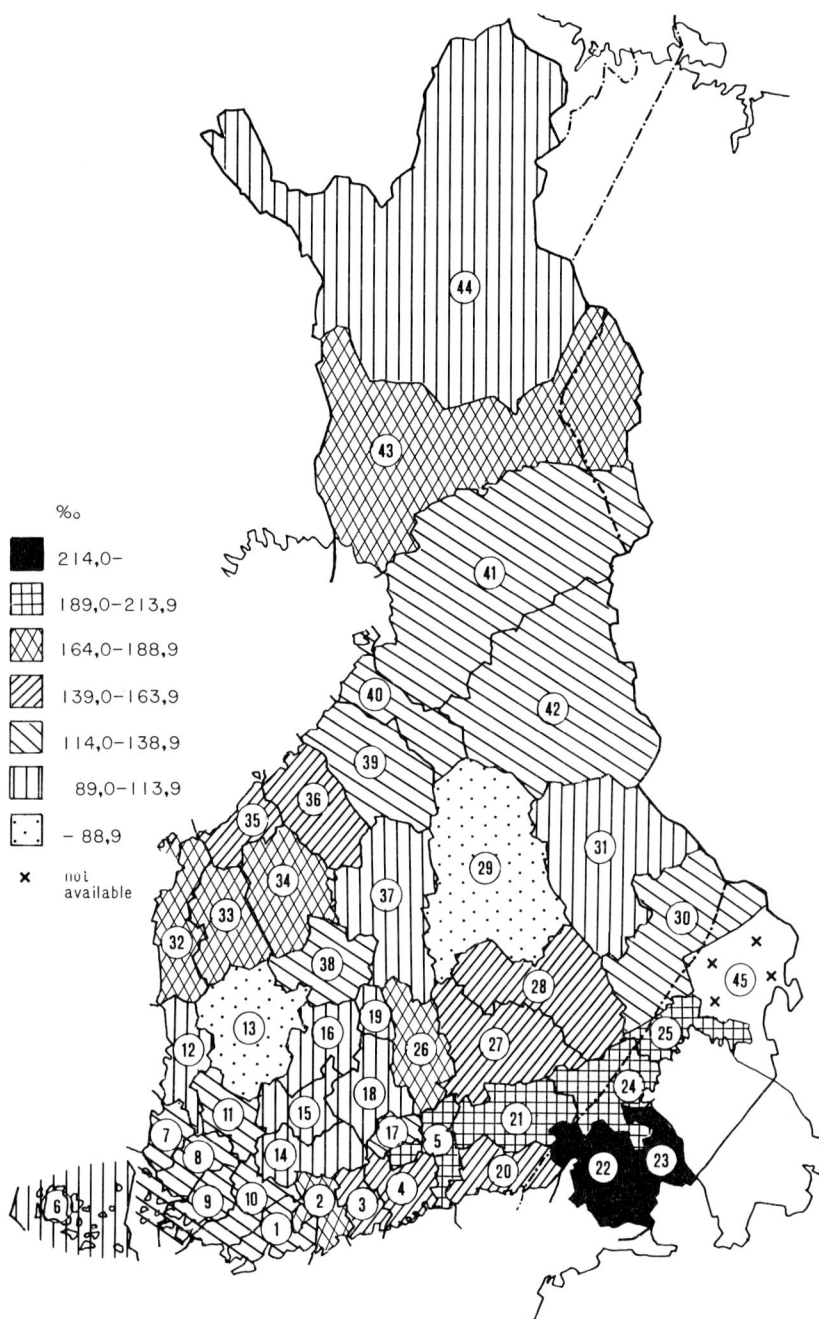

Map 6. Infant mortality in Finland 1869

Finland impoverished by succession of crop failures

At the opening of the 19th century Finland's population rose to about a million. In the mid-1860s the figure was near 1,800,000, so that in just over half a century there was an increase of 800,000.

This extra population settled mainly in the countryside. In the 1860's, in fact, Finland was still quite agrarian. The urban population was 6 % of the whole, and many towns were fully agrarian in character.[6]

A substantial part of the growing population settled the hinterland of villages and backwood areas. Independent farms were established, but the landless class grew even more. As a result of all this, settlement was more and more dispersed around Finland. Many regions of the centre and north received new inhabitants.

In the late 1850s there had been poor harvests, but the actual period of crop failure began in 1862. In many areas bad crops were recorded time after time. Most disastrous was the year 1867, when summer came, on the average, a month later than normal. As a result the growing season remained short, and the corn had no time to ripen. Night frosts in early September finally destroyed the corn harvest. The potato crop too was an almost total loss in many areas.

Several crop failures in succession reduced many farms to utter poverty. In autumn 1867 workers could be hired only to a very limited extent, and unemployment grew explosively. One farm after another went bankrupt and was sold by compulsory auction. All this increased the number of beggars greatly, in northern and central Finland especially. Population streamed from north to south, and at the same time the flood of beggars weakened the ability of southern Finland to provide a living for its own people. The consequence was an extraordinary state of poverty for the whole of Finland which reached the point of food shortage in many places.

To make matters still worse, imports of corn to Finland were nothing like adequate. The price of corn was also high—about twice the normal level — and the poor in particular were in great distress. Thus a kind of famine bread which included lichen, pine-bark and straw was used even in the south of the country.

Epidemics run riot

Spreading through Finland in 1866 was an infectious disease described as typhoid. Next year it was even more widespread and in 1868 it raged without restraint. It is highly probable that not merely typhoid was present but also spotted fever, relapsing fever, dysentery and perhaps influenza.

The spread of epidemics was markedly increased by general poverty and exceptional growth in the number of beggars. With these beggars disease passed from house to house and from village to village. In almost every municipality poorhouses were set up, partly as a means of solving the problem of beggars, and these very houses became hotbeds of disease. The situation became most catastrophic in the spring of 1868. Poorhouses were converted into sick quarters where death claimed many victims. The same happened in temporary hospitals. It was by no means rare for a third of the patients to die. Most were poor, but disease also struck wealthy farmers. Those who tended the sick were in particular danger. A tenth of Finland's doctors died in 1868.

Care of infants in the crisis

These two factors, poverty caused by crop failure and epidemics, in many ways increased the difficulty of tending small children including those less than a year old, as can be seen from the exceptionally high figures for infant mortality. At the same time regional differences in IMR for 1866-1868 deviated completely from their traditional state.

In 1865 IMR was still regionally similar to what it had been in the preceding decades. It was generally highest in areas where breast feeding was least common. The situation was changed in the following years by the large number of beggars and the death of many mothers of suckling infants from infectious diseases. There was an unusual increase in the number of orphans. When a nursing mother died, the child who had subsisted on that mother's milk soon died too. The direct reason for the death of the mother or the child was by no means necessarily starvation; rather it was to be found in the unhygienic, wretched conditions which prevailed in poorhouses and temporary sick quarters.

Conditions during pregnancy and childbirth were also extraordinarily poor in this period of crisis. Miscarriages and deaths in childbirth were appallingly frequent. When a mother succumbed to puerperal fever, for instance, the position of a newborn child was in many cases quite desperate. Death claimed many infants.

Infant care was also difficult because the poor food situation for mothers reduced the amount of their milk. Cow's milk as a substitute was by no means available to all households in winter, because cows were dry. Cessation of cow's milk was occasioned in turn by the very poor supply of cattle feed in 1867. Cattle had to be slaughtered either because feed was lacking for them or because they were needed as food for people who had nothing else. In this way infants received less and less cow's milk.

While the stream of beggars moved from north to south the regions of southern Finland were suffering want. They were obliged to feed growing hordes of beggars in addition to their own people. With the beggars spread many infectious diseases directly connected with the period of crop failure. One of these was smallpox, which killed children who at the age of a few months had lost the immunity received from their mothers. To increase the spread of smallpox still further, the inoculation programme could not be carried out to the usual extent during the crisis years.

After the period of crisis the regional differences in IMR returned to normal in 1869. The rate was lowest in the areas of central Finland where breast feeding was prevalent. The highest figures were recorded in coastal Ostrobothnia and south-east Finland. In these regions artificial feeding was still in use, but after some campaigning against this a change to breast feeding was steadily made. As a result IMR decreased and in the second half of the 19th century regional differences quickly levelled out.[7]

Appendix

Appendix Table I. Infant mortality in Finland 1865-1869

Deanery	1865	1866	1867	1868	1869
(1) Länsi-Raasepori	135.4	137.0	185.6	249.6	117.9
(2) Itä-Raasepori	167.4	193.2	232.5	350.8	164.0
(3) Helsinki	210.0	192.4	229.8	350.2	147.9
(4) Porvoo	160.5	155.0	160.2	417.0	161.4
(5) Iitti	188.6	247.9	177.4	383.6	192.7
(6) Ahvenanamaa	175.0	140.2	250.4	160.6	113.0
(7) Vehmaa	173.0	159.7	279.3	216.2	122.4
(8) Mynämäki	143.8	117.6	282.7	294.0	116.7
(9) Turku	152.2	180.3	277.7	187.3	131.1
(10) Perniö	150.9	140.8	200.6	250.2	119.5
(11) Ylä-Pori	163.9	141.7	354.7	237.8	125.5
(12) Ala-Pori	171.9	137.5	305.7	265.9	112.4
(13) Tyrvää	186.3	170.3	339.4	480.5	86.5
(14) Hämeenlinna	159.0	159.8	223.2	429.5	108.2
(15) Hattula	146.0	186.4	264.2	324.8	90.2
(16) Tampere	171.5	230.4	225.3	599.1	112.2
(17) Itä-Hämä	166.4	210.9	155.6	587.0	118.4
(18) Länsi-Hämä	140.5	205.6	124.3	342.8	97.4
(19) Jämsä	183.9	223.8	175.6	697.5	102.0
(20) Hamina	186.4	232.8	156.3	283.5	153.9
(21) Lappeenranta	197.5	226.3	197.1	280.3	196.4
(22) Viipuri	301.6	226.2	186.2	311.2	242.8
(23) Etelä-Käkisalmi	265.0	287.3	236.4	321.2	254.9
(24) Pohjois-Käkisalmi	241.2	231.3	196.2	316.7	206.9
(25) Sortavala	253.8	309.8	216.4	398.1	210.5
(26) Heinola	159.9	266.3	169.4	411.8	168.2
(27) Etelä-Savo	166.9	201.3	176.1	332.7	163.3
(28) Pohjois-Savo	174.2	235.9	161.9	446.4	158.5
(29) Kuopio	143.4	214.4	147.6	483.5	84.4
(30) Ala-Karjala	184.9	258.3	179.7	603.7	132.7
(31) Ylä-Karjala	207.1	187.5	181.5	629.0	94.5
(32) Ala-Vaasa	228.1	195.5	251.7	362.9	175.0
(33) Ylä-Vaasa	259.0	209.8	303.6	543.3	167.0
(34) Lapua	208.4	249.1	263.2	693.2	165.0
(35) Pietarsaari	177.3	205.2	322.8	453.5	162.8
(36) Kokkola	189.8	232.6	190.2	455.2	145.8
(37) Jyväskylä	164.0	272.2	233.9	467.7	104.1
(38) Keuruu	178.3	230.7	149.8	532.1	121.9
(39) Kalajoki	159.6	278.2	223.7	530.0	133.6
(40) Raahe	155.8	426.3	235.7	491.5	135.6
(41) Oulu	184.5	312.0	258.2	365.1	135.1
(42) Kainuu	107.0	343.4	229.6	390.7	134.8
(43) Kemi	245.6	268.2	346.2	247.9	184.3
(44) Lappi	156.2	148.6	144.4	234.9	95.2
All rural Finland	190.0	217.6	223.1	395.6	139.0
All towns	215.5	217.9	228.5	342.2	162.5
All Finland	193.7	217.6	223.4	391.7	140.5

Appendix Table 2. The number of deaths under 1 year in Finland 1865—1869

Deanery	1865	1866	1867	1868	1869
Länsi-Raasepori	117	113	131	157	77
Itä-Raasepori	182	199	221	255	123
Helsinki	180	152	171	187	101
Porvoo	199	179	187	359	142
Iitti	175	206	160	272	127
Ahvenanamaa	105	89	147	84	59
Vehmaa	178	157	237	155	122
Mynämäki	112	87	203	167	91
Turku	163	197	286	177	139
Perniö	219	194	269	271	157
Ylä-Pori	236	195	381	200	152
Ala-Pori	272	227	413	276	180
Tyrvää	503	426	689	504	217
Hämeenlinna	242	202	298	344	144
Hattula	146	183	232	152	77
Tampere	209	253	264	396	137
Itä-Hämä	94	108	87	199	49
Länsi-Hämä	165	226	141	254	100
Jämsä	98	107	92	219	60
Hamina	239	257	198	271	135
Lappeenranta	205	221	244	291	163
Viipuri	571	409	341	524	363
Etelä-Käkisalmi	313	346	292	423	236
Pohjois-Käkisalmi	241	251	238	343	186
Sortavala	266	317	248	334	157
Heinola	186	261	184	390	169
Etelä-Savo	302	343	313	554	278
Pohjois-Savo	321	384	282	608	252
Kuopio	550	857	568	1.321	353
Ala-Karjala	314	422	297	658	184
Ylä-Karjala	342	315	334	671	183
Ala-Vaasa	523	462	566	512	402
Ylä-Vaasa	568	482	647	628	373
Lapua	400	432	500	680	357
Pietarsaari	239	267	450	400	224
Kokkola	241	281	248	335	188
Jyväskylä	274	398	363	550	191
Keuruu	123	149	99	207	83
Kalajoki	252	382	330	513	220
Raahe	132	266	181	260	99
Oulu	283	429	361	391	175
Kainuu	131	274	183	327	89
Kemi	235	261	295	209	158
Lappi	30	26	26	35	18
All rural Finland	10 876	11 992	12 398	16 064	7 490
All towns	838	816	819	1 077	585
All Finland	11 714	12 808	13 217	17 141	8 075

Source: Population change tables in the archives of Central Statistical Office of Finland.

75

Notes

1. See for example: G. Broström, A. Brändström and L-Å. Persson, 'The Impact of Breastfeeding Patterns on Infant Mortality in a 19th Century Swedish Parish', *Newsletter No 1 from the Demographic Data Base* (Umeå 1983); O. Turpeinen, 'Infant Mortality in Finland 1749-1865', *Scandinavian Economic History Review,* XXVII, 1 (1979); A. Brändström, *"De kärlekslösa mödrarna". Spädbarnsdödligheten i Sverige under 1800-talet med särskild hänsyn till Nedertorneå.* With an English summary (Umeå 1984).

2. *Population change tables in Central Statistical Office of Finland;* Turpeinen (1979).

3. O. Turpeinen, 'Fertility and Mortality in Finland since 1750', *Population studies,* 33, 1 (1979); *Population and population change tables in the archives of the Central Statistical Office of Finland.*

4. O. Turpeinen, *Nälkä vai tauti tappoi? Kauhunvuodet 1866-1868,* (Was Hunger or Disease the Killer? Years of Terror 1866-1868) (Jyväskylä 1986).

5. *Population change tables in the archives of the Central Statistical Office of Finland and Vital Statistics VI, 3.*

6. O. Turpeinen, 'The Urban Population in Finland 1815-65'. *Yearbook of Population Research in Finland,* XX (1982).

7. Turpeinen (1986); P. Pulma and O. Turpeinen, *Lastensuojelu Suomessa 1750-1980* (Child Care in Finland 1750-1980) (manuscript 1987).

76

The Old in the New: Spatial Patterns in the 19th Century Demographic Change

Margareta Larsson

An important element in the model of demographic transition is the presence or absence of a parallel movement of fertility and mortality.[1] Thus, in the Swedish case, the combination of declining mortality with stable fertility during the greater part of the 19th century is used to demarcate a certain stage of that transition. At the end of the century, fertility started to fall and more of a parallelism emerged, this being interpreted as a new stage, a new objective situation called the fertility transition. According to Fridlizius, the mortality change acquired a new character (from the middle of the 19th century) in that it "did not return to the previous level", a consequence of the gradual but definite elimination "of the great secular epidemic cycles which cast their shadow over the pre-industrial community".[2]

The coupling of mortality and fertility within a process-oriented perspective, as implied by the model of demographic transition, is of interest as a starting point in understanding the fertility transition from the preceding stage in the population development. In this perspective, one crucial question is why fertility remained high for so long a period while mortality declined. To this, several answers have been put forward. In line with the increasing attention paid to the individual side of the transition within the field of historical demography, some of the concepts recurring in these discussions include lagged perception of the declining infant mortality[3], neglect of fertility limitation in spite of increasing survival resulting from adaptation to new economic circumstances[4], family limitation as a not yet perceived or accepted behavioural norm, and the lack of widespread knowledge of birth control techniques[5], etc.

Thus, the question as to why fertility remained high as mortality declined leads to further questions. What connection can really be expected between these variables? And what answers will be produced through analyses on different levels, such as the individual level, a level different from the one for which the questions was originally asked.[6] Against this background, the aim of this paper is to study the relationship between mortality and fertility during the stage preceding the fertility transition, by investigating the spatial pattern formed by the two variables. What follows is to be regarded as the product of work yet not completed.

Data and procedures

The regional analyses is based on the deanery *(prosteri)* tables of the *Tabellverk* (1759-1859), that is, yearly summaries of births and deaths and five-year summaries of age structure, occupational distribution, migration, etc. Parts of these tables—data for 1805, 1806, 1855, 1856—have been processed and computerized by the Demographic Data Base in Umeå.

Data comparable over time are given for rural deaneries only. Furthermore, depending on changes in the administrative boundaries between the beginning and the middle of the 19th century, some deaneries have been combined in the analysis. For the same reason, two deaneries situated in the northernmost part of Sweden have been excluded. The result is 168 units of varying area and population size (the population varies from around 2 000 to 40 000).

Though some uncertainty persists about the reliability of the *Tabellverk* data, the figures seem to be adequate for the descriptive analysis of regional differences in fertility and infant mortality to be presented here.[7]

As expected, the average fertility based on the 168 units/rural districts remains at about the same level with 172 live births per 1 000 women aged 20-45 years during the first period and 168 during the next. The corresponding rates for the country as a whole, are 171 for 1801-1805, 165 for 1806-1810, 171 for 1851-1855, and 181 for 1856-1860.[8] The picture of a relatively stable fertility is reinforced by the constant variation between the district rates: the standard deviations are 20 and 21. Also as expected, the average decrease in infant mortality is from 192 deaths before the age of one year per 1 000 live births 1805-1806 to 138 in 1855-1856, and the decline in standard deviation between the district rates is from 42 to 25. For the country as a whole, the infant mortality is 199 in 1801-1810 and, excluding the cities, 137 in 1851-1860.[9] Finally, it may be noted that there is virtually no synchronic correlation between the two basic variables, fertility and infant mortality. For 1805-1806 it comes out at +.14, for 1855-1856 at -.16, in both cases based on the 168 rural districts.

The limitation to four years, however, is of significance, especially for the infant mortality rates which not only, like the fertility rates, fluctuate from one year to another but also based on the lower numbers under risk. Although the means for two two-year periods have been used, the result suffers from uncertainties arising from temporary disturbances, mainly epidemics.

The variables have been subjected to cluster analysis, independent of geographical location, and the results have been transferred to maps. The clustering procedure used here groups the units/districts into clusters each of which have roughly the same degree of variance between the values of the variables.[10] At the present stage of work, cluster analysis has been used merely as an auxiliary technique in the geographical grouping of districts.

Bearing in mind the independence between the national rates, the spatial patterns of fertility and infant mortality will be analysed separately.

Regional change and national stability

According to its critics, the model of demographic transition is merely a description of the population development, the outcome of national rates of mortality and fertility, as experienced in a limited number of countries and, thus, with a restricted empirical applicability. A further problem is the existence of inter-regional difference in demographic rates, concealed by the highly aggregated picture of national rates.[11]

Returning to Sweden, Sundbärg found that the country could be divided into three main demographic regions, each geographically connected.[12] The distinctive feature from 1860 to 1900 was marital fertility. The validity of this division for the period 1890-1900 is confirmed by a study comparing 69 districts *(härader)*[13] scattered from northern to southern Sweden.[14] From this cross-sectional point of view and controlling for agrarian structure and geographical location, it was neither the influence of industry and agriculture on employment and economy, nor the secularization that was decisive for the differences in fertility pattern between the 69 districts. Instead, the fertility patterns in industrial districts were more similar to the patterns in neighbouring agricultural districts than to the patterns in distant industrial districts. And the significance of secularization turned out to be working within the characteristics of Sundbärg's main demographic regions. Obviously, there was a spatial relation of importance to consider; perhaps a space factor of the past resulting in a particular pattern of response within the productive sector to extraneous conditions and changes—regardless if they were of material or idealistic nature.

Consequently, a question of importance is whether these regional differences in fertility, found in the first decades of the fertility transition, can be related to a pre-existing spatial pattern.

Indicated by r^2, 65 % of the variation in the general fertility rates of the 168 districts (deaneries) in 1855-1856 remains when the influences from the differences in fertility 1805-1806 have been allowed for. Furthermore, the regional distribution of the residuals, as shown in Map 1, points to the presence of a spatial order or spatial autocorrelation. Thus, between the beginning and the middle of the 19th century, deviating from the national picture, the stability in fertility seems to be rather modest on the district level, at the same time as there appears to be a regional factor in the change.

A comparison of the regional situation for the years 1805-1806 and 1855-1856, shown in Maps 2 and 3, gives a more detailed information. Briefly, the picture created by the general fertility rates of the 168 districts at the beginning of the 19th century shows high fertility in Northern Sweden, low fertility in Middle Sweden, and variable yet mainly medium fertility in Southern Sweden. Upon closer scrutiny, there are also two low-fertility sub-regions in the South, one of high fertility, and many more or less isolated districts deviating from the dominant medium-fertility level. Of the two low-fertility sub-regions, one is situated in the counties of Halland, Älvsborg, Skaraborg, and Jönköping and the other mostly in the county of Kristianstad, while the high-fertility sub-region is located in the county of Blekinge and neighbouring areas in the counties of Kronoberg and Kalmar.

In accordance with the modest stability, mentioned above, this picture is still approximately valid fifty years later. Nonetheless, the changes are of great interest. Map 3 illustrates these changes as well as the demarcations which are drawn with some arbitrariness, between Southern, Middle, and Northern Sweden, based on the spatial pattern produced by the fertility rates of 1805-1806.

Starting from Southern Sweden, the deviant sub-regions as characterized by a high or a low fertility are reduced in size and the more or less isolated deviant districts are reduced in number, a reduction which favors an expansion of the already dominant medium-fertility level. With the boundaries drawn between Southern and Middle Sweden, there are 110 districts located in the South. Of these, the proportion of districts falling in clusters defined by low fertility decreases from 0.32 to 0.15, and those by high fertility from 0.23 to 0.15, while the proportion of districts falling in the cluster defined by a medium fertility increases from 0.45 to 0.70. Thus, in Southern Sweden, the variation in general fertility decreases somewhat from the beginning to the middle of the 19th century. While the mean remains the same, the coefficient of variation decreases from 0.10 to 0.08. In accordance with this vague tendency towards a more uniform picture, the earlier mentioned residuals as illustrated in Map 1 vary in distance and sign.

In Middle Sweden, there seem to be two simultaneous processes: on the one hand, a fall in the existing low fertility and, on the other, a reduction in the size of Middle Sweden as a low-fertility region. The first observation especially applies to the area surrounding the Lake of Mälaren where 21 of the 25 extremely low-fertility districts, found in the entire country, are situated in 1855-1856. Consequently, there is an accumulation of negative residuals here. The second observation, the reduction in size, is pronounced on the northern border of Middle Sweden. Here, five of the districts in question seem to form a transitional zone to the still high-fertility Northern Sweden. Further to the south, the reduction in size is more uneven and the resulting picture less coherent. Accordingly, parallel with the fall in fertility and shrinkage in size, the variation between the district rates for Middle Sweden shows a slight increase from the beginning of the century. The coefficient of variation rises from 0.08 to 0.12.

In Northern Sweden, the dominant tendency towards high fertility persists and becomes more consistent; the coefficient of variation sinks from 0.14 to 0.05, while the mean remains the same at 211. The residuals are positive in six of the seven districts constituting this northern part.

In conclusion, behind the national picture of a relatively stable fertility, the spatial pattern changes from the beginning to the middle of the 19th century.

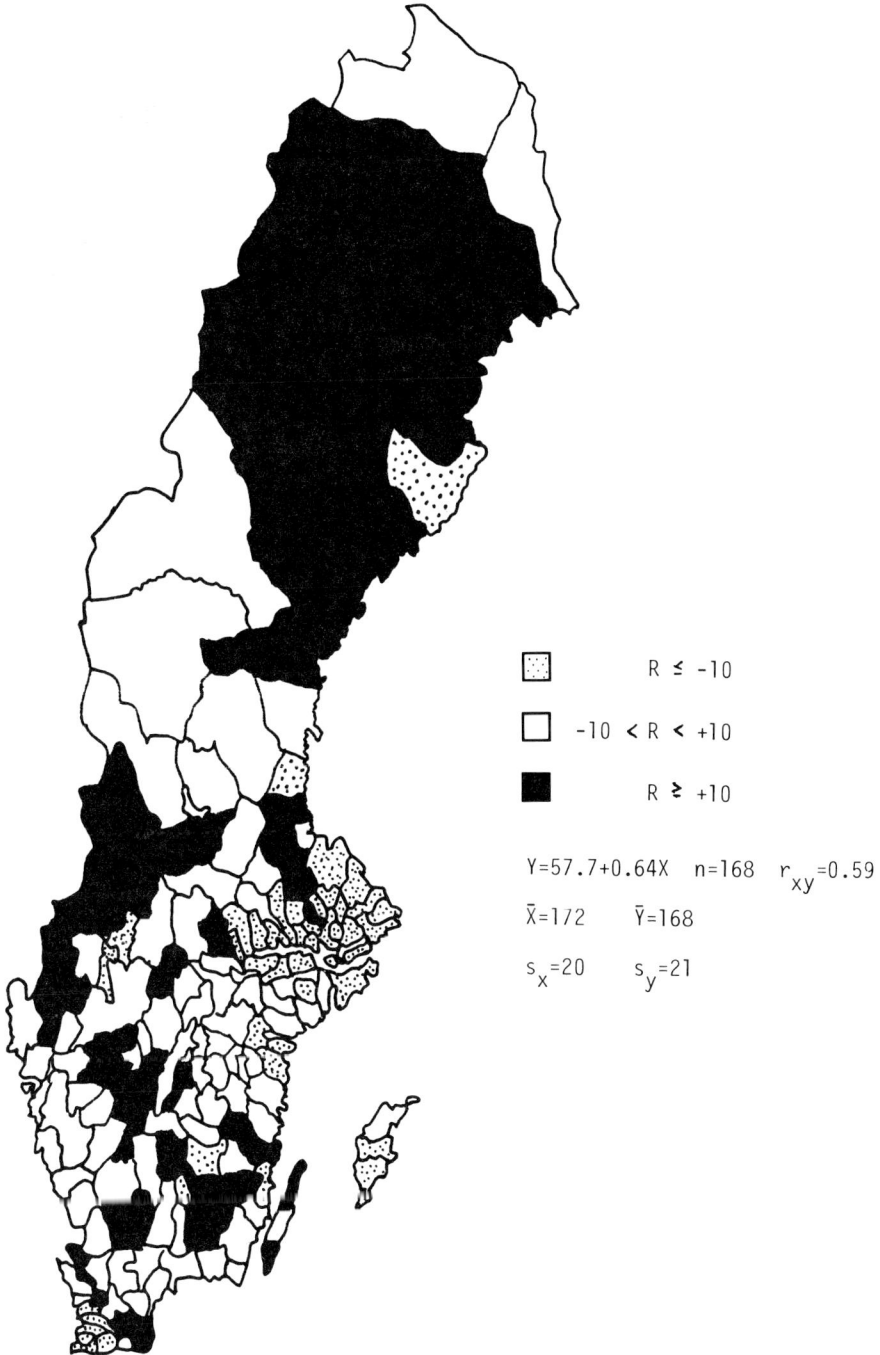

Map 1. The change in fertility between 1805-1806 (X) and 1866-1856 (Y) indicated by the residuals (R) from the line of regression.

R ≤ -10

-10 < R < +10

R ≥ +10

$Y=57.7+0.64X$ $n=168$ $r_{xy}=0.59$

$\bar{X}=172$ $\bar{Y}=168$

$s_x=20$ $s_y=21$

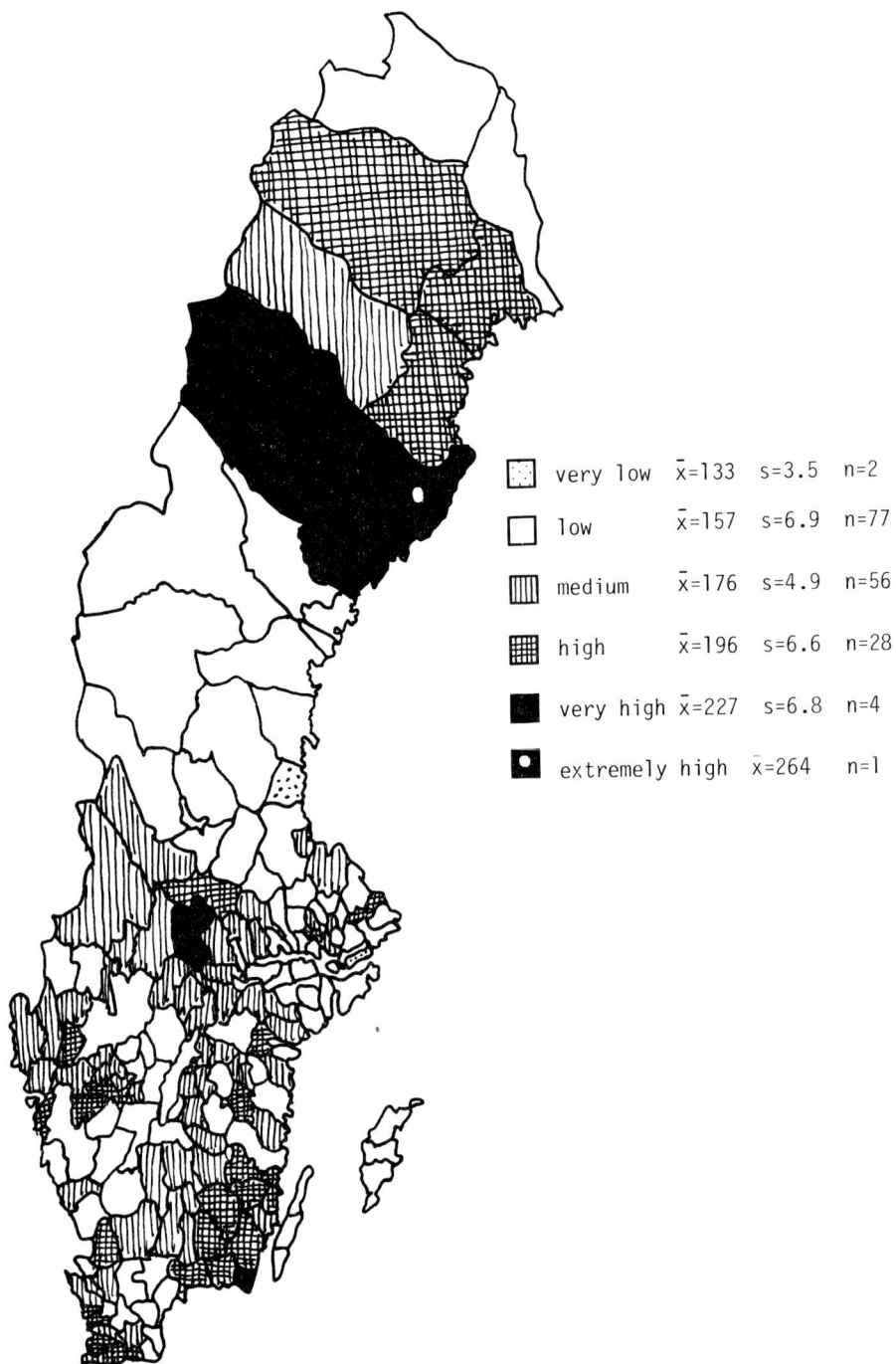

Map 2. Live born per 1000 women aged 20-45 1805-1806.

		$\bar{x}$=133	s=3.5	n=2
⬚	very low	$\bar{x}$=133	s=3.5	n=2
☐	low	$\bar{x}$=157	s=6.9	n=77
▥	medium	$\bar{x}$=176	s=4.9	n=56
▦	high	$\bar{x}$=196	s=6.6	n=28
■	very high	$\bar{x}$=227	s=6.8	n=4
◉	extremely high	$\bar{x}$=264		n=1

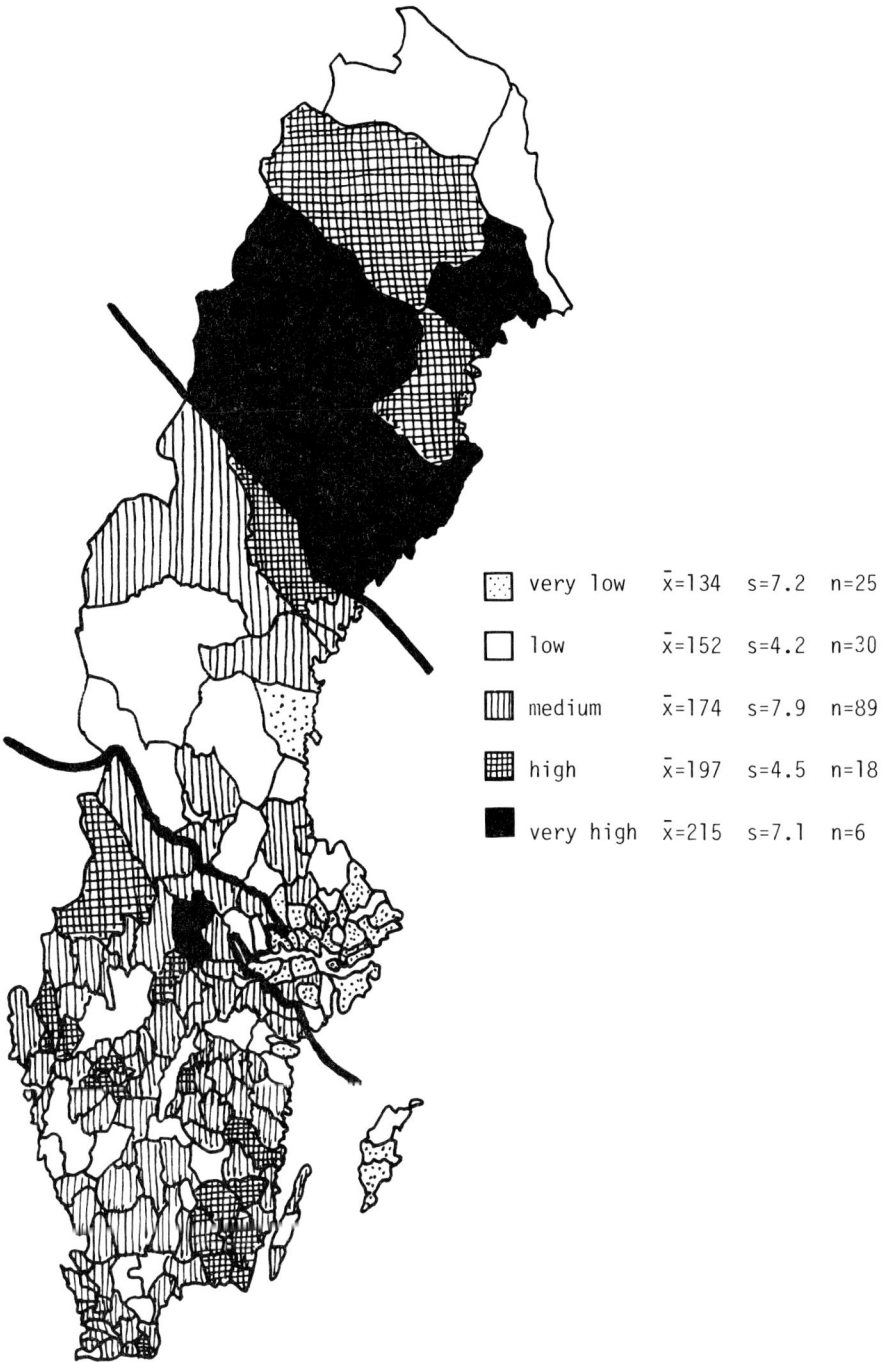

Map 3. Live born per 1000 women aged 20-45 1855-1856.

This result is in accordance with earlier studies, which point to the existence of regional differences underlying national aggregate, and it implies that the immediate validity of the model of demographic transition is limited at lower levels of analysis than the country as a whole. The regional changes in fertility levels also tend to strengthen a pre-existing pattern of spatial differences and to make it more distinct. Furthermore, the agreement between this spatial pattern and Sundbärg's three main demographic regions is obvious.[15] Consequently, the regional differences found in the first decades of the fertility transition, after 1870, should be regarded as an amplification of an old structure rather than something qualitatively new. And the background of these regional differences is to be looked for in circumstances, preceding the economic and ideological changes during the beginning of the transition.

A possible interpretation for this is that the space factor of the past manifest itself as a traditionally oriented behavior in Weber's sense, that is, through the habituation of a long practice.[16] From this point of view, Bourdieu's[17] concept of "habitus" is elucidating and combines the structural and individual level with the dimensions of time and space.[18]

Habitus, according to Bourdieu, is a system of dispositions, a product of history designating a way of being, a habitual state. As the principle of continuity, habitus is the "past which survives in the present and tends to perpetuate itself into the future by making itself present in practices..".[19] And as a cognitive and motivational structure, habitus enables the individuals to cope with changing situations within a limited frame of pattern.

Thus, as a space factor of the past, the presence of habitus will amplify or delay the regional differences in fertility rather than to contribute to a regional equalization.

Infant mortality—an uncertainty of everyday life

Characteristic of the infant mortality decline is "its regular and continuous nature" on the national level and "in all /sampled/ regions".[20] Reflecting the long-term fall, this picture is based on ten-year averages and mainly on comparably large regions (counties). An example of the variation behind this long-term fall is shown by the two-year averages of 1805-1806 and 1855-1856 for the 168 districts used here, probably expressing an environmental factor of relevance for everyday life.

The long-term fall, though relatively uniform across the country, must be seen together with the rather weak stability for individual small areas. Indicated by r^2 and based on the 168 districts, 84 % of the variation in infant mortality for 1855-1856 remains, when the influence from the differences 1805-1806 have been taken into account. Deviating from the fertility change, there is no sign of any reinforcement of the regional pattern formed by the infant mortality rates in the earlier period. On the contrary, the spatial distribution of districts defined by a comparably high infant mortality—that is, above approximately 200 during the first period and 140 during the latter—seems to become more disconnected. Map 4 illustrates this fact.

In the beginning of the century, the high mortality districts are concentrated in a small number of regions. One, containing 24 districts, is situated around the Lake of Mälaren in the middle-east, another is formed by 18 (or 21) adjoining districts, in the southernmost part of Sweden. The third obvious high-mortality region includes five districts in the counties of Ångermanland and Västerbotten in the north.

Fifty years later, the boundaries of these high-mortality regions are dissolved; while some of the old high-mortality districts have disappeared, others in the neighbourhood or at a greater distance have been added. The picture becomes more dispersed. At the same time, there are accumulations of positive residuals in the tracts of these high-mortality regions, shown in Map 5, although the presence of negative residuals should not be underestimated.

This shift to a seemingly more disconnected picture, together with the rather low regional stability, can be interpreted in more ways than one. Most probably, a combination of chance fluctuation and a more stable underlying pattern of structurally determined vulnerability is responsible. One common element behind both chance fluctuations (say, through epidemics) and structurally anchored high or low death rates, as environmental factors of relevance for the everyday life, is the lack of immediate and physical control over infant survival on the part of individual families. Death or survival is highly dependent on uncertain events or conditions during the first part of the 19th century. Although it is debatable whether these uncertainties were experienced more keenly in the high-mortality tracts than in low-mortality ones, it seems reasonable to assume that areas including high-mortality districts also experienced unusually large fluctuations. If it was so, the future was double unpredictable.

Hence, underlying the regular and continuous nature of the long-term fall in infant mortality, there seem to be variations. As far as these variations can be regarded as environmental factors of relevance for the everyday life, the resulting uncertainties on the part of the individual families probably made the even *and slow* long term fall hard to detect. Given a national average of 4.7 deliveries per woman, the number of surviving infants increased from 3.80 to 4.04, that is, a quarter of a child in fifty years.

Norbert Elias compares the transition of the code of behavior, during the process of the European civilization, to people with a double face—one looking backward and one forward.[21] The people are standing on a bridge. And there is a quite slow motion, problematic to observe in a single stage. Elias writes: "in observing a single stage, we lack a sure measure. What is accidental fluctuation? When and where is something advancing? When is something falling behind? /And/ are we really concerned with a change in a definite direction?" Most likely, also the double faced people standing on the bridge were lacking a sure measure, were lacking the overview which is possible

Map 4. Deaths aged 0-1 per 1000 live born 1805-1806 and 1855-1856.

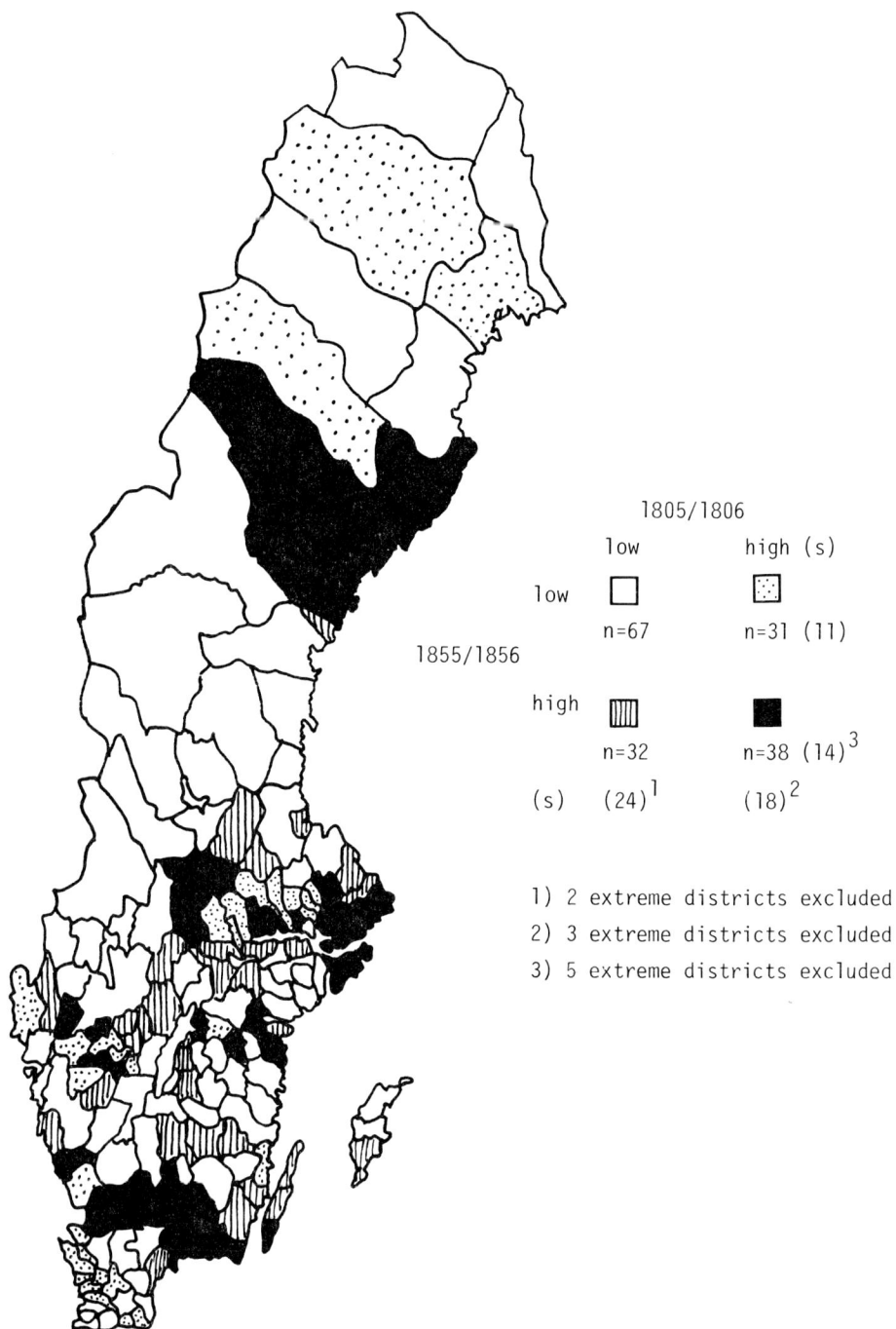

1805/1806

	low	high (s)
low	☐ n=67	⬚ n=31 (11)
high	▥ n=32	■ n=38 (14)[3]
(s)	(24)[1]	(18)[2]

1855/1856

1) 2 extreme districts excluded
2) 3 extreme districts excluded
3) 5 extreme districts excluded

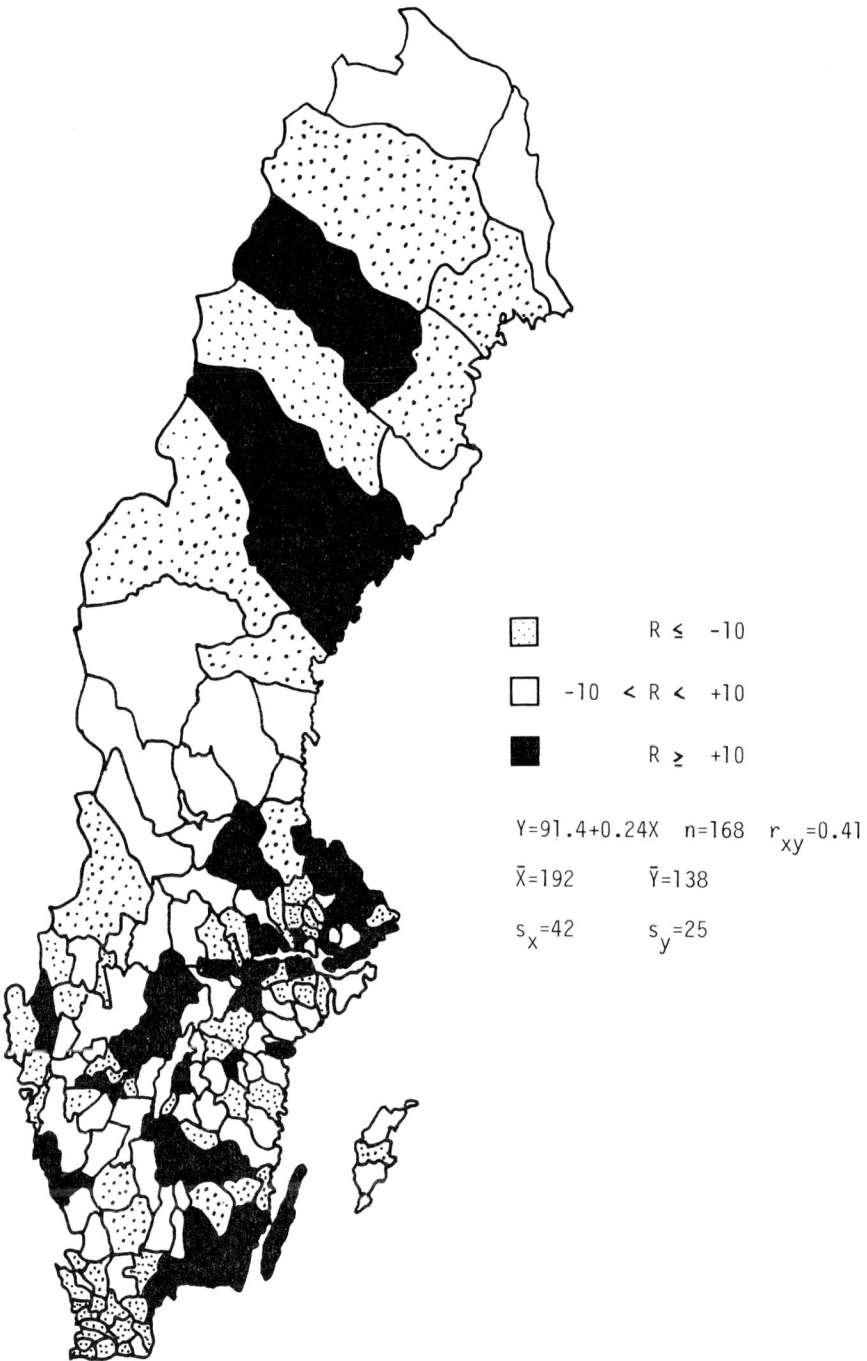

Map 5. The change in infant mortality between 1805-1805 (X) and 1855-1856 (Y) indicated by the residuals (R) from the line of regression.

$$R \leq -10$$

$$-10 < R < +10$$

$$R \geq +10$$

$Y=91.4+0.24X$ $n=168$ $r_{xy}=0.41$

$\bar{X}=192$ $\bar{Y}=138$

$s_x=42$ $s_y=25$

through time-series of means based on a large aggregate.

Thus, in agreement with Fridlizius'[22] general conclusion about the impact of the great secular epidemic cycles not yet eliminated, as well as with Carlsson's[23] hypothesis of stochastic perception, the infant mortality seems to constitute an uncertainty of everyday life, rather than a new lasting condition, during the first part of 19th century Sweden. That means a further limitation on the validity of the demographic transition model on levels of analysis lower than the national one. Consequently, the crucial question, as to why fertility remained at a high level while mortality declined, appears to be irrelevant from the point of view of the underlying spatial patterns.

Conclusion

In short, the regional analysis supports the result obtained from national data to the extent that fertility and infant mortality do not appear to be associated during the stage preceding the fertility decline. Changes in fertility give the impression of following a dynamic pattern of their own, not reducible to differences in mortality. Summarized by r^2 and based on the 168 rural districts, 97 to 98 % of the variation in fertility remains, both in the beginning and in the middle of the 19th century Sweden, when the influence from the differences in infant mortality have been allowed for.

There is a regional factor in the fertility change which tends to strengthen a pre-existing pattern of spatial differences. And the main demographic regions, found by Sundbärg in the first decades of the fertility transition, should be regarded as an amplification of an old structure—preceding the industrialization and secularization during the latter part of the 19th century—rather than something qualitatively new. A possible interpretation for this is the presence of "habitus" in practices (in Bourdieu's sense) mediating past and present in the space.

Regarding the infant mortality, the room for the effects of a regionally anchored "habitus" seems to have been smaller. Instead, the nature of infant mortality as an uncertainty of everyday life has been suggested. From the spatial and the limited time perspective used here, there were underlying variations in infant death rates probably obscuring the relatively slow, downward trend dominating the national picture. As mortality proceeded to decline, in the latter half of the 19th century, the fluctuations become less pronounced and the trend more visible in everyday life. Before that, a prominent condition was missing for the fertility to be dependent on the decreasing infant mortality. (In line with this and according to the above mentioned cross-sectional study of 1890-1900, the remaining variation in fertility, when the differences in infant mortality have been taken into account, decreases to 69 %).[24]

Thus, at levels of analysis lower than the national one, there are limitations in the immediate validity of the model of demographic transition as well as, from the viewpoint of everyday life, in the relevance of the question of why fertility remained high while mortality declined. And in the new stage of the demographic transition during the late 19th century, beside the old downward trend in infant mortality, the old spatial pattern in fertility was highly present.

Notes

1. 'United Nations, History and Population Theories'; 'The Determinants and Consequences of Population Trends', *UN, STISDA,* Ser A, 145 (1953).

2. G. Fridlizius, 'Sweden', R. Lee (Ed.), *European Demography and Economic Growth* (London 1979), pp. 340-405; G. Fridlizius, 'The Mortality Decline in the First Phase of the Demographic Transition: Swedish Experiences', T. Bengtsson, G. Fridlizius, R. Ohlsson (Eds), *Pre-Industrial Population Change* (Stockholm 1984), pp. 71-114.

3. G. Carlsson, 'The Decline of Fertility: Innovation or Adjustment Process', *Population Studies,* 20 (1966), pp. 149-174.

4. C. Winberg, *Folkökning och proletarisering* (Partille 1975).

5. J. Knodel, 'Family Limitation and the Fertility Transition: Evidence from the Age Patterns of Fertility in Europe and Asia', *Population Studies,* 31 (1977), pp. 219-249.

6. N. Ryder, 'Where Do Babies Come from', H.M. Blalock (Ed.), *Sociological Theory and Research* (New York 1980), pp. 182-202.

7. K. Lockridge, 'The Fertility Transition in Sweden—A Preliminary Look at Smaller Geographic Units, 1855-1890', *Report no 3 from The Demographic Data Base* (Umeå 1983, 1984).

8. G. Sundbärg, *Bevölkerungsstatistik Schwedens 1750-1900* (Stockholm 1907, 1970).

9. *Historisk statistik för Sverige,* I, (Stockholm 1969).

10. *SAS Users Guide:* Statistics (1982).

11. R. Andorka, *Determinants of Fertility in Advanced Societies* (London 1978).

12. G. Sundbärg, *Bidrag till Sveriges officiella statistik, serie A: Befolkningsstatistik* (Stockholm 1890, 1900).

13. An administrative unit, usually of somewhat smaller size than the deanery, used in the Swedish statistics after 1860.

14. M. Larsson, *Fruktsamhetsmönster, produktionsstruktur och sekularisering* (Stockholm 1984).

15. Following Sundbärg's division the corresponding coefficients of variation, based on estimated marital fertility rates, are 0.09 1805-1806 and 0.06 1855-1856 in Southern Sweden ("Western Sweden" in Sundbärg's terminology), 0.09 1805-1806 and 0.10 1855-1856 in Middle Sweden ("Eastern Sweden"), and 0.16 1805-1806 and 0.09 1855-1856 in Northern Sweden.

16. M. Weber, *Ekonomi och samhälle,* I (Lund 1918-1920, 1983).

17. P. Bourdieu, *Outline of a Theory of Practice* (Cambridge 1972, 1977).

18. See Giddens association between "habitus" and "duality of structures" in A. Giddens, *Central Problems in Social Theory* (London 1979, 1982).

19. Bourdieu (1977), p. 82.

20. Fridlizius (1979), p. 348 and Table 9:20.

21. N. Elias, *The History of Manners* (New York 1939, 1978).

22. Fridlizius (1978, 1984).

23. Carlsson (1966).

24. Larsson (1984).

Childcare—A Mirror of Women's Living Conditions. A Community Study Representing 18th and 19th Century Ostrobothnia in Finland

Ulla-Britt Lithell

Women play a substantial role in developing countries. This fact is obvious to most scholars and aid agencies in the world today. WHO has emphasized that the future for those countries depends to a large degree on the enrollment of women in different sectors of society.

> "It is the women who are expected to be health educators, to teach sound health practices to future generations; to create a home environment that is conducive to health (from clean water to nutritious food); to limit family size; to ensure the children are immunized and cared for during crucial years and to take them to the formal health care services when necessary; and to care for the elderly".

Women also assist as midwives and are volunteers at hospitals. Women

> "providing a giant's share of primary health care"[1]

If the living conditions for women become worse because of an increased work load this will lead to great difficulties for women, especially those in fertile ages. In most developing countries the amount of work performed by women is already extremely high. The balance therefore can easily be disturbed, and it is essential that all steps to involve women in further production should be taken with great caution. Intelligence and experience are needed to solve the problems of childcare, households duties, and involvement in production in a low socio-economic setting. Sometimes these different tasks are impossible to combine and become a matter of priority. In a poor environment it is easy to understand that the survival of the family household is the most vital issue. Single members of the family are of lesser importance.

There is strong evidence that the situation for women in the past was similar to that of women in the third world of today. A heavy work burden, many times combined with great difficulties in adequately solving the childcare problem, characterized the life of many women in the past.

The importance of mothers for the survival of children in the past has very clearly been shown by Ulf Högberg.[2] He has analyzed the effects of the death of the mothers during delivery on children's survival. Almost none of the children under the age of five survived. These findings show the great role the mother plays, especially in an environment in the past, characterized by ignorance and a low socio-economic level.

Scholars have stressed the possible effects of hard work on reproduction. In his paper "Women's work and child care in Prussia", W.R. Lee has presented extremely interesting data concerning child mortality in Germany during the 19th century. Some areas had higher child mortality than other provinces. Lee emphasized the probable effect of the changing working condition of women during the 19th century on child mortality.[3]

A.E. Imhof has stressed different attitudes towards infants as a factor influencing child mortality.[4] Brändström has examined the infant mortality in some Swedish parishes during the 19th century but can not find a direct relation between women's working conditions and increased mortality among infants.[5]

The aim of this paper is to present some new data and to discuss the background for and the effects of the extremely difficult situation which was the reality for many women during the period before 1900 in the Finnish province of Ostrobothnia.

Background

The area close to the Ostrobothnian coast was settled during the 14th century by a Swedish speaking population.[6] Beyond that area lived people who spoke Finnish.

Prior to the 17th century fishing and hunting seals were apparently the main sources of income in the coastal area. As a complement to these earnings the women cultivated land for grain production, and cattle were kept for milk and meat products.[7] Fish and oil from seal fat were transported to the Swedish capital, Stockholm, and served as tax payments and exchange commodities.[8] The population in the province needed cereals for bread; even during normal years the production of bread-grain did not meet the basic requirement.[9] Harvest failures were frequent, especially during the 17th century.[10] Even during normal years a great part of the population had to use bark bread or bread made from a mixture of cereals and straw.[11]

During the 17th century a "new" product increased in value for the people in Ostrobothnia. The demand for tar increased, and raw material for its production was abundant in the area. Tar had been produced during earlier periods in some of the most southern coastal parishes, such as Närpes.[12] Tar production increased during the 17th century, particularly in those areas which had a supply of raw material and short distances to ports.[13]

The tar production was very large, and in some areas the supply of pine forest decreased dramatically. The parishes which early started to produce tar were also those which already in the beginning of the 18th century, found that most of the forest useful for tar production had been wasted. In some of those areas even timber for buildings and for heating the houses was rare. New areas therefore became involved, and tar production shifted from southwest to northeast.[14] The abandoned areas depended on fishing, but there was also an increasing interest in cultivation of new land. At the end of the 18th century after the land and the forest had been distributed among the farmers in the province, tar production steadily decreased. Instead the cultivation of new land increased.

Authorities in the area welcomed the decreased tar production. For many decades representatives of the Swedish government had emphasized the negative effects on agriculture resulting from the interest in tar production. Governor Piper, for example, adopted this view and wanted to stop tar production.[15]

By the middle of the 19th century the number of parishes still engaged in producing tar had diminished, and these parishes were located in the interior. In some parts of the province the cultivation of land increased rapidly. In the beginning of the 19th century the Kyro valley was the main agricultural area, and the parishes of Ilmola, Vähäkyro, and Laihela were the most well-developed agrarian communities. The renowned Vasa rye was produced in these parishes, and Vasa was main port for the export trade.[16]

Division of work among men and women in Ostrobothnia

In 1749, when the registration of the population started in Sweden and Finland, it became clear to the Swedish government that there were pronounced differences within the country, especially in infant mortality. One area which was characterized by very high mortality among the smallest children was Ostrobothnia. In many parishes in this province one third of the infants died before the age of one year, while in other parts of Finland one fifth of the children died in that age.[17]

Government representatives who worked in the province stated that the reason for early death among infants was the effect of early weaning and poor nursing habits among mothers in the area. Some also made note of the extreme working conditions for mothers in this part of Finland, and emphasized that the harvest time was the most burdensome part of the year. The smallest children were left at home to be taken care of by elderly people, young siblings, or the children of other families.[18]

An increasing amount of work during harvest time must have been a common situation for most women during earlier periods in agrarian society. In Ostrobothnia the situation in most parts of the province was special.

It has already been mentioned that the men in the province, especially in the coastal area, were occupied by fishing and hunting seals in the Baltic sea during the first centuries following the settlement of the province. During that period the women were responsible for the cultivation of the farms.

During the 17th century the working situation changed for men and women in the province. The demand for tar increased the burden of work for both men and women in the western part of Finland. It seems as if most of the tar production was taken care of by men even though in some parishes women also participated in this production.[19]

During the 18th century the production of tar spread to new parts of the province because of the lack of pine forests in some of the communities which started their production early. During the first half of the 19th century some parishes in the interior of Ostrobothnia were still producing tar in large quantities.[20] The 18th century was also a difficult time for the people in the province in other ways. In the second decade of the century Finland and Ostrobothnia were occupied by Russian troops. During the first half of the 1740's a new Russian occupation hit this area. The effects of these wars were very negative in different ways for the province. Among other things there was a great loss of manpower, and many farms were deserted and destroyed. Cattle were killed, and horses and people were sent to Russia by the army.[21]

In the middle of this century after the wars, the clearing of new lands began. This work sometimes went on together with production of tar. The burden of work increased for both men and women and now with a decreased labor force.

The cumulative effects of the prevailing situation meant extremely severe conditions for women. In a great number of parishes this difficult working situation was combined with very poor living conditions. As mentioned earlier barkbread was the normal diet in much of the province. Women had to work hard and under severe environmental conditions. Work normally done by men, such as plowing, digging trenches, hay-harvesting, and slaughtering, were left to women. In some areas the women were responsible for 30-50 % of the hay harvest. On top of this women were also used as laborers in the tar production. In other areas the women were occupied in transportation of firewood and other goods.[22]

These different types of work were carried out in an environment distinguished by many hours of walking to reach the fields and frequent difficulties because of water-logged fields. It was necessary to stay over-night in small barns near to the fields during harvest time.

Working conditions for men and women in the province were extraordinary. However, the burden for women was greater because of their role in reproduction. The reality for most women was hard work and sometimes a low nutrition intake, factors which are inconsistent with pregnancy and lactation. The probability of great negative effects on reproduction are obvious.

Table 1. Infant mortality rate (IMR per thousand) for some coastal and inland parishes during 1840—1849.

Coastal parishes	No. of births alive	IMR
Himango	366	281
Kalajoki	1496	310
Korsholm	3766	291
Kronoby	1012	199
Petalax	2113	328
Sideby	603	187

Inland parishes		
Alahärmä	852	306
Östermark	1411	241
Kauhava	2475	238
Ätheri	633	123
Isokyro	2154	224
Vähäkyro	1478	216
Saarijärvi	2035	145

Source: Church records. Vasa local archives.

Demographic characteristics of Ostrobothnia

As already mentioned, infant mortality rate in the province was very high. Spatial and chronological variations could be seen as late as the 1840's (Table 1).

In some parishes the crude death rate is high mainly because of a high infant mortality rate. Early death in infancy accounts for 40-60 % of the total death rate. Some parishes characterized by high infant mortality also have high death rates for the rest of the population.[23]

The infant mortality rates also varied seasonally. Many parishes realized the highest mortality among infants during late summer. The seasonal pattern varied in different areas (Figure 1).

There is also a relation between infant mortality rates and birth intervals. The shortest birth intervals are related to the highest infant mortality rates. However, the opposite is not always true. For two parishes which have been analysed, Lappo and Övervetil, the infant mortality rate for families with mean birth intervals longer than 30 months was still very high.[24] In the coastal parish of Petalax infant mortality decreased while the length of birth intervals increased.[25] Similar observations have been made for a parish in the coastal area of Ångermanland in Sweden.[26]

Figure 1. Seasonal infant mortality rates (IMR) and the distribution of births (%).

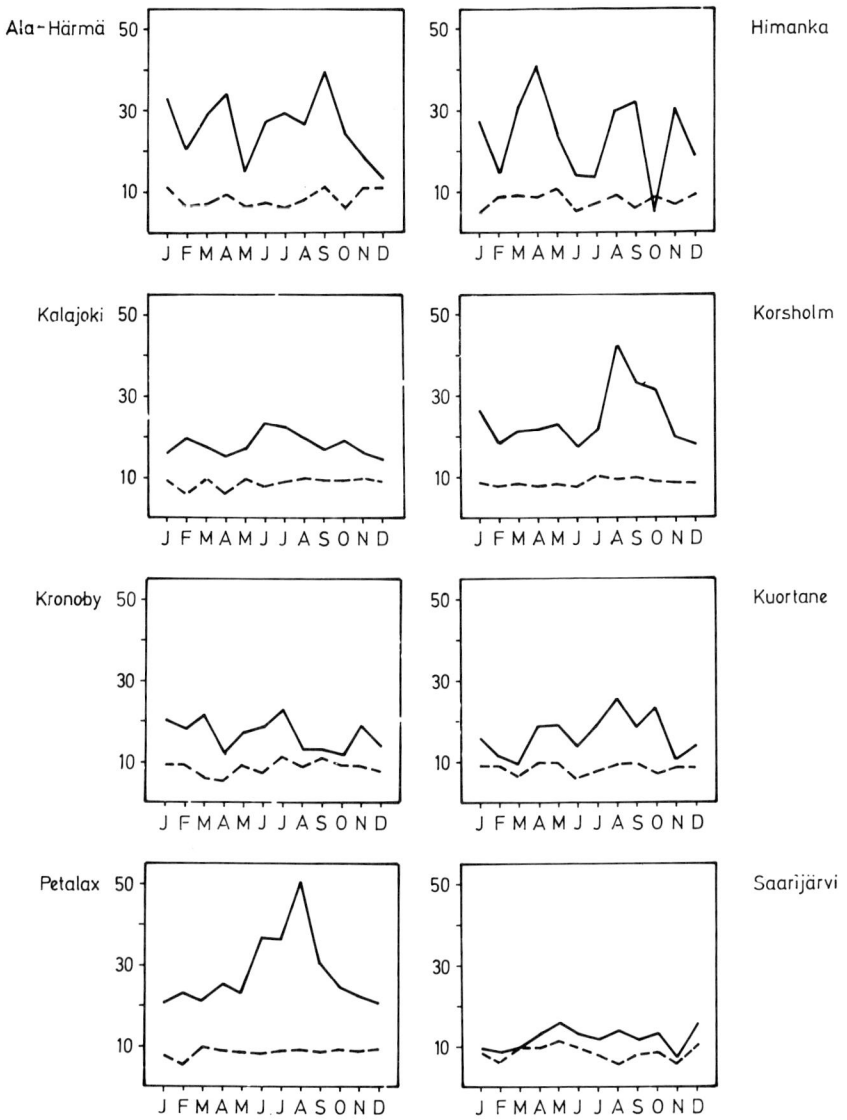

cont.

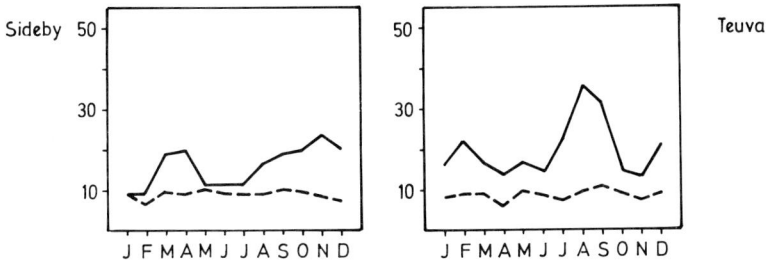

Source: U-B Lithell, Amning i svenska Österbotten under 1840-talet (Symposierapport 1985).

These findings have been interpreted as showing how differences in the standard of living in those parishes contributed to variations in mortality.

Another characteristic feature of the province is the overall high crude birth rates (Table 2). This is true even for the 1840's.

The high birth rate is seen as resulting from the lack of prolonged nursing among mothers in the province which thus meant early ovulation and a new pregnancy shortly after the delivery. The results support this interpretation, although there are reasons to expect that in some areas poor living conditions for certain groups of women resulted in fewer births. The overall mean length of birth intervals in the province seems to be moderate in spite of some groups of women who had very short spaces between deliveries.

The average length of the birth intervals in most parishes in the province was below 30 months which will result in comparably high crude birth rates.

In some areas the proportion of married women in fertile ages might be slightly higher, which will also have a positive effect on the crude birth rate

Table 2. Crude birth rates (per thousand) in some parishes in Ostrobothnia during the periods 1775—1784 and 1840's.

Parish	1775—1784	1840's
Lappo		48.1
Kauhava		42.4
Alahärmä		54.3
Ylihärmä		48.1
Isokyro	33.0	33.8
Ilmola	50.5	38.1
Vähäkyro	50.4	41.5
Korsholm		49.7
Kronoby		42.4
Petalax		55.5
Sideby		41.5

Source: Church records, Vasa local archives.

97

Social conditions in Ostrobothnia

Heikki Ylikangas in his book *Puukkojunkkareitten Esiinmarssi* has presented results from a research project with the aim of studying the extremely high rate of criminality in some parishes in southern Ostrobothnia. His main objective was to find factors which can explain the high frequency of homicides during the period 1790 to 1880. The highest frequency was found in the economically most well-off parishes within and close to the Kyro Valley. He stressed that the area known for the most violence was equal in all respects to the most well-known producers of cereals for export[27] The violence spread from southwest to northeast. The period characterized by high frequency of homicides started in 1790 even though the province for a long time had been known for social disturbances. Ylikangas stated that the violence was related to the economic development in the province. This development created competition between individuals and great socio-economic differences. These factors acted as "push-factors". His interpretation is that the reasons for the very long-lasting period of violence in the southern part of Ostrobothnia had social origins, because society accepted criminality and did not effectively prevent it.[28]

Ylikangas further discussed the criminality in Ostrobothnia and stated:

"The reason for the rise of the period of the "*knivjunkare*"(Nobility of the knife) should be sought long before the 1790's. Those elements which from the 1700's onwards committed crimes against human life had been preceded by a whole generation which committed illegal acts. The material investigated in general reveals the picture that criminality in many cases was inherited within a kinship group and became worse from generation to generation. It was not so much a question of corrupting influence of behavior pattern of close relatives, but rather of cumulative effects both of the total neglect of children and of liquor that tore family life to shreds. Among the "young nobles of the knife" of that period of violent crime, a hard-boiled, street mentality can be seen which may be assumed to have derived from circumstances of the type already mentioned while growing up. The picture is complemented by the dearth of labor which meant that children were also utilized economically in circles where the disruptive behavior was not significant. Only the scarcity of labor makes it possible to understand the surprising circumstance that the peasantry's willingness to allow their children to attend school decreased from the end of the 18th century. The combination of these things means that the frequent and often cliché-like contemporary statements concerning deficiency and neglect in child-raising can not be considered totally groundless and naive. It should further be noted that, according to contemporary reports, conflicts between children and parents were most common in southern Ostrobothnia".[29]

In the year of 1860 the county medical officer in Vasa wrote in his yearly report to the Medical Board that:

"The violence and the raw character of the native of southern Ostrobothnia goes hand in hand with and, to a great extent, has its roots in the cruelty to animals which occurs here more frequently and to a greater degree than elsewhere. From their earliest years the children of the peasantry are accustomed to assist women with delight in the slaughtering of the household animals, which is often done in a painful and inhumane manner.

It is no wonder then, becoming used to these scenes in childhood and growing up with such pleasures, that already at a youthful age, especially under the influence of liquor, with the knife that was always carried in the pocket, (a youth) sometimes in the most barbaric manner stabbed and tormented animals, usually horses, that belonged to someone against whom he held a grudge or blindly stabbed the first person he met in the chest, regardless of whether that person was a friend or an enemy, an acquaintance or a stranger".[30]

Ostrobothnia during earlier periods was in many ways different from other parts of Finland. It had so many strange features that persons of that day living in the region reacted and found it extraordinary. The parish of Vähäkyro was representative of this region and had all the above-mentioned characteristics including a high economic standard. Vähäkyro was one of the main parishes in the Kyro Valley.

The parish of Vähäkyro

The parish of Vähäkyro is situated in the Kyro Valley, the main rye-producing region in Ostrobothnia during the 19th century. During earlier periods tar production was the major source for cash income in the parish but already in the year 1792 most raw material for such production had been exploited.[31] Reports from the 1769-1770 stated that Vähäkyro parish did not produce any tar because of a lack of raw materials.[32] The property of the farmers had already been partitioned in the year 1768. During the five to six years following 1764, 64 acres of land had been cleared and cultivated. 5000 days' work had been used for ditching and clearing of the streams in the parish during the same period. In the year 1800 the military clergyman, Reverend Henric Wegelius, described the parish of Vähäkyro in a report and stated that there were 210 farms in the parish. A total of 1,230 acres and 5/8 *kappland* cultivated fields belonged to these farms while 4,707 acres of meadows, 11,020 acres of forest and 3,034 acres of swamps also belonged to the parish. The farms were in good condition.[33]

Wegelius stated that 2,600 people made their living from the farms and were able to produce goods for sale. He also mentioned that during the last decades of the 18th century 400 acres of land were cleared every year for new fields. According to him the busiest time of the year was the month of August when the rye and barley were harvested and rye was sown. Before and during the war in 1808-1809, the production of saltpetre became a main income source for Vähäkyro, but farming remained important.

The lack of raw materials for tar production increased the interest for farming in the region. The improvement of the farming therefore started early in Vähäkyro. C.C. Böcker, the secretary of the Finnish Agricultural Society reported from a tour of inspection in 1815 that Ilmola, Vähäkyro and Laihela parishes were the most developed farming regions in Ostrobothnia. Rye was exported from the region via Vasa. A great part, perhaps fifty percent, of the fields in Vähäkyro resulted from the clearing and reclamation of marshy bogs.[34]

In the beginning of the 19th century the parish of Vähäkyro was a rye-producing parish, and tar production was no longer a main income source. The population of the parish was in a state of *"jämn och medelmåttig välmåga"* (an average, good economic situation).[35]

The above-mentioned Böcker presented a compilation of economic data for different parishes in Finland and also information on the working duties for women in these areas. The information is given for the year 1835, and the collection is kept in the National Archives in Helsinki.

According to Böcker, Vähäkyro produced cereals for export during normal years. The largest part of the cash income (60 percent) came from this source. Other sources of income were the production of liquor (5 %), dairy products (15 %), and some forest products. The weaving of linen, wool, and hemp fabrics (1 %) was also mentioned. On the whole the economic situation during normal years in Vähäkyro was good. However, working conditions for women were harsh. The women were responsible for 75 % of all plowing, 15 % of the trench digging, and 50 % of the hay-making. Women in the parish were also required to give 2160 "day-works" per year as guards for the cattle. Children were also used for this type of work. In the information given by Böcker 4750 "day-works" were completed by children.[36]

In the year 1835 the women in the parish still had a very large burden of work on top of their role in reproduction, childcare and households duties. Feeding the animals was also their responsibility as well as threshing.[37]

On the other hand, it is obvious that the main source of income during that year was agriculture. Only 15-20 % of the cash income came from production outside farming. This might reflect the fact that men, to a large extent, were involved in agriculture.

The demographic data for Vähäkyro

In the year 1749 Vähäkyro parish had 1344 inhabitants, and by 1800 the population had increased to 2585 persons. During the period 1749-1800 4357 infants were born in the parish. The total number of deaths during that period was 3647. This period was known for its high crude birth rate (43.5 per thousand) and its high mortality (40 per thousand). In the year 1800 a total of 460 families lived in the parish, among whom there were 210 farmers and 67 crofters.

In the second half of the eighteenth century 80 children were born out of wedlock. Of the illegitimate children, 47.5 % were born during the last decade of the eighteenth century. The infant mortality rate for the period was very high: 375 per thousand, and the deaths among infants under one year were most numerous during two months of the year, July and August. During these months the infant mortality rate was 125 per thousand. Infants constituted 50 % of the total who died during these years. Children up to the age of ten made up 68 % of all deaths.[38]

Infant mortality has been charted for the period 1749 to 1850 (Figure 2). The diagram shows that the infant mortality rates were still very high until the middle of the 1830's. By the end of the 1830's mortality had dropped to nearly half the rates for the earlier periods. In the end of the nineteenth century Vähäkyro still had a markedly high frequency of death among the smallest children. Vähäkyro was one of a group of Ostrobothnian parishes which had an infant mortality rate exceeding 200 per thousand.[39]

Figure 2. Infant mortality rate (IMR) in the parish of Vähäkyro, 1749-1849.
* all parishes, including Vähäkyro, in Vasa Öfre prosteri
** figures for the year 1839 are missing

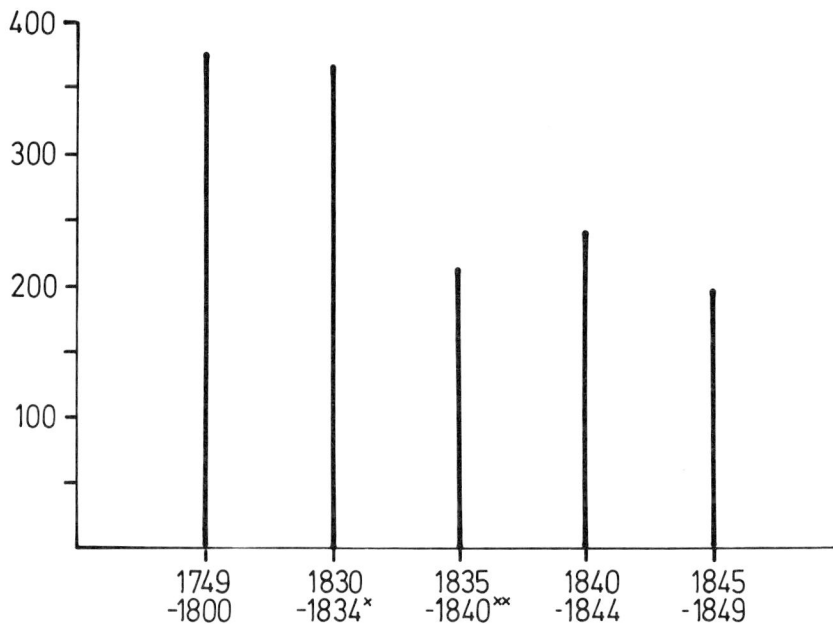

Source: Finska Hushållningssällskapet, Rapport från Vähäkyro 1800. Åbo Akademi bibliotek. Statistiska folkmängdstabeller, Local Archives of Vasa.

A report sent to the Finnish Agricultural Society *(Hushållningssällskap)* stated that decreasing fertility and increasing mortality characterized the development in Vähäkyro during the end of the eighteenth century. It was assumed that this was an effect of increasing population and a high population density.[40] During the period 1749-1800 the mean crude death rate was 35.7 per thousand, and the most frequent causes of death were intestinal diseases, smallpox, whooping cough, and tuberculosis. Together these causes made up 68.2 % of all deaths.[41]

The maternal death rate in Vähäkyro was 620 women per 100,000 live births,[42] a rate lower than the average for Sweden during this period.[43] However, maternal mortality was defined differently: the number of women dying in childbirth in Vähäkyro includes only those who died directly in conjunction with the birth of the infant. The figure for Vähäkyro therefore represents a minimum.

Two periods have been compared, 1775-1785 and 1840-1850. During these periods the infant mortality rates decreased from 393.7 per thousand to 223.9 per thousand. The crude birth rate also decreased from 47.5 per thousand to 37.0 per thousand. During the first period the major causes of death registered for children under one were intestinal diseases together with some smallpox and whooping cough. Infant deaths during the second period were most frequently recorded as "unknown". Intestinal diseases were not mentioned in the later period.

Both infant mortality and crude birth rates changed between the second half of the eighteenth and the first half of the nineteenth centuries. It is also clear that the major causes of death for the smallest children were different. Causes such as intestinal diseases are seldom or never mentioned in the church records, a fact which could be related to an improvement in the feeding habits for infants. However, the strongest evidence of such a change that can be associated with an improvement in child care is the decrease in the crude birth rates between the eighteenth and the nineteenth centuries.

Two major factors can influence the crude birth rate: the mean length of the birth intervals and the number of married women in fertile ages. The percentage of women per 1000 of the mean population has been calculated (Table 3).

As mentioned above the crude birth rate decreased from 47.5 per thousand to 37.0 per thousand between the period 1775-1785 and 1830-1840. This can not be explained with a decrease in the proportion of married women in the population. Therefore a factor which probably influenced this drop was a change in the length of the birth intervals. One possible explanation is that a larger number of women in the parish experienced an improvement in their working conditions and could therefore adequately nurse their children. This development could possibly be an effect of an increase in population which resulted in more workers being available per unit area in the parish. If more workers from other areas were employed because of an increase in the wealth of the farmers, this might also have influenced women's working conditions in the parish. As mentioned before, the main source of income was agricultural products. Most men were engaged in farming. All of these factors might have resulted in adequate nursing and also indirectly reduced the infant mortality and increased the intervals between births.

It is not possible to interpret the evidence from the infant mortality and the crude birth rate as showing a total lack of breastfeeding in the parish. However, during the first half of the period there were clear signs that the smallest children were not properly cared for. This was especially obvious in the summer season when deaths among infants increased. Even though the mortality rates dropped during the nineteenth century, the level is too high to indicate adequate child care. Some women still had great problems combining work and childbearing. The high mortality among the smallest children was especially notable in comparison with the high standard of living in the parish. One of the major agricultural regions in Ostrobothnia showed one of the highest infant mortality rates during the nineteenth century. Who were those women? Did women from the same socio-economic groups suffer from problems with living conditions during the different periods?

Table 3. The number of married women per 1000 of the mean population in the parish of Vähäkyro.

Year	Population	No married women	% women/ 1000 inhabitants
1775	1944	391	20.1
1780	2079	422	20.3
1785	2203	457	20.7
1830	3360	629	18.7
1835	3348	633	18.9
1840	3445	632	18.3
1845	3826	767	20.0
1850	3984	779	19.6

Source: Folkmängdstat. tables. Local archives of Vasa.

Table 4. Infant mortality 1820—1824 and 1845—1849 in Vähäkyro parish.

| | 1820 1024 | | 1845—1849 | |
	N	IMR	N	IMR
farmers	362	292.8	331	194.5
non—farmers	314	258.0	411	190.2

Source. Birth and death records, Vähäkyro parish. National Archives. Helsinki.

Infant mortality and socio-economic groups

A comparison has been made of the infant mortality rates in the two periods, 1820-1824 and 1845-1849. The first period represents a period of high infant mortality and the second a period of relatively low infant mortality. There seems to be little if any difference in infant deaths among the farmers and the non-farmers in the parish during the two periods analyzed (Table 4).

Both farmers and non-farmers had the same level of infant mortality during each period. The infant mortality was reduced and showed a lower level during the later period. How should these findings be interpreted?

There is evidence in the source material that the relative number of lodgers increased and that the infant mortality in this specific group exceeded that of others in the parish. Many farmers' wives still had difficulty solving the problem of child care, but the increase in the number of lodgers in the parish meant a decrease in the amount of work for some women. The lodging group *(inhyses)* was, of course, in a weak position in the parish. The decrease in infant mortality among the children of farmers might be an effect of a decreasing amount of work for their mothers. The work done by these women during earlier periods was now performed by the wives of lodgers. The negative effects could be shared and spread to an increasing number of lodgers in the parish.

The social characteristics of Vähäkyro and the nearby parishes

It was mentioned above that the parish of Vähäkyro belonged to a region known for violence and a high rate of homicides during the period 1790 to 1880. Ylikangas has emphasized that this type of violence was typical for the parts of Ostrobothnia that were most well-off. Furthermore, this region was also renowned for its well-developed agriculture. It was mostly the men who were involved in this violence and very often men from wealthy families, especially towards the end of the period.[44] Ylikangas has pointed out that this violent period did not start in 1790, rather violence had been common for generations.[45] In the areas where the most violence occurred the owners of farms were not willing to split their property among their children. This could lead to the relegation of younger sons to positions of lower status than those of their birth. This might be a factor which could contribute to violent behavior among young people who had been treated badly. It seems as if children many times received harsh treatment at the hands of their mothers and fathers.[46]

Ylikangas mentioned several factors which might have contributed to the problems in the region, and one of these factors was the lack of adequate child care. Many reports from different parts of Ostrobothnia mention the extremely difficult situation and state that, due to the severe working conditions for women, the smallest children had a hard life from the start. The infants were not breastfed, and they were generally left with the elderly or small children to look after them.[47]

Reports speak of the very poor hygienic standards in the parishes. The infants cradles were said to often be in very bad condition, worse than pigsties.[48] As late as the middle of the nineteenth century the county medical officers were sometimes unable to vaccinate the children against smallpox, because they were too scabby.[49]

Why was child care so poor in the province? It must be realized that the living conditions for women in the region far back in time were extremely severe because of the harsh environment and the lack of manpower. Women were used as laborers in all kinds of work. Priority had to be given to work in production for the survival of the family and the household. Great demands were made on the women in the region. "The women in Jeppo do not walk, they run" was an expression.[50] "A woman is not as good as a man when the ground is bare of snow, should not be respected, when she is ill, this could be an excuse" or "To nurse infants is just spoiling time" are both sayings from the past in Ostrobothnia.[51] During the busiest time of the year the men in most parishes were not at home. Fishing, sailing, and tar producing were work which was performed during the summer season. It is possible to assume that during this period there was very little time, if any, for kindness and for caring for the young children. All suffered from the hard conditions. Survival was the main objective. On top of this, the cash income and the willingness of the tar exporter to transform money into liquor did not create a better life for men and women.

Discussion

The importance of mothers for the well-being of children is obvious to people of today. It is possible to assume that in the past mothers in a pre-industrial environment characterized by ignorance played an equally important role. Högberg has shown how severe the effects of the mother's death were for the child's chance of survival. Even if the mother lived, but lived under such circumstances that she was not able to take care of her child properly, the child's health was in danger. Not only the physical health, but also the mental health might be affected. The children probably had many negative experiences, but very few positive ones.

The child was not protected by a high standard of living from illnesses, death, and poor mental health in an ignorant environment, if this standard was combined with severe working conditions for women. The situation in Vähäkyro and the parishes situated nearby can be described in a simplified model which makes assumptions about the relationship between women's living conditions and the effects of the health of society. Special attention is given to the children.

Summary

In this essay it has been assumed that the main reasons for the specific characteristics of Ostrobothnia are related to the severe living conditions for women in the province. This assumption is an effect of the knowledge of the situation in the third world countries of today. There is no reason to assume that women during earlier periods should have reacted differently to difficult working conditions. It is most probable that hard working conditions, sometimes low nutritional levels, and social disturbance increased the burden for women to such a level that it was no longer possible to prevent negative effects on reproduction.

In some areas the result was fewer children than expected because of a low nutritional level. In other areas nutritional levels were adequate, and more children were born.

In most parts of the province it was not possible for women to combine work with proper child care. High infant mortality, high fertility, poor health, and poor social relations prevailed in many parts of the province during the earlier periods.

The area close to the coast was probably the part of the province where women had the most severe working conditions for the longest period of time. It was also the area where the conditions early seemed to have changed for the better. When the production of tar began in the interior of the province, the situation for women in that part of the region also degenerated. It is likely that ever since the colonization period the women in the coastal region always had to give priority to work rather than to child care and breastfeeding. Artificial feeding was a way to solve child nursing problems and a cultural custom that originated in past centuries.

In the interior of the province tar production changed the breastfeeding pattern. Tar became a new important source of income. Priority was given to production, and substitutes had to be provided for nursing. These substitutes became a complement for nursing, but did not compensate for the lack of breastfeeding. The amount of work determined the number of women who nursed and the length of the period. The amount of work also determined the time women could spend together with their children. Women's participation in indoor activities was also related to their work burden. This affected the processing of food and the nutritional level of the children.

Notes

1. 'Women, Health and Development. A Report by the Director General', *WHO no 90* (1985), pp. 9-10.

2. U. Högberg and G. Broström, 'The Demography of Maternal Mortality — Seven Swedish Parishes in the 19th Century'. *International Journal of Obstetrics and Gynecology* (1985), p. 41.

3. W.R. Lee, 'Women's Work and Child Care in Prussia', J.C. Fout, (Ed.), *German Women In the Nineteenth Century. A Social History.* (London 1984), pp. 234-255.

4. A.E. Imhof, 'Unterschiedliche Säuglingssterblichkeit in Deutschland, 18. bis 20. Jahrhundert — Warum?', *Zeitschrift für Bevölkerungswissenschaft,* 6 (1981), pp. 343-382.

5. A. Brändström, *"De kärlekslösa mödrarna". Spädbarnsdödligheten i Sverige under 1800-talet med särskild hänsyn till Nedertorneå* (Umeå 1985).

6. *Svenska Österbottens Historia,* III (Vasa 1980), p. 5.

7. Ibid, p. 27.

8. Ibid, pp. 34-39, 45-46.

9. E. Birck, 'Om jordbruket med binäringar i 1700-talets Österbotten', *Österbotten 1970.* (Vasa 1970), p. 124.

10. Ibid.

11. E. Jutikkala, *Suomen Historian Kartasto. (Atlas of Finnish History). Rural Economic Conditions in the 1830's,* 48 (Helsinki 1949), pp. 122-124.

12. K.V. Åkerblom, *Lappfjärds Historia. Andra delen.* (Vasa 1952), p. 62.

13. Åkerblom (1952).

14. Birck (1970), pp. 132, 155-157.

15. Birck (1970), p. 42.

16. H. Ylikangas, *Knivjunkrarna* (Borgå 1985), p. 241.

17. K.V. Åkerblom, *Korsholms Historia,* 1 (Vasa 1941), pp. 636-637.

18. Report sent to the Medical Board from Provincial Medical Officers in Vasa, 1862, 1864. Local archives, Vasa.

19. E. Birck, 'Studier rörande Näringsliv och Befolkning i Pedersöre Härad, Österbotten, 1750-1850', *Fennia,* 79, 3 (Helsingfors 1955), p. 8.

20. Ylikangas (1985), p. 242.

21. E. Birck, *Om Österbotten efter Stora ofreden vid svensktidens slut. Ockupationen av Österbotten 1714-1721,* pp. 136-137.

22. E. Birck, *Näringsliv och befolkning i Österbotten* (Helsingfors 1955), pp. 35, 43.

23. U-B. Lithell (Own unpublished results).

24. U-B. Lithell, *Kvinnor som arbetskraft i preindustriella samhällen. Exemplet Österbotten i Finland under tiden före 1900.* (manuscript).

25. U-B. Lithell, 'Breast-feeding Habits and their Relation to Infant Mortality and Marital Fertility', *Journal of Family History. Studies in Kinship, Family and Demography* (1981).

26. U-B. Lithell, 'Premium Weaving in the 19th Century Parish of Nätra', *Historisk Tidskrift*, 4 (1985), p. 483.

27. Ylikangas (1985), p. 243.

28. Ylikangas (1985), p. 264.

29. Ylikangas (1985), p. 208.

30. Report from the Provincial medical officer in Vasa, A.E. Boden to the Medical Board in 1860. Local archives, Vasa.

31. Birck (1970), p. 156.

32. Birck (1970), p. 75.

33. Report from Vähäkyro sent to the Finska Hushållningssällskapet in 1800. Åbo Akademi Bibliotek.

34. Ibid.

35. H. Wegelius, 'Beskrivning över Vörå socken, Åbo Tidningar (1792)', K.V.R. Wikman (Ed.) *Meddelanden från Institutet för Nordisk Etnologi vid Åbo Akademi* (Åbo 1928).

36. Carl Christian Böckers samlingar. 1834-1835. National Archives, Helsinki.

37. Ibid.

38. Report from Vähäkyro sent to FHS 1800.

39. F.W. Westerlund, 'Om dödligheten bland barn under 1 år i Finland 1872-1886', *Finska Läkarsällskapets Handlingar*, XXXI (1886), p. 672.

40. Report from Vähäkyro to FHS 1800.

41. Befolkningsstat. tabeller, Local archives in Vasa.

42. Ibid.

43. U. Högberg, *Maternal Mortality in Sweden* (Umeå 1985), p. 11.

44. Ylikangas (1985), p. 262.

45. Ylikangas (1985), p. 208.

46. Personal communication with Prof. Heikki Ylikangas, University of Helsinki.

47. Report from the Provincial Medical Officer in Vasa.

48. C. Von Haartman, 'Om späda barnens uppfödande i vissa trakter af det nordliga Finland', *Hygiea*, 2 (1844).

49. Report from the Provincial Medical Officer in Kuortane.

50. Personal communication with Ass. Prof. Holger Wester, Jeppo, Finland.

51. Wegelius (1928), pp. 10-11; J.R. Aspelin, *Kertomus Maalahden pitäjästä. Suomi. Kirjoituksia isän-mallisesta aineista* (Helsingfors 1866), pp. 175-177.

The Development of Cause-of-Death Classification in Eighteenth Century Sweden. A Survey of Problems, Sources and Possibilities

Eva Nyström

Introduction

The cause-of-death statistics serve several different but closely related functions. In these statistics we have an important source of information for both medical and social research. Firstly, the statistics serve a descriptive function by providing information about the cause-of-death panorama, secondly it may generate hypotheses for epidemiological studies and other research, and furthermore the statistics are used for health political and social political purposes. Thus the cause-of-death statistics are of utmost importance not only as far as medical questions are concerned but also in social and political connections.

What kind of information do the causes of death provide? Recent research has shown that the cause-of-death statistics in fact involve a long row of qualified scientific problems of both medical and philosophical character and that we can not be certain of the reliability of the diagnoses given, their value of information and so on. An important question so far is the problem of selecting the principal cause of death and to determine how complications and other contributory causes should be recorded.[1]

When studying the state of health in a population in a historical perspective we usually use a mortality statistics which are based upon specific causes. That goes for both historical epidemiological studies and the historical demographic research. In that respect Sweden provides unique possibilities to research as we have from the middle of the eighteenth century a nationwide cause-specific statistics, up to the early nineteenth century including Finland, integrated within the well known vital statistics.

It is natural that our information about the growth or decline in a population or the occurrence of a specific disease or different diseases must build upon the cause-specific statistics and that this information must be based upon a quantitative analysis. From a historical perspective however, other questions are pertinent, such as: on what foundations are the cause-of-death statistics based? Wherefrom is the basis of divisions of diseases and injuries derived, and how has this classification changed over the time? What factors, external as well as internal, have contributed to this development? What kind of problems was the classification of cause of death afflicted with? Can comparisons be made with other countries, and if so, in what way is Sweden related to the international development?

The purpose of this paper is to give a brief orientation of an ongoing study and the possibilities to follow the development of the cause-of-death classification in Sweden with special concern to the questions named above. The period we are going to take a closer look at, is the time of the birth of the oldest Swedish cause-of-death statistics at the middle of the eighteenth century. We are also going to consider some of the questions to put, as to the in many ways intensive development that took place from 1860 to 1911.

The problems, sources and possibilities that are here outlined, I am at present investigating as a specific research task.[2] A central aim is to elucidate the conceptual foundations of cause-of-death statistics and how these have developed from the beginning in 1749 up to 1948, when Sweden joins the international collaboration work concerning causes of death. Consequently, this investigation deals with the development of cause-of-death statistics on a general level, not on the individual level, i.e., I am not studying the lethality in a specific disease, which requires an investigation of the death-books, the primary sources of the vital statistics. As it is not the factual mortality or the occurrence of certain diseases that are to be ascertained, this work differs from demographic investigations regarding aims, sources and methods. However, the results from the demographic research are important for such investigations. The primary sources, i.e., the death-books, ought to be used anyhow as a material of a comparative character. We will come back to that later in this paper.

Before we go further on, attention should be drawn to some basic problems. Even though the conceptual basis is in the centre of interest, we must not forget that organized statistics of this kind, always tend to respond to some kind of demands from the society. In Sweden in the middle of the eighteenth century the leading politicians were in demands of a complete view over the population, its size and conditions of health.[3] Due to the mercantilistic doctrines, a large and healthy population which was able to perform a productive work in the service of society, was tantamount to the wealth of a nation. In order to restrain the feared high mortality, a dangerous threat to the mercantilistic program, a basis for health political considerations was needed. This in turn was necessary for organizing and giving priority to preventive measures of different kinds. Naturally, any health service requires some kind of organized picture of the causes of ill health, and a prerequisite therefore was a general view of the diseases people died of. This demand was to be met by the cause-of-death statistics. Here we have a social condition and a social demand.

The impact of the results of the mortality statistics on health policy in

Sweden around the middle of the eighteenth century was of course enormous. A nationwide health organization was firmly established, and well organized with proportionally enlarged resources. Medical questions were discussed as problems of utmost economic and political value. Much stress has been laid upon the fact that mercantilism in this respect was fruitful for the development. In other words, that rather crass, economic principles drew attention to the medical scene. On the other hand, the increased knowledge about the cause-of-death panorama and mortality trends led to a deeper insight into the health conditions of the population, which together with the contemporary initiatives taken as to establish a Swedish epidemiology in the long run nourished not only social medical thinking in general, but also in connection to that growing humanitarian insights and ideals. Therefore, the history of cause-of-death statistics would benefit from being treated in a history of ideas context, where the social and political conditions will be paid attention to, and where references also will be made to functions and consequences for medicine and society.

Let us focus some other problems too. A statement of cause of death can in itself also be a definition of a certain disease category. But what then is a disease? Which are the factors that constitute its specific nature as a disease in relation to our conception of health? We know that our ability to discover and to identify a disease is dependent on the time and the society in which we are living. This of course also concerns our ability to diagnose the diseases and to treat them successfully. The cause-of-death statistics therefore reflect not only the connection between disease and society but also, and naturally, the scientific standards of the time, as well as attitudes and opinions to death and disease. A statement of cause of death is furthermore not only a definition of a disease category, but also a choice between different diseases. This ability to differentiate between various diseases is also of course due to certain factors. A precondition for discussing the nature and division of disease in terms of this, is of course a generally accepted form of conception, i.e., a nomenclature and a classification of diseases. The history of cause-of-death statistics is therefore intimately linked with not only the history of diseases but also with the history of disease classification and must be treated in these contexts. Nowadays, there is a generally applied uniform basis of division, the International Classification of Diseases (ICD), prepared by the World Health Organization, which consists of 17 different classes of diseases, injuries and causes of death. The ICD also contains rules for its application, for how the death certificates should be filled in, and how the causes of death should be registered in the statistics.[4]

From the historical perspective however, several questions may thus be posed. Regarding the situation during the eighteenth century, some of these I would like to put are: what or which kinds of "classification" were then used? Were there any distinction between causes-of-death classification and classification of diseases in general, so that there were two parallel systems side by side? Is it possible to study the selection of categories for the cause-of-death statistics during the eighteenth century compared to the contemporary conceptions of the disease panorama, and if so, what sources should then be used? In what way is it possible to study the reflections of the social and scientific conditions and demands?

The conditions for answering these questions will be discussed below; it should be mentioned though that no final results will here be presented, nor is there any claims laid to completeness, but the main purpose is to give a general outline of how the development of cause-of-death statistics can be investigated.

The eighteenth century background: no uniform classification of diseases

When cause-of-death statistics were initiated in Sweden during the middle of the eighteenth century, there was no uniform classification of diseases to start from. This lack of uniformity reflects the prevalent situation in the eighteenth century medicine. The first decades of the century in particular are often described as a period of crisis, characterized by conflicts between the old and the new and between different medical systems.[5] This split was very much a direct consequence of the great scientific revolution of the previous century.

The development of a mechanistic world picture of the scientific revolution had undermined the theoretical foundations of the prevailing medical philosophy, i.e., Galenism. When its theoretical basis, Aristotelianism, was threatened and superseded by the victorious mechanistic natural philosophy its dominating position was spoiled. In spite of this there were no great changes within medicine. The most remained within the old tradition. There was no all-embracing medical system to replace Galenism either. On the contrary, a new conflict, between on one hand a mechanistic conception on all organic functions and a vitalistic conception on the other, was soon established. The leaders of these schools soon worked out independent of each other, widely differing, very often rival systems, which was dominant from the end of the seventeenth century and during practically the whole of the eighteenth century. Within the framework of these closed systems all questions concerning the structure, the composition and the functions of the human body were to be solved and the view on diseases and how to treat them.

Initiatives were taken however, in trying to arrange and systematize the knowledge of diseases into very strict and uniform systems. During the eighteenth century the so called nosological systems based upon the symptoms of the diseases developed. However, none of these systems were to serve as a direct basis for the cause-of-death statistics. In spite of that, they can teach us a great deal about the medical world of the eighteenth century.

An important tradition leads from the English philosopher Francis Bacon (1561-1626), who had insisted upon a revival of the Hippocratic method to collect knowledge about different case histories and their different courses. Here were possibilities to solve the problems within medical science: viz. to avoid the theoretical systems, and in order to attain reliable results, follow the recommendations given by Bacon and rely on the experience and the knowledge that was made up by collections of clinical observations and systematically try to bring order in a material like that. The great attention focused on the symptoms of the disease has different explanations. The possibilities to try to understand what was going on within the body were of course limited before the era of pathological anatomy and clinical research. Therefore they had to rely on suppositions based upon observable signs and examinations of the symptoms of the patient. Important impulses which supported the doctrines of symptoms were also Bacons assumptions that medicine only would prosper as a science if, besides collecting case-histories, comparisons concerning pathological changes in the different organs were carried out at postmortem examinations with the observed and registered symptoms that characterized the disease before its course to death.

But most of all it was the methods from botany that came to be of utmost importance for the symptomatological classification of diseases. The botanists of the time were still working in an Aristotelian tradition, that taught that every species were once and for all given by God or by nature in an eternal and unchangeable pattern of genera and species. Therefore the botanists would study the nature very intensively and from that learn how to discover the species and distinguish them from each other with the help of their characteristic qualities. Thereafter he could give them names and systematize them into the classification system given by nature. When transferred to medical data this had important consequences. In the same way the nosologists thought that they could reveal the natural order, in which the diseases were organized. Therefore one should get as much information as possible about what was characteristic of the different diseases. Here the study of symptoms was to become very useful.

An important intermediary was the English physician Thomas Sydenham (1624-1689) at the end of the seventeenth century. Inspired by both Hippocratic medicine and the Baconian tradition, he argued for a systematic description of the diseases made upon their characteristic features. He meant that one should classify diseases in the same way as the botanists were classifying plants. The starting point was the careful observations of symptoms, because exactly as plants reveal similar patterns in their characteristic features, diseases manifest themselves with the same symptoms, though they appear in different individuals.

However, these ideas were not to be carried out until the middle of the eighteenth century, in the famous nosological systems of Francois Boissier de Sauvages (1706-1767) and Carl von Linnaeus (1707-1778). Characteristic for these systems were that similar symptoms were made the basis of classification of the diseases, which were split up into classes, orders and genera exactly as within the botanical science.

At the turn of the century, several systems of nosology built upon the criteria of symptoms, the most famous of which was the one of William Cullen (1710-1790), had developed, and even during the first decades of the nineteenth century similar systems were formed. For most of the cause-specific mortality statistics that we have not only in Sweden but also in other countries, these very complicated systems were of minor importance.[6] That means, that there was no connection between the cause-of-death categories, used for the statistical table forms, and the different nosological systems, even though the cause-of-death categories also of course were symptomatological in their character. They existed separately with their different purposes and functions.

The organization of collecting causes of death and the design of table II

Before going any further, we shall just recall the main features in the organization of collecting causes of death in Sweden in the older period. In 1749 a continuous compilation of tables in a national level, the so called *Tabellverket,* was founded, initiating the systematic production of population data. In 1755 a Statistical Committee, the *Tabellkommissionen,* was established, a forerunner to the National Central Bureau of Statistics.[7] The information collected was to include not only the number of births and deaths but also the causes of death. The obligation to report population data was laid upon the parish clergymen, who were to fill in the information required into the table forms. This meant that they transmitted the information from the church books to the table forms. Since the year of 1686, a special church act had imposed making parish registration for all Christenings, marriages, and burials compulsory. The information requested concerning causes of death was to be tabulated on the local level in a separate table, the so called table II. This information later reached Stockholm through a well organized network of administration, and was there collected as to serve as basis for the decisions of the authorities. Twenty-five years later a revision took place and during the first decades of the nineteenth century the table forms were revised furthermore, without though any important change taking place concerning the administrative rules. In 1831 the clergymen were released from the task to fill in the causes of death, with the exception of deaths from childbirth, smallpox, suicide and some other specified accidents. This was the situation up to the middle of the century.

The reasons for introducing cause-of-death statistics in Sweden are already referred to, but should be emphasized as they were of vital importance for the preparation of the cause-of-death table forms. When planning the compilation of statistical data concerns about the state of health in the population, influenced by mercantilistic thought, called for a registration of the mortality in a separate table, where the annual number of deaths should be reported, divided into age, sex and causes of death. Several objections were raised to this

114

proposal, for example the clergy assumed ignorance of medical issues. The Swedish clergy that was to establish and record the causes of death, was not expected by the opponents to manage this task. Other critics urged that the cause of death should be registered, but that it should be sufficient with a common popular terminology well known to the clergymen.

The leading politician behind the proposal that more information on the causes of death was needed, was J.A. Lantingshausen (1699-1769). On the table form he worked out by himself, no specification was requested though; general observations concerning the diseases with a supposed high mortality rate should, however, be commentated. In the late 1740's, with assistance from the Royal Swedish Academy of Sciences, where a discussion concerning the need of a vital statistics and the necessity of specified table forms for that purpose had been going on for some time, a table form which was to cover the mortality-rate and the diseases people died of, finally was set up. The task was to be fulfilled by Abraham Bäck (1713-1795), who in 1746 at the request of Pehr Elvius (1710-1749), the secretary of the Royal Academy of Sciences, had promised to be helpful in this matter. Bäck was then a newly graduated doctor of medicine, who was later to become the head of the *Collegium Medicum,* the forerunner to the National Board of Health, for a period of almost fifty years. Even Linnaeus, who had just started to develop his own classification system, was asked by Elvius to contribute, a proposal he rejected as an impossible task, claiming the Swedish clergy was not educated in medicine and probably never would be.

Unfortunately we know very little about the final discussions and decisions that formed the complete version of the table forms. As to the table II, we can only draw conclusions from the discussions that led to its preparations and the design it finally got; 33 headings were here tabulated with their Swedish names, from which 21 were diseases and 12 were casualties, i.e., accidental deaths of different kinds.[8] The fact that the diseases and injuries there tabulated were stated by their Swedish names and in the way they were familiar for most people, must be seen as a way to make it easier for the clergy. Health political demands, and practical considerations taking into account the fact that the clergy was to state the cause of death thus directed the preparation and the design of table II.

Sources and areas of investigation

The question is how to form an idea of the basis for the medical terminology used. Here I would like to propose the following procedure. As there was no uniform, generally accepted and applied classification of diseases and injuries to start from, the terms must have been drawn from a wider medical terminology. In order to solve that problem, we have to take into consideration what kind of sources to use for this kind of investigation.

The medical literature, the basis for selection of causes of death and the roots of the terminology

Here one have to go through the medical literature of the time and take a closer look at their scope and character.[9] There are different kinds of works to go through, medical textbooks, the more popular handbooks, and what could be called treatises of a more informative character, concerning communicable diseases called attention to by the authorities. There are also smaller treatises about individual diseases and the way to treat them. Furthermore, there are medical advice and information of different kinds in calenders and prognostic literature. These sources provide rich possibilities of comparisons. Bäck, who was responsible for working out the table II, has probably taken it for granted that the selection of the diseases tabulated should be well known to the clergy. As Britt-Inger Puranen has shown in her thesis on tuberculosis in Sweden, they were very familiar with the terminology of the medical literature mentioned above.[10]

To form an opinion about the selection of cause-of-death categories for table II, it is therefore necessary to examine how these conditions were described in the literature. From these descriptions the same kind of diseases or states of diseases could also be found, though perhaps mentioned with other names or similar names in the literature. In that way the diseases, selected from the literature to be tabulated in the table could clearly be defined. To this must be added complementary knowledge from the smaller treatises concerning certain individual diseases in order to explain further, or to fortify the pictures of the diseases.

An important problem concerns the roots of the terminology. How long back in time could we trace the medical terms in table II? We know already that there are registered notes about causes of death from the time of the church act in 1686, and of course there are notes even earlier. With the help of the medical literature that we have from the seventeenth century and notes about causes of death in the church books, it would be possible to first trace the terms back in time, and then turn again and follow the terminology through the first part of the eighteenth century and into the table. In that way it would be possible to define the "life-length" of the terminology if the names of the diseases have altered and so on. This is how "old" the diseases are, that are tabulated in the table II. It is in this connection it would be valuable to make comparisons with the primary sources, i.e., the death- and burial registers in order to estimate the scope of the terminology. So far the material and the possibilities to follow the "birth" of table II.

Another area of investigation is to consider the new more comprehensive medical terminology used in the table II 1774, the year when the revised version was introduced. The main problem here is to compare the table forms of 1749 with the new one as to the presence and differences of the cause-of-death categories. Here we also have possibilities to follow the prerequisites, in form of medical literature concerning diseases, for working out the new table.

Valuable information is also given by Bäck himself, who stated clearly in which medical handbooks further information can be found about the conditions (the cause-of-death categories) used in the new table.[11] From these and other books the development of the conceptual basis can be followed in the way that was described earlier; i.e., by considering the selection of categories in the table form compared to the diseases mentioned in the handbooks, treatises and so on and thus identifying the "new" cause-of-death categories and their relation to the "old" terminology.

As to the sources of the medical terminology of table II, it would in this way be possible to repeatedly compare the content of the table with the medical terminology of the popular handbooks that tried to cover the current disease panorama. That goes for not only the table form of 1749 and 1774, but also with addition of more literary knowledge for the revisions of 1801 and so on up to the 1830's.[12]

The application field of the mortality statistics and the selection of categories

Next question in this investigation consequently deals with the problem of selecting causes-of-death categories from this more widespread medical terminology. Beginning with the table form of 1749, which, as we have seen, was to be applied for a period of 25 years, it is possible to conclude which disease categories that were included. What decisions then, lay behind this process of selection? Again I would like to recall the connection between medicine and society at the time of the erection of the vital statistics. Here we have to take into consideration the application field of the cause-of-death statistics, their principle purpose being to provide the political authorities with a basis for health political considerations, in a state of fear that the population growth was to decrease due to the assumed high mortality. As was mentioned above, we lack foundations for the decisions which lay behind the concrete and final version of the table forms. Therefore we don't know whether Abraham Bäck was following special directives, or if he was acting entirely on his own when working out the table II. However one could create an opinion about the ambitions of the initiators of the vital statistics, and consequently which ideas Bäck in his turn should have been trying to put into practice. In the different documents, such as acts, letters and reports where the demand of vital statistics and their design was discussed, and which preceded the founding of the vital statistics, several arguments were put forward, directly or indirectly, as to the selection of causes of death.[13]

There were demands of what kind of diseases people died of in general, and which were the causes of the shifts in mortality, together with suggestions that the diseases with the supposed highest mortality-rate would be paid attention to in the first hand. The practical motives with a prospective cause-of-death statistics were emphasized throughout. The medical authorities were, it was expected, in this way to be guaranteed adequate knowledge of all kinds of damaging and epidemic diseases that threatened to be rampant. The information thereby collected should be used as a support to health political decisions, which would prevent the premature death of the people, not in the least amongst children. If we take it for granted that these demands and expectations in one way or another formed the starting point for Bäck and guided him in his choice, the ambitions could be summarized like this: the table form was supposed to give a survey of the mortality and its distribution into the diseases and injuries, which people generally died of, with a special attention to the diseases where the mortality rate was feared to be too high.

With this in mind one question to put is whether the excluded disease categories were considered as non-fatal, or was it assumed that the mortality rate was not so high in these diseases? In order to confirm whether the contemporary view on which disease, or states of diseases, that were supposed to lead to death, had to exclude some categories, we have again to take support in the medical literature. These problems though are not only connected with the level of contemporary medical thought, but also and unambiguously with contemporary attitudes and opinions to death and disease. Is it possible for instance, that the lack of certain categories of diseases in the table II were due to the fact that they shouldn't be paid attention to? In other words, what was then allowed to be seen, and what information was not allowed to be presented in the statistics and why was that so? In this connection it would be most valuable for this study to continuously check with the churchbooks for one parish or perhaps town and see what diseases or conditions that "disappeared" as disease-units when transferring to the table form, but might have still appeared with its figures in the table II, only tabulated by another medical term.

Now it remains to take the selected cause-of-death categories into closer consideration. Firstly, as was mentioned before, it is possible to follow the history of the tabulated categories back in time and in that way see what meaning and function they had in older Swedish disease-history. Further, with the help of the literature, which was used as a basis for the selection Bäck did, we could investigate to which extent the choice corresponded with the goal he supposedly had. The questions that then ought to be put are: which were the diseases? How could they be translated into modern terminology? Were the diseases chosen to be tabulated looked upon as prevalent or new occurring? Were there any suppositions about the mortality rate in this or that disease and were there any ideas concerning its rampaging different parts of the population; i.e., to what extent were the epidemic diseases feared to "hit" the young respectively the old people and how were these epidemics supposed to be regionally distributed? Which of the tabulated diseases were presumed to be the most dangerous as to the spreading, morbidity and mortality? Was there any ambition to take into account the social need such as diseases or conditions more or less directly resulted by poverty, famine and so on? Here again there is reason to consider the contemporary knowledge of and attitudes to the diseases.

118

Medical thought and the definitions of causes of death

As to the medical concept of disease, several of the tabulated diseases were not diseases in our modern sense but rather conditions, characterized by general symptoms, and thus differing from the modern anatomical-etiological concept of disease that was developed during the nineteenth century. The way of differing one disease from another is the next problem to consider, and also what factors determining that certain diseases in the table form could be unified and others would be divided, which put the question of the contemporary view on the mutual relationship between diseases. An account of the predispositions of the eighteenth century medicine, when it comes to the ability to create an opinion about diseases and how to define them, is therefore necessary.[15] Concerning the attitudes on the diseases we might, I would like to argue, try to broaden the outlook on the concept of disease and consider its social implications too. This should include not only what social conditions were supposed to determine the cause-of-death panorama, and what diseases that were assumed to be fatal for the wealth of the nation, but also in order to improve our understanding of this period, how these diseases were regarded by contemporary way of thinking as seen in relation to moral and religious conceptions, superstition and traditions in general.

Some of these questions lead unsoughtly to the problems the nosological systems tried to solve. Here there are rich possibilities to make comparisons between table II and for example the nosological system of Linnaeus, as to the selection of diseases and how they were specified. Another important material of comparison consists of the mortality tables that existed in other countries at the same time. Here we can compare with the sum of tabulated categories, the selection of diseases and injuries and their relation to other diseases of the table form and what categories are unified and which are not. In this way the table II of 1749 could be put in relation to both the seventeenth century and the contemporary disease panorama in Sweden and to similar initiatives in other countries.[16]

The revisions of table II

Regarding the revision of 1774, there are two factors to take into account. Firstly, as it was a question of a revision, there was the basis of earlier selection to consider. The main task is here to compare the table form of 1774 with the previous one as to the presence and absence of the old cause-of-death categories. Here we have to take into consideration the changes that the terminology underwent as to the number of entries and the exclusion and inclusion of old respectively new categories, and so on; i.e., a following up of the conceptual basis of the table form. In this way we might also connect to the question of the life-length of the table-terms that has been pointed out before, so that a line could be drawn from seventeenth century terminology and onwards up to the 1770's. As to the process of selecting categories to the formula, the same question as were put to the version of 1749 should of course be put even now, such as the concept of disease, the way of identifying and describing the diseases, and the contemporary level of and attitudes to the morbidity and mortality of the diseases. The possibilities to constant comparisons with the cause-of-death table forms in other countries and with the complicated nomenclature of the nosological system also remains.

This shouldn't be done, however, without putting the revised categories in relation to the suggestions of revisions, critical arguments and opinions in general that together with the new knowledge had collected during the years. That brings us to the second factor to consider when investigating the new design of table II. The first announcements of the figures of the mortality statistics caused both attention and reactions. Suggestions of measures that ought to be taken soon appeared and an increased watchfulness towards indicators of health and disease was generally ordered. This more observant attitude towards health conditions and its causes was reflected in the interaction between medicine, and the attention raised in the society as a whole from the 1750's and onwards, regarding the incidence and prevalence of certain diseases, the occurrence of "new" diseases and so on.

In the Statistical Committee for instance, a discussion took place with future revisions in mind early in the 1750's, and new suggestions with the same purpose were initiated in the years to come. There the necessity of maintaining, including and also excluding this or that category was discussed with the welfare of the state in mind.[17] Other influences are already referred to, such as the medical literature that focused on current problems and the attempts to picture the disease panorama in handbooks of various kinds. Another important basis for considering the future revision was of course the reports from the district local doctors.[18] Yet another factor worth considering, is the discussion concerning the reliability of the statistics not in the least the mortality statistics. In the correspondence of Bäck for instance, there are delivered many critical arguments that gives us important aspects of the problems that the cause-of-death statistics had occasioned.[19] That goes not only for the table form of 1749 but also for the revised formula of 1774. One problem often mentioned was the form the table II was given from the start. The number of entries for example, was too small, more should be added and a certain disease category should be replaced by some other, more frequent disease. It was also stated that the cause-of-death categories were not really reflecting the current situation, but gave a false picture of the mortality. Finally, there were critical arguments in the favour of the nosological system of Linnaeus, indicating that the preprinted table-form system was unadequate and that theoretical problems concerning the rules of classifying thus were observed.

These examples concerning our opportunities to follow the selection of causes of death from a yet not established classification of diseases will do for this older period. In the same way of course, we have to handle concerning the revisions which took place in 1801 and further up to the 1830's, but of course with new perspectives and by adding new sources.

Contemporary problems of the cause-of-death statistics

This leads us to another area of investigation. When studying the older cause-of-death statistics, the problems of historians today to interpret these old medical terms and translate them into a modern medical terminology are often put forward, the terms vagueness in character mostly ascribed to the symptomatological concept of the disease. But worth noticing, not in the least for interpreting the information given in the table forms, is also, I would argue, another problem of the cause-of-death registration. Hereby we have entered a new kind of selection problem called attention to in the paper by B.I.B. Lindahl in this volume, i.e., the problem of selecting the principal cause of death, and accounting for complications and contributory conditions in the individual case.

A comparison with the present situation can elucidate this problem. Nowadays, the specifications of causes of death are to be affirmed by certificates attested by a physician, where the principal cause, complications, and contributory causes can be stated. For the selection of causes of death there are the more uniform, generally applied ICD-classification to choose categories from, and a manual with guiding principles to help the physicians in their work of certifying. The certificates are used as a basis for the cause-of-death statistics, compiled at the National Central Bureau of Statistics. For the registrars who are to transfer the specifications given by the physicians in the certificates, there are also outlined rules for codifying the information into data, that are applicable to the international rules on cause-of-death statistics.

During the eighteenth century on the other hand, the clergymen whose duty it was to supply the authorities in Stockholm with information on the vital statistics, had a double responsibility. They were both to certify the cause of death (as physicians do today) and register the cause in the table form (the kind of work that the codifiers do nowadays). In order to put the correct diagnosis you might say that the clergymen were well taken care of. Several medical handbooks were compiled and published within the two first decades following the establishment of the vital statistics. In these books, which we have already referred to as sources when it comes to define the tabulated categories, the diseases were described with their characteristic symptoms, courses and sometimes even prognosis together with advice on cures and treatments. In the manuscripts left by Abraham Bäck there is also as we have already mentioned, a compilation of descriptions of the diseases tabulated in the revised table form that was announced in 1774, based on some of these handbooks, but with no more disease category to consider than these which were set up in the formula. None of these books however, and that goes for

Bäcks manuscripts too, included instructions in the modern sense, i.e., the way the ICD-classification is organized with its outlined registration rules and explicit definitions of basic concepts. The handbooks taught how to recognize the diseases and the way to treat them. When death occurred amongst the parishioners they were supposed to certify the cause-of-death in the churchbooks with the support of the descriptions given. No death certificates were issued, where the problems of tabulating one possible cause of death, in the case that two or more possible causes were identified, could be documented. Nor were any kind of testimony requested where they had to give an account for their procedure of ascertaining of this or that diagnosis. Yet the problems existed and were not seldom complained of in the correspondence of Abraham Bäck. The questions discussed concerned the index of terms settled beforehand and preprinted in the table forms, a limited terminology that did not allow for adding new disease categories from another classification, if there ever was one.[21] Further, the conceptual confusion within terminology itself must have been frustrating. Apparently there was a need for a generally applied, uniform basis of division, a nomenclature and classification of diseases, which could guarantee that one meant the same item everywhere, when discussing a tabulated disease category. Finally, the problems of causality that might occur and in some cases did, to the eighteenth century certifiers (the clergymen), only a radical change in the way of reporting and certifying the causes of death could alter the situation. That this in its turn implied that the problems concerning the design of the table form and the development of the classification of diseases also had to be solved, was to be shown in the middle of the next century.

The late nineteenth century: the same questions in a new medical and social context

Before concluding this paper, we shall just glance very quickly at the great changes that occurred in the nineteenth and early twentieth centuries, when several of the demands more or less clearly articulated in the earlier period, were to be fulfilled. As to the early decades of the nineteenth century the administrative methods of preceeding the compiling of tabulated data were just about the same, besides the fact that, due to the clergies complaints, the heavy task to report of the cause of death was cut down to cover only the deaths of childbirth, smallpox, suicide and some other specific accidents.

Great changes were made in the period between 1850 and 1860, The National Central Bureau of Statistics was instituted and an important statute was taken concerning cause-of-death statistics.[22] The Bureau of Statistics made it obligatory to give a specific report about the causes of death occurring in the Swedish cities. The reports should there, it was decided, be founded on death certificates signed by a physician. In the same year, 1860, a new classification of causes of death was instituted, and it was revised a couple of times during the last decades of the nineteenth century. A very important step was taken in 1911, when the original ambition was reassumed, that the statistical system was to cover the whole population. The obligation to register causes of death based on a physicians certificate was extended to apply not only to cities but also to boroughs and other densely populated communities. The clergymen in the country were again to report on the cause of death, even when there was no physicians certificate available. A new classification system was introduced the same year, and that was revised again in 1931. In 1949 Sweden accepted to follow an internationally applied system concerning medical statistics, which had begun to develop during the late nineteenth century and got its definite breakthrough in 1948, (the ICD-classification).

The conditions for reporting on cause-of-death statistics were changed radically during the nineteenth century.[23] The old medical systems were replaced by new knowledge of a quite different character. The medical revolution of the century, beginning with the birth of pathological anatomy in France and continuing with the breakthrough of cellular-pathology and bacteriology in the middle of the century, totally changed the conception of the nature of the diseases. On an international level initiatives were taken to establish a coordinated organisation of a classification of causes of death. Here the administrative demands from the society, to delineate the causes of bad health, i.e., the most occurring causes of death, and the internal, scientific demands of a generally accepted form of conception as to the meanings and divisions of the diseases, put forward by the physicians, finally got together.

In England important steps were taken by William Farr (1807-1883) at the General Registers Office, which was to register all causes of death from 1837. As there was no established nomenclature or classification of diseases to start from, he constructed a classification system of his own, which was to comply with both administrative and medical demands. He divided the causes of death into three main groups depending on in what way they "hit" the population. Farrs system was not generally applied however, but influenced the international development a lot. In the 1830's the large international statistical conferences started, where the classification of causes of death was an important task. After Farr the leading role was overtaken by Jacques Bertillon (1851-1922) in Paris. In 1893 he presented a classification, very much inspired by Farr, where the main principles of dividing the diseases were based on anatomical-topological foundations. The purpose was not mainly to reflect the scientific development, but to adjust the results of the statistics so it was easier to correspond to the health political demands. This system was generally accepted and applied and the basic principles we still have today in the ICD-classification, though of course it has underwent many changes in connection with the revisions, that are regularly taking place. An important step towards both an increased internationalization and an extension of the cause-of-death classification occurred in 1948 at a conference directed by the

WHO. With the UN involved and a great international forming, a suggestion of classification was accepted, including the whole range of diseases, causes-of-death and injuries, the ICD-classification.

Against this background I would like to put forward what kinds of research problems within the Swedish development that are to be investigated.[24] The main questions remain: what are the changes within the system of classification and what factors have contributed? What was the main distinction between the old classification put through in the older vital statistics and the classification that was released in 1860? Here we have the opportunities to follow again the development of the first tabulated diseases and see what happened to them in the first "modern" classification. What is the Swedish relationship to the international development mentioned very briefly above? How active were the Swedish participants at the statistical conferences, and to what extent were they influenced by the discussions going on there? In this connection it would be valuable to investigate the background of the changes that took place continuously as to the design of the death certificates. Another very important area of investigation is still the distinction between the classification of causes of death, its revisions included, and the contemporary classifications of diseases. Finally, to what extent is this development, as was the case in Sweden in the eighteenth century, and in England and France in the nineteenth century, adjusted to administrative health political conditions and demands. Here I would again refer to one of the basic problems in the introduction of this paper, i.e., the relations between medicine and society reflected in the application field of the cause-of-death statistics. The social demands on mortality statistics in eighteenth century in Sweden we have already treated. In the middle of the nineteenth century and onwards however, the relation between statistics and medicine, and medicine and society had changed in character. The ambition to survey the state of health amongst the population by an organized cause-of-death statistics still remained; the question is, adapted to what new circumstances? A couple of conceivable factors I will suggest below.

The advocates of the new scientific spirit, inspired by the development within natural sciences, and many of those were physicians, showed great confidence in science itself and its capacity to solve problems of any kind. That also included social problems, and bad health was indeed to be looked upon as one of these unsolved problems of society, though of course this attitude could develop into several directions. As to William Farr for example, the medical science could improve the social conditions of people, provided that the causes of bad health were investigated. Due to Farr, social conditions could be synonymous to health conditions and vice versa. Here cause-of-death statistics had a given function, to serve as a tool for a social oriented medicine. On the whole, the late nineteenth century medicine, so much based upon the natural sciences and their methods was prosperous and inspired to great expectations. In the investigation on the development of the cause-of-

124

death classification from the 1860's and onwards I intend therefore to discuss the selection of causes against this background and how they were to be certified, and to see if the ambitions raised, in for instance England, were reflected in Sweden and in that way try to picture the interaction between internal and external factors.

Conclusions

If we summarize what can be achieved by this investigation of the cause-of-death statistics, we find the following areas: as to the eighteenth century it is to reach and follow the roots of the terminology, i.e., the conceptual basis from its "birth" and onwards and the changes that it undergoes due to medical and social factors. We can observe that complicated problems of both practical and theoretical character were raised, and that complicated questions, debated today, were observed even then. When it comes to the definitions of the causes of death we might even shed some new light upon the problems of validity. As the problems of causality when selecting the causes of death were not carefully examined or documented, the reliability of the old diagnosis must be questioned, in the same way we are observing these problems today, and not only because the terminology is somewhat old-fashioned and hard to translate into modern terminology. Every judgment of the eighteenth century cause-of-death statistics must be seen against this background. In this way the final results might serve as a key to the medical definitions of the eighteenth century that the mortality trends are based on and lead to a better insight and understanding of the medical world of this period. In the same way the latter part of the investigation might form a firmer ground to our understanding of the registered health problems and the basis for epidemiology and their relation to the society in the decades at the turn of the last century.

Notes

1. A survey of cause-of-death validation studies in A. Royston and P.N. Gittelsohn, 'Annotated Bibliography of Cause-of-Death Validation Studies: 1950-1980', *Vital and Health Statistics, Data Evaluation and Methods Research*, Series 2, No. 89, (Hyattsville 1982); The problems of the theoretical and philosophical foundations of cause-of-death classification and statistics today, are treated in L. Nordenfelt, 'Causes of Death. A Philosophical Essay', *Forskningsrådsnämnden, Rapport 83*, 2 (Stockholm 1983); L. Nordenfelt and B.I.B. Lindahl, 'Om grunden för svensk dödsorsaksstatistik: Reflektioner kring grundbegrepp, regler och praxis', *Studies on Health and Society*, 4 (Linköping 1984); B.I.B. Lindahl, 'On the Selection of Causes of Death: An Analysis of WHO's Rules for Selection of the Underlying Cause of Death', L. Nordenfelt and B.I.B. Lindahl (Eds.), Health, Disease, and Causal Explanations in *Medicine, Philosophy and Medicine*, 16 (Dordrecht 1984) pp.137-152; B.I.B. Lindahl, 'Dödsorsaksstatistikens problem i modern tid', L. Nordenfelt (Ed.), *Hälsa, sjukdom, dödsorsak. Studier i begreppens teori och historia* (Malmö 1986), pp. 135-162; B.I.B. Lindahl, E. Glattre, R. Lahti, G. Magnusson and J. Mosbech, 'The WHO Principles for Registering Causes of Death: Suggestions for Improvement', *Department of Social Medicine, Huddinge University Hospital, Huddinge, Sweden* (manuscript 1987); see also the paper by Lindahl in this volume, 'On Weighting Causes of Death. An Analysis of Purposes and Criteria of Selection'; the problems of registering causes of death have also been studied in an empirical material by B.I.B. Lindahl, *Selection of the Principal Cause of Death. Studies on the Basis of the Principal Cause of Death. Studies on the Basis of Mortality Statistics for Rheumatorial Arthritis* (Huddinge 1985).

2. This research task is a work in progress and an extension of preparatory studies being done in a specific research project, Health, Disease, Causes of Death, supported by the Research Council for the Humanities and Social Sciences in Sweden. Project director has been Lennart Nordenfelt of the Department of Health and Society at the University of Linköping: other participants have been Øivind Larsen and Eric Falkum, Department of the History of Medicine at the University of Oslo, B.I.B. Lindahl of the Department of Social Medicine, Karolinska Institute, Huddinge University Hospital, and Eva Nyström, Department of History of Ideas, University of Stockholm; for further references and the directives on research within the project, see the contributions in Hälsa, sjukdom, dödsorsak. The project was initiated at the Department of Philosophy at the University of Stockholm and was later transferred to the Department of the Health and Society at the University of Linköping. The project being formally finished, I am now proceeding my research task according to the outlines I give in this paper at the Department of the History of Ideas at the University of Stockholm. The problems and areas of investigation discussed in the paper focus on the eighteenth century, a smaller space is given though to the late nineteenth century. The whole research task however is covering the period from 1749-1948.

3. For references on the establishment and early history of the vital statistics in Sweden, including the cause-of-death statistics, see footnote 7; the relations between mercantilism and medicine, society and cause-of-death statistics, and their impact on health political measures undertaken during the latter part of the eighteenth century, are discussed by H. Sandblad, *Världens nordligaste läkare. Medicinalväsendets första insteg i Nordskandinavien 1750-1810*, (Stockholm 1979), pp. 3-18; here Sandblad also points out the reflections of humanitarian insight and its further significance in the mercantilistic-influenced social-medical reform-programme laid out by Abraham Bäck (1713-1795); on the suggestions laid and the initiatives undertaken to decrease the mortality rate, see O.E.A. Hjelt, *Svenska och finska medicinalverkets historia*

1663-1812 (Helsingfors 1891-1893), vol. 1, pp. 155-165; for the beginning of a Swedish epidemiology, ibid., vol. 2, pp. 235-238; Sandblad (1979), pp. 10-12.

4. On diseases, causes of death and its classifications, see L. Nordenfelt and E. Nyström, 'Sjukdomsklassifikation i historisk belysning', Nordenfelt (1986), pp. 88-102; the revision applicable today is *Manual of the International Statistical Classification of Diseases, Injuries and Causes of Death, Based on the Recommendations of the Ninth Revision Conference, 1975, and Adapted by the Twenty-Ninth World Health Assembly,* 2 vol., WHO (Geneva 1977-78); on the ICD-principles for the selection of causes and outlined rules of registration and its application in Sweden, see L. Nordenfelt (1983), pp. 42-53; Nordenfelt and Lindahl (1984), pp. 7-34; B.I.B. Lindahl (1986), passim; ibid., 'On Weighting Causes of Death'.

5. L.S. King has discussed the problems of eighteenth century medicine in several books and articles, especially in *The Medical Thought of the Eighteenth Century* (1958, 2 ed. New York 1971); ibid., *The Philosophy of Medicine. The Early Eighteenth Century* (Cambridge, Mass. 1978); see also several passages in ibid., *Medical Thinking. A Historical Preface* (Princeton 1982); on the nosological systems, see also L. Nordenfelt and E. Nyström (1986), pp. 75-88.

6. Cause-specific mortality tables existed from time to time in several European cities and towns during the seventeenth and eighteenth centuries; to give a full report of them and their contents is an impossible task, some account of these is requested though; as to England for example, there is a compilation of the famous Bills of Mortality from 1657 to 1758, which reproduces all the annual bills for the years specified, in T. Birch (Ed.), *A Collection of the Yearly Bills of Mortality within the London district from 1657 to 1758, inclusive, ...,* (London 1759); see also footnote 16.

7. On the establishment of vital statistics and its early history in Sweden see A. Hjelt, 'Det svenska tabellverkets uppkomst, organisation och tidigare verksamhet. Några minnesblad ur den svensk-finska befolkningsstatistikens historia', *Fennia,* 16, (Helsingfors 1900); E. Arosenius, *Bidrag till det svenska Tabellverkets historia* (Sthlm, 1928); Hjelt (1891-1893), II, pp. 264-270; S. Lindroth, *Kungl. Svenska Vetenskapsakademiens historia 1739-1813* (Sthlm 1967), vol. I, pp. 370-374; a recent treatise is E. Hofsten, 'Pehr Wargentin och grundandet av den svenska befolkningsstatistiken', E. Hofsten, *Pehr Wargentin den svenska statistikens fader. En minnesskrift med sju originaluppsatser ur Kungl. Svenska Vetenskapsakademiens Handlingar för åren 1754, 1755 samt 1766* (Sthlm 1983), pp. 11-58; A survey on the causes of death statistics, mostly based on this literature is E. Nyström, 'Den svenska dödsorsaksstatistikens framväxt och tidiga historia', Nordenfeldt (1986), pp. 107-120; A short survey in English is given by Nordenfelt (1983), pp. 22-23; the table form suggested by Lantingshausen encloses his memorandum 'Nödvändigheten af närmare underrättelsers inhemtande om Rikets styrka i anseende til dess Inbyggares antal, tillväxt och afgång med mera', printed as supplement III, in Hjelt (1900), pp. 78-86; the participation of Bäck respectively Linnaeus as to the design of the cause-of-death table form is referred to and quoted by several of the authors named above; the engagement of Bäck is registered 8/11 and 13/12 1746 in 'Dagbok öfver Kungl. Vetenskapsacademiens ärenden och handlingar 1744-46', KVA; 'Linnaeus to Elvius, december 1746', T.M. Frics, et al (Eds.), *Carl von Linné. Bref och skrifvelser af och till Carl von Linné* (Sthlm 1907-43), I:2, pp.84-86.

8. The altogether five table forms that were issued from 1749 to 1830 are reproduced with their terms in A.E. Imhof and ø. Larsen, 'Sozialgeschichte und Medizin. Probleme der quantifizierenden Quellenbearbeitung in der Sozial- und Medizingeschichte', *Medizin in Geschichte und Kultur,* 12 (Stuttgart 1976), pp. 244-245; B-I.

Puranen, *Tuberkulos. En sjukdoms förekomst och dess orsaker. Sverige 1750-1980* (Umeå 1984), pp. 377-381.

9. In Hjelt (1891-1893), II, pp. 223-227 are listed medical handbooks and treatises of different kinds, that form the basis for this investigation.

10. Puranen (1984), pp. 53-72.

11. A. Bäck, 'Kårt Underrättelse til någon hjelp för Herrar Pastores, att kunna föra sjukdomarna, som stadna i döden, under sina titlar i IIa Tabellen', printed as supplement in H. Englesson, 'Dysenteristudien', *Acta Medica Scandinavica,* Suppl. LXXXIII (Lund 1937), pp. 277-288 and in Imhof and Larsen (1976), pp. 245-253; the works referred to by Bäck are, J.J. Haartman, *Tydelig Underrättelse, Om de Mäst Gångbara Sjukdomars Kännande och Motande, Genom Lätta och Enfalliga Hus-Medel; Samt et litet Res- och Hus-Apothek; Dem til tjenst som ej hafva tilfälle at rådfråga Läkare,* (1759, 2 ed. Åbo 1765); J.A. of Darelius, *Socken-Apothek och några Hus-Curer, utgifne under Kongl. Collegii Öfverseende och besörjande* (Stockholm 1760); S.A. Tissot, *Goda Råd och Underrättelse angående hälsan för dem, som bo på landet och som ej lätteligen kunna hafva någon förfaren Läkare at rådfråga* (Stockholm 1764); N.R. von Rosenstein, *Underrättelser om barn-sjukdomar och deras bote-medel: tilförene styckewis utgifne uti de små almanachorna, nu samlade, tilökte och förbättrade* (Stockholm 1764); N.R. von Rosenstein, Hus- och reseapoteque, på Hennes Kongl. Maj:ts nådigste befallning upsatt (Stockholm 1765); for the table terms appearing in the form of 1774, see footnote 8.

12. For the revisions of the table forms, see the terms reproduced in literature referred to in footnote 8.

13. These examples drawn from Elvius' memorandum on the size of the Swedish population, 'Svenska Vetenskapsakademiens betänkande angående folkmängden i Sverige och Finland' (1746), printed as supplement II in Hjelt (1900), pp. 75-; the proposal on establishing the vital statistics, 'Sekreta utskottets förslag om tabellverkets upprättande' (12/12 1747), printed as supplement IV in Hjelt (1900), p. 92; Lantinghausens memorandum, 82, 84; in the proposal from the Academy of Sciences turned down by Linnaeus, there was just a demand for 'a methodical catalogue of diseases by their Swedish names', Fries et. al. (1907-43), vol I:2, pp. 84-86.

14. The tabulated causes of death have been analyzed in several demographic accounts; contributions valuable for this investigation are given in Imhof and Larsen (1976), pp. 138-179; A.E. Imhof, *Aspekte der Bevölkerungsentwicklung in den Nordischen Ländern 1720-1750* (Stuttgart 1978), vol I, pp. 327-590; vol II, pp. 591-679; Ø. Larsen, 'Eighteenth Century Diseases, Diagnostic Trends and Mortality', *Scandinavian Population Studies, 5* (Oslo 1979), pp. 38-54; Puranen (1984), passim; for the meaning of the older Swedish cause-of-death terminology, see also G. Lagerkranz, Svenska sjukdomsnamn i gångna tider (1981, 2 ed.Eskilstuna 1983).

15. These problems discussed by Imhof (1978), pp. 338-339, pp. 478-479; Larsen (1979), pp. 46-49; Nordenfelt (1986), pp.75-80.

16. Cf. footnotes 5 and 6; Pehr Wargentin (1717-1783), secretary of the Academy of Sciences from 1749, discusses the mortality in relation to the selection of causes of death in the Swedish respectively English and German tables of mortality, see 'Anmärkningar, Om Nyttan af årliga Förteckningar på födda och döda i et Land', (Kungliga Vetenskapsakademiens Handlingar 6, 1755) printed in facsimile in Hofsten (1983), pp.127-139.

17. The first report on the figures of the compilation of statistical data were collected around 1755 and presented to the Swedish parliament where the high mortality in general and the mortality rate amongst children in special were mostly paid attention to as to the causes of death; in 1756 there was a parliamentary decision on an extension of the health services; next report from the Statistical Committee came in 1761, when the causes of death were discussed in an extensive chapter, every tabulated cause treated in connection to the figures collected; in 1763 the Collegium Medicum received new instruction with enlarged authorities and later in that decade several of the reforms suggested were carried out; in 1765 there was a third report from the Statistical Committee; for general surveys of all these, see footnote 3 and the literature there referred to; elaborated accounts on acts and sources of different kinds are given by Hjelt (1900), pp. 46-59; Arosenius (1928), pp. 15-28; the reports of 1755 and 1761 are edited in A. Hjelt, *De första officiella relationerna om Svenska tabellverket åren 1749-1757. Några bidrag till den svensk-finska befolkningsstatistikens historia* (Helsingfors 1899), the causes of death discussed at pp. 8-10 and pp. 91-132; at the same time Wargentin started to publish his treatises on the mortality statistics in 'Anmärkningar, Om Nyttan af Årliga Förteckningar', Kungliga Vetenskapsakademiens Handlingar, 1-6, 1754-1755), facsimile reprints in Hofsten (1983), pp. 59-139; cf. footnote 16.

18. The reports in Årsberättelser från Provinsialläkare, Riksarkivet, Medicinalstyrelsens arkiv, Coll. med. inlemnade handlingar; some of these reports that were initiated in 1755 were collected and put in order by P.J. Bergius, *Försök til de uti Swerige Gångbara Sjukdomarnas Utrönande för år 1754, 1755, 1756* (Stockholm 1755-1758); extracts and summaries later published by the Collegium Medicum in altogether three publications *Provincial Doctorernas til Kungl. Collegium Medicum inlemnade Berättelser, rörande Deras Ämbets förrättningar, desse senaste åren, i synnerhet sedan sista Riksdag* (Stockholm 1761); *Berättelser, inlämnade till Kongl. Collegium Medicum, rörande Medicinal-Werkets Tilstånd i Riket* (Stockholm 1765); *Berättelser till Riksens Högloftl. Ständer rörande Medicinal Werkets Tillstånd i Riket. Ingifne wid Riksdagen 1769 af Kongl. Collegio Medico* (Uppsala 1769); later this kind of publications were replaced by extracts in medical periodicals.

19. One example of that in Nordenfelt (1986), pp. 128-130.

20. See in this volume, B.I.B. Lindahl, 'On Weighting Causes of Death'.

21. Nordenfelt (1986), pp. 129-130.

22. This survey on the Swedish development is based on Nordenfelt (1983), pp. 23-28, who gives an account in English; see also Nordenfelt (1986), pp. 135-141.

23. On the international development, an account in English in Nordenfelt (1983), pp. 5-22; see also Nordenfelt (1986), pp. 94-105.

24. As to suggestions on further investigations, see examples discussed in Nordenfelt (1983), pp. 23-28 and pp. 135-141; there is a great deal of literature focusing on the relations between medicine and society in Europe during the nineteenth century; my suggestions on the function of cause-of-death statistics from the middle of the century and onwards are inspired by an excellent study on Farr, by J.M. Eyler, *Victorian Social Medicine. The Ideas and Methods of William Farr* (Baltimore and London 1979).

On Weighting Causes of Death. An Analysis of Purposes and Criteria of Selection.

B. Ingemar B. Lindahl

Introduction

Long term experience with the problems of identifying a single cause as *the principal cause of death*, i.e. the cause primarily tabulated in national statistics[1], coupled with the increasing proportions of deaths occurring in old age, where the complexities affecting selection are most evident, has led to the appropriateness of the traditional way of cause-of-death tabulation being seriously called into question.[2]

The task of selecting the principal cause of death is a problem that has followed cause-of-death statistics since its beginning. This problem is distinct from the diagnostic issue of establishing the causes of death. The selection procedure takes place after the causes have been established and is a matter of allocating relative importance, *weight,* to the causes already identified.

This task may seem relatively simple when death is caused by an acute condition, such as serious injury, infectious or communicable disease. The difficulties become far more obvious when a combination of concurrent and non-interdependent causes of death has been identified, which is not unusual in deaths occurring in old age.

A few countries have multiple cause-of-death statistics, yet still record a principal cause of death for every case.

The purpose of this paper is to show how the selection of the principal cause of death may be determined by different interests and that different causes in one and the same course of events may be pointed out depending on the purpose of the question: 'what was the cause of death?' However, which purposes may actually have guided the choice of causes in the history of cause-of-death statistics and how this could have influenced the statistics is left open.

The problem of selecting the principal cause of death will relate to a general discussion of how *the* cause of an event is determined in disciplines even outside medicine, such as social science, jurisprudence and historical research. Some central criteria of selection will be accounted for, and the relevance of selection criteria used in these disciplines to cause-of-death statistics will be examined. The overall purpose of the World Health Organization's principles for registering causes of death will also be discussed.

The development of the selection procedure up to today

In Sweden during the earliest compilations of cause-of-death statistics, 1749-1830, the selection of the principal cause of death was left entirely to the certifier, usually a clergyman. The problem of selection was facilitated by the fact that the national cause-of-death statistics were originally compiled at the parish level by the clergymen themselves. For this purpose table-forms with printed cause-of-death rubrics were distributed to the parish clergymen by the authorities. Therefore the clergymen, when acting as certifiers, knew what causes in a train of events leading to death could and which could not be tabulated. There could still be selection problems of course, for example when two causes both possible to tabulate were identified in a particular case. No official instructions for this selection seem to have existed.

From 1860 a new procedure was introduced for the cities with employed physicians: separate cause-of-death statistics were compiled, based on certificates attested by physicians. On these certificates, which were designed on the model developed in Great Britain, a distinction was made between "primär" (primary) and "sekundär" (secondary) cause of death; in 1892 these changed to "hufvuddödsorsak" (principal cause of death) and "bidragande dödsorsaker" (contributory causes of death).[3] This gave rise to a new selection problem: sometimes causes considered by the statistical registrars to be contributory causes were stated on the certificates as principal causes, and vice versa.[4] Should in such instances the registrars be entitled to register a "contributory" cause as the principal cause of death?

At the end of the 19th century several countries independently developed special rules for statistical registration to achieve a uniform tabulation of causes of death. At the turn of the century attempts were made to formulate rules that could be internationally adopted.[5] Three countries were to play a special role in this development: France, Great Britain and the USA.

The first set of rules to be adopted on a wide international scale was that compiled by Jacques Bertillon (1851-1922) for the first revision of the *International List of Causes of Death* in 1900.[6] In cases when more than one cause of death had been reported, the registrars should select the principal cause of death in the following way:

> Rule 1. If one of the two diseases is an immediate and frequent complication of the other, the death should be classified under the head of the primary disease.
>
> Rule 2. If it is not absolutely certain that one of the diseases is an immediate result of the other, we must see if there is a very great difference in the gravity of the two, and classify the death under the head of the more dangerous.
>
> Rule 3. When among the two causes of death there is a transmissible disease, it is preferable to assign the death to it, for statistics of infectious diseases are

132

particularly interesting to the sanitarian, and it is important that they shall be as complete as possible.

Rule 4. If a disease whose evolution is rapid is given in connection with another whose evolution is slow, it is preferable to charge the death to the first. Again, if a death is simultaneously attributed to a disease and to an external violence, it is usually proper to assign it to the latter.

Rule 5. Finally, if none of the preceding rules is applicable, the diagnosis most characteristic of the case should be selected.[7]

From the experience of applying these rules, The United States Bureau of the Census published in 1914 a handbook for its registrars, *Index of Joint Causes of Death*.[8] The basic principle of this handbook was rather simple. Conditions that might be reported as causing death in concurrence with other conditions were listed as a set of rubrics. Listed under each rubric were then the codes of those other conditions in concurrence with which the condition in the rubric might be reported to cause death. In the choice between a condition listed as a rubric and a condition under this rubric, the latter should always be selected. This handbook was used in several countries until 1948. A study in 1947 comprising 29 countries, showed that this handbook was used, with or without modifications and supplementations of other rules, in 12 countries.[9] The same number of countries, including Sweden, did not have any explicit rules at all. Three countries, including England, used only their own special rules. (The two further countries are not accounted for in the study.)

The handbook was revised in 1925, 1933 and 1940 to conform to the new revisions of the International List of Causes of Death. However, the 6th revision in 1948—the *International Classification of Diseases* (ICD)—was so thoroughgoing and amounted to such a considerable increase in number of categories, that it was no longer considered practical to adjust the handbook to the classification.[10] The handbook was discarded also for a more fundamental reason. It assigned the order of priority for *types* of conditions, but was not necessarily correct in the choice between *instances* of conditions in particular cases. For example, the physician's judgment in a particular case about the causal antecedence (the criterion of Bertillon's Rule 1) or the relative gravity of the conditions (Rule 2) might be contrary to the general experience on which the handbook was based. Dunn illustrates this with the example of a woman who was admitted to a hospital with coronary sclerosis and discharged as improved after ten days.[11] Four months later she was readmitted with myocardial infarction and after a week pulmonary edema developed, resulting in death the next day. This woman had been under treatment for syphilitic aortitis during the preceding ten years. Even if the physician in such case judged the pulmonary edema to have been mainly due to the myocardial infarction, and this in turn to the coronary sclerosis, the statistical clerk would have selected the syphilitic aortitis as the principal cause of death according to the handbook.

For these reasons new principles for selection of the principal cause of death were developed. The responsibility for this work was laid upon Percy

Stocks (1889-1974) at the General Register Office of England and Wales (GRO).[12] The GRO had used their own rules since 1901 and had developed a selection procedure by which the principal cause could be selected according to the certifier's judgment in the particular case.[13] In 1927 the GRO had introduced a new certificate form that enabled the certifiers to specify the way the principal cause had caused death and how this cause was related to other contributory conditions.[14] Up to then the certificate form did only distinguish between "cause of death" and "secondary (contributory) cause". The new certificate consisted of two parts, I-II. In part I it was possible to record on three lines respectively, an "immediate cause" and antecedent "morbid conditions, if any, giving rise to immediate cause", and in part II "other morbid conditions (if important) contributing to death but not related to immediate cause".[15] In this way the certifier could indicate the pathological history from the immediate cause of death back to the principal cause.

After slightly more than ten years experience of this certificate the GRO changed selection procedure and began in 1940 to register as the principal cause of death the condition stated as such on the certificate, provided of course that the certificate was not obviously inadequately filled out.[16] The rules for this selection procedure had been prepared by Stocks in 1939.[17] It was a modified version of these rules and this certificate form that was to become the new principles for selection adopted by WHO for the 6th revision of the ICD. The ICD has been revised three times since then, but the general content of the rules remain the same and the certificate form recommended has not changed.

The principal cause of death, in the ICD called *"the underlying cause of death"*, is defined as "(a) the disease or injury which initiated the train of events leading directly to death, or (b) the circumstances of the accident or violence which produced the fatal injury".[18]

In the ICD the basic principle for selection is that the cause stated on the last used line in part I of the certificate (Figure 1) should be selected for tabulation as the underlying cause of death. If more than one condition have been stated on this line or if it is highly improbable that this condition could have given rise to all the conditions mentioned as complications, the registrar should request the certifier for amplification of the course of events leading to death. If more information cannot be obtained, the registrar should apply the further rules of the ICD. These rules aim at a medically and causally correct interpretation of the information on the certificate, and at optimizing the usefulness and precision of the diagnosis selected for tabulation.[19]

In 1952 WHO published instructions for physicians on how the death certificate form should be filled out. A fourth edition of this booklet, *Medical Certification of Cause of Death, Instructions for Physicians on Use of International Form of Medical Certificate of Cause of Death,* was published in 1979.

134

Figure 1.

INTERNATIONAL FORM OF MEDICAL CERTIFICATE OF CAUSE OF DEATH

	CAUSE OF DEATH	Approximate interval between onset and death
I *Disease or condition directly leading to death* *	(a) .... due to (or as a consequence of)	. . .
Antecedent causes Morbid conditions, if any, giving rise to the above cause, stating the underlying condition last	(b) .... due to (or as a consequence of) (c)	. . . . . .
II *Other significant conditions* contributing to the death, but not related to the disease or condition causing it	....	. . .

* This does not mean the mode of dying, e.g., heart failure, asthenia, etc. It means the disease, injury, or complication which caused death.

135

To sum up, the main responsibility for the selection of the principal cause of death has been transferred from the certifiers to the registrars and back to the certifiers again. The difference being that originally the selection was entirely left to the certifiers, presumably without any official instructions, while today the certifiers' judgment is regulated by specific definitions, and rules internationally adopted.

Criteria for selection of the principal cause

The criteria of selection that can be discerned in the WHO concepts and rules resemble those employed when *the* cause of an event is stated in disciplines such as jurisprudence, social science and historical research.

The discussion of the problem of singling out as the cause one of several factors determining an event, such as death, can be traced back to John Stuart Mill, *A System of Logic,* 1843.[20] Mill objects to the whole idea of selecting one of the conditions jointly sufficient for the occurrence of an event and calling this "the cause" of the event: "The real Cause is the whole of these antecedents; and we have, philosophically speaking, no right to give the name of cause to one of them exclusively of the others".[21]

In his position, Mill presupposes a striving after what he calls scientific accuracy in the pointing out of the cause of an event. In common parlance on the other hand it is very common, according to Mill, that a single insufficient condition is denominated "the cause" and the rest of the antecedence as mere "conditions". Mill examines several criteria used when the cause is selected from among insufficient conditions and notices that there is no rule *always* adhered to; from this he draws the controversial conclusion that the selection is made capriciously.

Although this selection concerns, in Mill's terminology, choices between *conditions* (or *antecedents*) and not between *causes*, Mill's analysis is still relevant to cause-of-death statistics, because what Mill calls "conditions" are accepted as causes in the statistical context. WHO's concepts 'the underlying cause of death' and 'causes of death' allow both unconditionally *sufficient* and *in*sufficient conditions to be tabulated as *causes*. The choice among what WHO calls "causes" of death is often indeed a choice among, in Mill's terminology, "conditions" (or "antecedents"). Consequently, as long as the insufficient conditions satisfy the definition of '*causes* of death', used in statistics, it is of no practical significance that Mill (and others) chose to call all insufficient conditions, excepting the one selected as the most important, simply "conditions". (In the following, this difference in terminology, and sometimes also in concept, will be indicated by a differentiation in emphasis: *the* cause and *the* cause, respectively. The latter will also include cases when the distinction in the text referred to is uncertain.) WHO defines '*causes of death*' as "all those diseases, morbid conditions or injuries which either resulted in or contributed to death and the circumstances of the accident or violence which produced any such injuries".[22]

136

Mill points out the following criteria for selection between insufficient conditions: an insufficient condition is sometimes selected because it is (i) the condition "the fulfilment of which completes the tale, and brings about the effect without further delay", (ii) the condition "whose share in the matter is superficially the most conspicuous", (iii) the condition "whose requisiteness to the production of the effect we happen to be insisting on at the moment", (iv) the condition "being in closer proximity to the effect than any other of its conditions", and (v) the condition "which can be supposed to be unknown" to the hearer.[23]

Examples of selection of the cause of death according to the first criterion would be a person suffering in a particular case from congestive heart failure and who gets influenza, or a particular person with diabetes who gets bronchopneumonia. In such cases the condition selected, e.g. in the first case influenza and in the second diabetes, may be in the particular instance sufficient for death only provided some other condition(s) is (are) present, such as congestive heart failure or bronchopneumonia respectively. Let us call this criterion (1) *the criterion of conditional sufficiency.*

The second criterion is more ambiguously formulated, but in one interpretation examples of selection of the cause of death would be a person with malignant neoplasm of lung and myocardial infarction, or a person with ulcerative colitis and pulmonary embolism. The myocardial infarction and the ulcerative colitis could in such cases be the more conspicuous condition. Let us call this criterion (2) *the criterion of conspicuity.*

"Requisiteness" in the formulation of the third criterion can be interpreted in at least three ways: (a) the condition selected is in the particular situation non-redundant for the occurrence of the effect, (b) no other condition than the one selected could in the situation have completed the set of insufficient but jointly sufficient conditions for the occurrence of the effect, or (c) the condition selected is indispensable for every occurrence of the effect.[24] Examples of the first interpretation are selections of one or the other of the two conditions congestive heart failure and influenza in the first example or diabetes and bronchopneumonia in the second example of selection according to the first criterion. Depending on the situation, the same examples can be examples also of the second interpretation. Examples of the third interpretation are difficult, if at all possible, to find, at least regarding causes of death. If we chose for example cerebral hypoxia or cardiac arrest, the first can be viewed as a part of a definition of 'brain death' and the second as a part of the concept 'heart death'. Through these interpretations we get three criteria which we may call (3) *the criterion of non-redundancy,* (4) *the criterion of conditional irreplaceability,* and (5) *the criterion of unconditional irreplaceability.*[25]

A condition selected according to an interpretation of Mill's criterion (iv) would be, in WHO's terminology, the "direct cause of death", e.g.

postoperative shock or acute renal failure. Let us call this criterion (6) *the criterion of proximity.*

Mill's criterion (v), finally, we may call (7) *the criterion of ignorance.*

Collingwood asserts that the concept 'cause' endorsed by Mill, i.e., according to which a cause is always unconditionally sufficient for its effect, is not universally employed in science.[26]

Collingwood distinguishes between three senses of the term "cause" used in e.g. historical science; engineering and medicine; physics and chemistry; respectively. In the first sense, used in historical science, both cause and effect are human activities: "that which is 'caused' is the free and deliberate act of a conscious and responsible agent, and 'causing' him to do it means affording him a motive for doing it".[27] In the second sense, used in for example engineering and medicine and, in general, the "practical sciences of nature", a cause is something that can be *manipulated* and its effect a thing in nature: "that which is 'caused' is an event in nature, and its 'cause' an event or state of things by producing or preventing which we can produce or prevent that whose cause it is said to be".[28] In the third sense, traditionally employed in physics and chemistry and, in general, the "theoretical sciences of nature", both cause and effect are things in nature: "that which is 'caused' is an event or state of things, and its 'cause' is another event or state of things standing to it in a one-one relation of causal priority: i.e. a relation of such a kind that (*a*) if the cause happens or exists the effect also must happen or exist, even if no further conditions are fulfilled, (*b*) the effect cannot happen or exist unless the cause happens or exists, (*c*) in some sense which remains to be defined, the cause is prior to the effect".[29]

Mill's concept 'cause', Collingwood maintains, is compatible with the third sense of "cause", but not with the second.[30] In the second sense a cause "is never able by itself to produce the corresponding effect".[31] According to Collingwood, which insufficient condition a person points out as *the cause* of a given effect depends on *this* persons ability to produce or prevent the different conditions, and if a person is not able to produce or prevent any of the conditions, there is no cause, for *this* person, in the second sense of "cause".[32] Therefore, in this sense of "cause", *the cause* is not arbitrarily pointed out, Collingwood objects, but the identification is made according to a criterion, which we can call (8) *the criterion of manipulability.*

Hart and Honoré go a step further than Collingwood in their critique of Mill's concept 'cause' and its alleged relevance to science.[33] They assert that Mill's concept is unattainable both in practice and in principle: "To meet such a standard there would have to be evidence that 'everything' (*all* other things, events or states) apart from the set of conditions specified in the generalization was irrelevant, so that the specified conditions would be unconditionally and invariably sufficient".[34] Instead, Hart and Honoré maintain, insufficient conditions are often pointed out as *the cause*, and this without knowledge or concern for what other conditions are required for the effect to follow 'invariably'.[35] Hart and Honoré acknowledge that sometimes this identification of *the cause* is made according to what we have called the ignorance or manipulability criterion, but at the same time they assert that these criteria are subordinate to a more fundamental principle: the condition regarded as *the cause* of an event (e.g. a person's death) is a condition that *makes a difference* from what normally characterizes either the particular phenomenon in question (i.e., in the case of a person's death, the normal life of this particular person) or the type of objects which this phenomenon instantiates (i.e., in the case of a person's death, the normal life of persons in general or persons of the same sex, age, etc).[36] Let us call this criterion (9) *the criterion of abnormality.*

However, there are cases, Hart and Honoré point out, in which this principle is overridden, and that is when the effect (e.g., a person's death) was determined by a voluntary human action intended to bring about this effect, and in the manner in which it took place: "when the question is how far back a cause shall be traced through a number of intervening causes, such a voluntary action very often is regarded both as a limit and also as still the cause even though other later abnormal occurrences are recognized as causes".[37] Thus in such cases the cause may be traced through later abnormal conditions, but according to Hart and Honoré the cause is not traced through the deliberate action, e.g. an act of homicidal poisoning: "though we may look for and find an explanation of why the poisoner did what he did in terms of motives like greed or revenge, we do not regard his motive or speak of it as the cause of the *death* into which we are inquiring, even if we do (as is perhaps rare) call the poisoner's motive the 'cause' of his action".[38] Let us call this criterion (10) *the criterion of human action.*

Martin calls attention to the difference between weighting *instances* of causes leading to effects in particular cases and weighting *types* of causes leading to certain effects in general—the distinction we saw was taken into account in the abandonment of the Manual of Joint Causes of Death in 1948.[39] Martin notes that there is a skepticism among philosophers regarding the propriety of weighting instances of causes leading to effects in particular cases, whereas many consider it meaningful to weight types of causes leading to certain effects in general. Martin objects to a view in a similar vein of thought, accounted for by Nagel[40], according to which the weighting of instances of causes leading to effects in particular cases implies a *frequency* claim about other conditions of the same type as the causes and effects in question: "that (roughly) it may be said of particular factors, A and B, which were each a cause of a particular factor, P, that A was a more important cause of P than was B, if the frequency with which a factor of type-A has been a cause of a factor of type-P is greater than the frequency with which a factor of type-B has been a cause of a factor of type-P".[41] Let us call this criterion (11) *the criterion of frequency.*

Instead of this criterion, which Martin shows to be untenable, he proposes another criterion: "(D1) A was a more important cause of P than was B, if (1) A and B were each a necessary cause of P, and (2) there is some appropriate state, ϕ, such that: (i) A, B, and P are each deviations from ϕ, and (ii) on the occasion in question, had A occurred as it did and B occurred as in ϕ, a result would have occurred more similar to P than had B occurred as it did and A occurred as in ϕ ".[42] The first two parts of this criterion, (1) and (2) (i), do not seem to add much to our list of criteria: by "necessary" Martin here means what we earlier called conditionally irreplaceable in criteria 4, and "appropriate state" may, according to the example given by Martin, be interpreted as a previous state of the same individual, e.g., what normally characterizes the particular individual in question; c.f. the criterion of abnormality. The third part, (2) (ii), however, introduces a new aspect of the weighting problem. The expression "a result would have occurred more similar to P", means according to Martin, that "more, less, or the same amount of the result explained, P, would have occurred".[43] If we allow not only direct causes but also *indirect* causes to be selected as the principal cause, Martin points out, we are able to select a cause according to this criterion even when the effect to be explained is not itself quantifiable, for example in cases of weighting causes of death. The effect quantified is then not death, but an immediate cause of death, e.g., "a deterioration (of the sort that led to death) of that individual's health".[44] Let us call this criterion (12) *the criterion of causal efficacy.*[45]

Martin also examines some criteria for selection between a relatively permanent condition and a more substitutable condition jointly sufficient for the effect:

Perhaps the weighting distinction among causes that is most frequently encountered in historical studies is that sense in which the more important cause is often (but not always) a relatively permanent feature of the situation under investigation, and it is supposed that given the more important cause and the 'prevailing circumstances', it was likely that had the less important cause not occurred, a 'substitute cause' would soon have been present, and a result similar to the actual result would soon have occurred.[46]

Different criteria may be used for this selection depending on what aspects are taken into account. If the permanency of the more important cause is left unanalyzed, the selection criterion used may simply be called (13) *the criterion of durability.* Nagel formulates the distinction in terms of the more important, relatively permanent, condition being "contingently necessary" and the less important condition defined in terms of its frequency of occurrence;[47] a formulation which Martin finds untenable. (The selection could then be seen as a mere example of choices according to what we have called the criterion of conditional irreplaceability.) Instead Martin proposes that the difference between the more important, what he calls the "underlying" or "dispositional" cause and a less important "precipitating" cause is formulated as a difference in making the occurrence of the effect probable: "(D2) A was a more important cause of P than B if for any factor, X, such that A, B, and X were each a cause of P, and were each a non-redundant member of the set of factors, (A, B, X), which set both occurred and was sufficient for P, the probability was greater, given A and X, than it was, given B and X, that a factor of type-P would occur during an appropriate temporal interval".[48] Let us call this criterion (14) *the criterion of probability.*

White[49] sees in Nagel's six interpretations of how 'the most important' determinant is selected in historical and social science, attempts to find an objective ground for this selection—'to eliminate the element of 'subjectivity' in picking out the cause".[50] It is of a similar reason, White maintains, that Mill reaches the conclusion that there is no "scientific ground" for the selection, but that it is made capriciously.[51] According to White, a reason why Mill failed in his efforts to find a distinguishing feature always employed when an insufficient condition is pointed out as the cause, and a reason why other writers have not been able to present a criterion necessary or sufficient for the selection of the most important cause, is that they assume that the distinguishing feature must be *intrinsic* to the cause—i.e., a feature "that the cause has independently of the context and independently of how the investigator views the situation".[52] Examples of such criteria, pointed out by White, are what we have called the criterion of human action and a version of the criterion of durability, according to which the relatively permanent condition is a *state* and the precipitating condition an *event* or *episode.*[53] According to White, this 'absolutistic' view on how *the cause* is selected in historical science is based on overgeneralizations: although conditions such as a human action or a state are sometimes identified as *the cause*, intrinsic properties are neither necessary nor sufficient as reasons for the selection.[54] The criterion actually employed on most occasions in historical science, White insists, is the criterion of abnormality: even in cases when the cause is selected according to intrinsic properties, such as being a human action or an underlying state, the more general principle guiding the selection is often that the (decisive) cause is the abnormal contributory cause.[55]

In contrast to the property of being a human action or a state, abnormality is, as White and Hart and Honoré point out, a relative property, dependent upon context and on how the investigator views the situation—it is what we may call an *extrinsic* property. Other extrinsic properties are those that are the basis of the criterion of ignorance and the manipulability criterion. The criteria based on extrinsic properties are relativistic in the sense that one and the same criterion may be applied differently in different situations and by different investigators; e.g. what "makes a difference" in one context or in comparison with one person's reference values can be "normal" in another context or when compared with another person's reference values, etc.[56] The basis for selecting *the* cause of an event is relative also in another sense. Different criteria may be used, depending on the *purpose* of the selection. As Mill points out: "However numerous the conditions may be, there is hardly any of them which may not, according to the purpose of our immediate discourse, obtain that nominal pre-eminence [of being denominated 'the cause']".[57] But, as Hart and Honoré, White and other writers have shown, an admission that the basis for the selection of *the* cause is relative does not entail—neither in the first nor in the second sense of 'relative'—that the choice is made without ground, capriciously.

Finally, it should be noted that the principal cause of death in the vital statistics context is selected not only because of the characteristics of the condition itself (whether intrinsic or extrinsic) but also because of the semantic qualities of the *diagnosis*. This is apparent from Bertillon's Rule 5. In the present WHO rules priority is given to more precise (Rule 5), inclusive (Rule 7) and specific (Rule 8) diagnoses.[58] The WHO Rules 5 and 7 concern choices between diagnoses denoting different conditions, whereas Rule 8 concerns choices between diagnoses denoting one and the same condition. Therefore, at least Rules 5 and 7 are relevant to the choice between *causes*. Let us call this criterion (15) *the criterion of completeness*.

The purpose of the selection

At least five of the purposes of causal accounts, commonly referred to in causal theory in general, are relevant to selections of causes of death: (i) to *describe* what caused death; (ii) to *explain* why death occurred; (iii) to identify causes, the manipulation of which would *prevent* untimely death; (iv) to identify risk factors, which make it possible to *predict* untimely death; and (v) to *adjudge personal responsibility* for a death.

Consider the following example: *A cold winter day Mr Smith, the caretaker of the house in which the 91 year old Mrs Jones lives, has neglected to sand the icy pavement outside Mrs Jones' front-door. Due to this fact, Mrs Jones slips down and fractures the femural neck in her left leg. She is admitted to hospital and operated on. But due to the fracture being comminuted, Mrs Jones' immobilization is extended up to five days and she develops bronchopneumonia, leading to her death two days later.* Depending on the purpose of the selection, different answers can be given to the question: 'what was the cause of Mrs Jones' death?' Let us consider some possible answers from the five purposes mentioned.

Description

Presumably the overall purpose of the selection of the principal cause of death for mortality statistics has never been purely descriptive, even if a possible lack of official instructions for this selection during the earliest compilation of cause-of-death statistics might suggest this.

142

Figure 2.

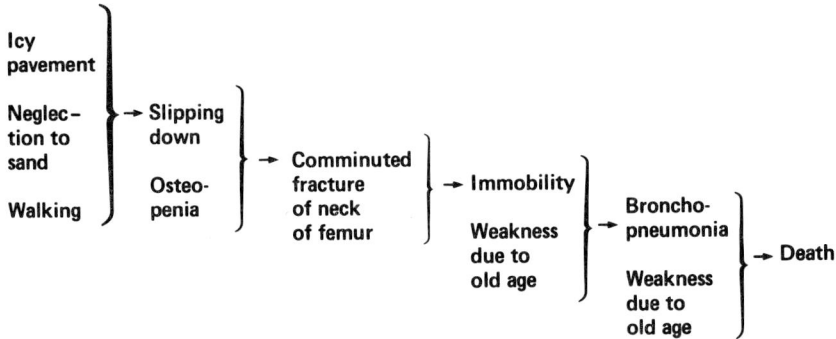

Though the WHO's instructions for the modern cause-of-death statistics makes clear that description is not the main purpose of selection of the *underlying* cause of death, the definition of *contributory* causes of death does not seem to have any other purpose. Since the selection of contributory conditions may determine the coding of the underlying cause of death, the purpose(s) of selecting the contributory conditions is relevant to the registration of the underlying cause. The purpose(s) of registering contributory conditions is also important to note as a part of the purpose(s) of multiple cause of death statistics.

Contributory conditions are "*all* other diseases or conditions believed to have unfavourably influenced the course of the morbid process and thus contributed to the fatal outcome but which were not related to the disease or condition directly causing death".[59] This demand for *completeness* — "all other diseases or conditions" — is other than for example the one Mill insists on. As an illustration of this, consider the following preliminary characterization of the course of events leading to Mrs Jones' death.

Since each link in the course of events leading to death may only be accounted for by *one* condition and since none of the insufficient conditions in this example can be linked under one code (and in that way form *one* condition, according to the ICD), it is not possible to state any link in this chain by an unconditionally sufficient condition in Mill's sense. From this observation, it could seem plausible to assume that the information of contributory conditions is supposed to supplement this incomplete information about the sufficient conditions, and that "contributory conditions" should be interpreted as (i) the insufficient conditions which, *together with an insufficient condition stated as part of the principal course of events leading to death* (i.e. in part I of the certificate) form an unconditionally sufficient condition directly or indirectly causing death. But, obviously, this is not a correct interpretation, since the contributory conditions may not be "directly part of the fatal sequence" and may not be "related to the disease or condition directly causing death".[60] For example, if the following sequence is judged to be the principal course of events in the case of Mrs Jones' death, bronchopneumonia, 2 days, due to immobility, 5 days, due to comminuted fracture of femoral neck due to fall on same level from slipping, the osteopenia or old age weakness may not be stated as contributory conditions, because the old age weakness is directly related to the bronchopneumonia (the disease directly causing death) and the osteopenia is indirectly related to this condition.[61] This exclusion of conditions from the certificate is of less significance, of course, in cases like this, where the conditions left out may be inferred from the circumstances (Mrs Jones' age), than for example it would have been if the fracture had occurred in a forty years old person, where the osteopenia was due to liver cirrhosis.

The exclusion of conditions "related to the disease or condition directly causing death" in the definition of 'contributory conditions' precludes as well, of course, the following interpretation of "contributory conditions" (ii) the causally redundant conditions which, *independent of any condition in the principal course of events leading to death*, causes the direct cause of death. In other words, no parallel chain of events leading to the direct cause of death in the principal chain may be entered as 'contributory condition'.

The part of the original definition of 'contributory conditions', which delimits these conditions as "not related to the ... *antecedent* causes",[62] could in one interpretation of "related", be understood to exclude even the following interpretation of "contributory conditions" (iii) the conditions not causing the direct cause of death in the principal course of events, but which may be *caused* by a condition stated in the principal course of events. Examples of contributory conditions in this sense would be: Mrs Jones' immobility leading to venous thrombosis, causing multiple pulmonary embolism, and the pulmonary embolism being judged not to have influenced the bronchopneumonia (Figure 3).

Figure 3.

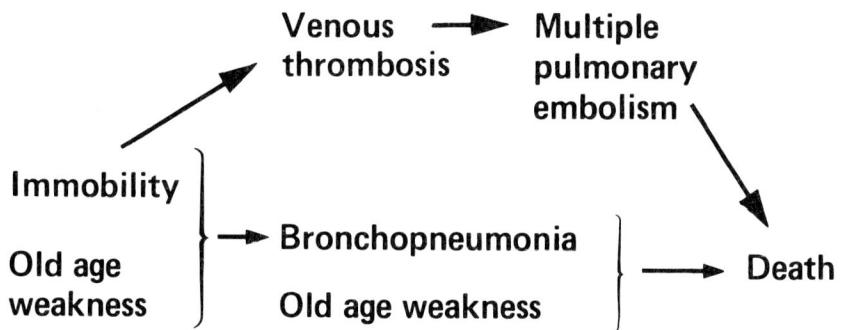

If "related" is only interpreted in the way that a 'contributory condition' may not *cause* any condition in the principal course of events (i.e. may not be a direct or indirect cause of the direct cause of death in the principal course of events), then both the venous thrombosis and the bronchopneumonia may be entered on the certificate (one as part of the principal course of events and the other as contributory cause). However, if "related" is interpreted in the way that a 'contributory condition' may not *be caused* by any condition in the principal course of events, then only one of the conditions, the venous thrombosis *or* the bronchopneumonia, may be entered on the certificate—and, thus, the interpretation (iii) of "contributory conditions" is precluded.

Even if WHO's definition of 'contributory conditions' is not intended to exclude contributory conditions in the third interpretation (iii), the definition does seem to allow only causally redundant conditions, without significant explanatory, predictive or preventive value, to be entered as contributory conditions. It is difficult to see that these conditions are tabulated for any other purpose than a purely descriptive.

In practise, the information of contributory conditions is often used to improve the coding of the underlying cause of death. Information about contributory conditions (rightly or wrongly entered on the certificate, according to the definition) often modifies the coding of the underlying cause of death, and a more informative code can be selected for the underlying cause. An example of this is the linkage of two conditions under one code in Rule 7. The descriptive relevance of this and other rules, such as Rule 7 and Rule 8 (i.e. rules selecting the underlying cause according to the criterion of completeness) is evident.[63]

However, in Mrs Jones' case, when we have all the information given in Figure 2 and 3, these Rules 5, 7 and 8 do not give sufficient guidance for selecting the underlying cause of death. They do not tell us which cause should be selected. But if we had had less information, let us say only "bronchopneumonia and weakness due to old age", preference would have been given to bronchopneumonia.

If any of the other criteria could be said to serve (only or mainly) a descriptive purpose, it may be the criterion of conspicuity; a commonsense criterion, which has no explicit support in the WHO rules.

Explanation

Without going into the general issue concerning the distinction between descriptions and explanations, we may note that at least in the context of commonsense and clinical medicine, the mere citing of a single cause—a disease or injury—is often sufficient as an explanation of a particular death. Therefore, in such cases, explanations are a kind of descriptions, e.g., descriptions pointing out the *abnormal* conditions, or the conditions *unknown* to the addressees;[64] and whether such a description is a sufficient explanation or an explanation at all, depends on the context and the addressee. 'Explanation', in the following, will be used in this somewhat restricted sense.

In another version of the formal definition of 'the underlying cause of death' than the one cited above (in the second section), it appears that "the train of events leading directly to death" is supposed to be a "train of *morbid* events";[65] (as to the rest, these two versions are identical). Besides these two versions of the formal definition, the concept 'the underlying cause of death' is also characterized in WHO's instructions as "the condition that started the sequence of events between *normal health* and death".[66] This indicates that "the train of morbid events" is supposed to have been preceded by "normal health".

Taking this into consideration, 'the underlying cause of death' is (a) the disease or injury which initiated the train of morbid events leading directly to death (i.e. *the first condition in the fatal sequence of morbid events)*, or (b) the circumstances of the accident or violence which produced the fatal injury (i.e. *the external cause of the fatal sequence of morbid events*). The WHO's definition obviously leaves open which condition should be selected, the first condition or the external cause.[67]

According to the first part of the formal definition, (a), 'the underlying cause of death' may be characterized in terms such as Hart's and Honoré's, as the first condition in the fatal sequence of morbid events that "makes a difference" between normal health and fatal morbidity. This indicates the relevance of the abnormality criterion in the selection of the underlying cause of death.[68] From this criterion the question of the cause of Mrs Jones' death can be formulated: (A) 'what was the first condition in the train of morbid events leading directly to death, that made a difference between the normal health and the fatal morbidity of Mrs Jones?'

According to the second part of the formal definition, (b), the question of the cause of Mrs Jones' death could be formulated: (B) 'what was the external cause producing the injury initiating the fatal train of morbid events leading to Mrs Jones' death?'

An immediate answer to the second question, (B), could be: the slipping down. The osteopenia could not be selected, since it was not an *external* cause of the injury. But what could be a correct answer to the first question, (A)? If we restrict the choice to the conditions mentioned in Figure 2, should the osteopenia or the fracture be considered the first condition in the train of morbid events? The answer obviously depends on whether or not the osteopenia is to be considered compatible with normal health. An immediate answer to this is, of course, that it is compatible with the normal health of Mrs Jones being 91 years old, but that it would not have been so, had she been much younger. One might say that osteopenia is a natural old age infirmity and must be considered compatible with normal health among the elderly, if aging shall not be considered a morbid process.

The osteopenia could be rejected as an explanation also from the criterion of ignorance. Since it is common knowledge that persons of Mrs Jones' age suffer from osteopenia, to single out that condition would not add anything to our knowledge of Mrs Jones.

A third criterion of relevance to an explanatory purpose is the criterion of proximity. Bohrod points out that it can be relevant for the purpose of research to select as the principal cause of death a physiological condition which made the person die at one particular point of time.[69] From this criterion the question of the cause of Mrs Jones' death could be put: (C) 'what condition made Mrs Jones die at one particular point of time and not earlier or later?' In which case an answer could be, bronchopneumonia.

Prevention

Regarding the purpose of the formal definition of 'the underlying cause of death' WHO states: "From the standpoint of prevention of deaths, it is important to cut the chain of events or institute the cure at some point. The most effective public health objective is to prevent the precipitating cause from operating".[70]

It is easily recognized that the criteria of irreplaceability (conditional and unconditional) are relevant to a purpose of prevention of untimely death: for the prevention of a cause to prevent an effect the cause must be indispensable for the effect. It is not clear what is meant in the ICD by "to prevent" the cause from operating. In one interpretation it may be the occurrence, in another it may be the progress of the condition, that should be counteracted.[71] However, in both interpretations the underlying cause ought to be manipulable—directly or indirectly.

Consequently, from a purpose of prevention the question of the cause of Mrs Jones' death could be formulated in at least two ways: (D) 'the manipulation of what cause of death would most effectively or to the greatest extent have prolonged the life of Mrs Jones?' or (E) 'which of the causes of death would have been easiest to manipulate in a way that would have prolonged the life of Mrs Jones?' Ideally, the cause to be selected should be both the easiest to manipulate and the manipulation of which would be comparatively the most effective way to prevent untimely death.

It would carry us too far to discuss here which of the conditions in Mrs Jones' case could be considered—in some interpretation of the situation—most appropriate to select according to the criterion of conditional irreplaceability (i.e. which condition is such that it is least likely that in its absence another condition could, in the situation, have completed the set of insufficient but jointly sufficient conditions for death). Let us simply note the fact that this criterion, as well as the non-redundancy criterion and the criterion of unconditional irreplaceability are relevant to a purpose of prevention. However, the latter two hardly give any guidance in the choice between the conditions mentioned in Figure 2 and 3.

Prediction

A central criterion in the ICD is the *seriousness* of the conditions. In a choice between a condition unlikely in itself to cause death and "a more serious" condition, the first condition should not be selected and in a choice between two stages of the same disease "the more advanced stage" should be selected according to the ICD.[72] The seriousness of the conditions has been a recurrent criterion of selection in the rules for registration of causes of death since the turn of the century.[73] For example, the second of Bertillon's rules considers "the gravity" of the conditions.

'Seriousness' can be interpreted in several ways.[74] Some of the criteria mentioned earlier can be regarded as interpretations of 'seriousness': the criteria of causal efficacy, conditional sufficiency, durability, frequency, and probability. These criteria are all relevant to a purpose of predicting a certain effect, e.g. untimely death. From a predictive purpose, a general formulation of the question of the cause of Mrs Jones' death, not taking into account the different interpretations of 'seriousness', could be: (F) 'which cause was the greatest threat to Mrs Jones life?'

Different causes may be selected on each of the criteria as the principal cause of death in one and the same course of events. For instance, according to the criterion of conditional sufficiency the slipping down may be selected in Figure 2—it was all it took to fracture the brittle skeleton of Mrs Jones—or the bronchopneumonia—which was all it took for the old and weakened Mrs Jones to not get through the immobilization.

The difference between the predictive and the preventive perspective on the selection of causes is clarified by the way certain conditions, e.g. osteopenia and weakness due to old age, are likely to be viewed. For a predictive purpose, one of these conditions may be selected as the principal cause, because it is the most durable, and therefore it makes the fracture and respectively the death likely to occur.[75] For a preventive purpose, the osteopenia and old-age weakness are the least interesting, because they are the least manipulable.

Though the WHO concept 'the underlying cause of death' is defined for the purpose of preventing untimely death, the possibility to manipulate this cause and thereby counteract untimely death is not a criterion of selection emphasized in the international instructions for physicians or in the ICD-rules. The main purpose of selection seems rather to be to try to identify important risk-factors for untimely death, i.e. prediction.

However, though it can be questioned whether a serious condition initiating a fatal sequence always is the most effective point at which "to cut the chain of events or institute the cure" in order to prevent untimely death, information on such conditions can still be of value for the epidemiological search for factors best suited for prevention.

Adjudging personal responsibility

In legal and ethical situations the selection of the principal cause of death is guided by an interest in establishing personal responsibility for the death. The question of Mrs Jones' death could for such purpose simply be formulated: (G) 'was anyone responsible for Mrs Jones' death?' A possible, but perhaps somewhat far-fetched, answer could be: yes, Mr Smith, the caretaker who neglected to sand the icy pavement outside Mrs Jones' front-door.

Personal responsibility is decisive in insurance cases and when death was caused by an error or accident in medical treatment. Regarding deaths due to errors or accidents in medical treatment, WHO has changed policy between ICD-8 and ICD-9. According to ICD-8 the complication and misadventures in therapeutic procedures and complications of medical care should not be selected as the principal cause of death, if the condition for which the treatment was given is known, whereas according to ICD-9 the accident or misadventure should be selected.[76]

Summary

The fifteen selection criteria accounted for in this article are each relevant to different purposes (Table 1).

Concluding remarks

The quality studies that over the years have appeared on cause-of-death statistics and the measures employed to improve such statistics have focused predominantly on data validity and the reliability of registration procedures, while the *relevance* of the data obtained has received comparatively little attention.

Hitherto, the definitions of basic concepts, the criteria of selection employed and their respective appropriateness to the purpose(s) of statistical data have been insufficiently analysed. In other words, we are unsatisfactorily informed of what content of the question, 'what was the cause of death?', the statistical material intends to extract.[77]

This paper has recounted a philosophical debate on causal selection that has gone on for some time within such disciplines as jurisprudence, social science, and historical research, but which is insufficiently known to medicine.

It appears that a principal cause may be selected according to at least fifteen different criteria; that different criteria suit different purposes; and that the relativism characterizing both the choice of criteria and the practical application of these criteria, is not necessarily tantamount to the principal cause being selected capriciously.

Table 1. Selection criteria listed according to relevant purposes.

Purpose	Criteria
Description	
	Completeness
	Conspicuity
Explanation	
	Abnormality
	Ignorance
	Proximity
Prevention	
	Irreplaceability
	conditional
	unconditional
	Manipulability
	Non-redundancy
Prediction	
	Causal efficacy
	Conditional sufficiency
	Durability
	Frequency
	Probability
Adjudging individual responsibility	
	Human action[1]

[1] Depending on the ethical theory implied, this criterion could be replaced by the purpose, motive or consequences of the action.

This analysis of criteria and purposes of causal selection is simply an initial step in a thorough study of this complexity of problems. The author has consciously not considered here that selections can be made for more than one purpose simultaneously. Nor has the interrelationship of the different criteria been illuminated, whether they presuppose, overlap or exclude one another. A considerable work of defining the purposes, the selection criteria, and the various interpretations of the question, 'what was the cause of death?', remains.

Notes

1. Traditionally only one condition for each death has been tabulated in the cause-of-death statistics. This cause of death has been given different names in different countries and at different times in mortality statistics: "primary cause", "primitive disease or primary cause", "primary underlying cause of death", "principal cause" or simply "cause of death". See A.H. Sellers, 'The Physician's Statement of Cause of Death', *American Journal of Public Health*, 28 (1938), pp. 430-444. Sometimes the difference in terminology corresponds to a conceptual difference, sometimes not. In this paper the expression "the principal cause of death" simply refers to the cause of death considered most important to point out. It will be used as a general name for this cause, regardless of how it is selected and how it may be further specified. Thus, the concept 'the principal cause of death' will include, for example, the WHO concept 'the underlying cause of death' used elsewhere in this paper.

2. See e.g. A. Angrist, 'Certified Cause of Death—Analysis and Recommendations', *The Journal of the American Medical Association*, 166 (1958), pp. 2148-2153; H.F. Dorn and I.M. Moriyama, 'Use and Significance of Multiple Cause Tabulations for Mortality Statistics', *American Journal of Public Health*, 54 (1964), pp. 400-406; C.L. Erhardt, 'What is "The Cause of Death"?', *The Journal of the American Medical Association*, 168 (1958), pp. 161-168; I.M. Moriyama, 'Development of the Present Concept of Cause of Death', *American Journal of Public Health*, 46 (1956), pp. 436-441; I.M. Moriyama, 'The Eighth Revision of the International Classification of Diseases', *American Journal of Public Health*, 56 (1966), pp. 1277-1280; C.S. Petty, 'Multiple Causes of Death. The Viewpoint of a Forensic Pathologist', *Journal of Forensic Sciences*, 10 (1965), pp. 167-178; A.E. Treloar, 'The Enigma of Cause of Death', *The Journal of the American Medical Association*, 162 (1956), pp. 1376-1379; World Health Organization, Epidemiological Methods in the Study of Chronic Diseases. Eleventh Report of the WHO Expert Committee on Health Statistics, *World Health Organization Technical Report Series*, No. 365 (Geneva, 1967), ch. 2.1.

The potential for multiple cause-of-death data has been explored in several studies. See R.A. Israel, H.M. Rosenberg, and L.R. Curtin, 'Analytical Potential for Multiple Cause-of-Death Data', *American Journal of Epidemiology*, 124 (1986), pp. 161-179.

3. See B.I.B. Lindahl, 'Dödsorsaksstatistikens problem i modern tid', L. Nordenfelt (Ed.), *Hälsa, sjukdom, dödsorsak. Studier i begreppens teori och historia* (Malmö 1986), pp. 135-162; L. Nordenfelt, *Causes of Death—A Philosophical Essay* (Stockholm: Swedish Council for Planning and Coordination of Research, Report 83:2, 1983).

4. See e.g. W. Winther, 'Några ord om dödsattesters affattande och inregistrering', *Eira* (1901), pp. 461-466.

5. See Nordenfelt (1983), ch. 1.1.5.

6. United Nations *Demographic Yearbook 1951* (New York 1951), ch. II, pp. 18-26; World Health Organization, *Manual of the International Statistical Classification of Diseases, Injuries, and Causes of Death*, Sixth revision, Vol. 1 (Geneva: World Health Organization, 1948), p. XXXIV.

7. United Nations *Demographic Yearbook 1951* (1951), p.20. Cf. Nordenfelt (1983), ch.I.1.5.

8. World Health Organization (1948), p.XXXIV. Starting with the second edition, this handbook was called *Manual of Joint Causes of Death*.

9. World Health Organization, *Sixth Decennial Revision of the International Lists of Diseases and Causes of Death. International Conference. Problem of Joint Causes of Death. Final Report of the United States Committee on Joint Causes of Death. Addendum 1* (Geneva: World Health Organization. Unpublished document WHO.IC/MS.ll/Rev.1/Add.1, 30 March 1948), pp. 47-49.

10. Moriyama (1956); World Health Organization, *Expert Committee for the Preparation of the Sixth Decennial Revision of the International Lists of Diseases and Causes of Death. Second Session, Geneva, Switzerland in Combined Meetings with the Index Sub-Committee. Problem of Joint Cause Selection. Recommendation by the Government of Canada* (Geneva: World Health Organization. Unpublished document WHO.IC/MS/16, 16 October 1947), pp. 1-3.

11. H.L. Dunn, 'The Doctor and the New International List of Diseases and Causes of Death', *The Journal of the American Medical Association,* 140 (1949), pp. 520-522. Cf. J.V. DePorte, 'Mortality Statistics and the Physician. An Argument for Classifying Deaths According to Informed Medical Judgment', *American Journal of Public Health,* 31 (1941), pp. 1051-1056.

12. Lindahl (1986), p. 141.

13. *Manual of the International List of Causes of Death as Adapted for Use in England and Wales, Scotland and Northern Ireland,* Fifth revision (London: H.M. Stationery Office, 1940), pp. VI, XXXVI.

14. *Ibid.,* p. VII. A similar form of certificate was recommended for general international use in a League of Nations report in 1925. League of Nations, 'Report of the Group Entrusted with the Study of the Causes of Death' [T.H.C. Stevenson and S. Rosenfeld. Geneva, March 14th, 1925; *(C.H.288) (C.588.M.80.1925,* pp. 80-85).][Examined by the Health Committee, League of Nations. Fourth Session, April 20-25, 1925]. See also Sellers (1938), pp. 432-433.

15. Sellers (1938) pp. 432-433.

16. *Manual of the International List of Causes of Death as Adapted for Use in England and Wales, Scotland and Northern Ireland,* Fifth revision (1940), pp. VII-VIII.

17. Lindahl (1986), p. 141.

18. World Health Organization, *Manual of the International Statistical Classification of Diseases, Injuries, and Causes of Death,* Ninth revision, vol. 1 (Geneva: World Health Organization, 1977), p. 763.

19. *Ibid.,* pp. 699-737.

20. J.S. Mill, *A System of Logic,* First published in 1843, (London 1889), Bk. III, ch. V. As Hart and Honoré point out, this problem was also recognized by Jeremy Bentham (1748-1832). H.L.A. Hart and A.M. Honoré, *Causation in the Law* (Oxford 1959), p. 16; see C.K. Ogden, *Bentham's Theory of Fictions,* Second edition (London 1951), pp. 39-49.

21. Mill (1889), Bk. III, ch. V, sec. 3. It should be noted that Mill speaks of the selection problem in terms of distinguishing between the *cause* and the mere *conditions* of an event. According to Mill, an antecedent determining the occurrence of an event may be called a "condition" but not a "cause" of this event, unless the effect follows "invariably and unconditionally" on this antecedent. Mill (1889), Bk. III, ch. V., sec. 6.

Consequently, a selection between *causes*, in Mill's sense, can only take place in instances of overdetermination, i.e., when two simultaneous antecedents are, each independent of the other, unconditionally sufficient for the occurrence of the effect. In all other instances there is, by Mill's definition, only *one* cause bringing about the effect. (Mill points out, however, that causes, in his conception, are not always *necessary* for the occurrence of their effects: effects of the same kind may occur due to causes of many different kinds. Mill (1889), Bk. III, ch. X., sec. 1).

22. World Health Organization (1977), p. 763. Furthermore, it should be noted that WHO includes as causal relations not only "sequences with an etiological or pathological basis" but also "sequences where an antecedent condition is believed to have prepared the way for the more direct cause by damage to tissues or impairment of function, even after a long interval". World Health Organization, *Medical Certification of Cause of Death. Instructions for Physicians on Use of International Form of Medical Certificate of Cause of Death* (Geneva: World Health Organization, 1979), p. 8; cf. World Health Organization (1977), p. 700.

23. Mill (1889), Bk III, ch. V, sec. 3, including the footnote.

24. Cf. the three interpretations of "necessary condition" in M. White, *Foundations of Historical Knowledge* (New York and London 1965), pp. 155-160.

25. Cf. Nordenfelt (1983), ch. III.1.4, III.2.2.

26. R.G. Collingwood, *An Essay on Metaphysics* (Oxford 1940).

27. Collingwood (1940), pp. 285-286.

28. Collingwood (1940), pp. 285-287, 296.

29. Collingwood (1940), pp. 285-287.

30. Collingwood maintains that Mill's "formal definition of the term 'cause' is a definition of sense III". Collingwood (1940), p. 301. Taking into account the understanding of Mill's concept 'cause' in the parenthesis in n. 21, Collingwood's condition (b) of his sense III ought to be interpreted in terms of non-redundancy or conditional irreplaceability, and not as unconditional irreplaceability.

31. Collingwood (1940), p. 301.

32. Collingwood (1940), pp. 304, 306.

33. Hart and Honoré (1959).

34. Hart and Honoré (1959), p. 42.

35. Hart and Honoré (1959), p. 42.

36. Hart and Honoré (1959), pp. 30-41.

37. Hart and Honoré (1959), p. 39.

38. Hart and Honoré (1959), p. 40.

39. R. Martin, 'On Weighting Causes', *American Philosophical Quarterly*, 9 (1972), pp. 291-299.

40. E. Nagel, *The Structure of Science. Problems in the Logic of Scientific Explanation,* Fourth impression, (London 1974). Nagel distinguishes between six senses, designated a-f, of "*A* is a more important (or basic, or fundamental) determinant of *C* than is *B*" used in for example historical and social science. Nagel (1974), pp. 582-588.

41. Martin (1972), p. 292. In Nagels own words: "Suppose that the joint presence of *A* and *B* is not a necessary condition for the occurrence of *C*, but that *C* occurs either when *A* is present conjointly with *X* or when *B* is present conjointly with *Y*, where *X* and *Y* are otherwise unspecified determining factors; and suppose also that *A* in conjunction with *X* occurs much more frequently than does *B* in conjunction with *Y*. In that case, *A* might again be said to be a more important determinant of *C* than is *B*". Nagel (1974), sense d, p. 585. (In one of Nagel's examples "*A*", "*B*" and "*C*" signify types of determinants, in another instances.)

42. Martin (1972), pp. 292-293. This criterion is developed from a criterion presented by Nagel: "Assume once more that *A* and *B* are both necessary for the occurrence of *C*. But suppose that there is some way of 'measuring' the variations in each of the variables *A*, *B*, and *C*—at least in the limited sense that, although the magnitudes of changes in one variable may not be comparable with the magnitudes of changes in the other variables, the changes in any one of the variables can be compared. Let us assume further that a greater proportional change in *C* is produced by any given proportional change in *A* than by an equal proportional change in *B*. In consequence, *A* might be assigned a higher degree of importance as a determinant of *C* than would *B*". Nagel (1974), sense b, p. 584.

43. Martin (1972), p. 293.

44. Martin (1972)., p. 294.

45. This name has been suggested for Nagel's sense b (see n. 42) in L. Nordenfelt, Causation. An Essay, *Filosofiska småtryck*, No. 11 (Stockholm 1981), p. 42.

46. Martin (1972), p. 295.

47. Nagel says, "Suppose next that *A* is a contingently necessary condition for *C*, and that, although *B* is not, it nevertheless belongs to a set *K* of mutually independent factors $(B, B_1, \dots B_n)$ such that the presence of some one member of *K* is a necessary condition for *C*. Suppose also that the various members of *K* occur with about the same frequency, the frequency of occurrence being in each case considerably greater than the frequency with which *A* is present. Accordingly, since the frequency with which some member of *K* occurs is greater than the frequency of *B*'s occurrence, then, even if *B* should not be present when *A* is present, the necessary conditions for *C* may nonetheless be realized because of the presence of some other member of *K*. These stipulations specify a sense of 'more important' that is perhaps most frequently intended when *A* is said to be more important than *B*". Nagel (1974), sense c, p. 585.

48. Martin (1972), p. 298.

49. White (1965).

50. White (1965), p. 130.

51. White (1965), p. 160. See Mill (1889), Bk. III, ch. V, sec. 3.

52. White (1965), p. 160.

53. White (1965), pp. 134-147, 160.

54. White (1965), pp. 150, 180.

55. White (1965), pp. 107, 150.

56. How the choice of objects of comparison (reference class) may be decisive in the selection of the principal cause calls attention to in G. Hesslow, 'Explaining Differences and Weighting Causes', *Theoria*, 49 (1983), pp. 87-111; G. Hesslow, 'What is

a Genetic Disease? On the Relative Importance of Causes', L. Nordenfelt and B.I.B. Lindahl (Eds.), *Health, Disease, and Causal Explanations in Medicine* (Dordrecht 1984), pp. 183-193; and in G. Hesslow, 'The Problem of Causal Selection', D.J. Hilton (Ed.), *Contemporary Science and Natural Explanation. Commonsense Conceptions of Causality* (Sussex, 1987), pp. 11-32.

57. Mill (1889), Bk. III, ch. V, sec. 3.

58. The rules read:

"*Rule 5. Ill-defined conditions.* Where the selected underlying cause is classifiable to 780-796, 798-799 (the ill-defined conditions) and a condition classifiable elsewhere than to 780-799 is reported on the certificate, re-select the underlying cause as if the ill-defined condition had not been reported, except to take account of the ill-defined condition if it modifies the coding."

"*Rule 7. Linkage.* Where the selected underlying cause is linked by a provision in the classification [or]in the Notes for use in primary mortality coding on pages 713-721 with one or more of the other conditions on the certificate, code the combination.

Where the linkage provision is only for the combination of one condition specified as due to another, code the combination only when the correct causal relationship is stated or can be inferred from application of the selection rules.

Where a conflict in linkages occurs, link with the condition that would have been selected if the underlying cause initially selected had not been reported. Apply any further linkage that is applicable."

"*Rule 8. Specificity.* Where the selected underlying cause describes a condition in general terms and a term which provides more precise information about the site or nature of this condition is reported on the certificate, prefer the more informative term. This rule will often apply when the general term can be regarded as an adjective qualifying the more precise term." World Health Organization (1977), pp. 707-710.

This descriptive purpose is also discernible in some of the *Notes for use in underlying cause mortality coding.* World Health Organization (1977), pp. 713-721. See B.I.B. Lindahl, 'On the Selection of Causes of Death: An Analysis of WHO's Rules for Selection of the Underlying Cause of Death' Nordenfelt and Lindahl (1984), pp. 137-152.

59. World Health Organization (1979), p. 8, my italics; cf. World Health Organization (1977), p. 700.

60. World Health Organization (1979), pp. 6, 8.

61. "directly related" is understood here to mean 'related without intermediate condition'.

In the first edition of WHO's instructions for physicians, it is made clear that the contributory conditions may not even be indirectly related to the direct cause of death: the contributory conditions are described as the conditions "not related to the direct or *antecedent* causes". World Health Organization, *Medical Certification of Cause of Death. Instructions for Physicians on Use of International Form of Medical Certificate of Cause of Death* (Geneva: World Health Organization, 1952), p. 5, my italics.

62. See n. 61.

63. See n. 58.

64. A controversial view in this debate is Ernst Mach's, briefly accounted for in P. Alexander, 'Mach, Ernst', P. Edwards (Ed.), *The Encyclopedia of Philosophy,* Vol. 5, Reprint edition (New York 1972), pp. 115-119.

65. World Health Organization (1977), p. 700, my italics; World Health Organization (1979), p. 6, my italics.

66. World Health Organization (1979), p. 8, my italics.

67. In Sweden two causes, both the injury and the external cause, are registered as the underlying cause in cases of accidents or violence.

68. The criterion of abnormality may perhaps also be discerned in WHO's exclusion of certain conditions from the definition of 'causes of death' as *modes of dying*. See Lindahl (1984).

69. M.G. Bohrod, 'The Meaning of "Cause of Death"', *Journal of Forensic Sciences*, 8 (1963), pp. 15-21; see also J. Orth, 'Was ist Todesursache?', *Berliner Klinische Wochenschrift*, 45 (1908), pp. 485-490.

70. World Health Organization (1977), pp. 699-700.

71. See Lindahl (1984).

72. The rules read:
"*Rule 6. Trivial conditions*. Where the selected underlying cause is a trivial condition unlikely to cause death, proceed as follows: (a) if the death was the result of an adverse reaction to treatment of the trivial condition, select the adverse reaction. (b) if the trivial condition is not reported as the cause of a more serious complication, and a more serious unrelated condition is reported on the certificate, re-select the underlying cause as if the trivial condition had not been reported."
"*Rule 9. Early and late stages of disease*. Where the selected underlying cause is an early stage of a disease and a more advanced stage of the same disease is reported on the certificate, code to the more advanced stage. This rule does not apply to a 'chronic' form reported as due to an 'acute' form unless the Classification gives special instructions to that effect." World Health Organization (1977), pp. 707-708, 710-711.

73. See Nordenfelt (1983), ch.I.1.5..

74. See Nordenfelt (1983), ch. III.2.2.

75. It should be noted here how closely related the criterion of probability is to the criterion of efficacy: the more osteopenia, the more likely a fracture (the criterion of probability): the more osteopenia, the more comminuted the fracture, even when the bone is subjected to the same mechanical force (the criterion of causal efficacy), providing an increased likelihood of prolonged immobilization and its consequences (the criterion of probability).

76. See the *Notes* for E930, E931 and N997-N999 in World Health Organization, *Manual of the International Statistical Classification of Diseases, Injuries, and Causes of Death*, Eighth revision, Vol. 1 (Geneva: World Health Organization, 1967), p. 432, and Rule 12 World Health Organization (1977), p. 712.

77. For an analysis of practical consequences of these uncertainties for cause-of-death registration, see B.I.B. Lindahl, 'In What Sense is Rheumatoid Arthritis the Principal Cause of Death? A Study of the National Statistics Office's Way of Reasoning Based on 1224 Death Certificates' *Journal of Chronic Diseases*, 38 (1985), pp. 963-972.

Recent Trends in Mortality among the Elderly in Sweden

Dan Mellström

Introduction

For more than a century epidemiologists have noticed that marriage seems to increase longevity.[1] Studies of vital statistics have shown that life expectancy is shorter in those who have never married or are divorced, as well as in widowers and widows compared with that of married men and women.[2] Mortality in affluent society nowadays mostly afflicts the aged. In Sweden, 82 per cent of all deaths in 1982 occurred in the age-class 65+. Nevertheless, most epidemiological studies of risk factors of ill health and mortality have dealt with people under 65 years of age, at ages when the incidence and prevalence of many diseases as well as of mortality are comparatively low. Only 50 years ago the age pattern of mortality was quite different. The life expectancy in Sweden increased in a parallel way from 1900 to 1950 for women and men. The difference between men and women in this period was about 3 years. After 1950 there has been a rapid increase in the difference of life expectancy between men and women to 6 years (Figure 1).

Studies of mortality and specific causes of death according to marital status could only be regarded as a relative and indirect measurement of the influence of the social network on mortality. Surveys on the relation between occupational risks and longevity have most often in a similar way been restricted to age groups below the age of 60. In our studies, we have used the longitudinal population study of elderly in Göteborg as a generator for hypotheses of the relation between occupation social network and marital status and its relation to social class and life style factors. These hypotheses could then be tested on the total population in Sweden. The greatest advantages by studying mortality trends of marital status groups in vital statistics are that such studies require controlled surveys of a very large population and over a long period of time. In the Scandinavian countries, information of the exact day of death and change in marital status is considered to be quite accurate.

Figure 1. Life expectancy at birth in Sweden 1900-1980.

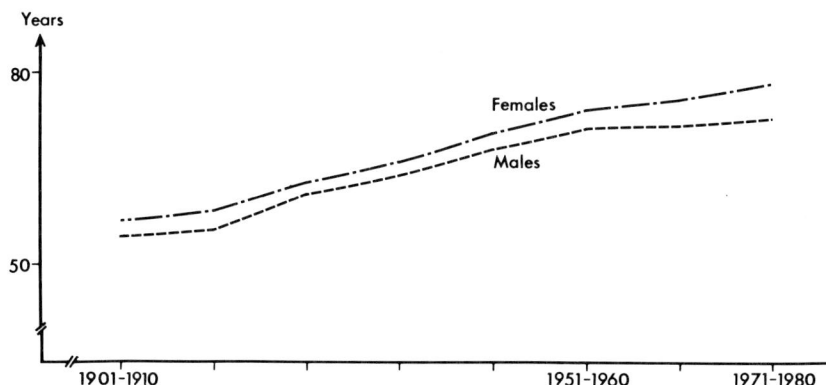

Population and methods

Data is presented from a study of the secular trend of mortality in Sweden during 1970-1979. We had access to a data-base that covered the total population of Sweden as well as deaths, distributed by sex and marital status, in one-year classes. We also had individual data of all people who became widowed or divorced during that period of time.

Another study that will be presented is from the pooled research-register of the Census 1960 and the register of causes of death 1960-1970. The aim of this study was to examine the influence of former occupational belonging to longevity among the elderly.

The longitudinal population study of elderly in Göteborg has been presented earlier.[3] This study consists of three longitudinal 70-year-old cohorts which started in 1971, 1976, and 1981. A non-parametric trend test described by Mantel was used when testing differences.[4]

Secular trends in mortality in Sweden 1970-1979

The age-standardized mortality trend was markedly different between the sexes. In Table 1 the mortality rate is given in different age-classes, showing that the decline in female mortality is most impressive. Meanwhile, the picture for males is quite different with no significant change in most age-classes except for a decline in mortality among children and also a significant increase in mortality in the 40-59 year age-class. By subdividing the population by marital status and in ages above 35 it was evident that female death rates were significantly declining in all marital status groups, but among males there was only a significant decline in married males while mortality rates in other male marital status groups increased during the decade studied (Table 2). This finding was perhaps not expected because the differences in mortality rates, for

Table 1. Mortality trends in Sweden 1970-1979. A significant change is indicated: + increase, - decrease, 0 = unchanged. The level of significance is less than 1 per cent. The numbers within brackets indicate the annual change.

Age	Males	%	Females	%
0-14	-	(5.1)	-	(4,8)
15-39	0		-	(1,3)
40-59	+	(0,55)	-	(1,0)
60-74	0		-	(1,8)
75 +	0		-	(1,4)

Table 2. Mortality trends in Sweden 1970-1979 in marital status groups. A significant change is indicated: + increase, - decrease, 0 = unchanged. The level of significance is less than 1 per cent. Age class 35 +.

Marital status	Males	Females
Married	-	-
Never married	+	-
Divorced	+	-
Widowed	+	-

instance between married males and divorced males in 1970 in the 35-50 year age-group was three times higher for divorced males and in specific causes of death, like accidental falls, ten times higher for divorced males than for married males.

During the 1970's, the demographic trend in Sweden was quite dynamic. One of the most significant trends was the rapid increase of divorces which resulted in an increase of divorced males from about 105,000 in 1970 to about 220,000 in 1980. The increased mortality in the 40-59 year age-class among males in Sweden could be expressed in an excessive number of deaths in specific causes. The total excessive number of deaths was 1100 and the most common single increasing cause of death was ischemic heart disease 800, followed by cirrhosis of the liver 450, and cancer of the lung 200. The most frequent decreasing causes of death in these age-classes were deaths in motor vehicle accidents and in cerebrovascular disease (Table 3).

In contrast to the development in most western societies, like the US, Canada and Finland, the risk of death in ischemic heart disease was increased in Sweden during the last decade. When subdividing the death rate in ischemic heart disease among males 55-59 years of age into marital status groups, it is evident that the risk for death from ischemic heart disease increased for all marital status groups, but much more for the unmarried groups.

Table 3. Secular changes in the pattern of specific causes of death in Sweden 1970-1979. Age standardized annual percentual change. * = P<.01.

CAUSES OF DEATH	MEN	WOMEN
Cardiovascular disease	-0.2*	-2.0*
Ishemic heart disease	+0.2	-1.8*
Cerebrovascular disease	-1.2*	-2.0*
Neoplasms	+0.9*	-0.2
Lung cancer	+2.9*	+3.1
Smoking related cancer	+1.6*	+1.1*
Peptic ulcer	-4.7*	-4.7*
Cirrhosis of the liver	+4.7*	+2.2*
Accidents and suicides	+0.1	+0.5
Suicides	-1.2	-1.2
Traffic accidents	-3.6*	-3.1*
Accidental falls	+3.1*	+1.0*

It is obvious that the increasing risk of ischemic heart disease among unmarried men, and their increasing number during the 1970's, is in some way related to the increasing mortality in ischemic heart disease in Sweden. Another important demographic factor, related both to social network and the increasing risk of deaths in ischemic heart disease, is immigration. During the 1960's the annual number of immigrants to Sweden was very high, up to 2/3 of the nativity rate. The majority of the immigrants were from Finland, predominantly males. In several urban societies in Sweden, male Finnish immigrants could be up to 15 per cent of the total male population between 40 and 59 years of age. In Finland, death rates in ischemic heart disease are much higher than in Sweden, but are decreasing over time. The total risk of death among Finnish male immigrants in the age group 35-59 was about 30 per cent higher compared with Swedish males, and in ischemic heart disease much higher.

In the gerontological study of elderly in Göteborg, three longitudinal cohorts of 70-year-olds were started in the beginning, middle and the end of the period 1970 and 1979. Comparative studies of these cohorts have indicated that there is a secular trend to a general improved health,[5] to better performance in intellectual functions,[6] a very rapid improvement of the odontological health status[7] and also indications of a declining prevalence of diseases like peptic ulcer disease. However, the prevalence in most diseases was markedly higher among males than females. There was a similar trend towards better general health among married people compared with the unmarried. This trend was stronger among men indicating a greater gradient between married and unmarried men than females. There were no great differences in the socio-economic levels between the female marital status groups. In the male marital status groups, never married males tended to have a much lower socio-economic status than the others. Divorced males were registered at the Temperance Board twice or more in 46 per cent, compared to 6 per cent in married males.[8] This indication of a greater alcohol consumption was validated by dietary enquiries. Divorced males and widowers also had a higher percentage of tobacco smokers than married males.[9] In contrast, the percentage of never married males who had been non-smokers was significantly higher, 42 per cent compared to 24 per cent among married males. Women in this cohort were current tobacco smokers in about 10 per cent of the cases compared with current male smoking in about 35 per cent. It seems that the relation between social class, social network and life style factors was complex in this Swedish generation. In contrast to studies in Finland and Great Britain, it could be shown that never married males who tend to have a much lower socio-economic level than married males in Sweden had a 40 per cent lower mortality in lung cancer, obviously related to smoking habits.

In the longitudinal population study it was found that 24 per cent of all females, and 12 per cent of all males, perceived a feeling of loneliness which was related to a higher consumption of drugs and health care. On the other hand, it was not possible to find a higher morbidity in the group with a feeling of loneliness. The most significant background factors for the perceived feeling of loneliness was widowhood and lack of close friends.[10] At the follow up study at the age of 82, 33 per cent of males who had a feeling of loneliness at the age of 70 survived, compared with 53 per cent in the contrast groups (p < 0.01). In females there were no differences between the groups in survival rate.

Mortality trends in the 70-79 year age-class during 1970-1979

In order to compare the cohort effects of general health studied in the population survey with regard to mortality trends in mortality in the total population of Sweden were studied. The decline in mortality for females in the age-class 70-79 years in the decade was 19 per cent, which was much greater than earlier projected, and the total number of deaths was about 8000 fewer than expected. A decrease by 9 per cent is of the same magnitude as the total mortality in all cancers in that age-class. In this age-class during this decade the mortality for males was unchanged (Figure 2). For females, the age-standardized mortality declined in a parallel way for both married, widows, divorced and never married females (Figures 3 and 4). In males, there was an unexpected trend that elderly widowers and divorced and never married showed an increasing mortality rate, while the mortality rate among married men was decreasing (Figures 5 and 6). The difference in life-expectancy at the age of 50 years between married and not married men is most impressing compared to women (Figure 7).

Figure 2. Age standardized mortality trends in Sweden 1970-1979 ICD 8. Age group 70-79. 100 000 person year.

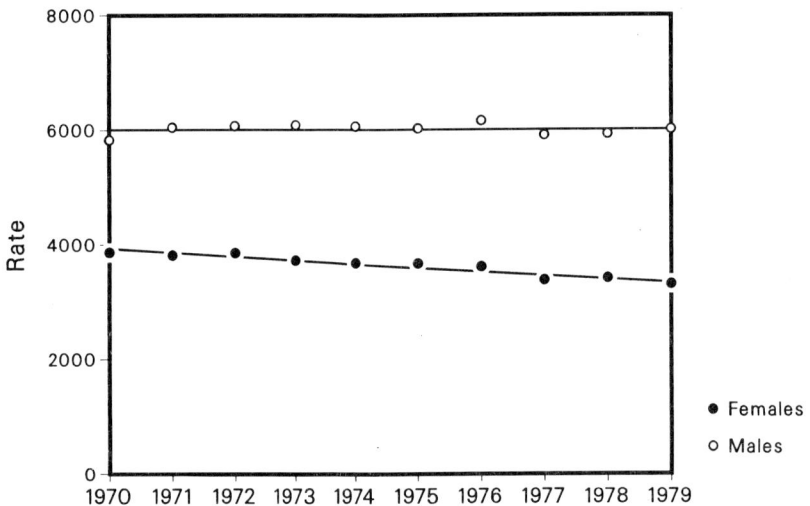

Figure 3. Age standardized mortality trends in Sweden 1970-1979 ICD 8. Age group 70-79. 100 000 person year.

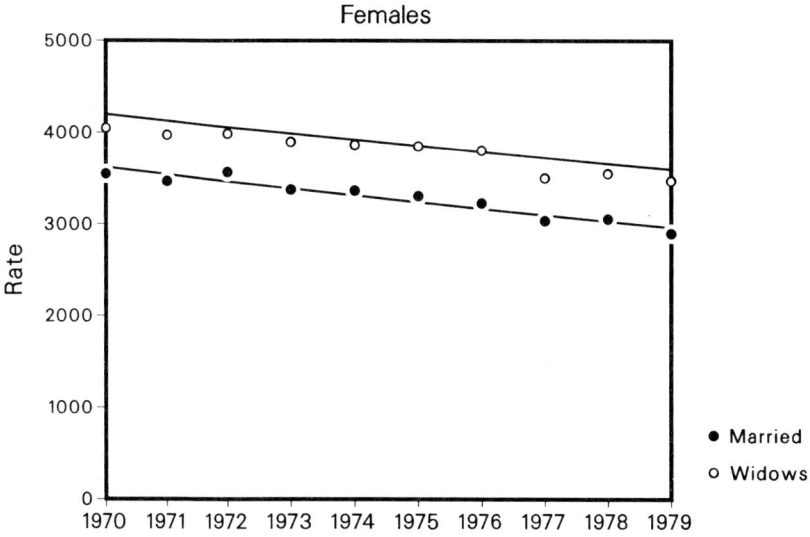

Figure 4. Age standardized mortality trends in Sweden 1970-1979 ICD 8. Age group 70-79. 100 000 person year.

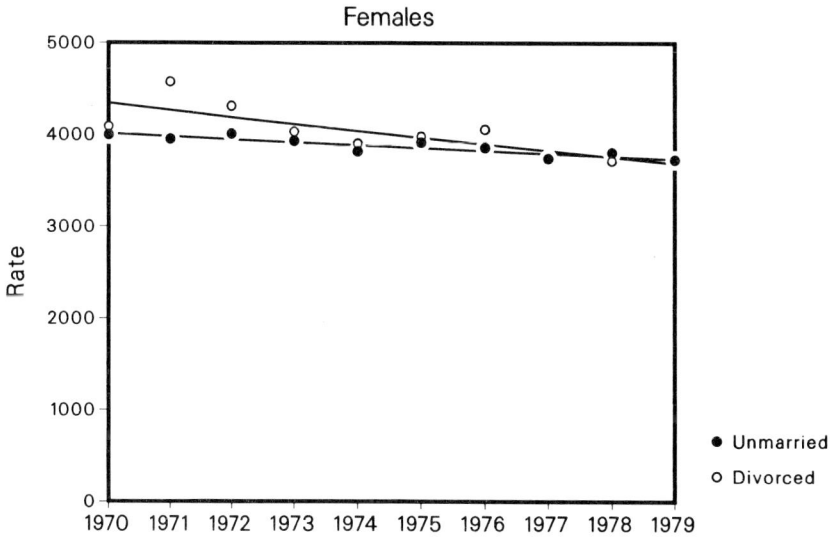

Figure 5. Age standardized mortality trends in Sweden 1970-1979 ICD 8. Age group 70-79. 100 000 person year.

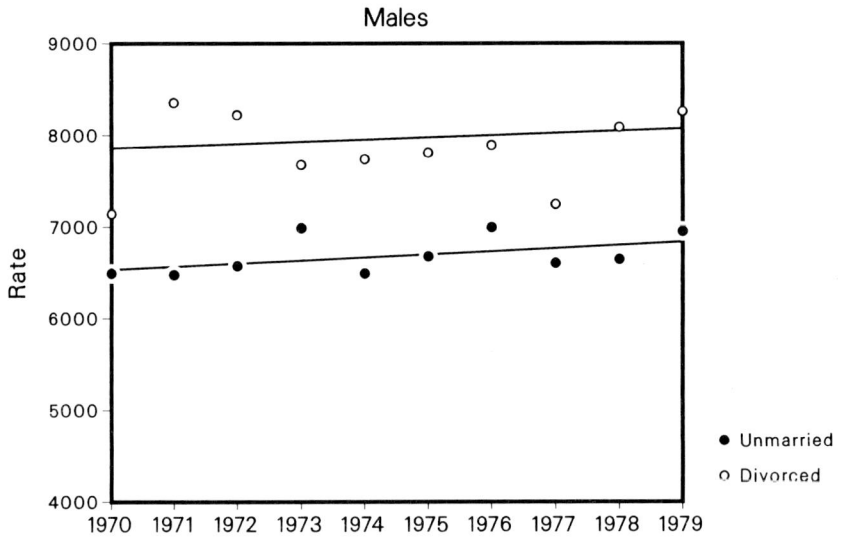

Figure 6. Age standardized mortality trends in Sweden 1970-1979 ICD 8. Age group 70-79. 100 000 person year.

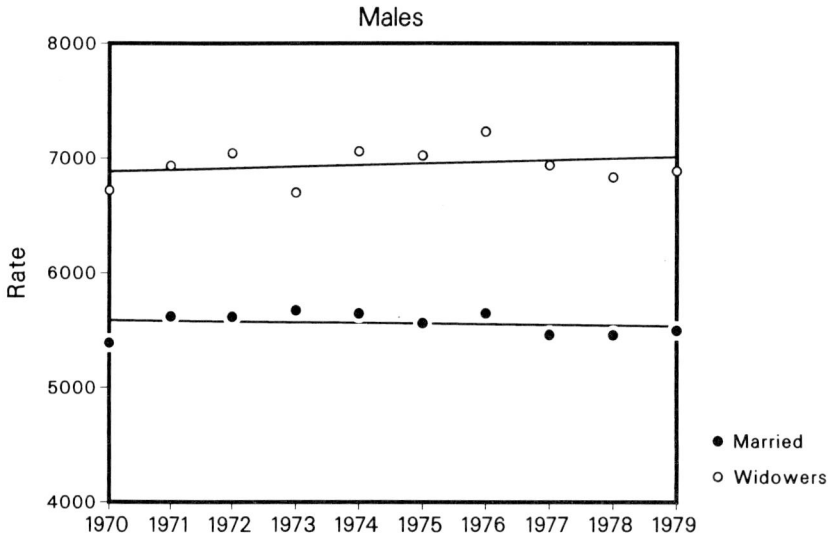

Figure 7. Differences in life expectancy at 50 years, measured in years, in Sweden 1978 distributed by marital status and sex with married men as the level of comparison.

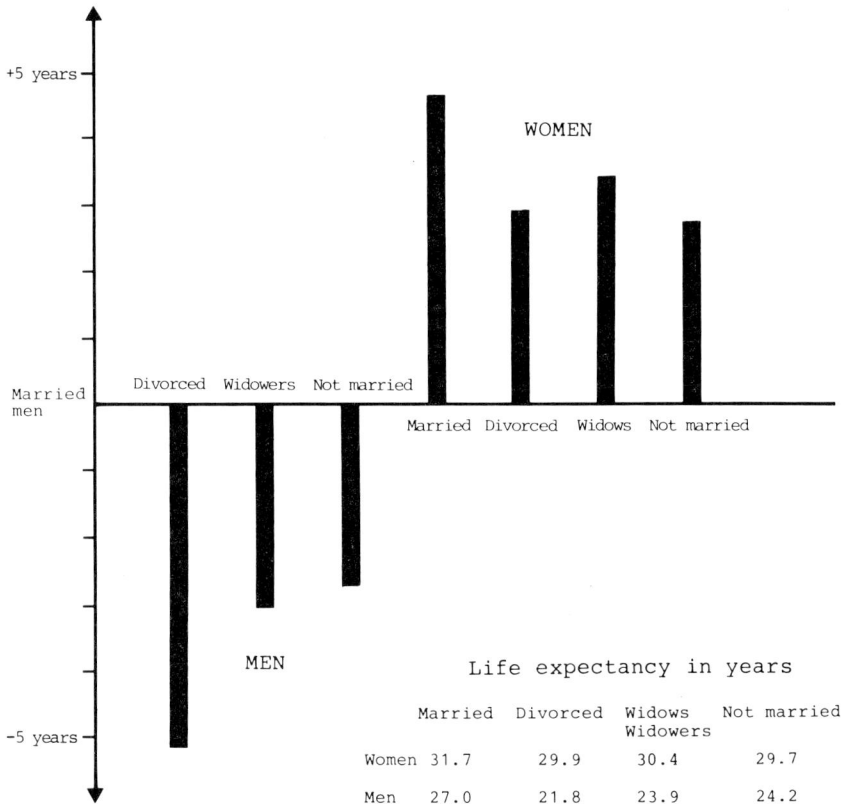

Life expectancy in years

	Married	Divorced	Widows Widowers	Not married
Women	31.7	29.9	30.4	29.7
Men	27.0	21.8	23.9	24.2

Mortality trends in newly bereaved and divorced people

Several studies indicate that the duration after changing marital status is of importance for health and mortality. An earlier study from our group including all bereaved people in Sweden (370,000) showed that the excess mortality among males was 48 per cent three months after the death of the spouse and the equivalent figure for females was 22 per cent.[11] In a recent study, individual data of all bereaved people in Sweden from 1968-1981 was included (460,000). It was found that in various age-groups, from 50 years of age up to 75 years of age, the most common specific causes of death causing the excess mortality were suicides and accidental falls. The risk gradient for suicide tended to increase up to ten-fold during the first three months period for widowers when compared with the standard married population. A similar study was performed of all newly divorced males in Sweden during 1968-1982. The excess mortality compared to married males is much higher in younger

165

groups but is also in contrast to that of widowers much lower than that of the total group of divorced males during the first year. In the gerontological population study it could be shown that very few elderly widowers remarry and less than 10 per cent live together with children or other cohabitants. In the case of divorced males, the remarriage rate is much higher because of the lower mean-age. It could be suspected that there is an ongoing accumulation of high risk men in the divorced population of Sweden.

Bereavement could be seen as a natural experiment causing a severe prolonged stress which increases stress hormones like cortisol and adrenalin but decreases testosterone. The immune response is lowered in newly bereaved people. Furthermore, the heart rate and blood pressure could be changed during long periods giving a rationale for the expression "broken heart".

Females tend to have better coping strategies after severe social stress than males and it could be stated that marriage is more of a benefit for males than for females. A most interesting finding is that the mortality rate is increasing over time for males while it is decreasing for females.

Mortality and occupation among the elderly

Studies of the relation between life-expectancy after the age of 70 and previous occupation in the longitudinal population study in Göteborg did not reveal significant differences when the male population was subdivided in SEI-groups. In the population study the number of people was comparatively small. In order to test hypothesis generated in the population study the mortality of all Swedish males was studied during the decade 1960-1970 in relation to occupation. This study was based on the census 1960 which has been coordinated with register of causes of death.

The mortality did not follow strict socio-economic levels indicating that life-style factors and other environmental factors could have great importance (Figure 8). The difference between low-risk and high-risk occupations seemed to be more pronounced after retirement (Figures 9 and 10).

Farmers have the longest life-expectancy and also a comparatively low cancer incidence. Very few elderly farmers have divorced or are tobacco-smokers. There are differences in longevity also between female occupational groups but on a much lower level than in males.

These data indicate that the influence of socio-economic factors on mortality is lower than 50 years ago.

Figure 8. Age standardized mortality index for some selected occupations; men born 1895-1920 in Sweden.

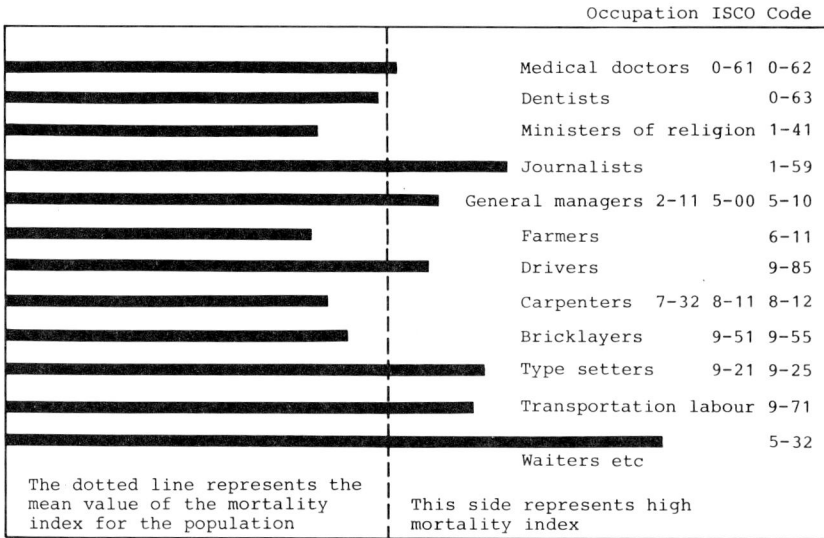

```
                                    Occupation ISCO Code

                           Medical doctors   0-61 0-62
                           Dentists                0-63
                           Ministers of religion  1-41
                           Journalists             1-59
               General managers 2-11 5-00 5-10
                           Farmers                 6-11
                           Drivers                 9-85
                           Carpenters    7-32 8-11 8-12
                           Bricklayers        9-51 9-55
                           Type setters       9-21 9-25
                           Transportation labour 9-71
                                                   5-32
                           Waiters etc

The dotted line represents the
mean value of the mortality        This side represents high
index for the population           mortality index
```

Figure 9. Mortality among low-risk and high risk occupations in Sweden 1960-1970.

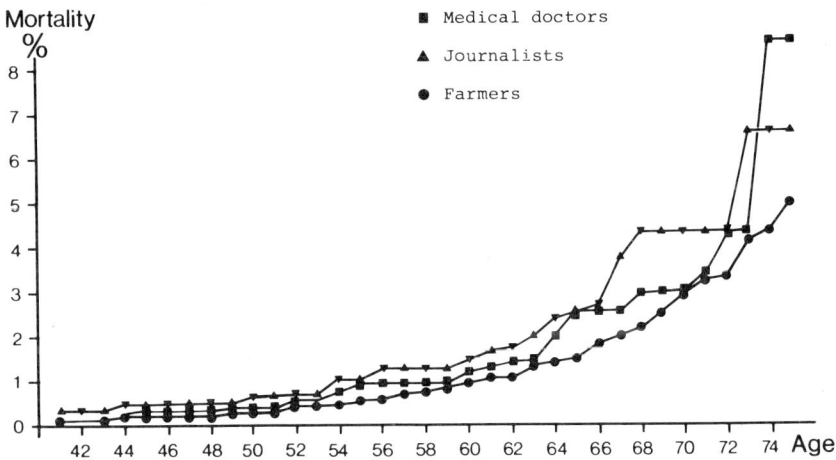

167

Figure 10. Mortality among low-risk and high risk occupations in Sweden 1960-1970.

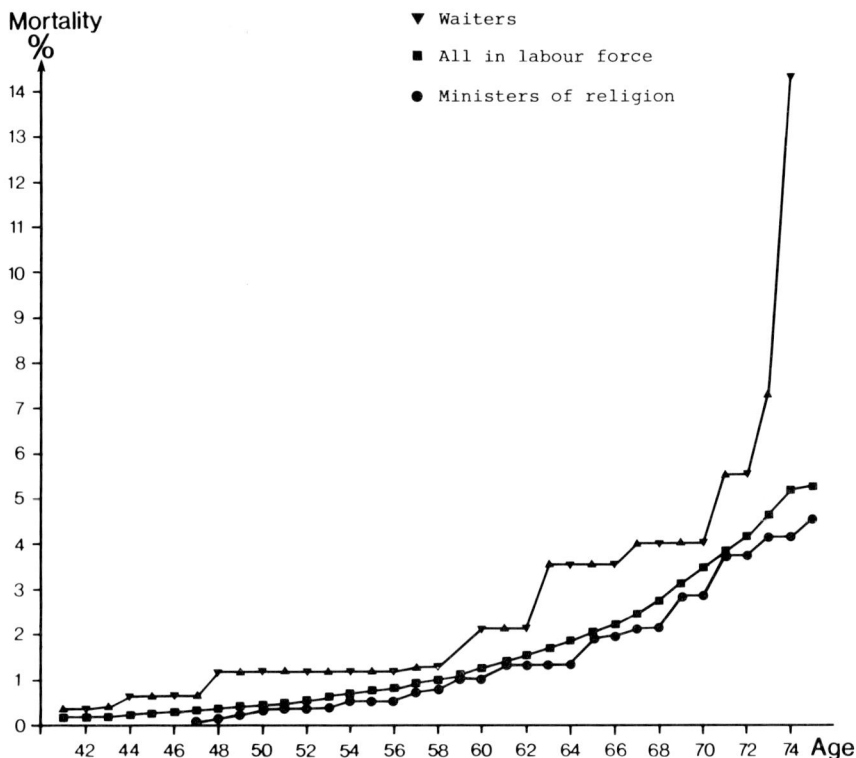

Recent trend of mortality in accidental falls

Several common specific causes of death has in recent years decreased in the Scandinavian countries, like cerebrovascular disease and peptic ulcer disease. Accidental falls are, as cause of death, increasing rapidly in Sweden; mostly because of a demographic change with a rapid increase in the 80+ group. In a study with individual data of all people with accidental falls in the decade of 1970-1980 (N=16,200), it could be shown that more than 80 per cent of all deaths in accidental falls were linked with hip fractures. Most often the immediate causes of death were pneumonia and thromboembolic disease. The time trend showed that the risk is increasing much faster for males than for females (Figure 11). This data well corresponds with several studies from Oslo, Copenhagen, Stockholm, Göteborg and Malmö; indicating that there is a rapid increase in the incidence of hip fractures in Scandinavia. In Göteborg, the annual increase of the incidence of hip fractures is calculated to about 6 per cent.[12] When subdividing, the risk of death in accidental falls into marital status groups it is obvious that unmarried males have a greater risk in both accidental falls and in accidental falls linked with hip fracture (Figure 12). When relating the multiple causes of deaths, it was found that divorced

168

males in this age-group were classified as chronic alcoholics in 24 per cent of the cases compared with 4 per cent in married males. In the gerontological population study, it was found that the bone mineral content in the right calcaneus measured by dual photon absorptiometry was 26 per cent lower in 70-year-old divorced males compared with those of married males (p<0.001). Furthermore muscle strength was worse in divorced males. However, inadequate nutrition and a lower degree of physical activity seem to be more common among divorced males, compared with married males. It is obvious that this life style also increases the risk of falls among the divorced males. In a prospective study of 868 patients with hip fracture in Göteborg, it was shown that living alone and tobacco smoking were two of the most important risk factors for hip fracture among males.

Figure 11. Time trend of accidental falls with Hipfracture as the nature of the injury.

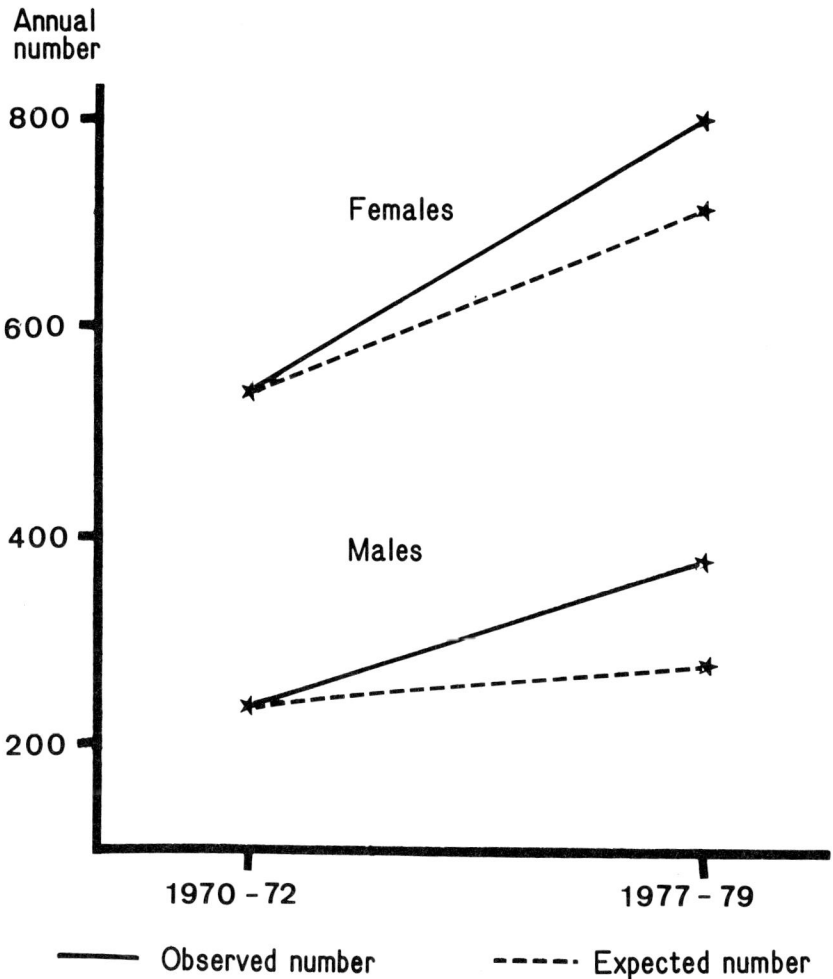

Figure 12. Mortality in accidental falls in Sweden 1970-1980. Age 70-74. AE 141. ICD 8.

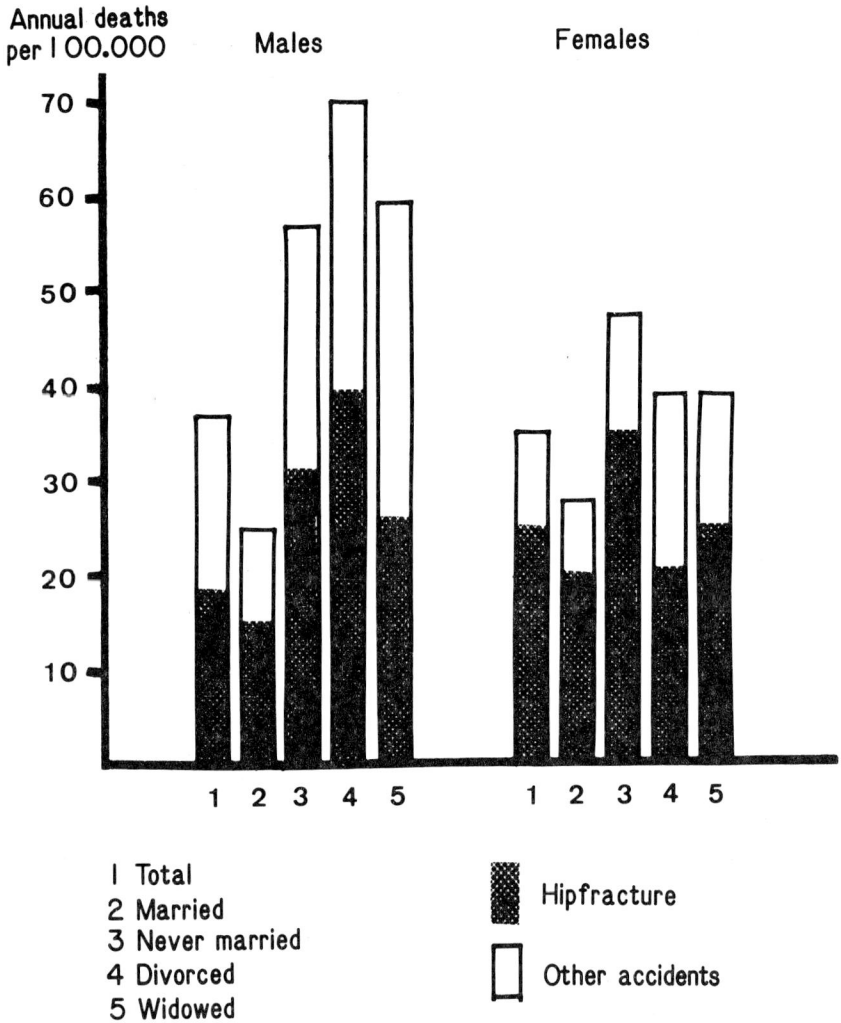

Conclusion

It seems that the social network has an increasing relation to the mortality pattern in Sweden. It is also obvious that this demographic change affects males more than females. A certain degree of the differences between the marital status groups could be explained by differences in life style factors. However, just living alone is often, especially among elderly men, an indicator of high risk. Since second World War the difference in life-expectancy between women and men has increased from three to six years. Differences between the sexes in social stress, occupation and life-style factors could partly explain this secular trend. Marital status and cohabitation are variables that could be used in demographic studies in order to explain changes in longevity.

A noticed time trend in a certain cause of death could more fully be understood if the demographic study is based on epidemiological data.

Acknowledgements

The author is indebted to professor Alvar Svanborg for cooperation and advice and to the National Bureau of Statistics in Sweden for providing the background data.

The population studies became possible through grants from the Delegation for Social Research within the Ministry of Health and Social Affairs, the Gothenburg Administration of Social Services, the Gothenburg Medical Services Administration, the Swedish Medical Research Council and the Wilhelm and Martina Lundgren's Foundation.

Notes

1. M. Susser, 'Widowhood: A Situational Life Stress or a Stressful Life Event', *American Journal of Public Health, 71* (1981), pp. 793.

2. J. Berksson, 'Mortality and Marital Status. Reflections on the Derivation of Etiology from Statistics', *American Journal of Public Health,* 52 (1962), pp. 1318; A-M. Bolander, 'Mortality as Indicator of Health at Present and in Long-Term Perspective', *Committee for Future Oriented Research. FRN* (Stockholm 1980); O. Horowitz and J. Weber, *Marital Status and Mortality. I. All Denmark, Ugeskr. Laeg.* (1973), pp. 1089.

3. L. Rinder, S. Roupe, B. Steen and A. Svanborg, 'Seventy-Year-Old People in Gothenburg. A Population Study in an Industrialized Swedish City. I. General Presentation of the Study', *Acta Medica Scandinavica* (1975), pp. 397-405; A. Svanborg, 'Seventy-Year-Old People in Gothenburg. A Population Study in an Industrialized Swedish City. II. General Presentation of Social and Medical Conditions', *Acta Medica Scandinavica,* Supplement 611 (1977), pp. 5-37.

4. N. Mantel, 'CHI-Square Tests with One Degree of Freedom; Extensions of the Mantel-Haentzel Procedure', *Journal of the American Statistical Association,* 58 (1963), pp. 690-700.

5. A. Svanborg, S. Landahl and D. Mellström, 'Basic Issues of Health Care', H. Thomae and G.L. Maddox (Eds.), *New Perspectives on Old Age* (New York 1982), pp. 3-53.

6. S. Berg, 'Psychological Functioning in 70- and 75-Year Old People', *Acta Psychiatrica Scandinavica,* Supplement 288, vol. 62 (1980).

7. T. Österberg, B. Hedegård and G. Säter, 'Variation in Dental Health in 70-Year-Old Men and Women in Gothenburg, Sweden. A Cross-Sectional Epidemiological Study, Including Longitudinal and Cohort Effects', *Swedish Dental Journal,* 7 (1983), pp. 29-48.

8. D. Mellström, Å. Nilsson, B. Odén, Å. Rundgren and A. Svanborg, 'Mortality among the Widowed in Sweden', *Scandinavian Journal of Social Medicine,* 10 (1982), pp. 33-41.

9. D. Mellström, Å. Rundgren, R. Jagenburg, B. Steen and A. Svanborg, 'Tobacco Smoking, Aging and Health among the Elderly: A Longitudinal Population Study of 70-Year Old Men and an Age Cohort Comparison', *Age and Aging,* 11 (1982), pp. 45-58.

10. S. Berg, D. Mellström, G. Persson and A. Svanborg, 'Loneliness in the Swedish Aged', *Journal of Gerontology,* 36 (1981), pp. 342-349.

11. Mellström, Nilsson, Odén, Rundgren and Svanborg (1982), pp. 33-41.

12. C. Zetterberg and G. Anderson, 'Fractures of the Proximal and of the Femur in Göteborg, Sweden, 1940-1979', *Acta Orthopaedica Scandinavica,* 53 (1982), pp. 419-426.

Comments on the Session Urban Disease and Mortality

Hans Norman

"The rise of population and the associated transformation of health are among the great themes in history, in interest and importance perhaps second only to the origin of life".[1]

These solemn words by Thomas McKeown illustrate the significance of mortality decline in the western world during the last two, three hundred years, which is one of the most discussed problems in demographic research. In this context the health conditions and the mortality of the people in the cities are matters of utmost importance for the general pattern of mortality. Urban mortality was often dramatic compared to the rural mortality but many times surprisingly speedy in its decline, once the down-turn had begun.

The five papers presented here are rather different in character, but together they give good insights into urban mortality and its decline. I have read them with great interest and I will now recapitulate and comment on some of the findings.

According to the presented papers, typical characteristics of urban mortality in pre-industrial and newly industrialized societies include:

1. Mortality in urban milieus has mostly been higher than mortality in the countryside.

2. Examples from Stockholm show that mortality there rose even during the first half of the nineteenth century (1820-1850), when the general trend of mortality was falling.

3. Sex differences were more pronounced in the cities than in the countryside. Men in working ages had higher death rates than women, a fact which has been clearly illustrated by Gunnar Fridlizius. Especially terrifying are the very high death rates of unmarried men in urban milieus. During the years 1821-1830, the mortality excess of unmarried men in rural areas was 25 percent, whereas it was as high as 175 percent in Stockholm during the same period. In these decades the Swedish capital was one of the European cities with the highest mortality rates. During the 1820's, when the figures reached

their peak, the male mortality was two or three times higher than in most European cities.

4. Infant mortality was also higher in the cities than in the countryside, a fact which is shown in the paper by Castensson-Löwgren-Sundin.

5. Compared to the rural areas and to the total figures, the urban mortality rates decreased quickly in many places during the second half of the nineteenth century, eventually becoming lower than in the rural areas. It is important to observe, though, that urban mortality varied, both with regard to the type of cities and between regions. Gerry Kearns emphasizes that mortality many times differed more over space than over time, and there was a notable difference in the cities' mortality rates depending on their size. The bigger they were, the higher mortality. In Sweden, on the other hand, the highest mortality was in the cities in the Mälar Valley, big as well as small, while it was lower in the cities in the northern and southern parts of the country.

A general explanation of the high mortality in the cities is found in the bad sanitary and hygienic conditions, where infectious diseases, such as tuberculosis, easily spread. The fact that many people lived in small areas contributed to these detriments. In addition these urbanites had proportionally many contacts with other places and were therefore more exposed to diseases than people in the countryside.

A city like Mainz found itself in a special situation with an important military location and great numbers of soldiers in its fortress. Walter Rödel mentions the frequently occurring crises because of sieges, as for example during the 30-years war, when first the Swedish armies and later the imperial troops under Tilly occupied the city. The same happened several times during the Napoleonic wars. At such occasions, as e.g. in 1793, mortality reached very high figures, since blockading, food shortage as well as epidemic dysentery had to be met. This caused 1800 people to die that year, with as many as 800 in August. As was usual in connection with sudden demographic crises, the after effects in Mainz included a rapid drop in mortality, a sharp rise in the number of conceptions and marriages and also a high rate of re-marriages, a pattern which has also been observed during the first years following sharp crises in Sweden in the 1700's.[2]

Scholars studying the factors behind the mortality decline soon realize that it is a very complex problem. Most seem to object to McKeown, who stresses better nutrition, that is an improved economy and thereby an improved nutritional situation, as almost the only explanation. These objections are, for example, eloquently formulated in the paper about Linköping, where the authors discussing the cause of the decline of the urban mortality rate to the level of the countryside, state that "it is not at all evident that this process was caused by a step from a lower to an equal level of economic prosperity among the inhabitants of the towns compared to their neighbours in the countryside".

174

The construction of urban water supply systems and the subsequent improvement in water quality, as well as the installations of sewage systems, which are discussed in two of the papers to this session, must in the long run have been of great value. This was especially important in fighting dysentery, typhoid fever and other diseases spread with water. Important for the general decline of mortality was also improved information and help to people and their willingness to accept this information from doctors, midwives, the church and other authorities about medicine, diversified food etc. which has been illustrated in studies by Anders Brändström and Britt-Inger Puranen. One example is the medical care in paternalistic iron foundries, as has been shown by Jan Sundin and Lars-Göran Tedebrand. Even if it is true that for a long time the hospitals were rather ineffective, they at least helped to isolate sources of infections.[3]

The paper by Castensson et al. emphasizes the significance of health problems and health conditions in the political discussion during the nineteenth and early twentieth centuries. Special attention were given to the improvements of health conditions in the growing cities. Medical experts of that time also showed great interest in what contributed to healthy or unhealthy rural areas, often discussing if they were situated in high, forested districts with a good supply of fresh water, or if they were plainlands and lowlands with swampy areas, where malaria was much spread.[4]

In the long run the change in the authorities' attitude towards people was of greatest weight, a fact which is emphasized by Jean-Pierre Goubert. This changing mentality meant a cultural un-blocking, where the state began to intervene in the public and private life and to influence people to accept news, as ''almost nothing can advance without the agreement from concerned people''.

Although the causes of urban mortality stands out as a complex subject, several of the authors in this session have preferred to concentrate the analysis on particularly one variable. Concentrating on the mortality sex differentials in Stockholm Gunnar Fridlizius attempts an interesting explanation of men's high mortality by focusing on the enormous consumption of alcohol. As the statistics and arguments are presented, I find this to be a very probable interpretation. As a complement it would also have been of great value to get information on the contemporary medical view on the risks connected with alcohol consumption. It is mentioned in the paper that a new liquor legislation was passed in the 1850's after long discussions. To get a wider perspective on this problem it is of interest to know how much the medical experts of the time knew of diseases and mortality connected to alcohol customs and also what measures the authorities took to remedy the situation.

In two of the papers the effects of the construction of water supply and sewage systems on mortality are discussed. Castensson-Löwgren-Sundin have done a study of the city of Linköping in Sweden and Jean-Pierre Goubert one of French cities. Of course these installments must have been of great importance in the long perspective, but it seems to be difficult to measure the effects in the short run. In the cities in France, for example, only a few per cent of the population really got water in their houses during the first years after these water pipes were constructed. As late as in the beginning of the 1890's only about 3 per cent of the people had access to the water network and sewage systems. This means that few had it installed in their homes and a very reduced part of the population — only a small privileged minority — was served by the water network.

Much evidence indicates that the situation was about the same in Swedish cities. It is therefore not surprising that it is difficult to see any direct effects on the mortality rates in Linköping and in the three other cities compared (Jönköping, Malmö and Norrköping) by the creation of water and sewage systems. This is especially true as the installment of the water system in two of them (Jönköping and Malmö) occurred a couple of years before the crisis of the catastrophic years of the late 1860's in the Nordic countries. During these years people suffered greatly in the cities as well and there was a sharp peak in the mortality rate. A general impression of the discussion in the paper about the mortality rates in Linköping and its rural parish (St. Lars) is, that it should be more closely connected to the demographic crises of the period, both that one in 1773, which was one of the hardest hunger crisis ever in the country, as well as that during the time of the war 1808-1809.

The fact that infant mortality usually constituted a very important part of the total mortality is underlined by Gerry Kearns in his technically very well performed paper, where concerning the rise of population it is stated that the saving of young children is more important, than to prolong retirement with a few years. It had therefore been of great value to get more of discussion on this problem and an explanation of the rates in figures 2 and 3, especially as infant mortality does not seem to have been reduced between the periods 1851-1860 and 1891-1900. Are these figures representative for the situation in English cities at that time? What did the economic and social structure of these cities look like and how much do the social circumstances explain the high infant mortality? A high infant mortality rate as late as in the 1890's also appears in Walter Rödel's expose of the demographic structure of Mainz during the last 300 years. An attempt to explain the figures had also been of interest here, especially since, according to Arthur Imhof's studies, Mainz was situated in an area in Germany with comparatively low infant mortality rates.[5]

One of the purposes with this demographic conference must be to get perspectives on how to study health and urban mortality with a broad approach, especially as the Demographic Data Base have plans to do investigations on both the Sundsvall and Linköping areas. Studies in this field are often of a complicated nature. Many factors are involved, and they are often connected with each other. Furthermore the many variables to examine often belong at different levels of society.

One way to handle this kind of a problem could be to make an inventory of all conceivable variables on the various society levels and then choose a few, who are considered to be most significant.[6] Some examples of these variables could be on the country level: ordinances for epidemics, vaccinations, liquor regulations and poor relief, on the city level: city plans, water and sewage systems and hospital building, on an unofficial city level: associations for sick and poor, organizations for temperance and sports, and on the individual level, finally: interest in anatomy, in personal hygiene, in sports and in taking care of the body, in nutritious food and in acceptance of medical care.

Presumably, the most easily accessible variables are those originating from the authorities, both on the country and city levels. It will be more difficult to get hold of data telling about the individual's efforts to take care of his life.

Notes

1. T. McKeown, *The Modern Rise of Population* (New York 1976), p. 4.

2. A-S. Ohlander, and H. Norman, 'Kriser och katastrofer. Ett forskningsprojekt om nöd svält och epidemier i det förindustriella Sverige', *Historisk tidskrift*, 2 (1984), pp. 163-178.

3. A. Brändström, *"De kärlekslösa mödrarna"*. *Spädbarnsdödligheten i Sverige med särskild hänsyn till Nedertorneå* (Umeå 1984); B-I. Puranen, *Tuberkulos. En sjukdoms förekomst och dess orsaker. Sverige 1750-1980* (Umeå 1984); J. Sundin and L-G. Tedebrand, 'Mortality and Morbidity in Swedish Iron Foundries 1750-1875', A. Brändström and J. Sundin (Eds), *Tradition and Transition, Studies in Microdemography and Social Change, Report no 2 from the Demographic Data Base* (Umeå 1981).

4. H. Norman, 'Svält och epidemier. Krisåren 1773 och 1808-1811 i Örebro, Stora Mellösa och Hällefors. Omfattning, dödsorsaker och demografiska följder', *Bebyggelsehistorisk tidskrift*, 5 (1983), pp. 13-14.

5. A.E. Imhof, 'Unsere Lebensuhr. Phasenverschiebungen im Verlaufe der Neuzeit', P. Borscheid and H.J. Teuteberg, (Eds), *Ehe, Liebe, Tot. Studien zur Geschichte des Alltags* (Münster 1983), p. 191.

6. Compare S. Edvinsson, Hälsa-sjukdom-död i svenska städer1800-1900—en ansats till ett forskningsämne, *Unpublished paper, Dept. of History. University of Umeå* (1986), pp. 7-9.

Sanitary Standard, State Policy and Town Involvement: The Example of Water in 19th Century France

Jean-Pierre Goubert

Hot and cold running water has become ever so common in our daily life that we do not think about it any more. Reality should prevent us from considering as a norm our western habits and from forgetting how recent the conquest of water in fact is: how much it affected the prudish feelings of our most immediate ancestors, and how much it cost in terms of persuasion, labour and money. Yet, in France only it was in the 19th century that everything changed and this conquest, which up to then had been unthinkable, became a reality and developed until the eve of the second world war.

This development was founded on scientific knowledge, was spread through public education and media, and could expand owing to the support of a few town councils from the beginning of the 18th century. Then the Third Republic decided to have public water supply supervised (from 1884) by the "Conseil Supérieur d'Hygiène Publique de France" (High Committee of Public Hygiene in France).[1] In 1902 the important law on Public Hygiene provided financing through grants for works concerning water conveyance and drainage.

Nationwide action was then undertaken in France only at the very end of the 19th century, at a time when bacteriology was developing and the Republican State began intervening in citizens' public and private lives. Improvements in the sanitary standards spread quite fast, even if they remained rather limited between 1890 and 1910. The increase of life expectancy thus seems to be primarily linked with progress of a scientific order and with a change in the State's attitude towards the people. Nevertheless, other factors, both social and cultural, should not be overlooked. For in the field of health and more precisely of water quality, nothing or almost nothing can be done without the agreement of all concerned. Lastly, even if the culture of a people should be regarded as eminently significant, the social and economic background should be considered too.

During the second half of the 19th century the standard of living improved. Private fortunes in France, in this period of stable currency, doubled from

1851 to 1911. During the same fifty years, the index of industrial salaries went up from 52 to 100; that of agricultural salaries from 67 to 100. Even though social inequality increased in the 19th century it is still true to say that "the standard of living ... rather than the way of living created (for the 1868 conscripts) the contrast of physical anthropology"[2].

The rise in calorie intake as well as a more diversified diet and better quality water largely account for the improvement which physical anthropologists could measure among conscripts. Although efficient social medical care really did not exist, an improvement of public hygiene gave good results just as it had done in England somewhat earlier. The decrease of the death-rate concerned "the two categories of population which up to then had given death the largest share, (these were on the one hand the very young children and on the other elderly people)"[3].

The above mentioned factors, both economic and social, do not, however, entirely explain the changes recorded by the demographic "barometer". The explanation—to our mind—is rather to be found in what Philippe Ariès as early as 1948 called: "one of the deepest revolutions that mankind went through in the Western World: the revolution of death and life". From the end of the 18th century in France, and somewhat earlier in Northern Europe, the main priority of the western man was no more "to maintain the order of the world" but "to enter this world and rule it to his advantage".

A deliberate plan was then devised which drastically changed the uses and "production" of water which was expected to be clean and even drinkable. It included, too, a change in man's relation to Nature: water being one of the four elements, along with air, fire and earth according to an old Indo-European tradition. It also had something to do with the link between man and his own body. In both cases, "the situation of water" was modified.

The difference between the stagnant putrid water, which was the source of the economic life of the Middle Ages, and the clear running water of the modern and contemporary era was vivid[4]. Nature was radically altered; the industrial Revolution could step in. At the same time a new concept of the body slowly emerged between the 16th and 19th centuries. The cosmological and Christian images which are essentially fatalistic, due to their submission to the order of the World or/of God, were then challenged by the scientific image; which, being deterministic, sees Man as a new Prometheus.

Thus the living being became an intricate machine; anatomy then pathology, physiology and microbiology could now examine how the body worked. As far as nature was concerned, a similar change occurred. Nature is scrutinized by, among others, physicists, geologists, chemists and hydraulicians. So then, the western man was no longer afraid (or at least less afraid) to intervene in the order of the World on a massive scale: by spreading the small-pox vaccine, for example, or by modifying the composition of water.

It was favoured by enlightened despots for whom an interventionist policy meant a population increase, tax revenues and armed forces. This cultural "unblocking" appeared at the same time as the France of the Ancien Regime was slowly dying. Here we can find this cultural seed which at the end of 19th century blossomed with the settling of a true health policy concerning public hygiene and later a medical care for everyone.

Before the State started to intervene (at the end of the 19th century) into research for quality water and hydraulic equipment, town councils were already active according to their inclinations, their local policy and their wealth. With the French Revolution, town councilors and mayors (1790) were obliged to keep watch over public hygiene and mainly over water quality as it was so important for nutrition, health, economic life, fire-fighting and — incidentally — cleanliness.

Little by little, often sparingly, hydraulic equipment in France changed during the course of the 19th century: but the big changes happened only at the end of this period thanks to State intervention (1902-1940).

The necessary investment was quite high. Between 1824 and 1833, the first cities to become involved were big ones such as Paris, Lyons, St-Etienne and Montpellier. At the end of the century things had changed: of course big cities were still involved, but lesser cities started to acquire such equipment too, such as Annecy, Arcachon, Castres and Annonay.

The sort of works necessary and therefore the amount of money required, were, of course, linked to the size of each town: Amiens borrowed 600 000 F in 1843 for "the cost of works of water supplies in various districts", Dijon borrowed 220.000 F "a sum ... meant to be used to finish off the water supplies in various districts of the town". Chartres borrowed 240 000 F in 1844 for "the cost of raising and supplying water from the river Eure to the highest part of the city"[5]. At the end of the century, one can add to the problem of this basic equipment that of dealing with the improvement of the already existing water supply network, as a town's population increased and its network had to be adapted. By the end of the 19th century, people turned their attention to a matter which, up to then, had seemed subsidiary, namely the drainage system. More and more towns became interested in this and after the new laws in 1902, even the rural "parishes" prepared thick files which were asked for by the administration. They were sent to the bureau in charge at the Ministry of Agriculture only the items necessary to obtain the longed for grants.

These files are, indeed, a first-class help for historians[6]. They point out the link between the timing of hydraulic equipment and the relief, climate, type of cultures and the economy of the regions concerned. Some "parishes" did understand how interesting water supplies were, while others did not perceive it, owing to their economic resources and their own cultural modes.

There was a sizable gap between what a big or middle-sized city needed and what rural parishes required. It could amount to several thousand francs, even sometimes tens of thousands of francs of that time. Between 1920-1940 for the hamlet of Fenières in Ferté-Chevresis — Aisne, with a population of 983, the total cost was 8,805 F. On the contrary, in gold-francs and for a preceding period (1830-1850), several hundred thousand francs were necessary for such towns as Lyons, Grenoble, Mulhouse, Saint-Etienne, Dijon, Poitiers and Besançon. The cost could even be far higher for unusually important works. This was the case for Marseilles, which borrowed money several times to build the Durance canal: 10 million in 1839, 7 million in 1844, 9 million in 1847 and 2 million in 1853. Or to a lesser degree for Metz which borrowed 1,446,000 F in 1857 for a new water supply and Bordeaux in 1852 which needed 4,800,000 F.

As could be expected, the expenditure varied according to the size and desires of the urban areas. For the same basic equipment (public fountains, water mains, sewers) it seems to have been less high *per person* in big or middle-sized towns, except for a few cases such as Marseilles because of the necessary works on the river Durance and its inconvenient geological site. One must bear in mind that the financing of these expenditures relied on borrowing made possible by new taxes. Quite often the parishes, although really keen on such developments, gave the matter a second thought before asking the voters. On the other hand, it is easy to see that the so-called hierarchy of towns was respected, as the first to get their water and sewerage plants were the bigger ones.

In 1880 Besançon borrowed 700,000 F at a rate of 5 %, repayable in 16 years starting in 1853 taken from its ordinary revenues. Thanks to this loan, it could partly pay (700,000 F of 1,250,000 F) for "the conveyance and supply of water from the spring of Arcier to different districts and the completion of the already started sewers". As this town had no previous debts and its yearly surplus budget reached 131,308 F, its application was accepted at once and getting into debt raised no problem.

As regards the city of Beaune on the other hand, which was already deeply in debt and had had to resort to local rates in order to cover its 1849 deficit, it could only achieve the building of public fountains by further increasing its debts: it borrowed 150,000 F at a rate of 5 % repayable in 10 years, and started paying back from 1852 by creating new local rates. For similar reasons, Vannes only planned in 1856 the building of a water main between Meucon and the fairgrounds. In the same year, Grenoble was already borrowing to add "various drainage sewers".

This priority shown to thriving towns with multiple economic interests gave them a notable lead over other cities and even more so over rural communities. By the end of the 19th century (around 1880-1900), they were already improving the conveyance of water and the sewerage network. This was the case in Caen, Calais, Castres and Béziers in 1888: for between 1851 and 1881 the urban population and the number of middle-sized towns (from 20 to 50 000 inhabitants) rose sharply.

However, the study of the applications which enables us to make these observations only concerns the "communes" which resorted to a state loan.

In fact, a minority of these were real forerunners and became very early in the 19th century involved in the conveyance of public drinking water, since the hygienists were many and attentively listened to and so great had been the fear provoked throughout the population of the 1830's and 1850's by the outbreaks of cholera.

The investigation which was carried out by engineer Bechmann in 1892 concerns about 691 towns of more than 5,000 inhabitants. It reached a similar conclusion and stated the time when the first water supply works took place:

—   7 towns had a water supply before 1700,
—   8 water supplies were built between 1700 and 1800,
—   4 water supplies were built between 1800 and 1820,
— 23 water supplies were built between 1820 and 1840,
— 11 water supplies were built between 1840 and 1850,
— 55 water supplies were built between 1850 and 1860,
— 94 water supplies were built between 1860 and 1870,
— 74 water supplies were built between 1870 and 1880,
— 92 water supplies were built between 1880 and 1892.

If the yearly average number is calculated for every 10 years, the increase is quite spectacular. A terrific increase between the 18th and 19th century is clear. This development took place during the whole of the 19th century, speeded up quite remarkably between the first and second half of this period, in spite of a temporary slowing down between 1870 and 1880 which was probably caused by the fall of the Empire, the war and the "Commune".

We should not conclude from this that all French citizens had access to a water supply and a drainage system. First of all, until 1900 water had not been installed in peoples' homes except for a small privileged minority. Secondly, a very reduced part of the population was serviced by the water network ... when there was one! Indeed in 1892 only 290 towns of 691 were supplied with pressurized water. These 290 towns represent 4,512,941 inhabitants among whom only 127,318 subscribers could be numbered. Even if we suppose that public places such as barracks, boarding-schools, convents, hospitals ... may have been considered as *one* subscriber the number of subscribing homes remained very inferior to that of lodgings.

Still according to Bechmann's survey, the sewerage system was far less developed than the water supply network. Of 691 towns only 90 could use sewers for which there were only 156,050 subscribers. Finally, the draining of waste, according to an engineer like Bechmann, was not entirely satisfactory. In fact, the great majority of towns used their rivers and brooks in which to dump their sewage: this was the case for 354 towns of a total number of 420 that answered the survey on this matter. Only 17 towns (representing 225,913 inhabitants) of 313 towns (7,158,316 inhabitants) used a proper sewerage system whereas most of them, 294 towns that is to say 6,928,226 inhabitants used fixed cesspools and a tiny minority used movable ones—2 towns (14,170 inhabitants). Lastly, a very reduced number of towns resorted to a steam sewerage system, in other words a water-tight one! For a very long time to come, water supplies and waste drainage would remain precarious and poor, almost non-existent.

The case of towns

The Paris pattern

As neither doctors nor the administration of "communes" and "départements" were interested, the opinions expressed by scientists often came to a nothing, the famous exception being that of Paris. By 1800 Paris, whose population was about 600,000, provided 8 000 cubic metres of water every day which represented 13,3 litres per inhabitant; the town owned 26 kms of sewers which meant 1 km for every 23,000 inhabitants. In 1900, the year of the World Fair Exhibition, Paris numbered about 2,700,000 inhabitants and actually used 249 litres per day and person (the loss is estimated at around 50 litres). Its sewerage network spread over 1,113 kms, which meant one kilometre for 2,240 inhabitants.

This explains why the authors of *"Annuaire sanitaire de France"* enthusiastically exclaimed: "the smallest claims to fame of our nineteenth century will not be to have created this great sanitary implement which can be used in a way which honours those who conceived and achieved it.."[8]. It was during the second half of the 19th century that meaningful progress was made as Haussman was the "préfet" of Paris and Belgrand, an ambitious organizer and innovator.[9]

Before this, only works for a slow extension took place without any change in the old principles and "erring ways". Girard had increased the volume of water to be supplied owing to the opening of the Ourcq canal as had Dupuy, too, owing to the rebuilding of the Chaillot fire pump apparatus. As for Mary, he had improved the service by establishing new reservoirs. Emmery, Loic and Dulan had developed the sewerage network and Dupuy had introduced the new egg-shaped pipes which had lately appeared in England.

But around 1860 as Belgrand and his successors were in charge, two new great principles were stated and applied. These consisted of:

1. improving the quality of water already in use, which was low;

2. making progress with regard to river manholes and to substitute a new course for the natural one.

Instead of water from the Seine or the Ourcq canal, spring waters whose clarity and taste were enjoyed, were distributed for private use. The manholes were then moved away from Paris walls, further down-stream in the Seine valley and further progress was expected such as putting an end to the dumping of sewage in dry weather and making usual the purification of used water by spreading it over fields.

Big and middle-sized towns[10]

The study of how the water works evolved in big and middle-sized towns points out clearly that Paris is not only a model but also an exception. In fact, in these towns works were so slow and started so belatedly and even then only partially that they could not catch up with the increase in the population and the general economic expansion.

Marseilles

In comparison with these, Marseilles appeared as an exception. Its biggest sanitary problem concerned water supply and as soon as 1821, the "conseil général" began to study a plan for a canal. On July 12th 1834, the town council encouraged by Consolat, the Mayor, declared that: "the building of a canal has been decided irrevocably; whatever might happen, whatever it might cost, the canal will be achieved"; and "the Sémaphore de Marseille" supported this idea in its July 15th 1836 issue. This canal which took a long time to be finished, was the huge task undertaken by engineer Franz Mayor de Montricher. It was 82 kms long, of which 67 kms were in the open and 15 in tunnels underground. It meant the in-migration of a large French and foreign labor force. It was started in 1838 and solemnly opened on November 29th 1849 in front of an audience of about 15-20,000 people. However, it was only towards the end of the 19th century that the cleansing network became efficient. As it had not been expected to be used by large suburbs whose population swiftly rose, it quickly proved to be inadequate.

Angers

In Angers, though several doctors and some local medical societies insisted upon it, a conservative and thrifty town council remained reluctant to realize important works for the supply and cleansing of water even after the 1832 outbreak of cholera. Then endless arguments took place; which water was better, that of the Maine or that of the Loire? Even chemical analyses could not settle these so easily.

At long last, the plans were carried out but not until 1854, the year when cholera recurred. At first there were merely a hundred fountains, then little by little homes could be supplied owing to the setting up of a second steam engine. From 60 litres a day in 1856, the delivery per inhabitant went up to 150 litres in 1860, and to 270 in 1892, then down to 100 litres in 1900 and later up again to 182 in 1933. This means that the Paris figures dating from 1900 (per day and per inhabitant consumption) were reached later and only sporadically here. Demand, mainly from horticulturists and market-gardeners, soon became once again higher than supply. In 1907, 5,700 consumers could be numbered, which meant half the town households which is quite a good figure. This service spread from the centre of the towns to suburban districts but remained strictly within the limits of the "commune" in the 19th century. This town delayed getting a cleansing network which is always costly. So the old habit of dumping all waste in the river was carried on for a long time. Sanitation in Angers, which was achieved reluctantly, belatedly, parsimoniously and mainly in the rich districts in the centre of the town is a typical example of conservative ideas not concerned with public health.

Bordeaux

The Bordeaux sanitary policy reminds us, in some respects, of that of Angers. In Bordeaux, however, the works undertaken by the "intendants" and carried on during the First Empire had stipulated precise social limits: particularly the "Chartrons" quartier and a part of St Peter's parish even though the town spread greatly in the 19th century. Just as in Paris and many other French towns, the First and Second Empires were the times when great urban works took place. The threats hanging over Bordeaux and already pointed at in 1810, connected with its situation and the nature of the ground, led the local authorities to decide they had to get rid of "pernicious fevers" and fight against "rotten gases" which, in the summer, came up from marshes and rubbish tips.

During the First Empire, brooks had been cleaned out, ditches of old fortifications filled in and the first sewers built, mainly in the "Chartrons bourgeois" neighbourhood. As they were for economic liberalism, the town councils of the time of parliamentary monarchy decided, under the pretense that the cleaning up of the "Pengue" had caused some apprehension, that they could not find the necessary funds for the sanitation of the town despite the opinion of opposition members and the local medical society. So when, in 1852, the Empire was reintroduced, old plans reappeared trying to draw profit from the favourable political and economic circumstances: the town council went far into debt though they were opposed from within. At this time, the town began to collect springs and a sewerage system gradually took shape. Yet it was only in 1887 after seven years of works and high expenditures (5 million) that the solution of the provision of meters was found. By the same time, the cleaning up of the town was also completed. For it was built in a place which, naturally, could not make for an easy development. Bordeaux had a rather belated sanitation system: the gap between the idea and its realization was remarkable since it was widened by social conservatism and economic liberalism, both caring little about changing an order and thereby bringing about their own decline.

Rennes

The site where Rennes was built was no better after it spread to the other side of the "Vilaine" at the end of the 19th century. However, drainage had been accomplished, for the main part, in the first half of the 19th century and during the Second Empire. In the First Empire, the "Mail" district and the area surrounding Bourg-L'Evêque' had been cleaned up. In Louis Philippe's time, the "Vilaine" had been canalized and, later, the building of a district near the station had meant the filling in of a river branch. The problem of drinking water had been solved at the beginning of the 18th century; it became acute again between 1720 and 1880.

The architect Gabriel restructured the water supply network. But the works which started in 1727, were soon to be interrupted. They began again only sixty years later.

The fire which occurred at the beginning of the 18th century destroyed the former water supply network. Though Gabriel started to build it again (in 1727), the water supply network did not become a reality until the end of the 19th century. Marteville wrote in 1848 in his *"Histoire de Rennes"*:"The town, in its present state, definitely lacks any real water supply network either for drinking or irrigation, and we can't perceive when and how it may get out of this unthinkable situation!" Not until 1890 was this problem tackled. Among the different plans, that was drawn up by the architect Martenot, one was adopted: it consisted of the collecting of two springs, "la Minette" and "la Loyzance". On April 25th 1874 the town council agreed on this plan and on April 13th 1878 voted in favour of a loan of 4 million to carry out these works. On July 14th 1882, Le Bastard, the Mayor of Rennes, opened the first water supply system. Just as in Angers 30 years before, the appeal to succeed in a showy way, as well as the need to reassure taxpayers their money had been well used, led the same town council to build a temporary pond with a fountain in the Town Hall Square and then another, which remained, in the Palace Square.

Drinking water was not available until 1883. Water came by gravity all along a 45 kms long pipe which used the difference in level between the place where it was collected and the highest place in the city. It was kept in a 15,000 m^3 reservoir, then a second was built in 1889 which contained 20,000 m^3 and in 1919, a third containing 27,000 m^3 was added. The daily supply reached 12,000 m^3 in 1883, which meant about 180 litres per inhabitant and day. This first water supply network was sufficient until 1933. Then it quickly became inadequate; in 1931 the daily supply per capita only reached about 135 litres because of the population increase. In 1933 a water processing works came into use at Mézières-sur-Couesnon and processed 15,000 m^3 more water every day. As for the network itself, it grew from 37 kms in 1882 to 82,6 kms in 1919 and nearly a hundred in 1939. A growing proportion of the townspeople could thus be supplied. So in 1930 Rennes could have 25,000 m^3 water every day, this meant 400 litres per capita and day. In fact, as in most cases, the loss all along the way happened to be quite significant. Add to this the weather dependence which diminished water pressure and did not enable people living on the top floors of the buildings in the city centre to get water in 1939.

Water had not only to be supplied, it had to be drained and if possible purified too. The 1875 report from Brière, an engineer at the "Ponts-et-Chaussées" underlined the negative effects of the severe lack of sanitation: the sewers in Rennes were too few and ill conceived, the "poisoned" wells whose water people used for drinking and washing, for waste water and refuse carried by these few old sewers were directly poured into the "Vilaine" without any filtering. Quite logically, the first cleansing network was, according to the demands made by Doctor Perret, to be made in the public interest in 1887 shortly after the first supply network was built. It served almost exclusively with the town centre alone, just as in Angers, Paris and Bordeaux at different dates. Here again (as in Angers) the building-rate of drainage sewers and pipes was very slow indeed: in 1890 only 27 kms had been built; in 1919, 51 kms; in 1933, 69 kms. Connected with two big mains on each side of the "Vilaine", as in Paris, the sewers then met in a big main which poured the waste water into the "Vilaine" about 2 kms from the town. Here just as in Paris, a common system had been made which was used for waste water and rain. So it had an important drawback as it mixed both of these together and led them to the water processing factory which then had a great quantity of water to purify. The Paris model had, then, here again the upper hand and the conquest of water could only take place slowly just as in Nevers.

The installation of running water increased slowly and cost a great deal but it had two assets. It gave the growing population good quality water and at a fairly reasonable price at that time of economic development.

The countryside[11]

Few French rural places had, before the end of the 19th century, a modern water works. Even fewer were those that used a waste water draining system. The old system of dumping all waste in streets or rivers still prevailed for a long time to come. Yet the need to get pure water was felt. Some fountains and wells were well-known by villagers for pleasant-tasting water, others were celebrated for their qualities in the cooking of vegetables and for washing— lastly, water in which to clean oneself was also among their concerns if only to a very minimal extent.

Equipment was, of course, centuries old and carefully kept in good condition: though of a simple kind, it was necessary for the rural community, mainly in cattle-breeding areas where water supply was a continuous concern. In the "Doubs" department, the need to give cattle their daily 30 or 40 litres pushed some rural "communes" into planning as early as the 1860's for a water supply system in a very careful way. Both household and agricultural needs concurred so that country people did not hesitate to build a drinking-trough or a wash-house. Sometimes they not only paid for these out of their own pockets but also lent their teams or their own strength to repair or rebuild this or that building.

188

This equipment, however, remained of the traditional type in the "Belle Epoque" time. Every village had its own watering place, even if it was sometimes rather far away. Most villages had a wash-house, a small number had a relatively high population and were almost market towns, the middle course between a village and a city.

Water supply was, then, a typically urban phenomenon. Initial costs and maintenance expenditures made it unrealistic for rural "communes". In the country, wells or old fountains, somewhat improved, were predominant. Wells were given stronger copings, pails were no longer wooden ones but often zinc, ropes were replaced by chains. In some cases the water had even been analyzed by some local chemist as some enlightened people had demanded. As soon as it was proved efficient, the idea of hygiene was adopted by wise country people who cared for their cattle and their health. So water-catchment was often improved, wooden pipes were made of a more resistant material, the surroundings of the fountain were protected from animals by iron gates.

Inversely, the waste water drainage network remained undeveloped. The emptying, carrying and removal of fauces was only carried out in big villages which imitated the cities. In other places, refuse was "recycled", it was used as fertilizers for fields or vegetable-gardens. When it was not used in this way it went into the ground or underground. Ponds, rivers, brooks, underground water and well water then became natural dumping places. It was exceptional to see a cesspool or pits (especially watertight ones) that could receive human or animal refuse and excrement. Wells were often situated near manure heaps, which alarmed hygienists. The fact should here be emphasized that for country people excrement was neither disgusting nor connected with death. The idea of pathogenic germs was entirely unfamiliar to them and remained so for a long time: all the more so as they had always witnessed the good effects of excrement in the cultivation of plants.

In spite of these old habits, things eventually changed little by little in the second half of the 19th century. Many mayors asked for and received help from local hygienists. Many country people felt concerned with defects that the "Conseil Supérieur d'Hygiène Publique" pointed out to them from 1900 onwards: a lack in water quality and quantity, a too remote watering-place and bad or lacking equipment. After 1902 mayors of rural "communes" could, by using State grants, apply for a better quality water supply and they industriously filled up thick files in which one could find everything from chemical and bacteriological analyses to the planned outflow including the type of supply pipes and the planned financing.

Contrary to widespread opinion, this modernism was not the characteristic of towns. According to a sample survey for 1892, a majority of "communes" had less than 1,000 inhabitants and these were the ones asking for modern water equipment.

In the "Ain" department, market towns and hamlets got their networks between 1910 and 1930 (in round figures). Versonnex (161 inhabitants) is an example of this. Not content with "pumps next to stables, cowsheds and manure-heaps ... which were a real danger for public health", this "commune" made up its mind to catch two springs, divert 3 litres a second and to supply 1 600 litres per inhabitant. With the agreement of the water service engineers, the local council accepted to take only 90 litres a minute which meant 800 litres per inhabitant. This figure was not very high as farm animals (cows and horses) need about 20 to 50 litres a day each. Planned in 1911, given agreement and grants in 1914, this project was launched in 1922, given other grants in 1923, revised in 1926 and finally carried out from 1927 to 1930. This case is not unique. The French revanchist tendency also favoured, in some cases, water supply, mainly near military forts and all along important railway routes.

On September 25th 1908 for example, the War Minister asked the Minister of Agriculture to create "water supplying in Montreuil-sur-Ille station, so as to ensure for a future mobilization a high traffic of military trains between Rennes and St-Malo".

Between 1920 and 1940, however, works concerned mainly the creation, improvement and extension of a drinking water supply network. There were still numerous new plants created in "backward" departments of the Centre and West specially in market towns. Ménétreols-sous-Vatan (Indre), for example, asked in 1939 for a grant in order to build a trough with a 600 m^3 supply reservoir using two springs; for "the market town is presently only supplied with water coming from some wells whose flow is not sufficient in a dry period. To make up for this, farmers have to bring water — in large casks so as to fulfill their agricultural and family needs and so they have to travel long distances". The plan which was agreed on October 9th 1940, by the "*Conseil Supérieur d'Hygiène Publique*" did not receive the granted loan until 1946 ... by which time it was already carried out!

Installations in "deep France" have been carried out slowly, year after year, at the same pace as positivism entered people's minds and thanks to obvious successes that scientists, technicians and entrepreneurs achieved[12]. Progress was made by thousands of plans which remain unknown, unlike the big and sometimes showy realizations that took place in great cities. A drinking-trough, a wash-house, a pump, a diversion, cast-iron pipes with more branches, a few well-placed fountains, a connection with the nearest city network: all these are works that were achieved on a small scale but which gave birth to a true revolution in everyday life and represent change in peoples' minds. The level of sanitation which France reached in 1930 is the evidence of this "silent revolution". State intervention speeded it up, but it could only become effective insofar as the type of civilization had progressively changed and, at the same time, Man's relationship with water.

Notes

1. The "Conseil Supérieur d'Hygiène Publique de France" was created in 1822 and revised in 1848 and 1902. The September 30th 1884 order demanded the "Conseil Supérieur" to give its opinion about any plan concerning water supplies in each town, which had more than 2 000 inhabitants. The order of the 5th September 1884 exacted a water analysis and distinguished between four quality levels (very pure, drinkable, suspicious, bad).

2. N. Bernageau and E. Le Roy Ladurie, 'Etudes sur un contingent militaire (1868): mobilité géographique, délinquance et stature, mises en rapport avec d'autres aspects de la situation des conscrits', *Annales de Démographie Historique* (1971), p. 337.

3. A. Armengaud, *La population française au XIXe siècle* (Paris 1975), p. 112.

4. See A. Guillerme, *Les temps de l'eau. La cité, l'eau et les techniques. Nord de la France. Fin IIIè-début XIXè siècle* (Seyssel 1983).

5. Sources: Archives Nationales (Paris), C 838 and C 852 (specially).

6. Archives Nationales, F10 2225, 2228, 2254 (specially).

7. G. Bechmann, 'Enquête statistique sur l'hygiène urbaine dans les villes francaises', *Revue d'Hygiène* (1892), pp. 1062-1069.

8. 'Notice sommaire sur l'état actuel de la distribution d'eau et l'assainissement de Paris', *Annuaire sanitaire de France* (Paris 1900), p. 1.

9. About Paris, see G. Jacquemet, 'Urbanisme parisien: la bataille du tout-à-l'égout à la fin du XIXe siècle', *Revue d'Histoire Moderne et Contemporaine,* t. XXVI, oct.-déc. (1979), pp. 505-548. For a technical point of view, see also G. Dupuy and G. Knaebel, *Assainir la ville hier et aujourd'hui* (Paris 1982), pp. 5-35.

10. We can find the sources and the bibliography for the 'big and middle sized towns' in my book: *La conquête de l'eau. L'avènement de la santé à l'âge industriel* (introduction by E. Le Roy Ladurie) (Paris 1986), pp. 203-214. To be published in English by Polity Press, Cambridge (May 1988)

11. For the countryside, see, in the same book, pp. 222-236.

12. For more information, see J.-P. Goubert, *La conquête de l'eau. Analyse historique du rapport à l'eau dans la France contemporaine (1830-1940),* doctoral States Examination, typewritten ex., Paris, University - VII (1984).

Urban Mortality and the Population's Health: Mainz from the Seventeenth to the Beginning of the Twentieth Century

Walter G. Rödel

The survey to be made here of mortality in the City of Mainz over a time span of more than three hundred years makes it necessary to divide the period into two. To begin with we shall deal with the situation in the seventeenth and eighteenth centuries as that period must be regarded as belonging politically to the *ancien règime,* demographically to the "old type of population", and with regard to sources to the pre-statistical period. In a second main chapter conditions in the nineteenth and early twentieth centuries will be examined with special attention being devoted to the question whether signs are to be found in that period of a demographic transition or its initial stages. However, before turning to these questions we must first take a look at the political, economic, ecclesiastical and also military situation of the City of Mainz in the modern period in order to provide the necessary framework and background for our findings on the health and mortality of the inhabitants of Mainz. This also includes a brief account of the sanitary and hygienic conditions, as also of the facilities available for health care and the medical personnel.

Survey of the situation on the city of Mainz in the modern period

In 38 B.C., the Romans, who always had a good eye for the strategic potentials of a site, established a legionary camp on a piece of high ground directly opposite the point where the Main flows into the Rhine. This *Castrum Maguntiacum* developed into a settlement located between the camp and the river, which was surrounded by a wall at the end of the third century as a protection against attacks from Teutonic tribes. After weathering the storms of the Age of the Migration of the Peoples, this settlement developed into the medieval city. The area of 110 hectares (= approximately 260 acres) enclosed by the city wall hardly changed in size from the Roman period right down to the eighteenth century, with just a small suburb's being included within the ring of wall in the thirteenth century. The fortification system with its huge bastions erected in the early modern period, with work beginning during the Thirty

Years' War, only meant a very insignificant increase in the size of the city. It was only with the demolition of this fortification system, which had been repeatedly strengthened and improved over the years, that it became possible to construct new parts of the town at the end of the nineteenth and beginning of the twentieth centuries.

Thus, in connection with our topic, we may first observe that, over the past 2000 years, Mainz has always been of great strategic importance. From the seventeenth century on, the fortifications were constantly strengthened making it into the strongest German fortress on the left bank of the Rhine.

The populace of Mainz had to endure many sieges and some conquests, and always had to live together with a garrison, whose strength varied between 700 and 30,000 men. Life was even more difficult when the city was occupied by foreign troops.

From the historical-demographic research point of view, a further important factor is that the city hardly changed in size on account of its function as a fortress, meaning that the study deals with a constant unit.

As far as the political and ecclesiastical status of the city is concerned, Mainz was the seat of a bishop from the fourth century on, and was raised to an archbishopric in the eighth century. The archbishops also became the rulers of the city. The successors to the first archbishop, the Englishman St. Boniface (+ 754), claimed—in competition with the archbishops of Cologne—the dignity of being the most eminent prelate in the Holy Roman Empire. As *"Archicancellarius per Germaniam"*, the archbishop of Mainz also held the highest secular office in the imperial administration and was responsible for organising the elections of emperors, whence later came the dignity of being one of the imperial electors. Thus Mainz was not just the residence and territorial capital of one of the many archbishops in the Empire, it was also the seat of the most senior representative of the Estates which always had strained relations with the Emperor.

In 1462, after a disputed election for a new archbishop, and after the victor had successfully taken the city by storm, all municipal privileges were abolished; the archbishop became the unrestricted lord of the city, and appointed a *"vice-dominus"* as his senior administrative official. The patricians—including the family of Johannes Gutenberg, the inventor of the art of printing—were for the most part expelled from the city and had no chance of regaining their former leading position within the city. Consequently until the end of the archiepiscopal rule in 1797, the citizens had hardly any say in the administration of the city. Many noble families settled in the city, from among whose ranks the highest secular and ecclesiastical offices in the administration and government of the city, archbishopric and electorate were filled.

Just like the archbishop's court and the noble families, the numerous ecclesiastical institutions in the city gave many citizens employment and a source of income, and some of them also the chance of climbing up the social ladder.

Admittedly, from the economic aspect, despite its function as a residence and its favourable location on major trade routes, Mainz was only an intermediate centre, and was very much in the shadow of the neighbouring trading metropolis of Frankfurt am Main.

The third function to be mentioned is that of university city which Mainz had been since the foundation of the archiepiscopal university in 1477. Professors, students and other university employees formed a further foreign element in the city population, alongside the soldiers of the garrison and the noble families.

A further point which should be mentioned is that until the end of the rule of the archbishops-electors in 1797, Catholicism was, in effect, the state religion. No non-Catholics could acquire citizenship or be admitted to a guild. At the end of the eighteenth century, there were only 100 Jewish families and about 600 tolerated Protestants in the city. This situation makes it relatively easy for a researcher to deal with the entire population in the period prior to the introduction of official statistics by evaluating the Catholic church registers. The earliest of them began in 1582. Despite some gaps, it is possible to produce a good survey of the development of the population in the seventeenth and eighteenth centuries. When the French authorities, in what was then the French département Mont-Tonnerre, introduced civil registration in summer 1798, all the church registers were confiscated. They contained the data of some 244,000 persons in 46 volumes. Thus, on the basis of 94,267 burials, it is possible for me to report on mortality in the seventeenth and eighteenth centuries. Censuses were introduced from 1799 on. After the city passed to the Grand Duchy of Hesse in 1816, these censuses were conducted every three years.

To recapitulate briefly: Mainz, with its functions as a fortress, residence and university city, cannot be compared with the majority of other German cities. These three functions had a great influence on the population and on the development of natality, nuptiality and mortality. These same three functions also made Mainz especially attractive for newcomers, provided they were Catholics.[1]

The situation changed fundamentally in the nineteenth century. Mainz lost its position as a residence, and declined into a provincial town. The university had also been abolished by Napoleon, and was not re-established until 1946. Only the function of fortress was retained until the end of the nineteenth century. Until 1866, the garrison was made up equally of Prussian and Austrian troops.

The episode of French rule from 1798 to 1814 had an enduring effect on the city's social structures. The previously predominant nobility and the senior clergy recruited from among their number had lost their position and also did not return to the city again after 1814. From 1802 on, Mainz was only the see of a bishop; the numerous noble foundations and commanderies of chivalric orders were disbanded. The Protestant community grew steadily in size after

195

1802; the proportion of Jewish inhabitants also grew considerably after the restrictions imposed on them in the early modern period had been removed. The *haute bourgeoisie*, which had not existed in Mainz under the *ancien régime*, began to establish itself and took over the positions previously held by the nobility.[2] As a result of the state and customs frontier along the Rhine established by the French, economic life in Mainz had been paralysed and only recovered slowly. It is only possible to talk of the beginnings of a certain degree of industrialisation after the middle of the nineteenth century. The wine trade still played a predominant role, and was soon joined by sparkling wine (*"Sekt"*) production. The establishment of steamship navigation on the Rhine and the opening of the railway along its banks helped to make Mainz, among other things, the starting point for the Rhine journeys so popular in the nineteenth century. This also had an effect in the catering sector and in the hotel trade. It was not until the demolition of the city fortifications at the turn of the twentieth century allowed the construction of new inner suburbs (the city's area increased in size from 125 ha to 338 ha, thus by 186 %) that space was created for the steadily growing population. From 1816 to 1864, the number of houses within the ring of fortifications had only increased by 11 %, whereas the population figure increased by 70 % during the same period.[3] It was only when the fortifications were completely dismantled in 1920, as required under the Treaty of Versailles, that all restrictions on the city's expansion were removed. However, 80 % of the city was destroyed by the air raids of the Second World War. After a long and arduous period of reconstruction and the establishment of new suburbs, Mainz nowadays has a population of something over 180,000.

The public health service and medical personnel

Living conditions for the people of Mainz within the massive ramparts of the fortifications were very cramped and were further restricted in the seventeenth and eighteenth centuries by the completely unbalanced distribution of landed property. The nobility and clergy, who accounted for about 5 % of the population, together owned over 57 % of the built-up area, whereas the citizens and denizens were crowded together in the remaining 43 % of the built-up space; 80 % of all residential buildings were located here.[4] The majority of streets and alleys were narrow, crooked and dirty; it was not until between 1830 and 1860 that all the roads were paved. The buildings themselves were a conglomeration of noble palaces, splendid churches and monasteries, impressive bourgeois town houses, small shops and wretched hovels. It was not until the Surveyor's Office Ordinance of 1755 that it was decreed that in future houses were to be constructed in stone, or that the ground floor at least was to be built of that material, that only tiles or slates were to be used for roofs and that every house was to be provided with a toilet, which should not, however, be located too close to the house well.[5]

Within the city area there were only three springs so that the water supply had to be taken mainly from the ground water, the quality of which had long been described as bad and had repeatedly led to outbreaks of illnesses. Two piped water supplies were constructed in 1678 and 1728 to bring spring water from outside the fortifications into the city. It was only from 1863 on that work began on laying a modern mains water supply, and even as late as 1895 over 700 houses in the city were still without a supply.

A further source of risk to health came from the graveyards located around the ten parish churches in which the dead were buried in a very restricted space. Their bones were exhumed soon after and put into charnel houses. Numerous interments were also made within the churches themselves. From 1760 on, repeated attempts were made by various bodies at having these crowded graveyards abandoned and replaced by cemetaries outside the city walls. Despite a report submitted by the faculty of medicine in 1782 in which the custom of burial inside the churches and in the graveyards within the city was described as extremely dangerous to health and as a source of infection, the clergy were able to resist any change. Not until 1803, at the order of the French Prefect, was a central cemetery established outside the city.[6]

It goes without saying that all species of domestic animals were kept within the city, that the disposal of waste and rubbish was extremely unsatisfactory and that increased attention was only devoted to these matters in times of raging epidemics. The waste from butchers, tanners and other trades was "disposed of" into the Rhine, into which river the French also threw their dead in the siege of 1689.

After this sketch of conditions in Mainz, which were further complicated in times of armed conflicts by the billeting of troops, who occasionally even exceeded the population in number, we should like to take a brief look at the hospitals to be found here. There were a whole series of hospitals in the city derived from various foundations, the oldest having been established in the year 1000. They served the most varied purposes, such as almshouses for the clergy or domestic servants, as hostels for the destitute, as inns for pilgrims and foreigners, for the care of destitute patients, as a lepers' hospital, as an orphanage, as a military hospital and as a hospital for plague victims and the elderly infirm.[7] In the course of improvements in the care of the poor, the St. Rochus Hospital was established as a central institution in 1721-1728 with the task of caring for poor patients. It contained a section for the sick, an orphanage and a section for the poor who were here intended to contribute towards their livelihood by work; it had accommodation for over 300 inmates.[8] This modern establishment by eighteenth century standards had its own parish church, a number of male and female nurses and a physician whose salary was paid by the city. He was obliged to make regular visits. After the establishment of the municipal home for invalids in 1848, the St. Rochus Hospital devoted itself exclusively to the care of the sick as a municipal hospital until 1914, then becoming a military hospital. Nowadays it serves as an old people's home.

The *"Accouchement"*, a maternity home with training facilities for midwives, established in 1785 as a university institute, survived the dissolution of the old university of Mainz and was integrated into the newly established university gynecological clinic in 1946. In addition to the military hospital which had first served as the university hospital from 1788 to 1793 and continued to exist until 1895, there was a further military hospital (1814-1841), a war hospital (1843-1903), a garrison hospital (from 1892 on) and a home for invalids. In addition to the St. Rochus Hospital, the civilian population was served by the Vincenz- und Elisabeth-Hospital from 1850 on. Further hospitals were opened in 1892, 1906, 1912 and 1914.

When considering the medical personnel available to the inhabitants of Mainz in the seventeenth and eighteenth centuries, a distinction must be made between the physicians who were trained at the university and the surgeons organised in a guild. The latter tended open wounds, put fractured limbs into splints and carried out operations, whereas the physicians were concerned with the diagnosis of internal disorders and the prescription of remedies. Thanks to the existence of the faculty of medicine, the prerequisites for medical care were not bad in Mainz. In addition to physicians engaged in free general practice, of whom five are named for 1683, there was also an officially appointed City Physician from the mid-seventeenth century on at the latest. Apart from caring for the sick, his task was to supervise the surgeons and midwives, as well as the three apothecaries, and to assist the city council as medical consultant. From 1773 on there were two, then from 1784 four city physicians who had to treat the poor free of charge in four practices. In addition to these officially appointed and freely practising physicians, there was also a garrison physician, a physician to the cathedral chapter and the professors of the faculty of medicine, who for the most part also acted as personal physicians to the elector or had a general practice in the city in addition.[9] There was thus no lack of physicians in Mainz in the early modern period, the only question which remains is how many of the inhabitants ever consulted a doctor in their life and were also able to pay for his services.

The surgeons, whose fields of activity were defined in the new Surgeons' Guild Ordinance of 1673, were supposed, according to the university reform of 1784, to attend lectures and courses at the university in surgery for three semesters and obstetrics for two semesters, but they also did not want to forego their traditional craft training. According to the guild lists, their number varied between 12 and 17 in the eighteenth century.

At the beginning of the nineteenth century, as medicine's possibilities for life-preservation and life-prolonging began to become apparent, the care of the sick was raised to a higher degree of efficiency. The number of doctors with practices in Mainz also increased; the garrison was given increased medical care, and a district physician appointed by the Grand Duchy of Hesse-Darmstadt supervised the public health system. He was also responsible for the preparation of the statistics which were also required to record the causes of death exactly from 1869 on. Admittedly, the head of the District Medicinal Office in Mainz, Dr. A. Helwig, noted from 1869 to 1873 *"mors ex causa ignota"* in 762 cases out of a total of 7425 deaths and adds, by way of an explanation, that this heading includes all those deaths which occurred "without a physician's having seen or treated the deceased during his illness".[10] They included 570 children less than one year of age and 91 aged between 1 and 5 "who all without exception died without their parents' considering it worth their while to call in a physician" as the district physician complains. In 1908 there were then just 16 (including 13 children) out of 1870 deaths for which no cause of death could be given because no doctor had been called in.[11] One may be allowed to draw conclusions from this changing attitude to medical care about a change in the mentality of the inhabitants of Mainz.

Mortality in the seventeenth and eighteenth centuries[12]

Firstly, let us take a brief look at the monthly and seasonal fluctuations. As a basis for this, the data of the four largest of the seven territorial parishes were taken and evaluated for the entire period and also for detailed studies covering 25 years each.

In general terms, this produces the following picture:

1.	March	9.19 %	7.	December	8.14 %
2.	April	9.09	8.	October	8.09
3.	September	9.01	9.	February	7.78
4.	August	8.99	10.	November	7.66
5.	May	8.54	11.	June	7.55
6.	January	8.53	12.	July	7.43

The two mortality peaks in late winter/spring and in late summer can be readily recognised. The months of March and April are at the top of the scale, slightly ahead of September and August. The winter months proper are much further down the scale than might have been expected. The months of June and July are the periods of minimum mortality in Mainz too. The seasonal situation in the seventeenth century differs very considerably from that of the eighteenth if a breakdown of the figures is made on the basis of quarter centuries. The minima and maxima are much more clearly marked, something which is to be explained by the crisis situations which we shall be dealing with in more detail later. The eighteenth century shows a flattening of the curve; the late summer maxima recede more and more. All in all, a normalisation becomes apparent, which is only disturbed by the year 1793—a siege of the city followed by a dysentery epidemic. Admittedly, this development, as will be shown in a moment, is not to be explained by a lower child mortality rate, which is traditionally held responsible for the so-called "summer peak" in mortality.

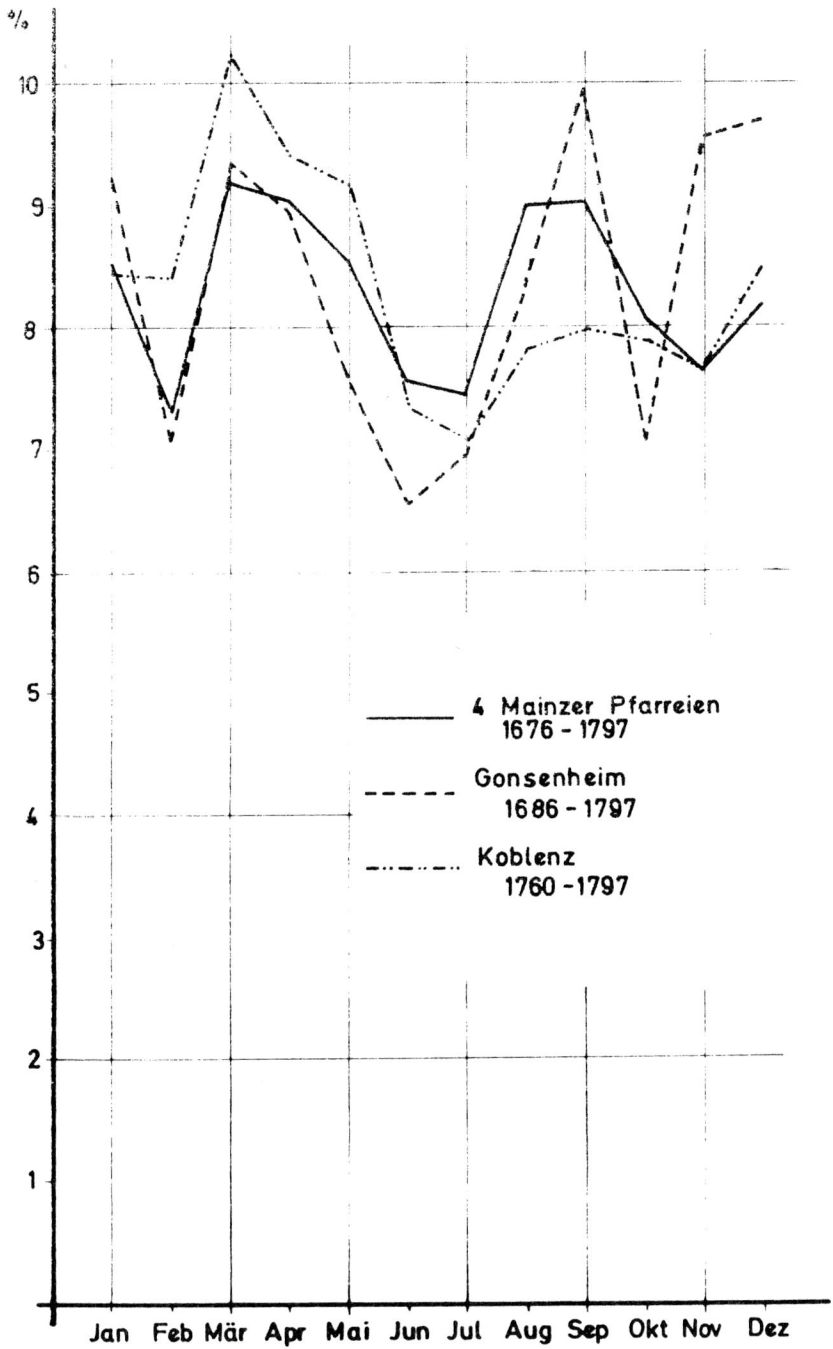

Figure 1. Seasonal fluctuations in mortality.

When studying the mortality rate for babies, children and adults, we encounter considerable problems as the registers only seldom contain exact details of age. In the final analysis, it is only possible to differentiate the age groups 0-10 years and "over 10 years of age". If all the 94,267 burials are classified for the entire period, then there is a percentage distribution of 49.58 % children aged between 0 and 10 and of 50.42 % people aged over 10. For the eighteenth century, for which there are no significant gaps, the ratio can be calculated as about 55 % children and 45 % older persons. If an evaluation is made on the basis of individual decades, this overall figure fluctuates very considerably between 60 % for child mortality and 40 % for people over 10 years of age. The results from the family reconstitution may be taken as a corrective. Admittedly, these can only provide minimum estimates, as many of the dates of the deaths of older people cannot be established. However, they do provide a fairly exact picture in the field of babies' and children's deaths.

0-1 m.	1 m.-1 y.	1-5 y.	6-10 y.	11-20 y.	21 y—	Total
8.36%	13.73%	16.01%	3.06%	1.85%	56.99%	100.00%

The mortality rate for babies (0-1 y.) thus totals 22.09 %; this value can be confirmed by Arthur Imhof's studies for Giessen (22.04 %). Admittedly, in Mainz they would appear to have increased rather than decreased in the course of the eighteenth century, because the values fluctuate in the individual decades between 20 and 26 % and increased in the second half of the century. It can also be shown in the case of Gonsenheim, a village close to Mainz, and for the city of Koblenz, for which we have studies, that the mortality rate for babies and children did not decrease in the eighteenth century. It is not possible to determine a turning point which might be taken as indicating the beginning of a demographic transition—at least in this Catholic area of Germany.

Demographic crises and crisis-like developments

"A peste, fame et bello, libera nos, Domine" our ancestors would implore, if their existence was once again threatened. This fervent prayer was particularly applicable for Mainz, because in view of the city's special situation, its population was often afflicted, not just by famine and plague, but also by armed conflicts.

These periods of crisis, which were especially frequent in the seventeenth century, have attracted much interest and a very differentiated analysis among those engaged in historical demography. As I am talking to specialists here, I do not need to go into the various definitions of "crisis". Following Pierre Guillaume and Jean-Pierre Poussou: Demographie historique[13], I have endeavoured to define a demographic crisis as follows: A demographic crisis occurs if the number of deaths rises sharply and suddenly, so that the number of dead over a period of at least three months is twice, three or four times the average number of deaths in the preceding or following years. The population losses caused by such a crisis may amount to 10-15 %, or 20-25 % or even more of the total population. At the same time as this maximum mortality rate, it is also possible to observe a marked reduction in the number of conceptions and marriages. The end of the crisis is marked by a decrease in the number of deaths, and parallel to that there is a temporary increase in the number of conceptions and marriages. Until normal conditions return, in so far as it is possible to speak of such in the seventeenth and eighteenth centuries, an increased number of births is to be observed, accompanied by a simultaneous fall in the number of deaths. I shall not attempt any typology of the crises here according to the ratios of the various age groups and the effect on the population as a whole, and shall just limit myself to presenting some characteristic crisis periods affecting the population of Mainz.

For the seventeenth century, which was particularly richly endowed with crises for the people of Mainz, the following events may be taken: After the occurrence of the plague in 1606/07, 1611, 1613 and 1623, whereby the latter instance was preceded by a dysentery epidemic, the city was afflicted by famine, plague and siege in autumn 1632 after the Swedes under Gustav Adolf had established their rule in the city. Mortality rose tenfold, so far as can be established on the basis of the very incomplete church register entries. The same was also true for the siege by Imperial troops in summer and autumn 1635, which were able, under the command of Tilly, to force the Swedish garrison to capitulate, after repelling a French relief army. All in all, the population of Mainz was probably reduced by half, i.e. some 6,500 inhabitants. The last epidemic of plague in 1666, which had also raged in London in the preceding years, brought a further loss of some 2,300 persons. The population was able to recover again, thanks to the city's functions, as mentioned above, and thanks to the generously exercised policy of repopulation implemented by Archbishop Philipp von Schönborn (1647-1673), who busied himself with the reconstruction of the city after the Thirty Years' War, and was also largely responsible for the erection of the bastion fortifications around the city. Admittedly, this marked growth—the population figure at the end of the seventeenth century was about 15,000—is also to be ascribed to the population's own great readiness to recuperate, in keeping with the Catholic church's teachings, and the large influx of newcomers.

The events in the War of the League of Augsburg (1688-1697), in the course of which Mainz was captured by the French without a battle and then had to be laboriously reconquered by Imperial troops in 1689, meaning that the inhabitants had once again to endure a long siege, did not have any long-term effect on the population figure. Despite the losses in the course of these armed conflicts and in the years of famine during the general European crisis in 1694-1696, which had a particularly serious effect in France, the population of Mainz was at least able to maintain its level, or increase slightly. The numerous deaths were compensated by a boom in births beginning after the recapture of the city in 1690. The function as a fortress had a positive effect on the population development in this case; whereas the whole of the Palatinate and other areas along the left bank of the Rhine had been completely ravaged by French troops following the new system of "burnt earth", Mainz was spared this fate on account of its strategic importance, which also made it a desirable corner stone for the French for their eastern chain of fortresses. After its reconquest by Imperial troops, the French did not succeed again in regaining this important point.

After the seventeenth century with its serious demographic crises, the eighteenth century at first began very positively for the development of the population. In the first three decades, despite the constantly high mortality rate, it was possible for those surpluses to be attained on which the city was then able to draw for the whole century. All in all, the vital statistical balance sheet for the eighteenth century closes with a slight deficit of 947 persons. This positive development may be explained by the fact that there were no further occurrences of the plague, and that the fortress city of Mainz was not directly affected by any of the wars of the century until the events following the French Revolution. We do, it is true, find peaks in mortality in the vital statistic curves. These increase in number in the second half of the eighteenth century and are especially marked in the parishes with a population of low social status. These were due to severe winters, such as in 1740, smallpox or influenza epidemics, etc. Smallpox would appear to have occurred with a certain degree of regularity every 5-7 years, claiming its victims especially among children aged 0-7. The epidemic of 1766 may be taken as a particularly outstanding example which, with its ratio of 69 % children in the total number of deaths, brought the highest rate of child mortality in the century (832 children compared with 372 adults). This caused mortality to increase by 28 % by comparison with the mean value for the preceding decade; admittedly, by comparison with the following decades it was 50 %. But if only the group of children aged 0-10 were to be included in the calculation, then there would be a crisis as in the old days with a doubling of the number of deaths, as so often occurred in the seventeenth century.

Even the years of famine occurring in the whole of Western Europe after the bad harvest of 1770, which in many places led to severe losses in the population, may at the worst be described as a *"crise larvée"*, as defined by our French colleagues, in the case of Mainz. Although the price for bread-cereals more than tripled between 1769 and 1771 (from 3 fl. 38 kr to almost 8 fl. (1771), with a peak price in May 1771 of over 11 fl. per *Malter* (= 106 7 litres)), the worst was prevented thanks to imports from Danzig via Amsterdam arranged by the archbishop. In Mainz in the eighteenth century, people no longer died from starvation; the cereal price and mortality curves no longer correlate with one another. As the above example shows, the improved possibilities of transport and the cultivation of new useful plants, combined with improved agricultural techniques may be regarded as being the explanation for the absence of subsistence crises.

Figure 2. Baptisms and burials in the parish of St. Ignaz in Maintz 1631-1636 (monthly in absolute figures).

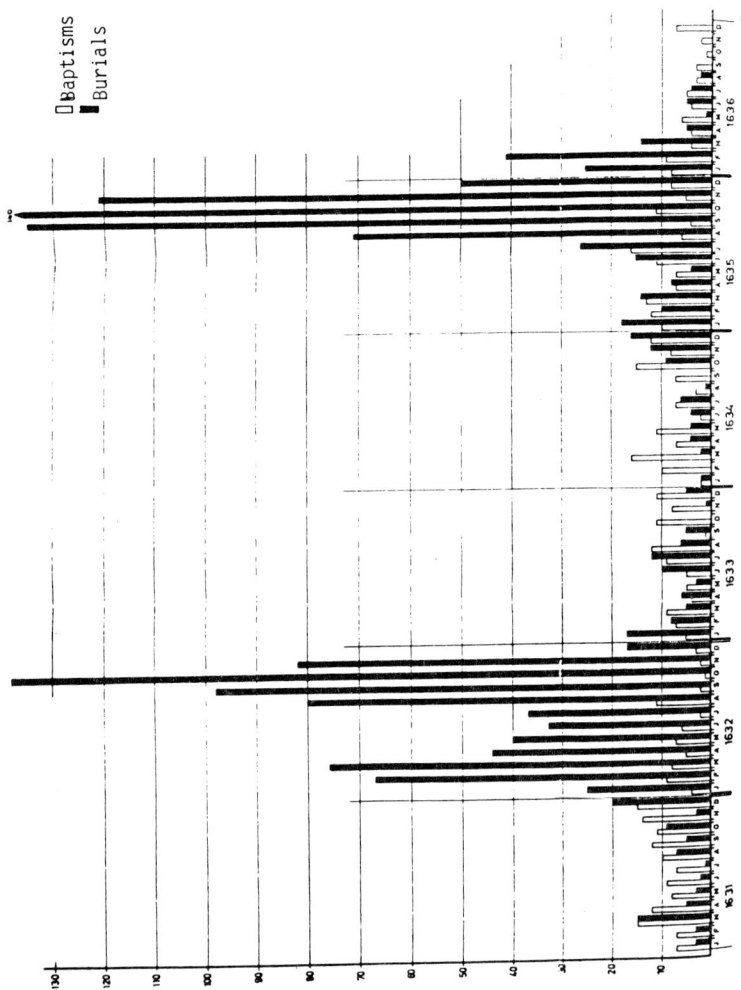

Figure 3. Vital statistics for the parish of St. Emmeran in Maintz July 1688 to June 1690 (monthly).

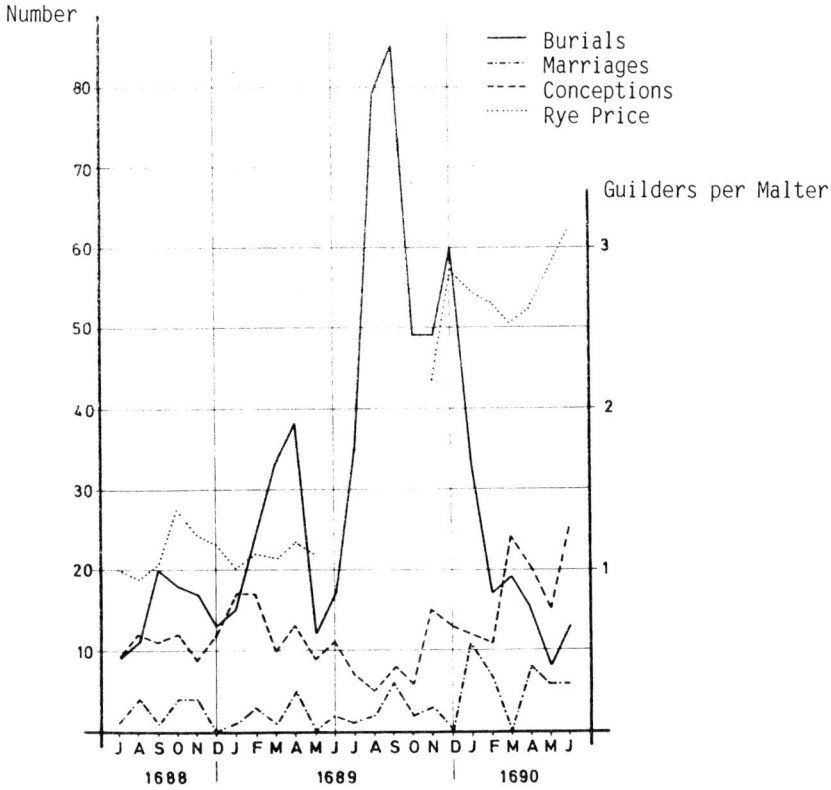

Figure 4. Adult and child mortality in Maintz 1765-1767 (monthly in absolute figures).

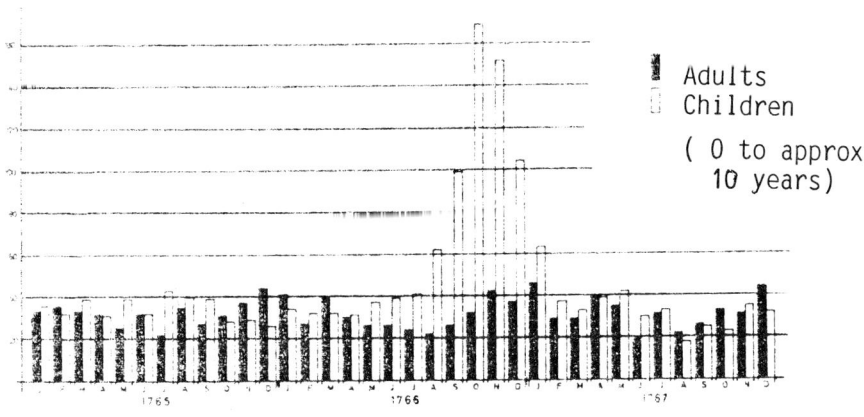

Figure 5. Adult and child mortality in Mainz 1760-1765 (annually in absolute figures).

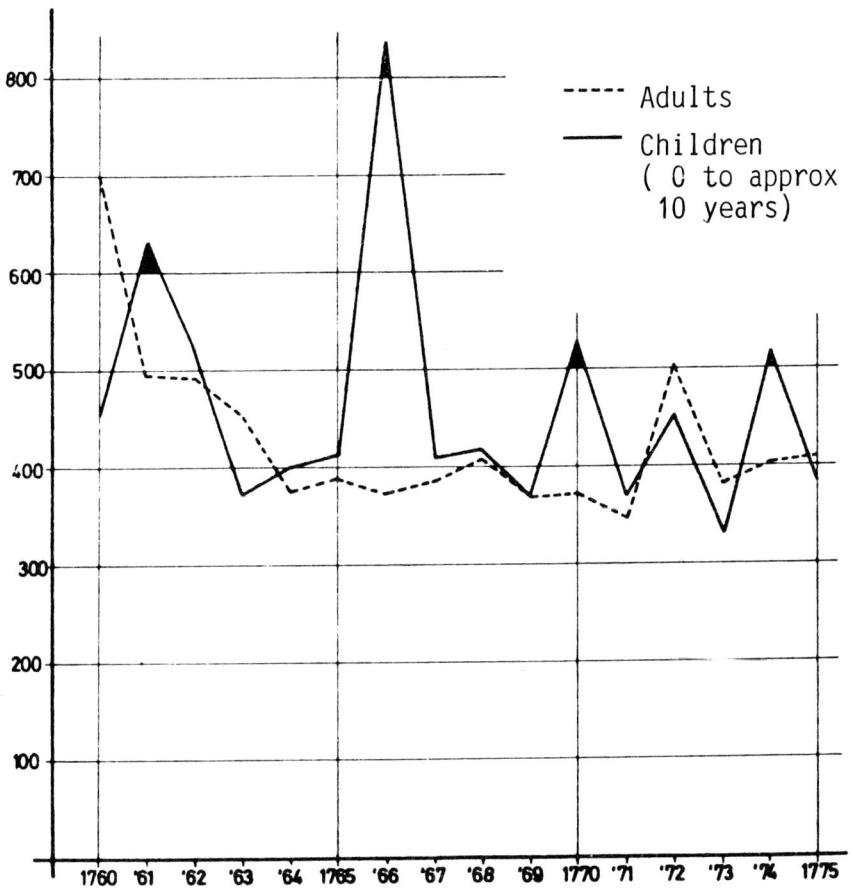

Admittedly, at the end of the eighteenth century there was one great exception to the conditions of life described here which again led to crises of the "old style". The attendant circumstances were once again comparable with those of the crisis years 1635 and 1689: capture of the city by French revolutionary troops under General Custine, an occupying garrison of 23,000 men, the burden of billeting for the citizens, shortage of food, blockading and siege of the city by German troops (14th April—24th July 1793) with a heavy bombardment, as well as a dysentery epidemic from the end of May until the end of September 1793. Some 1800 people from a greatly reduced population died in 1793, 800 of them in August alone. The rate of increase compared with the average value of the preceding decade was 114 %. The after-effects too, rapid drop on mortality, sharp rise in the number of conceptions and marriages, high rates of re-marriage, are a clear indication of the old style of crisis,

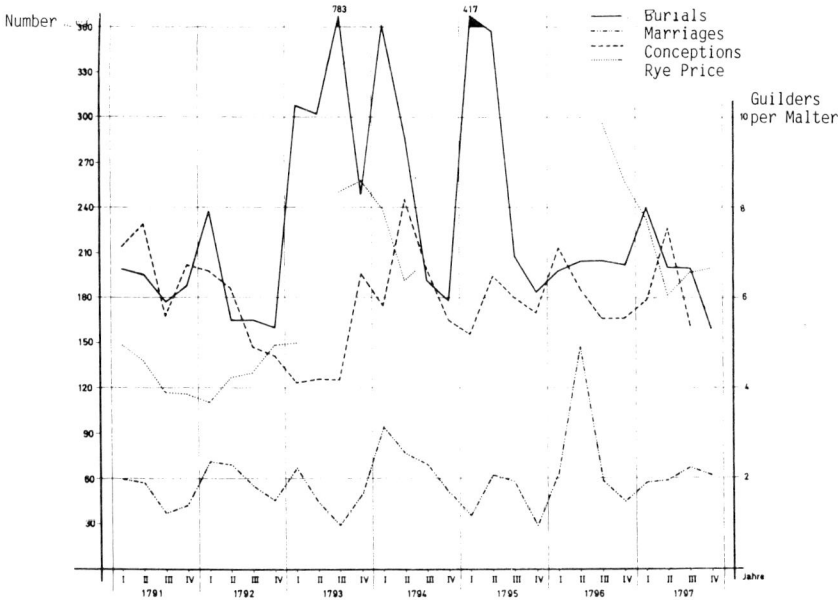

Figure 6. Vital statistics for the urban parishes in Mainz 1791-1797 (quarterly).

especially as the three factors war, epidemic and famine were involved in the deficitary demographic development, even if in varying density. A similar situation occurred in 1795 during a further siege, which was this time conducted unsuccessfully by the French. As the conditions were somewhat more favourable, only 1281 people died in that year, although it is still possible to talk of an at least crisis-like situation. After a long period of peace, Mainz was once again called on to fulfill its function as a fortress, with a return of virtually the same conditions again as had prevailed in the seventeenth century.

The special character of this important fortress also meant that even at the beginning of the nineteenth century the population of the city was once again afflicted by an old style crisis. At that time, Mainz had some 25,000 inhabitants and a French garrison of 30,000. After the Battle of Leipzig in 1813, some 100,000 of Napoleon's troops passed through Mainz on the retreat. A typhus epidemic which raged in the city from November 1813 until the end of April 1814 claimed the lives of 2,485 civilians and over 17,000 French soldiers. In 1814, with 1,979 deaths out of a population of 23,302, it is still possible to calculate a mortality rate of 85.29 per thousand.

If we consider the net result of mortality under the *ancien régime,* then it may be stated that Mainz, thanks to the Catholicity of its inhabitants, was able to make good mortality, which remained at its old level, by a high birth rate (34.5 -28.5 from 1700 to 1780), and maintain the size of its population.

207

Table 1. Mortality in Mainz

Year	Inhabitants	Diseases	Death rate
1800-01 (IX)	21218	742	34.97
1801-02 (X)	22325	663	29.98
1803-04 (XII)	21583	726	33.64
1806	23505	1257	53.47
1809	24142	858	35.54
1814	23202	1979	85.29
1815	23881	733	30.69
1816	25251	824	32.63
1819	25390	790	31.11
1822	26800	960	35.82
1825	28409	818	28.79
1828	28439	921	32.38
1831	30234	1015	33.57
1834	31535	1142	36.21
1837	31702	1180	37.22
1840	32142	966	30.05
1843	33826	1098	32.46
1846	36656	1160	31.64
1849	35140	1187	33.78
1852	36741	1013	27.57
1869	44000	1381	31.38
1871	47483	1901	40.03
1873	48000	1270	26.50
1890-96 Ø p.a.	74650	10632	20.35
1908	108000	1870	18.00

Owing to the brisk influx of newcomers, an important growth in population was indeed achieved in the course of the eighteenth century (in 1700 approx. 15,000, in 1786 approx. 26-28,000 inhabitants). As we only know the exact numbers of inhabitants in the pre-statistical period for three years by chance, namely for 1694 (15,000), 1771 (26,753) and 1786 (some 28,000), but we are unable to quote the complete number of deaths for 1694 on account of the incomplete register, it is only possible to calculate the mortality rate for 1771 with 28.7 per thousand, and for 1786 with 28.4 per thousand. That certainly does not provide an answer to questions about an increase or decrease in the mortality rate in the eighteenth century. However, on the basis of everything we know about the vital statistical material, mortality probably did not decrease, either among children or adults in the course of the eighteenth century.

Mortality in the nineteenth and early twentieth centuries

In the nineteenth century, Mainz remained a fortress, first under the French, then under the German Confederation and finally under the German Empire,

208

and normally had a garrison of over 4,000 men. However, it had lost its other functions: in Hesse, undergraduates went to the Grand Ducal university in Giessen to study, and the residence of the Grand Dukes of Hesse-Darmstadt was in Darmstadt.

As far as mortality is concerned, we are far better informed, as we can now consult the material on the censuses and statistics which were taken and compiled regularly from 1799 on.

We are thus able to give exact details on the development of the mortality rate.

From the figures presented here it can be seen that down until the period after 1870 the mortality rate moved back and forth in great bounds and only rarely dropped below 30 per thousand. Admittedly, the figure of 40.03 per thousand for 1871 must be regarded as atypical as in that year a smallpox epidemic broke out among the 36,000 French prisoners of war being held in Mainz which also claimed 295 victims from among the civilian population. Although the French authorities had made smallpox vaccination compulsory in 1801, people had become careless again in the meantime: almost all the children who died in 1871 aged between 0 and 5 years of age had not been vaccinated!

It was not until the last third of the nineteenth century that the mortality rate figure dropped noticeably, even if there were still marked differences. Thus for the years 1890 to 1896, which we have shown in the table as average values, the figures were 22.08, 19.25, 21.98, 22.65, 18.79, 19.42 and 18.44 per thousand. Thus Mainz would seem to lie in the national trend, as the figures for the mortality rate in the German Empire, so far as they have been determined up to now, lie between 29.0 and 30.8 per thousand.[14] Peter Marschalck in his history of Germany's population in the nineteenth and twentieth centuries probably dated the beginning of the fall in the mortality rate a little too early with 1865.[15] For the period 1815 to 1865 he determined an average natality rate of 37 per thousand and a mortality rate of about 26 per thousand, whereby he, like R.W. Lee[16] before him, draws attention to the great regional differences to be found (natality rate 30-45 per thousand, mortality rate 22-35 per thousand).[17] In the last third of the nineteenth century— according to Marschalck—there was a marked increase in life expectancy (of about 10 % between 1850 and 1881/1890, and a further 20 % between 1881-1890 and 1901-1910), not admittedly due to any reduction in infant mortality; the latter was still rising after 1850, and did not reach the mid-century level again until about 1885, to then drop again by 17 % by 1910.[18]

The figures for Mainz may thus be linked as follows: Of every 1000 deaths, the number of infants (0-1 year) was

1835—1872	328
1869—1873	325
1890—1896	292

for 1908 the figure was 15.7 infant deaths per 100 live births.[19]

The drop in infant mortality was thus clearly marked, and together with the general increase in life expectancy (which, according to Marschalck, was 37.0 years for the German Empire in 1871-1880, but already 46.6 years by 1901-1910[20]) led to the demographic transition which laid the foundation for the further explosion-like rise in the population figure.

In conclusion, we should like to take a brief look at the illnesses which contributed especially to mortality in the second half of the nineteenth century. The health authorities repeatedly issued ordinances on the prevention and containment of epidemics, and thus, for instance, in 1894 declared smallpox, typhoid fever and fleck-typhus, Asiatic cholera, scarlet fever, diphtheria and croup, epidemic cerebrospinal meningitis, puerperal fever and trichinosis to be notifiable diseases. This ordinance was extended in 1911 to cover leprosy, Oriental bubonic plague, anthrax, spinal infantile paralysism rabies, conjunctivitis and food poisoning.[21] Admittedly, that only included the spectacular diseases which could lead to a rapid death. The statistics compiled by the District Physician for 1869 to 1873, mentioned above, report on the practice. He determined on the basis of the causes of death that smallpox was then only causing deaths in a few cases. Scarlet fever, on the other hand, was still a widely spread children's disease occurring epidemically, and in 1873 it caused 40 deaths in combination with diphtheria which previously only had been rarely observed. Measles were also constantly occurring in epidemic form, but only caused deaths in combination with diphtheria. An average of 22 children died annually of whooping cough *(tussis convulsiva)* in the period under consideration, whereas the victims of diphtheria numbered some 18 annually. Some 29 people fell victim annually to abdominal typhus *("vulgo nervous fever")*, mainly in the 15 to 30 age group, while a total of 1154 died of tuberculosis in the five years from 1869 to 1873 (out of a total of 7425 deaths) giving an average annual figure of 17.4 %. If the other diseases of the respiratory organs are also added, they account for a total of 26.6 % of mortality as a whole.[22]

It can be calculated on the basis of the list of causes of death for 1896 that tuberculosis, with 14,78 %, and diseases of the respiratory organs, with 13.65 %, again lay to the fore among the causes of death. These were followed by enteritis in children with 13.0 %. For the first time, cancer and cancer-like neoplasms also appeared accounting for 5.98 %; in 1908 this heading accounted for 5.60 %. Tuberculosis, which in 1908 was the cause of 36 % of all cases of death in men aged between 20 and 50, had decreased slightly with 13.4 %; this was also true for diseases of the respiratory organs which with 218 out of 1870 cases still accounted for 11.7 % of the total mortality.[23]

Summary

To sum up, it may be said that mortality in Mainz had hardly declined at all up to the beginning of the last third of the nineteenth century. The causes of death had, it is true, changed: instead of the plague, which had last claimed victims in 1666, and smallpox, which raged in the eighteenth century, other diseases had appeared. Tuberculosis is probably the most difficult to record, as its effects on mortality in the early modern period can scarcely be calculated. It was only in the nineteenth century that medical statistics were able to supply information on how great the share was of those who died of this protracted disease. The old type of population with high natality and high mortality was not past with the political demise of the *ancien régime* in Mainz, but continued for a further seventy years. With the decrease in mortality, in which admittedly infant mortality lagged somewhat behind, the gap between the natality and mortality curves opened—with initially still a constantly high rate of fertility (still 29.8 per thousand on average for 1890 to 1896)—leading to the explosive growth in population. The demographic transition also began in Mainz from 1870 on, thus showing the city to be little different from the other regions in the German Empire.

Notes

1. Cf. W.G. Rödel, *Mainz und seine Bevölkerung im 17. und 18. Jahrhundert. Demographische Entwicklung, Lebensverhältnisse und soziale Strukturen in einer geistlichen Residenzstadt* (Stuttgart 1985).

2. F. Dumont, 'Vom kurfürstlichen zum hessischen Mainz', C. Jamme and O. Pöggeler (Eds.), *Mainz "Centralort des Reiches". Politik, Literatur und Philosophie im Umbruch der Revolutionszeit* (Stuttgart 1986), pp. 42-76.

3. L. Falck, 'Mainz', *Städtebuch Rheinland-Pfalz—Saarland* (Stuttgart 1964), pp. 254-291.

4. Rödel (1985), p. 32.

5. 'Bau-Ambtsordnung in der Stadt Mayntz', *Churfürstlich-Mayntzische Land-Recht und Ordnungen* (Mainz 1755), Tit. VII, pp. 65-73.

6. N. Adler 'Die Bemühungen um die Verlegung der Mainzer Friedhöfe vor die Stadt in der zweiten Hälfte des 18. Jahrhunderts', *Mainzer Almanach* (1963), pp. 60-73.

7. Rödel (1985), p. 55 et seq.

8. G. Krummeck and W.G. Rödel: 'Das Hospital St. Rochus in Mainz und seine Insassen. Ein Beitrag zur sozialen Schichtung und Mortalität in Spitälern des 18. Jahrhunderts', *Beiträge zur mittelrheinischen Landesgeschichte* (Wiesbaden 1980), pp. 230-259.

9. H. Terhalle, *Das Kurmainzer Medizinalwesen vom Spätmittelalter bis zum Ende des 18. Jahrhunderts,* Phil. Diss (Mainz 1965).

10. A. Helwig, *Beiträge zur Mortalitätsstatistik der Stadt Mainz. II. Die Sterblichkeit in den Jahren 1869 bis 1873* (Mainz 1874), p. 12.

11. Stadtarchiv Mainz 70/187 Jahresbericht des Grossherzoglichen Kreisgesundheitsamtes Mainz für das Jahr 1908.

12. Cf. Rödel (1985), pp. 194-249.

13. P. Guillaume and J.-P. Poussou, *Demographie historique* (Paris 1970), p. 145 et seq.

14. A. Kraus (Ed.), *Quellen zur Bevölkerungsstatistik Deutschlands 1815-1875* (Boppard 1980), Tab. 57.

15. P. Marschalck, *Bevölkerungsgeschichte Deutschlands im 19. und 20. Jahrhundert* (Frankfurt 1984), p. 41.

16. R.W. Lee: 'The Mechanism of Mortality Change in Germany 1750-1850', *Medizinhistorisches Journal,* 15 (1980), pp. 244-268.

17. Marschalck (1984), p. 34.

18. Marschalck (1984), p. 41.

19. Helwig (1874), p. 8.—Stadtarchiv Mainz 70/187 Tabelle der in der Stadt Mainz Gestorbenen 1890-1896.—Stadtarchiv Mainz 70/187 Jahresbericht des Ghzgl. Kreisgesundheitsamtes für 1908.

20. Marschalck (1984), p. 164.

21. Stadtarchiv Mainz XVII/9 Ansteckende und gemeingefährliche Krankheiten 1892-1937.

22. Helwig (1874), pp. 9-12.

23. Stadtarchiv Mainz 70/187.

(Translation: John M. Deasy, Mainz)

The Urban Penalty and the Population History of England

Gerry Kearns

This paper presents some speculations on the significance of urban mortality for the study of what McKeown christened "the modern rise of population".[1] One school of development-studies presents the links between population growth and wider social and economic changes within a model of the demographic transition. For these scholars, modernisation is associated with technological changes which in turn allow industrialisation, urbanisation, demographic transition and population growth. Technology is considered central because in raising agricultural productivity it releases people from the land. They can devote themselves to working at other things than producing food and may even move into towns to do so. At the same time, the easier availability of food may relax the positive check on population growth allowing a change from a high-pressure demographic régime of high-fertility/high-mortality to a low-pressure one of low-fertility/low-mortality. If the improvements in mortality are realised before the compensating fall in fertility, then, population growth will accompany the lagged transition.

Population growth and urbanisation over the "long" eighteenth century, 1670-1820

As a highly generalised model of the economic and demographic history of western Europe since 1700 and of more recent changes in the poor countries of today, the theory of the demographic transition is superficially attractive and promises to forge a link between economic history and development studies. Of course things were and are not quite this straigthforward and economic historians have drawn attention to a number of problems with the theory of the demographic transition. On one hand, they point out that pre-industrial Europe was never characterised by the sort of demographic systems now prevailing in many poor countries. Fertility was never persistently at what we would now recognise as high levels and, in the medium term, neither was mortality. Well before the industrial revolution, Europeans held back population growth, accumulating goods during better times and restraining fertility during worse. This control was exercised through nuptiality with Europeans having high rates of celibacy and marrying relatively late. Pre-industrial Europe was, as Jones concludes, already a low-pressure demographic régime compared to contemporary and modern Asia.[2]

A second source of empirical embarrassment for the theory of the demographic transition follows on from this and comes with the finding that English population changes in the period 1541-1871 were fuelled more by variations in fertility than by fluctuations in levels of mortality. Indeed, the leap in the total English population from about five million in the 1670s/1680s to about eleven-and-a-half million in the 1810s/1820s, the first leg of England's modern rise of population, was produced by a rise in fertility rather than by a lagged fall in mortality and then fertility: "the fertility rise contributed about two-and-a-half times as much to the rise in growth rates as the mortality fall."[3] Wrigley and Schofield show further that this rise in fertility was brought about by falls in both the age at first marriage and in the level of celibacy. In thus stressing the preventive rather than positive check on population growth, Wrigley and Schofield conclude that the economic history of pre-industrial England must now be looked at in a more positive light than when the period was seen as one in which people were pressed against the subsistence limit, buffeted by the impersonal forces of bugs and breezes.

Wrigley and Schofield's findings change our understanding of both the behavioural and the economic context of the population dynamics of pre-industrial England. If population changes were determined by autonomous fluctuations in mortality, then, the prime moves in the demographic system appear to have been beyond human choice and the pre-industrial English population could faithfully be presented as ground down between biological urges and environmental scourges. Should the relations between economy and demography run along the tracks of preventive rather than positive checks, then, the English people chose their own adjustment to available resources rather than having one imposed upon them. In decisively shifting the weight of evidence towards the second of these sets of possibilities, Wrigley and Schofield have restored the dignity of choice to the people of pre-industrial England. Turning from behaviour to economy, the implications here are equally profound. It is clear that the sustained rise in the rate of population growth in the eighteenth century was something very special. It implies such dramatic improvements in agricultural productivity that people were repeatedly able to choose higher fertility when, as Jones suggests, they had a general predilection for chattels over children during times of plenty. It was also achieved without bringing in its train a compensating rise in the cost of living, such as might have been expected to reverse the gains of the early eighteenth century. Yet population growth and stable prices were not the only evidence of increased productivity for they were accompanied by a significant rise in the share of the population not directly engaged in producing food. This is of both economic and demographic moment. Economically, the crucial variable is the ratio between people who produce food and those who do not. Leaving aside the question of age-specific dependence (the dependency ratio), the non-food-producers of pre-industrial England may be divided into a rural and an urban group. The rural artisans formed, suggests Wrigley, an increasingly substantial part of those living in the countryside, rising from 20% of the rural population in 1520, to 30% in 1670, to 50% in 1801.[4] In addition, practically all town-dwellers produced little or no food and to the rural non-food producers may be added the proportion of the total population living in places of 5,000 inhabitants or more, 5.25% in 1520, 13.5% in 1670 and 27.5% in 1801. In other words the food producers made up approximately four-fifths of the population in 1520, three-fifths in 1670 and one-third in 1801, leaving the rest to follow other pursuits. The demographic importance of this fall in the share of the people producing food relates to the different characteristics of urban and rural populations. This is where the debate over the role of mortality in English population growth might be re-opened.

On the face of it, the current state of scholarship in economic/demographic history appears to relegate mortality to a very lowly position in the explanation of English population growth. Of course, this directly challenges the long-held view of McKeown that declines in mortality were central to the modern rise of population. Wrigley and Schofield are in no doubt where their work leaves McKeown's arguments and note at one point: "the view that mortality played the dominant role in determining changes in population growth rates, whose most recent champion has been McKeown, must now be set aside so far as English demographic history in early modern times is concerned."[5] Certainly, McKeown's argument was rather simplistic and was spread across the whole period from 1700 to 1940.[6] Nevertheless, it is worth reconsidering the status of McKeown's conclusions in the light of the works summarised above since they have such wide currency.[7]

McKeown's argument is quite straightforward. In pre-industrial Europe, levels of fertility were at the biological maximum leaving no room for fertility-induced increases in population growth. Consequently, the European beginnings of the modern rise of population must have been the result of some relaxation of the mortality constraint. In other words, levels of mortality in pre-industrial Europe must have been substantially higher than those of the early nineteenth century. Yet while McKeown thus placed great emphasis on questions of health and disease in accounting for demographic development, in explaining declining mortality he laid little of the credit at the door of the medical profession. For whatever period he considered, the conclusion was the same: mortality has been more strongly influenced by diet than by medical care. McKeown said that he proceeded on the basis that "when we have eliminated the impossible, whatever remains, however improbable, must be the truth."[8] The problems for McKeown begin with the very first elimination in the argument. McKeown said nothing about marriage. Although he considered and dismissed abstention from intercourse in marriage, prolonged lactation, mechanical birth control, abortion and infanticide as effective controls on fertility in pre-industrial England, he ignored celibacy and age at marriage altogether. Hajnal has subsequently shown these to be the axes of a distinctive European marriage pattern.[9]

There is, it seems, no basis for continuing to accept McKeown's dismissal of the possibility of the preventive check in pre-industrial England. If the case for considering mortality when explaining population growth is to be established by elimination then it must fail. On the other hand, Wrigley and Schofield have made a very strong positive case for giving pride of place to fertility for the "long" eighteenth century. A positive case can be made, however, that mortality's importance is under-estimated in their work because they model a national population which in fact consisted of at least two distinct régimes (urban and rural), the relative weights of which changed substantially over this period. The rise in English population from 2.4 millions in 1520 to 5 millions in 1670 to 8.7 millions in 1800, on Wrigley and Schofield's estimates, was accompanied by substantial urbanisation, as detailed above. It is also apparent that urban living carried with it a significant demographic penalty. Rates of mortality in towns were sometimes substantially greater than those of the countryside. As Wrigley and Schofield remark: In the past, high density frequently brought high mortality in its turn. The absolute level of the mortality rates in Hartland /a rural coastal parish in Devon/ and Gainsborough /a market town in Lincolnshire/ differed by a factor of between two and three for the most part, a remarkable example of the variable incidence of mortality in pre-industrial England. Translated into rough estimates of expectation of life at birth, the two sets of mortality rates suggest that in Hartland in 1600-1749 it may have been 50 years or more at a time when it was only 30 years in Gainsborough.[10]

This geographical variability is greater than the improvement of aggregate mortality during England's eighteenth-century growth spurt: "Expectation of life at birth, which averaged only 32.4 years in the 1670s and 1680s at the start of the "long" eighteenth century had risen to an average of 38.7 years in the 1810s and 1820s at its end."[11] The geographical variability is also persistent and in 1861 is of the same order as in 1600-1749.[12] It is the relative stability of mortality in the aggregate which is striking when set alongside internal variations. Variation across space is more significant than variation over time. In relative terms one can speak of a low-mortality rural system and a high-mortality urban system. If urbanisation was associated with no change in the severity of the urban penalty, then, other things being equal, since a greater share of the population would be living in high risk areas, aggregate mortality should rise. Whereas if urbanisation is accompanied by relatively stable levels of aggregate mortality, then, it is possible either that rural mortality is falling to compensate or that the urban penalty is decreasing in severity.

216

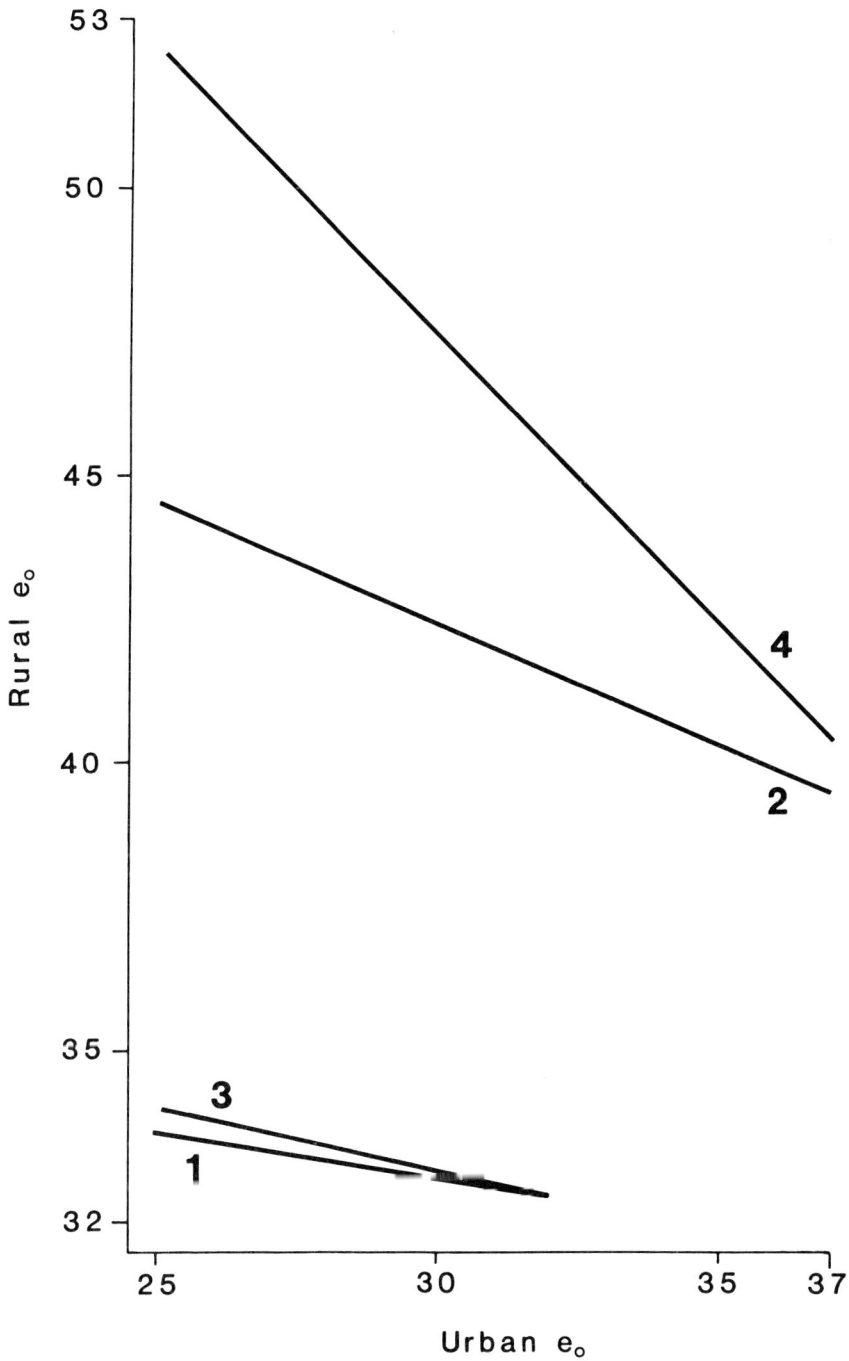

Figure 1. Some possible combinations of urban and rural life expectancies for different levels of urbanisation.

Hartland was clearly exceptional in 1600-1749 and there was certainly some scope for movement of general levels of rural mortality towards this low value over the eighteenth century. Gainsborough had a population of less than 5000 in 1600-1749 and has not even featured in the figures for urbanisation given above. If the urban penalty is paid in places of fewer than 5000 inhabitants then the proportion of the population in high risk areas obviously increases. For example, if Law's cut-off point of 2,500 is taken, then the urban share of 27.5% for places of 5000 or more in 1801 rises to 45% on this more generous definition.[13]

Given that the national life expectancy is the average of the rural and urban values weighted in proportion to their respective shares of the total population, the reasonable range of values of urban and rural life expectancies is easily estimated. Four situations are shown in Figure 1.

1. With national expectation of life at birth 32.4 years and 13.5% of the population living in towns, this illustrates the possible relations for 1670s/1680s on the assumption that the urban penalty is paid only in places with 5,000 inhabitants or more. Here the bulk of the population is rural and rural life expectancy can not depart too much from the national figure showing just how remarkable Hartland would have been at the time.

2. Should the proportion urbanised increase to 30% and the national life expectancy rise to 38.7 years (the situation by the 1810s/1820s if 5,000 is again the cut-off point), the likely combinations are dramatically changed. The rural share can reasonably be allowed to fluctuate a little further from the national average. If, for example, the urban life expectancy remained at 30 years over the "long" eighteenth century, to produce the observed rise in national life expectancy the rural value would need to have changed from 32.7 to 42.4, that is, about half as much again as the national improvement and the rural-urban differential would have gone from 2.7 years to 12.4 years. Woods gives a rural life expectancy of 42 years for 1821 for England and Wales, using 10,000 as the population defining urban areas, so that the improvement in rural mortality indicated by these assumptions is at least plausible.[14] Perhaps the rest of rural England was indeed catching up with Hartland and thus offsetting the urban penalty.

3. and 4. If, however, the urban penalty is paid in places of as few as 2,500 inhabitants, the rural improvement needs to have been even more dramatic. In the 1810s/1820s the share of the population in such towns was about 50% and if we guess at 18% for 1670s/1680s (18:13.5 = 50:30; although in fact the precise guess made makes little difference to the calculations for the earlier period), over this period a constant urban life expectancy of 30 years would have needed a rural improvement from 32.9 years to 47.4 years to secure a national change in life expectancy equal to that observed. This would have taken up all the slack between Hartland and the rest of rural England and is an almost incredible amelioration of mortality extending rural life expectancies by more than twice the national average.

Table 1. Some possible contrasts between urban and rural demographic régimes. * Assumed, □ read from graph.

	Quinquen. fertility mortality		Weighted average			Urban values			Rural values (Urban > 5,000)			Rural values (Urban > 2,500)		
	GRR	e_o	GRR	e_o	r	GRR	e_o	r	GRR	e_o	r	GRR	e_o	r
1676	1.906	36.37												
1681	1.935	28.47												
1686	2.170	31.77												
1674-1688			2.004	32.23	-0.18□	2.004*	30*	-0.40□	2.004*	32.57	-0.16□	2.004*	32.71	.0.14□
1816	3.056	37.86												
1821	2.981	39.24												
1826	2.885	39.92												
1814-1828			2.929	39.06	1.75□	2.959*	30*	0.90□	2.959*	42.94	1.95□	2.959*	48.12	2.20□

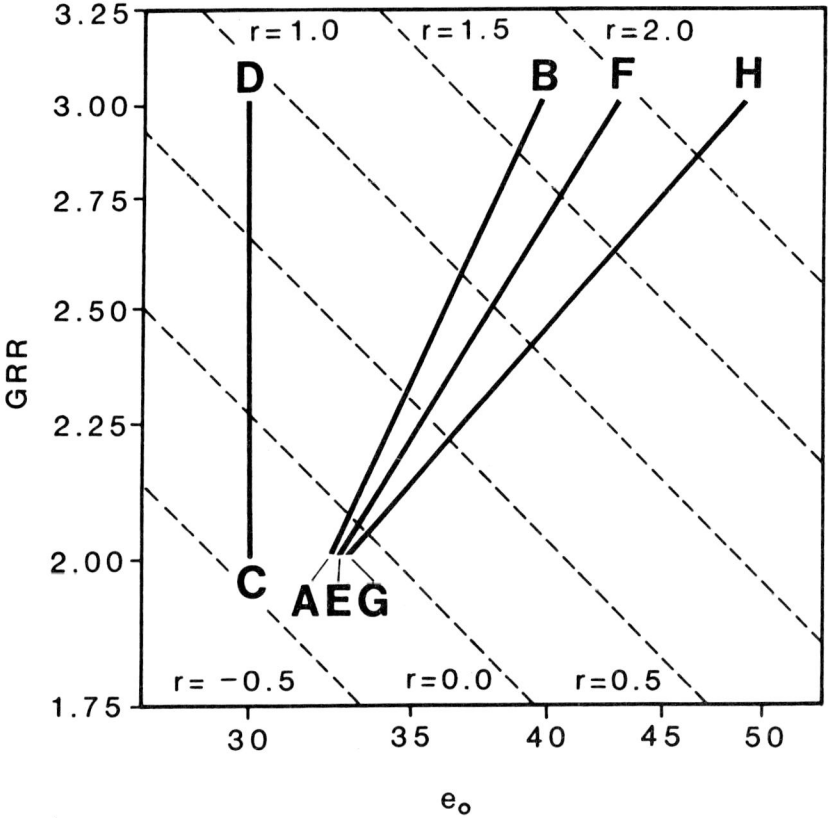

Figure 2. Mortality, fertility and population growth, some possible combinations 1670-1820.

Figure 2 is a simplistic attempt to illustrate some implications of these alternatives. AB is the national change in vital rates (GRR — gross reproduction rate; eo — expectation of life at birth) over the "long" eighteenth century taking a 3-point weighted average of quinquennial rates centred on 1681 for its start and 1811 at its close, using Wrigley and Schofield's data and their ingenious graph.[15] The gradient of the line is 2 so that fertility contributed about twice as much as mortality to the observed change in growth rates (r — intrinsic rate of growth). If the same fertility rates are ascribed to urban and rural populations but we make adjustments to their respective rates of mortality, it is possible to show some of the possible consequences of the argument above. If urban life expectancy remains unchanged at 30 (CD), then, the rate of intrinsic rate of growth of this group would of course have been lower than the national total at both the beginning and the end of the period (see Table 1). Two alternative rural trajectories are shown on the basis of a cut-off point for the urbanised population of 5,000 (EF) and, more generously, 2,500

(GH). The assumption of common rates of fertility means that the higher than average rural life expectancies take the intrinsic growth rate of the rural population way past the national total by the end of the period. More intriguingly, these assumptions change the gradient of the line so that on a modest definition of the urban share, with no significant improvement in urban mortality and comparable fertility in urban and rural areas, the change in rural intrinsic rates of growth would still have been based more on fertility than mortality, but now in ratio 1.5:1. However, the broader definition of urban, with the same assumptions about general fertility and urban mortality, requires that the change in rural growth rates be the product equally of fertility and mortality improvements.

Urbanisation, therefore, poses certain problems for studies of the population changes of national aggregates. National averages are valid summary measures in synchronic studies and in many cases are the only parameters which can be reliably calibrated given the lack of information of internal migration. In diachronic studies they are at best a convenient fiction applying to a different entity at different times. It is likely that if England is modelled as one population over the period of its impressive growth spurt, the "long" eighteenth century, then, the significant changes in the mix of high- and low-risk peoples in this aggregate hides the true importance of mortality changes in relation to changes in fertility. If rural and urban fertility differ to a markedly lesser degree than do rural and urban mortality, then it will indeed be specifically the mortality variable which is passed-over too lightly in national studies. For English population history in the early modern period, the importance of changes in mortality in fuelling population growth, therefore, is perfectly compatible with significant contemporary shifts in fertility and even with such shifts being apparently more significant at the national level.

Mortality changes and urbanisation in the nineteenth century

If the rate of urban mortality at the start of the nineteenth century was similar to the national average for rural and urban England in the late seventeenth century, then, the increase in the level of urbanisation over this period leads the national figures to understate the improvement in rural mortality. For the first half of the nineteenth century, the aggregate mortality improvement is comparable to that of the whole eighteenth century. On Woods' estimates, this now downplays a more signficant decline in urban mortality. The national life expectancy at birth for England and Wales, according to Woods, was extended from 38 years to 41 years during the period 1811 to 1861. Londoners experienced a more dramatic improvement, their life expectancy rising from 30 to 37 years. For large towns (with populations of over 100,000), the figures were 30 and 35 and other towns (populations of between 10,000 and 100,000) saw a change from 32 to 40. Only the rural (residual) areas (1811: 41; 1861: 45) appear to replicate the more sluggish national figures. The urban leap forward is pulled back by the transfer of a larger share of the population into these high-risk areas. The urban areas have to run if the national figures are even to stand still. Figure 3 is a simple illustration of this. The line going from the lower left-hand part of the graph to the upper-right shows the progress of national life expectancy at birth from 38 to 53 over the century 1811 to 1911.[16] The other lines present national averages based on the respective mortalities of the four groups (London, large towns, other towns, rural) at different dates applied to the changing proportions of the population actually in those groups at different times. Thus if the share of the population in towns grew as it did over the nineteenth century but the urban penalty had remained constant, then, the national average life expectancy would have deteriorated in line with the transfer of people into high risk areas. By 1911 urbanisation would have reduced life expectancy at birth from the 38 of 1811 to 33, whereas in fact it actually rose to 53. Similarly, if the mortality rates of 1911 had coincided with the lower urban shares of 1811, then, eo would have been greater than 53 but, because the urban penalty was so much lower by 1911, the improvement induced by shifting people out of relatively-high risk areas is less dramatic and eo would have risen only by a further two years.

Figure 3. The interaction of urbanisation and life expectancy at birth; England and Wales, 1811-1911.

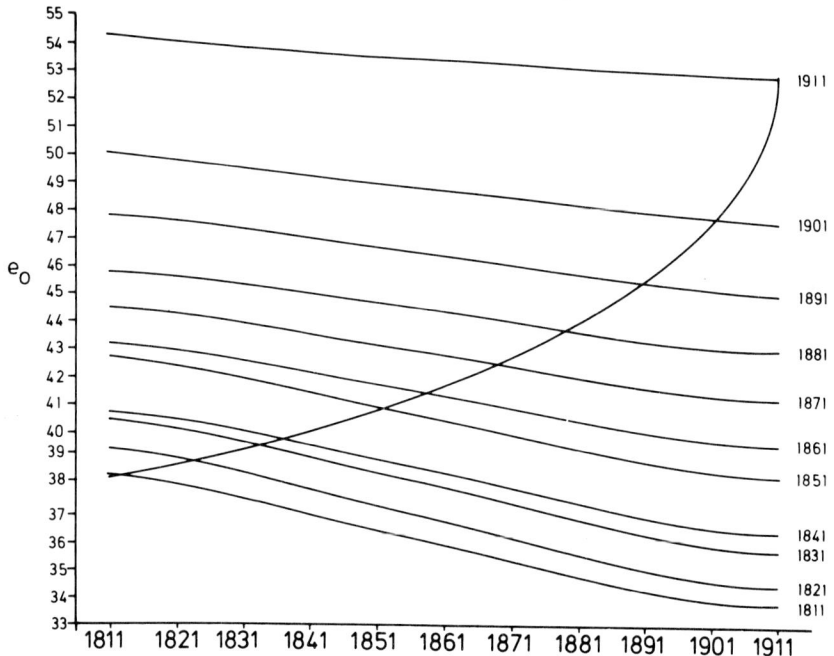

222

A central feature of any explanation of mortality changes over the nineteenth century must be an account of the near removal of the urban penalty. In 1811 when people in urban areas (over 10,000 in population) had a life expectancy of 31 years, rural areas were ten years better-off at 41, by 1861 the gap was seven years (38 and 45 years) and in 1911 it was only three (55 and 52). Yet when McKeown and Record consider the matter they conclude that general economic conditions as they affect diet and nutrition were primarily responsible for at least half the decline in national mortality over the second half of the nineteenth century. This implies either that the specifically urban penalty is poor diet or that the mortality changes of rural areas were so overwhelmingly diet-based that they swamped the specifically urban developments. As a prelude to exploring these issues, the rest of this paper considers how McKeown and Record establish a conclusion which is widely accepted as an axiom by sociologists, economists and historians.

McKeown and Record's approach is engagingly direct. For England and Wales in two decades (1851-1860 and 1891-1900), they provide death-rates for various causes standardised to the age structure of the population of 1901. They give the share of certain causes in the aggregate decline. They associate sets of causes with particular controlling factors and thereby establish the priority of certain factors in accounting for the decline in mortality in England and Wales over the second half of the nineteenth century. McKeown and Record compute the fall in standardised mortality to be about 3 per thousand over this period and the fall in tuberculosis rates to be equivalent to one half of this, and thus diet is set in place as primum mobile. After this comes the sanitary revolution with a third of the decline accountable to fevers and diarrhoeal diseases. A fifth is due to a spontaneous change in the virility of a disease organism (scarlet fever). Finally, medical intervention (vaccination) is credited with the one-fifteenth of the fall set down to smallpox. Doctors are relegated behind bread, brushes and bugs.[17] Have McKeown and Record correctly identified the salient features of the mortality decline and have they explained them adequately? An analysis along the broad lines they propose is certainly attractive which is why their approach is worth refining. The scope of these comments is more modest still because they are methodological rather than substantive.

Tables 2 and 3 present the age-specific death rates in England and Wales for the different causes of death identified in the Registrar General's Decennial Supplements of 1851-1860 and 1891-1900.[18] It is possible to present them separately for the two sexes but only their respective age-specific rates are given here. Male, female and total cause-specific rates were standardised to the total age structure of 1901 and these are the basis of Table 4 and Figure 4. The final column of Table 4 is what McKeown and Record base their analysis on and the table is arranged so that their key diseases rise to the top and the residual groups are arranged according to the reverse order in which they were dropped from the analysis. The table also shows the ratio between the male

Table 2. Age/cause-specific death rates (per million living), England and Wales; 1851–1860.

Cause of death	0	1-4	5-9	10-14	15-19	20-24	25-34	35-44	45-54	55-64	56-74	gt.-74	Total
a. Smallpox	1602	801	257	73	93	130	93	55	38	24	18	14	222
b. Measles	2158	2885	275	38	13	9	6	4	2	1	1	2	412
c. Scarlatina	1736	4814	1995	495	150	73	44	31	19	15	10	7	877
d. Diptheria	288	458	254	104	42	20	13	12	10	10	13	16	109
e. Whooping cough	5916	2707	174	10	2	1	1	0	0	0	1	1	504
f. Typhus	904	1523	1009	782	944	814	649	623	713	965	1413	1543	909
g. Cholera	14125	2110	229	106	111	175	257	347	477	934	2196	5136	1082
h. Other zymotic	6334	2204	459	179	187	189	261	396	545	878	1734	3093	834
i. Cancer	28	19	9	9	17	28	104	390	862	1414	1964	2085	317
j. Scrofula	3633	1271	283	233	208	170	139	111	117	140	165	113	408
k. Phthisis	2032	1007	573	1027	2964	4182	4321	4102	3475	2848	1987	809	2683
l. Hydrocephalus	4024	1937	364	102	31	10	7	6	6	7	7	8	398
m. Brain	33404	2910	583	359	403	437	583	1024	1837	3963	9353	16180	2745
n. Heart	662	285	228	257	338	370	561	1064	1988	4364	8841	11665	1249
o. Lungs	21936	6137	597	231	339	476	673	1283	2572	5807	12149	19704	3025
p. Stomach	3368	556	252	207	288	369	520	916	1639	3007	4769	4948	1006
q. Kidneys	51	50	35	39	60	86	140	220	339	617	1396	2114	215
r. Generative	11	4	0	1	8	25	52	109	153	167	179	149	55
s. Joints	58	51	62	78	76	58	52	59	71	103	141	115	70
t. Skin	462	54	11	9	10	11	13	22	37	80	197	370	49
u. Childbirth	0	0	0	0	72	323	465	465	36	0	0	0	164
v. Violent	1760	1085	536	469	508	516	542	652	810	976	1225	2248	735
w. Other	49508	3269	291	166	184	208	270	448	845	2618	14110	89585	4132
Male	168404	36512	8523	4931	6696	8836	9578	12506	17996	30951	65474	165528	23081
Female	138930	35758	8432	5062	7394	8542	9934	12180	15240	27075	58777	155574	21360
Total	153999	36136	8477	4974	7047	8681	9764	12339	16586	28937	61869	159899	22200

224

Table 3. Age/cause-specific death rates (per million living), England and Wales; 1891-1900.

Cause of death	0	1-4	5-9	10-14	15-19	20-24	25-34	35-44	45-54	55-64	65-74	gt.74	Total
i. Smallpox	55	20	10	3	5	11	16	18	13	10	10	8	13
ii. Measles	3319	3120	221	18	7	4	4	3	2	1	1	0	413
iii. Scarlet F.	290	979	353	81	33	22	15	8	4	2	1	0	157
iv. Diptheria	457	1584	679	125	36	20	16	14	12	14	12	9	263
v. Whooping C.	5810	2060	96	3	1	0	0	0	0	1	1	3	376
vi. Typhus F.	0	1	1	2	2	2	3	4	4	2	1	2	2
vii. Enteric F.	24	97	127	162	256	271	283	189	144	112	69	29	174
viii. Continued F.	23	17	7	4	3	3	3	3	4	5	9	13	6
ix. Diarrhoea	17521	1169	33	9	7	9	18	31	70	204	675	2035	712
x. Cholera	462	41	4	1	2	2	4	8	15	29	32	29	25
xi. Cancer	22	31	16	16	29	44	138	644	1828	3651	5594	6129	756
xii. Tabes Mes.	3721	661	103	68	57	46	38	34	30	27	21	9	216
xiii. Phthisis	561	345	206	367	1141	1726	2129	2585	2355	1876	1152	436	1388
xiv. Other T.B.	3573	1471	415	234	194	160	129	115	101	99	88	65	402
xv. Nervous	21745	2061	382	222	244	237	381	932	1910	4456	10501	19583	2166
xvi. Circulatory	502	88	169	266	334	336	541	1232	2634	6121	12958	19613	1653
xvii. Respiratory	27727	6778	587	173	277	380	647	1425	2900	6637	14476	29677	3401
xviii.Digestive	14186	1457	225	162	218	247	307	636	1226	2160	3540	5063	1190
xix. Urinary	246	145	71	56	77	118	203	438	812	1544	2936	4672	460
xx. Generative	43	9	1	2	10	22	47	87	106	104	149	176	46
xxi. Puerperal F.	0	0	0	0	24	155	220	134	5	0	0	0	68
xxii. Childbirth	0	0	0	0	25	131	240	255	16	0	0	0	84
xxiii. Violent	3029	748	357	224	326	362	447	647	875	118	1450	2560	659
xxiv. Other	50178	1364	307	307	412	422	600	1040	1644	3212	11254	61656	3523
Male	167775	24312	4309	2447	3782	5046	6738	11466	18894	34852	70286	159692	19272
Female	138360	23688	4370	2565	3658	4449	6065	9566	14702	28361	60606	146063	17101
Total	153326	24248	4340	2506	3720	4730	6384	10485	16711	31385	64931	151768	18152

and female standardised rates at each date and the proportionate change in the standardised rate for each cause over the period.[19] Figure 4 shows some of this information graphically. The height of the histograms corresponds to the standardised mortality rate in 1851-1860, broken down into some of the major causes of death on the left and into age-groups on the right.[20] The shaded area depicts the decline in mortality over the period and shows the proportionate reduction in standardised rates for each cause- and age-category.

On the same basis a deterioration in specific mortality will take any particular cause- or age-group beyond the boundary of the 1851-1860 histogram. In this way, the area shaded for each category is proportional to its contribution to the overall fall in national standardised mortality. With this figure and these tables, two comments might be made on the analysis by McKeown and Record. They make little use of sex-specific mortality, age-specific mortality and mortality from their groups of "others" for diagnostic purposes. Furthermore, some questions remain about their identification of the causes they do have recourse to.

In both these decades, life was shortest for men. For 1861 Preston, Keyfitz and Schoen give an expectation of life at birth of 40.5 for males in England and Wales and 43.1 for females; for 1901 their respective figures are 45.3 years and 49.4 years.[21] The gap is increasing at a time of general improvement in mortality. In explaining mortality decline, therefore, our account must be compatible with the improvements it identifies being most particular visited upon females. Table 4 shows that male mortality was worst for most causes and that female mortality was improving faster for most causes. For some of the major causes of death, the relative sluggishness of male rates is quite marked. In the case of respiratory tuberculosis, the male standardised rate in 1891-1900 is 61% of the 1851-1860 figure while the female rate is only 42%. This ought to have some bearing on how reasons are assigned for the decline in mortality, both as a whole and as regards the contribution of particular causes.

As figure 4 shows there is no improvement in infant mortality over this period and there is a deterioration in the mortality of the elderly; if 45 for men and 55 for women is not too inappropriate a cut-off point for the use of this term. This pattern is relatively consistent between the sexes with the female improvement being significantly greater than the male in adulthood (15-44). It is clear from Tables 2 and 3 that the mortality improvements are concentrated in the middle years of life whereas the greatest mortality was found among the old and the young. In this respect the one-third fall in child mortality is especially striking. Indeed a fall in the standardised rate resulting from a decline in child mortality will have a much greater impact on the survivorship curve and thus on life expectancy than will a fall of the same magnitude caused by falling adult mortality.

226

(1)	(2)	(3)	(4)	(5)	(6)	(7)
	1851-1860		1891-1900		Change	
Cause of death	s.m.r.	Male/Female	s.m.r.	Male/Female	(4/2)	(2-4)

A. Communicable diseases contributing greatly to mortality decline

Resp. T.B. (k;xiii)	2760	94	1410	133	51	1350
Other T.B. (j,l;xiii,xvii)	685	123	570	116	83	115
Typhus (f;vi,vii,viii)	890	100	183	132	21	707
Scarlet F. (c;iii)	775	102	150	100	19	625
Diarrhoeal (g;ix,x)	923	106	631	111	68	292
A. Total	6033		2944			3089

B. Certain other communicable diseases

Smallpox (a;i)	195	117	13	149	7	182
Whooping C. (e;v)	408	78	338	79	83	70
Measles (b,ii)	349	101	385	105	110	-36
Diptheria (d;iv)	98	89	251	95	256	-153
B. Total	1050		987			63

C. Certain other causes distinguished in McKeown and Record

Brain (m;xv)	2410	118	2054	118	85	356
Heart (n;xvi)	1272	95	1665	107	131	-393
Lungs (o;xvii)	2767	123	3249	125	117	-482
Stomach (p;xviii)	992	102	1116	108	113	-124
Kidneys (q;xix)	219	286	463	179	211	-244
C. Total	7660		8547			-887

D. Other causes

Cancer (i;xi)	328	48	764	72	232	-281
Other zymotic dis. (h)	748	124				(748)
Generative (r;xx)	57	4	47	8	82	10
Joints (s)	68	135				(68)
Skin (t)	44	113				(44)
Childbirth (u;xxi;xxii)	173	0	156	0	90	17
Violence (v;xxiii)	715	307	649	264	91	66
Other (w;xxiv)	3606	106	3270	114	91	336
D. Total	5739		4886			853
All causes	20482	108	17364	115	85	3119

Figure 4. Mortality decline in England and Wales, 1851-1860 to 1891-1900.

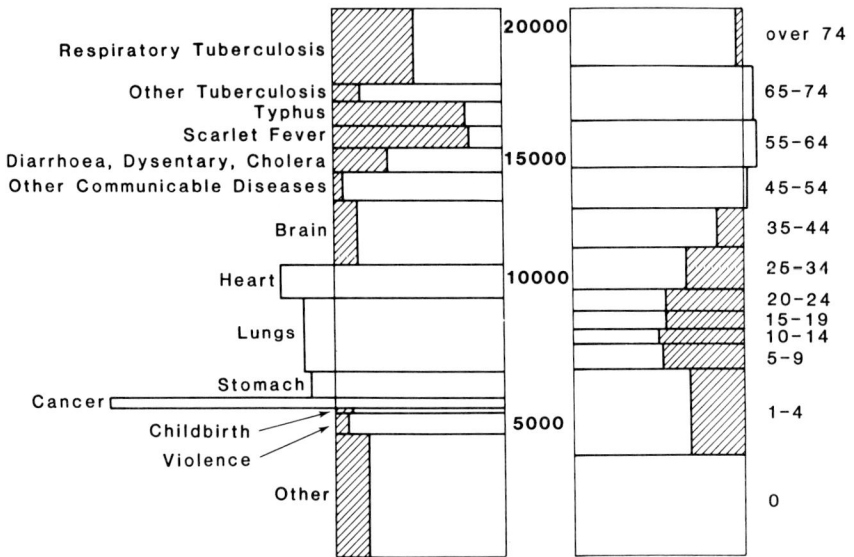

In measuring the mortality decline, age- and sex-specific factors are only touched on implicitly by McKeown and Record insofar as those factors come out in the wash of aggregate rates due to the five selected causes. Taking up the question of measuring the mortality decline due to specific causes, the first point to be made is that McKeown and Record discard most causes of death from their analysis. The five sets of causes on which they focus (Group A in Table 4) make up about one-third of the standardised mortality in 1851-1860 and a sixth in 1891-1900. They argue that these causes are identified as significant by their contribution to the mortality decline. With the standardised rates for England and Wales going from 20482 per million living to 17364 per million and these causes going from 6033 to 2944, they seem to more than adequately account for the mortality decline. Table 4 attempts to show the effect of thus comparing gross falls from specific causes to the net fall from all causes. Broadly speaking, the category "other" holds a host of diverging mortalities, some improving some deteriorating. These others by no means equal the changes identified by McKeown and Record but the relative stability of the "others" category is an arithmetic fiction. We can easily illustrate this. In Groups B, C and D the final column shows eight sets of causes deteriorating in mortality and ten improving. Some of these causes are only given for one decade so the comparison is probably meaningless. Nevertheless, the sum of the positive changes is quivalent to a change in the standardised mortality rate of 1897 per million, not insignificant when set alongside the net change of 3118 per million and certainly raising questions about dismissing "other" causes as a relatively stable residual.

Part of the problem, as McKeown and Record recognise, arises from disease classification, misclassification and reclassification. The disease classification recognised three main categories of disease: those which "ferment" in the body quickly, feverishly dispatching it from this life; those which work slowly, wearing the body down; and those which are malfunctions of particular cogs in the mortal motor. Yet symptoms were often ambiguous guides in thus distributing deaths. McKeown and Record are right to remind modern readers that contemporaries were a good deal more familiar with these diseases than is the modern European physician. Yet if one wished to be mischievous one might begin by questioning three of the five sets of causes on which McKeown and Record hang their analysis.

First, their own discussion raises doubts about the distinction between scarlet fever and diptheria in 1851-1860 since they complain of "the confusion between scarlet fever and diptheria until 1855".[22] This would be less significant were it not for the fact that scarlet fever declines while diptheria increases. If there is some diptheria in the scarlet fever figures for 1851-1860, then, the fall in scarlet fever has been overstated. The net fall from scarlet fever and diptheria combined is 472 per million and the stated fall from scarlet fever is 625. Even on this, the least helpful assumption for their argument, their conclusion about scarlet fever seems safe.

A second disease category worth looking at is typhus. Leaving to one side the different histories of typhus and typhoid, it is clear that the fevers as a whole present problems.

McKeown and Record equate the typhus of 1851-1860 with three separate categories in 1891-1900: typhus, enteric and simple continued fevers. Yet if we are looking for that complex of fevers which contemporaries associated with environmental improvements (the purpose of isolating typhus), one might ask where the "other zymotic diseases" of 1851-1860 have gone. Certainly, contemporaries noted a great improvement in these but this is lost, firstly because they are not separately distinguished in the decennial table for 1891-1900 and secondly because McKeown and Record sweep them up with the residual "other causes" in 1851-1860. If enteric and simple continued fevers are to be added to typhus as a fevers-complex in 1891-1900, a reasonable case might be heard for adding some of the "other zymotic diseases" in 1851-1860. The consequences are of moment. Typhus alone (if the bulk of the 1851-1860 figure refers to this) falls from 890 to 2 per million, adding in enteric and simple continued fevers for 1891-1900 reduces the fall by 181 but adding in other zymotic diseases increases it by 748. We have a fall in the fevers-complex which ranges from 707 to 1455 per million. The latter figure is greater than that set down to respiratory tuberculosis and if the sanitary revolution were measured by the diarrhoeal and fevers sets of causes, it would only require three-fifths of the "other zymotic" category to be added to the fevers before the environmental factor would give a fall equal to that of McKeown and Record's tubercular diet and nutrition factor.

Figure 5. Change in age-specific mortality rates for respiratory tuberculosis, chest diseases and other causes.

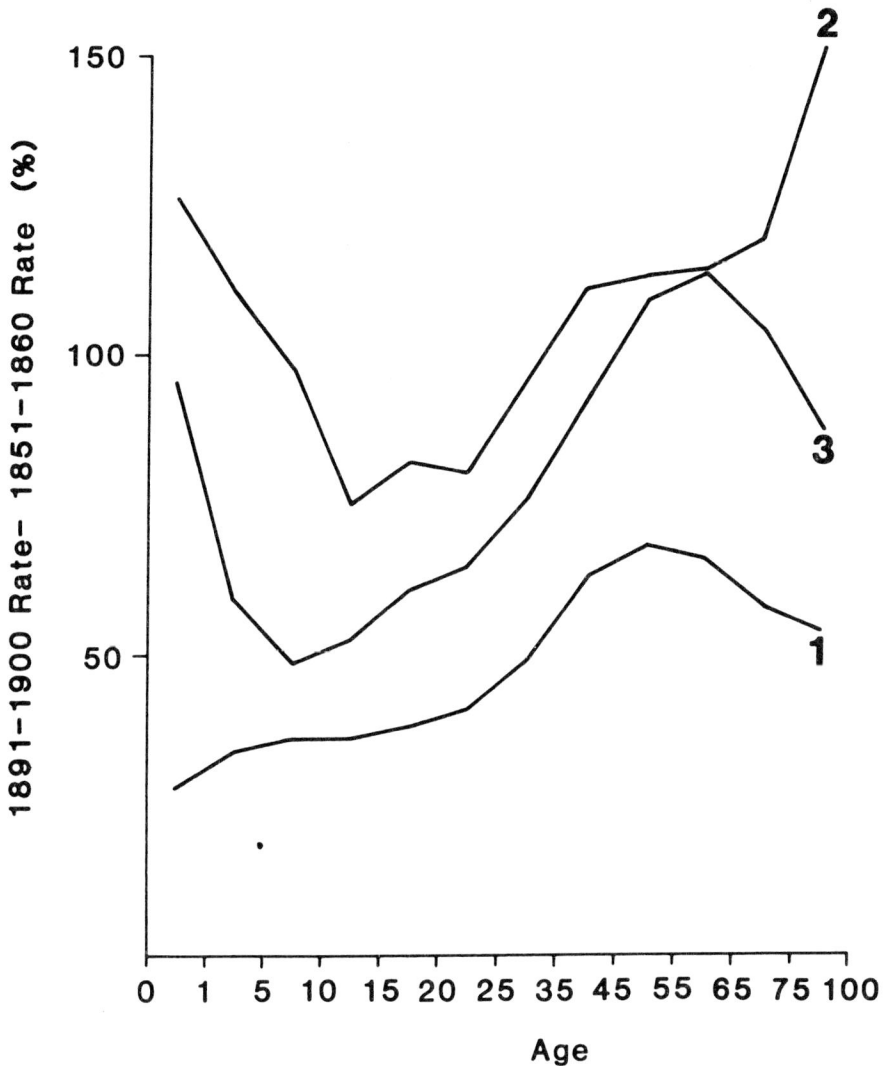

The third set of causes we might reconsider is respiratory tuberculosis. The fall in respiratory tuberculosis was accompanied by a rise in diseases of the lungs. The first point to make is that, as can be seen from Table 4, the fall in standardised rates due to respiratory tuberculosis (1350 per million) far outstrips the deterioration in diseases of the lungs (482 per million). Secondly, from Tables 2 and 3, it is clear that diseases of the lungs are afflictions of the young and old but respiratory tuberculosis stalks the relatively healthy years of adulthood, being responsible for 41% of all deaths between the ages of 15 and 45 in 1851-1860. There is little evidence here that the two disease categories are equivalent. Over time, their distinctiveness becomes even more pronounced which may suggest some confusion in the earlier period. Figure 5 shows the proportionate change in mortality at the different ages for respiratory tuberculosis (1) and diseases of the lungs (2); equivalent data for all other causes (3) is given for comparison.

Between ages 5 and 55, the two diseases share the general pattern of improvements in mortality being concentrated in early adulthood but the changes for the young and old are divergent for the two causes. Although the disease was primarily an adult-killer, one-fifteenth of all phthisis deaths in 1851-1860 were registered to those under five years of age, whereas in 1891-1900 the figure was one in twenty-eight. The changes in mortality due to respiratory tuberculosis at these ages are commensurate with the increases assigned to diseases of the chest, and similarly for the oldest age groups. The worst case would be to suggest that the bulk of the improvement in respiratory tuberculosis among the under-fives and the over-sixty-fives can be explained by a greater tendency in the later period for deaths in these age-groups to receive the less-specific label "diseases of the respiratory system" rather than the more precise term "phthisis". This would wipe-out one-sixth of the fall in standardised rates displayed by respiratory tuberculosis. If we confine our skepticism to the younger age group the effect is less and about one-fourteenth of the improvement is removed. In terms of the balance between the factors explaining the mortality decline, any adjustment along these lines will narrow the gap between the nutrition factor and the sanitary revolution. There is at least a prima facie case for looking again at the statistics of respiratory tuberculosis.

When all is said and done, considerations such as those above will only put wider margins of error around any conclusions we may draw on the basis of cause of death statistics, we can obviously never replace a historical and messy set with a modern and tidy one. We have to work with what we have got. The main attraction of McKeown and Record's analysis has been that they used cause of death statistics to say something definite about the factors controlling mortality. It has been hinted above that age and sex might also be powerful diagnostic tools and question marks have been placed against the relative sizes of the falls associated with their environmental and nutrition factors. Their measurement of mortality change needs its possible margins of error spelling out. When that is done there is still the matter of interpretation. In at least two respects their equation of causes and factors may be queried. First, there is their claim that the primary control on tuberculosis was exerted by nutrition. Secondly, there is the question of the interaction between causes of death.

So much depends on McKeown and Record's interpretation of the decline in tuberculosis mortality that it is worth looking at this factor again. Tuberculosis, they suggest, was primarily responsive to changes in the quality of diet: "incomplete as it is, the evidence for the nineteenth century is at least consistent with the view that diet was the most significant environmental influence in relation to the trend of mortality from tuberculosis."[23] By this, they do not mean that they have found evidence that the quality of diet advanced faster in places where tuberculosis fell dramatically, nor do they mean that the chronology of mortality decline follows that of certain indicators of real income. Rather, they fail to turn up evidence for other hypotheses and are left holding this one. Livi-Bacci has recently commented on the simplistic way historical demographers turn to nutrition in explaining long term trends in mortality and there is certainly a body of evidence to suggest that respiratory tuberculosis is not one of those diseases where nutrition exerts a strong influences on rates of fatality.[24] With a respiratory disease, one might expect a primary control to be exerted by contact with infected persons and among other things one would might pay close attention to overcrowding. In the nineteenth century, McKeown and Record inform us, "new building of houses did little more than keep pace with the increase in the size of the population, and the number of persons per house decreased only slightly (from 5.6 in 1801 to 5.3 in 1871)."[25] Despite these statistics, it is hard to believe that in certain cities the problem of overcrowding did not fluctuate in ways which might allow one to re-examine the claim that diet was the primary determinant of receding rates of respiratory tuberculosis. Certainly, the development of new bye-law housing in cities such as Liverpool over the second half of the nineteenth century may have diluted the problem of overcrowding for the working class. McKeown and Record also countenance no improvement in the quality of milk before the 1922 Ministry of Health Order on the pasteurisation of milk yet city authorities were aware of the problem of infected milk and at least towards the close of our period made efforts to control the milk supply drawing particularly on districts which they felt to be relatively free from infection. In addition the vigorous campaign against urban cowkeepers conducted throughout this period may have improved the salubrity of dairies offering some prospect of falls in bovine tuberculosis. With this, as with other diseases, a multiplicity of factors may be at work and the aim of the analysis should be to explore these through comparative analysis of different places and periods. McKeown and Record's residual reliance on nutrition indicates that the issue is still open.They have not proved that general economic improvement rather than specific medical or sanitary interventions was the primary motor of progress.

If it is difficult to assign a unique factor to a single disease it is also hard to confine a particular factor to a solitary disease. McKeown and Record proceed as if the effectiveness of any intervention may be limited to falls in the disease it immediately touches upon. One needs to distinguish here between using changes in the mortality from certain diseases as indicative of certain improvements and using those changes as measurements of the contribution of those improvements. McKeown and Record have followed the latter and more difficult path. There are certain problems involved with thus considering diseases in isolation. If we consider the consequences of the sanitary revolution and of medical intervention which they associate with fevers plus diarrhoeal diseases and with smallpox respectively, we can easily appreciate the problem. Cleanliness obviously reduces exposure to certain of the infections producing both respiratory and bowel complaints; it is difficult to understate the importance of clean hands. McKeown and Record look to fever and diarrhoeal diseases to register the sanitary revolution in water supply, drains and sewers. As indicators that improvements have been made, this seems helpful and a comparative study of different cities along these lines might be instructive. However, as a measurement of the consequences of the sanitary revolution this is potentially misleading. Diseases obviously interact and a generally lower level of infection might save individuals from debilitating complaints which lay them low before the depredations of some other, unrelated killer. The same goes for smallpox and their medical factor. The practical eradication of smallpox over this period points to the success of a variety of control strategies and by investigating the geography of this conquest one might begin to evaluate those strategies. Yet the importance of smallpox extended beyond the immediate deaths it claimed to the scores more who bore its disfiguring marks for the rest of their lives and to those whose constitutions were permanently impaired by an attack of this vigorous disease at a time when their young bodies should have been developing apace. In other words, McKeown and Record's hypotheses and methods are suggestive rather than conclusive and their air of precise accounting is deceptive. The causes of death which capitalised upon victims weakened by early smallpox or repeated stomach or chest infections may well appear in boxes far removed from the "sanitary revolution" or "medical intervention" but it is these two latter developments which have deprived them of their mortality tribute all the same.

A lot of the issues raised in this consideration of McKeown and Record's account of the decline in mortality in nineteenth-century England and Wales are almost impossible to explore with aggregate data at a national level. Data on individual life histories would be ideal but there is a halfway post which is worth exploring further. Given the importance of the geographical redistribution of people between rural and urban areas and given the relations which may exist between labour markets and sex- and age-specific mortality, there may be a lot to be gained in following a comparative approach in comparing rural and urban mortality and in looking at the histories of individual cities.[26]

Urban mortality and the context of population change

This paper has considered two issues. First is the claim that the population history of England in the early modern period resonates to an economic rhythm heard mainly through the preventive check. In this respect, urbanisation and urban mortality pose some difficulties for attempts to isolate mortality and fertility effects at a purely aggregate level. Some playful alternatives have been proposed all of which rely on urban mortality being more sluggish in improving than rural mortality in eighteenth century England. The second claim which this paper has reconsidered is that mortality changes in the nineteenth century can largely be set down to changes in diet and that, as such, they are an almost unconscious benefit of economic development in general rather than a tribute to specific interventionist measures. Here, it has been suggested that the matter is far from closed because the identification, apportionment and interpretation of the mortality decline might still be subject to contention. In particular, the sorts of measures one associates with better urban management may have contributed to the decline in respiratory tuberculosis, their effect on mortality from fevers may have been understated and the effects of changes in employment patterns have not yet been explored.

In terms of general economic history restating the importance of the urban penalty might have a number of consequences. First, it may reinforce the view of the rapid development of British agriculture in the eighteenth century. Ironically, it appears to leave open the door for an exploration of dietary improvements in rural England, operating as a long term trend rather than through short-term crises. Alternatively, it may return our attention to the towns as ecological gatekeepers with rural areas sharing in the benefits of a more effective exclusion of infectious or epidemic disease from the country. This is a theme which could extend over the whole period 1500-1940 and which requires that we explore the correlations between cause-specific mortality declines across countries with very different economic histories.

Acknowledgements

I want to thank John Rogers, Lars-Göran Tedebrand, Paul Laxton and Robert Lee for their encouragement and advice as well as seminar groups at Liverpool, Nottingham, Uppsala and Umeå for their constructive criticism.

Notes

1. As McKeown defines the term, "it will be taken to refer to the growth of population which began in the late seventeenth or early eighteenth century and has continued to the present day"; T. McKeown, *The Modern Rise of Population* (London 1976), p.1.

2. E.L. Jones, *The European Miracle: Environments, Economies and Geopolitics in the History of Europe and Asia* (Cambridge 1981).

3. E.A. Wrigley, 'The Growth of Population in Eighteenth-Century England: a Conundrum Resolved', *Past and Present*, 98 (1983), pp. 121-150, p. 131. See also R.S. Schofield, 'The Impact of Scarcity and Plenty on Population Change in England, 1541-1871', *Journal of Interdisciplinary History,* 14 (1983), pp. 265-291. These two articles present some of the main findings of their book, E.A. Wrigley and R.S. Schofield, *The Population History of England, 1541-1871: a Reconstruction* (London 1981).

4. These and the other statistics in this paragraph are taken from E.A. Wrigley, 'Urban Growth and Agricultural Change: England and the Continent in the Early Modern Period', *Journal of Interdisciplinary History,* 15 (1985), pp. 683-728.

5. Wrigley and Schofield (1983), p. 484.

6. The main works are as follows: T. McKeown and R.G. Brown, 'Medical Evidence Related to English Population Changes in the Eighteenth Century', *Population Studies,* 9 (1955), pp. 119-141; T. McKeown and R.G. Record, 'Reasons for the Decline of Mortality in England and Wales during the Nineteenth Century', *Population Studies,* 16 (1962), pp. 94-122; T. McKeown, R.G. Record and R.D. Turner, 'An Interpretation of the Decline in Mortality in England and Wales during the Twentieth Century', *Population Studies,* 29 (1975), pp. 391-422; T. McKeown, R.G. Brown and R.G. Record, 'An Interpretation of the Modern Rise of Population in Europe', *Population Studies,* 26 (1972), pp. 94-122; T. McKeown, 'Food, Infection and Population', *Journal of Interdisciplinary History,* 14 (1983), pp. 227-247.

7. For a recent review of McKeown's arguments see R.Woods and J. Woodward (Eds.), *Urban Disease and Mortality in the Nineteenth Century* (London 1984).

8. McKeown (1983), p. 227; and elsewhere.

9. J. Hajnal, 'The European Marriage Pattern in Perspective', D.V. Glass and D.E.C. Eversley (Eds.), *Population in History* (London 1965), pp. 104-106.

10. E.A. Wrigley and R.S. Schofield, 'English Population History from Family Reconstitution: Summary Results', *Population Studies*, 37 (1983), pp. 157-184, pp.178-179.

11. Wrigley (1983), p.129.

12. This is clear from the maps presented in R. Woods, 'The Structure of Mortality in Mid-Nineteenth Century England and Wales', *Journal of Historical Geography,* 8 (1982).

13. C.M. Law, 'The Growth of the Urban Population of England and Wales, 1801-1911', *Transactions of the Institute of British Geographers,* 41 (1967), pp. 125-143.

14. R. Woods, 'The Effect of Population Redistribution on the Level of Mortality in Nineteenth Century England and Wales', *Journal of Economic History,* 45 (1985), pp. 645-651.

15. Based on figure 7.12 (p.243) and Table A3.1 (pp. 528-529) in Wrigley and Schofield (1981).

16. All the data are taken from Woods (1985).

17. McKeown and Record (1962).

18. The population at risk for age 0 is the total number of births in each ten year period. The other ages are estimated as the geometric mean of the values given for that age in the decennial censuses bordering the period, 1851, 1861, 1891, 1901. This estimate of the population at risk is not the best possible and could be improved on. In 1851, the age group 0-4 is not broken down into its component years and here it is assumed that those in ages 1-4 made up the same proportion of the 0-4 group in 1851 that we know they did in 1861. This approximation depends on the infant mortality rate being roughly constant between the two dates and is certainly capable of refinement.

19. The numbers and letters in the tables refer to the following lists of causes of death, abbreviated in tables 2 and 3. '1851-1860: a.smallpox, b.measles, c.scarlatina, d.diptheria, e.whooping cough, f.typhus, g.cholera,diarrhoea,dysentery, h.other zymotic diseases, i.cancer, j.scrofula, tabes mesenterica, k.phthisis, l.hydrocephalus, m.diseases of the brain, n.heart disease and dropsy, o.diseases of the lungs, p.diseases of the stomach and liver, q.diseases of the kidneys, r.diseases of the generative organs, s.diseases of the joints, t.diseases of the skin, u.childbirth and metria, v.violence, w.other. 1891-1900: i.smallpox, ii.measles, iii.diptheria, iv.whooping cough, v.typhus, vi.enteric fever, vii.simple continued fever, viii.diarrhoea and dysentery, ix.cholera, x.cancer, xi.tabes mesenterica, xii.phthisis, xiii.other tubercular and scrofulous diseases, xiv.diseases of the nervous system, xv.diseases of the circulatory system, xvi.diseases of the respiratory system, xvii.diseases of the digestive system, xviii.diseases of the urinary system, xix.diseases of the generative system, xx.puerperal fever, xxi.childbirth, xxii.violence, xxiii.other.

20. The age-specific mortality rates are standardised to the population distribution of 1901. Since both the 1851-1860 and the 1891-1900 rates are standardised to the same age structure, the ratio of any given age-specific rate between the two dates will be the same as the ratio of the unstandardised age-specific rates. The statistics on tuberculosis used by McKeown and Record come from a 1949 Ministry of Health Report but inspection of the data suggests that the definition adopted here gives similar figures and has the virtue of being compatible with the rest of the tabulated data.

21. S.H. Preston, N. Keyfitz, and R. Schoen, *Causes of Death. Life Tables for National Populations* (New York and London 1972), pp. 224, 226, 240, 242.

22. McKeown and Record (1962), p.95.

23. McKeown and Record (1962), p.115.

24. M. Livi-Bacci, 'The Nutrition-Mortality Link in Past Times: a Comment', *Journal of Interdisciplinary History,* 14 (1983), pp. 293-298. See the review essay, D.N. McMurray, 'Cell-Mediated Immunity in Nutritional Deficiency', *Progress in Food and Nutrition Science,* 8 (1984), pp. 193-228. On the basis of the literature cited therein one can only conclude that there may be some diseases where the replication of the disease in the body and thus its ability to overwhelm the system is prejudiced by under-nutrition. Respiratory tuberculosis could be one such disease and thus the well-documented lack of immune response with under-nourished children is an unreliable guide to their prospects of surviving an attack.

25. McKeown and Record (1962), p.113.

26. At the conference some very early results were presented for the twenty-two largest English cities, to which Hans Norman makes brief reference in his commentary. This discussion has been excluded from the present article and I hope to develop the analysis of the individual cities in a later paper.

Sex-Differential Mortality and Socio Economic Change. Sweden 1750-1910

Gunnar Fridlizius

Introduction

The interest in the problem of sex-differential mortality is a quite recent one. So is the case for international as well as for Swedish research. For the 19th century, studies on this topic have been concentrated to the age between 10 and 20 years. In that interval, the excess female mortality during the second half of the century has been the object for the development of certain theories.[1] For other age groups, the sex-differential mortality has been almost neglected by researchers.[2] This is a problem as there is no doubt that studies on sex-differential mortality give important contributions to our understanding of socio-economic development during the century. They also make possible a more reliable interpretation of the mortality decline during the Demographic Transition. An analysis of this based only on averages of male and female rates of mortality may conceal important facts. This— among other things—will be demonstrated in this paper.

However, our purpose is neither to develop any theories in these matters, nor to start from postulated correlations between sex-differential mortality patterns and various socio-economic and biological factors. In the first place our aim has been to systematize and differentiate a large and complicated material into as homogeneous series as possible in order to create a more solid basis for generalizations and perhaps new theories. This is performed on different levels of aggregation for rural and urban Sweden during the period 1750-1914. In this paper, I restrict myself to a presentation of comprehensive series on sex-differential mortality for rural Sweden, urban Sweden and Stockholm.[3]

Irrespective of aggregation level, the same main pattern emerges; for childhood a transition to a clear excess female mortality during the latter part of the century; for the working population an increasing excess male mortality during the first part of the century especially regarding the towns, notably Stockholm; during the latter part of the period a decrease in this excess male mortality, much more pronounced for the rural areas than for the towns, for the former also manifest in an excess female mortality in the lower age-groups.

It is, however, difficult to analyze the sex-differential mortality without a close connection to the general mortality development. This makes our task more complicated, as we as yet know little about the Swedish mortality decline and its causes during the last century. For this and other reasons, the causal explanations presented may sometimes be rather tentative.

Reasons for the excess female mortality during childhood at the end of the 19th century

At the end of the 19th century, the sex-differential mortality development led to an excess female mortality in the age-groups 5/20 years (Figure 1). This pattern is not unique for Sweden. It can be found in many European countries, and often earlier than in Sweden.[4]

In her article "Differed infanticide", Sheila Johansson introduces a model for interpretation of this excess mortality during childhood.[5] In short, her thesis, which she claims is confirmed by "the Swedish example", says that in the old agrarian society there was no discrimination of women and, consequently, no excess female mortality in childhood. The latter was a phenomenon connected to the commercialization of the agrarian sector and the general change towards "cash economy". As a result of these changes, boys were valued higher than girls and, consequently, they were offered better nourishment. For that reason, the mortality rates for boys were lower than for girls, and excess female mortality had become a reality.

This pattern is assumed to have been accentuated further as tuberculosis, the dominant cause of death at the time, was highly sensitive to changes in nutrition. However, the pattern was to change again in the early period of industrialization. Women were offered better opportunities to enter the labour market and participate in the cash economy. For that reason they were beginning to be valued higher than before. However, due to the exceptionally rapid economic development at the end of the 19th century, the stage of commercialization covers a very short period of time in Swedish economic history. Consequently, the phase of female excess mortality was very short and not very accentuated, in comparison with many other countries.

Considering Sweden, however, I think that this thesis can be questioned. Swedish economic development does not, in fact, follow the pattern suggested. The thesis is based on the popular idea that practically nothing had happened in the Swedish economy prior to 1870, but that when the change did occur it came that much faster.[6] Not unexpectedly, this picture has been disproved by recent research showing that Swedish economic growth measured in GNP per capita was approximately in parity with the European average during the 19th century.[7] In addition, the modernization of agriculture began very early, and so did the urbanization and commercialization of society. As early as the second half of the 18th century, there was a considerable degree of market integration in the Swedish economy.[8] In this process of expansion of the market economy the women were given a role that was far from passive. This has been shown, for instance, by studies of the process of proto-industrialization in Sweden.

Figure 1. Sex differential mortality rates for rural Sweden (A) and Stockholm (B) in different age-groups 1751/1760-1901/1910. Females = 100.

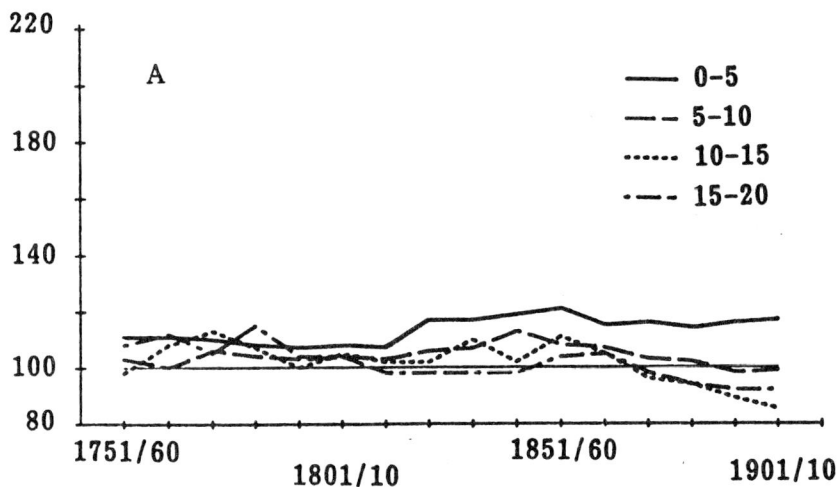

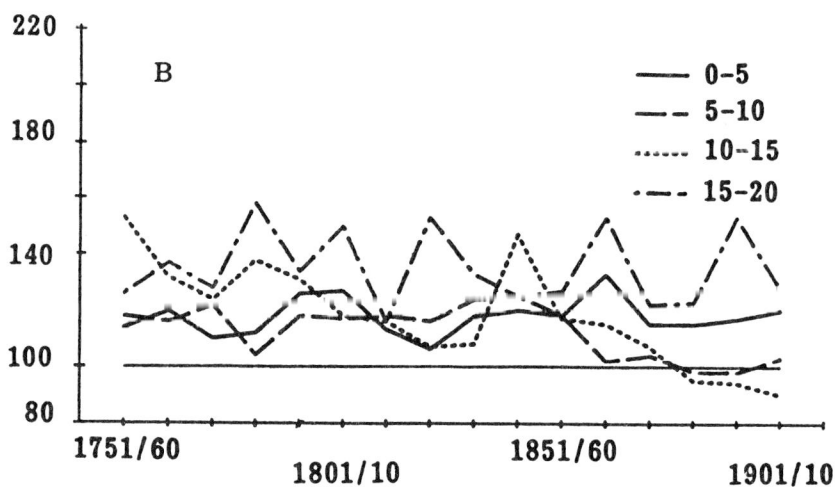

The thesis is questionable from another point of view as well. If it is correct, we would find no excess female mortality in tuberculosis in an early stage of development when there was no cash economy and no discrimination of women. According to my interpretation this is not the case (Tables 1 and 2).

Table 1. The mortality in tuberculosis in percent of total mortality in different age groups in rural Sweden (A), urban Sweden (B) and Stockholm (C).

		Males			Females	
	0/5	5/10	10/20	0/5	5/10	10/20
A						
1779-82	1.6	2.7	7.2	1.5	3.0	9.9
1821-30	2.4	4.7	13.5	2.8	8.3	18.5
1911-14	1.1	5.6	26.0	1.4	8.5	40.4
B						
1821-30	4.5	9.5	16.0	5.2	13.3	27.3
1881-90	2.6	9.8	30.3	2.7	13.3	41.0
1911-14	2.6	8.7	33.3	2.7	14.2	46.0
C						
1781-90	2.5	8.3	13.6	2.3	8.9	14.8
1821-30	4.5	16.1	20.8	6.0	21.1	26.9
1891-00	3.4	11.7	35.6	3.4	13.9	42.8

Table 2. Sex-differential mortality rates in different age groups in rural Sweden (A), urban Sweden (B) and Stockholm (C). Female = 100.

		Tuberculosis			Others	
	0/5	5/10	10/20	0/5	5/10	10/20
A						
1779-82	120	92	78	111	106	112
1821-30	100	59	73	118	108	106
1911-14	100	67	61	120	104	118
B						
1821-30	97	86	81	113	126	168
1881-90	110	75	79	116	101	107
1911-14	110	67	77	116	109	106
C						
1781-90	121	97	136	111	105	150
1821-30	100	88	117	106	121	163
1891-00	118	82	104	118	99	141

In fact, the results are the same for the modern "cash economy" as for the old agrarian system. As the share of tuberculosis in total mortality was larger at the end of the period, its influence on mortality was far greater than earlier. A standard calculation reveals that if the share of tuberculosis in total mortality in the age-groups 10/25 had been the same in 1821-1830 as in 1911-1920 there would have been an excess female mortality in the former period as well. Thus, her interpretation appears to be based on statistical fiction. This, however, need not imply that the Swedish example could not possibly confirm the thesis; in fact it could, if one could find a different mortality pattern prior to the phase of commercialization.

The "discrimination thesis" can also be questioned from other viewpoints. A discrimination of females ought to be manifest also in the age group 1/5, an age at which children are particularly sensitive to infections, which means that changes in the nutritional standard will be visible very soon. However, this is not the case. Furthermore, how could a discrimination of girls lead to a large excess female mortality in tuberculosis only and not in any other disease? And why do we find the same pattern in the towns as well where, according to the thesis, there was no discrimination of girls?

What, then, are the reasons for this excess female mortality in tuberculosis in these age groups? Probably, this is not primarily a matter of nutrition. Tuberculosis does not appear to be connected with nutrition to the great extent that has often been assumed.[9] On the other hand, tuberculosis is a typical "crowding" disease. It is very sensitive to housing and working environment.

There is reason to believe that girls were, in fact, discriminated but in a different sense than suggested by the "discrimination thesis". The boys were outdoor workers and spent more time out in the open, breathing fresh air. The girls, in contrast, assisted their mothers with indoor occupations and spent a lot of time in dusty bedrooms and kitchens. As a result, they were much more exposed to tuberculosis hazards than boys. Perhaps it is symptomatic that no excess female mortality could be found in the age group 0/5, for which the conditions in this respect were the same for boys and girls.

So far, the discussion has been restricted to the age group 10/20. A differentiation into age groups 10/15 and 15/20 adds some interesting aspects to the issue. As can be seen from Table 3, in all regions studied, excess female mortality was particularly pronounced in the lower age group. A tentative explanation could be that when boys and girls entered the labour market, the differences in living conditions between the sexes were levelled out. The excess male mortality for Stockholm in the age group 15/20 could possibly be explained in this way, especially as we know that the labour conditions in the capital were extremely disadvantageous for males and that the in-migrants to a surprisingly large extent were recruited from the age group 15/20.[10]

After this analysis of the sex-differential mortality level of tuberculosis, the main question must be: Why did the mortality in tuberculosis develop in a way

Table 3. Sex-differential mortality rates in different age groups in rural Sweden (A), urban Sweden (B) and Stockholm (C). Female = 100.

	Tuberculosis		Others	
	10/15	15/20	10/15	15/20
A				
1779-82	80	77	110	113
1911-14	40	69	108	109
B				
1901-10	49	79	102	134
C				
1781-90	91	189	148	154
1891-00	58	129	113	181

that differed from all other causes of death, thus leaving the possibility that there was a specific sex-differential pattern related to tuberculosis which could influence the total age-specific differential mortality pattern? As both sexes were involved, it cannot be interpreted in terms of discrimination. On the whole, at this stage of research, it is difficult to give any satisfactory explanation to the phenomenon. As can be seen from Table 7, we find the same mortality pattern also in the age groups just above 20. We know that from a biological point of view there was a peak in mortality related to tuberculosis around this particular age. Would it be reasonable to suggest that the disparate development of the mortality related to tuberculosis reflects an autonomous, biological process, a sort of adjustment to more "natural" mortality pattern, away from the high mortality era before the middle of the century?[11]

The male mortality hump in rural Sweden

As shown in Figure 2, there is an increase in excess male mortality in working ages from the beginning of the 19th century. A peak was reached in the period 1820-1850 whereupon a deterioration began. The pattern is repeated on disaggregated levels although on different sex-differential mortality levels.

A convenient point of departure for analysis is to contrast our result with the study by Arthur Imhof concerning the situation in Germany during the 19th century.[12] Imhof starts his analysis with data from a sample of four parishes. For the period covering the second half of the 19th century, he has added data on national level. On both levels, he finds a clear excess female mortality in the age groups that are relevant here. The excess female mortality is explained by an alleged high mortality rate of mothers in child-birth, the repeated pregnancies and births, the care of men and children with infectious diseases, the suppression of the women's own illnesses as long as possible, and the transition to a more labour-intensive type of agricultural production.

There is no reason to assume that the situation of women in rural Sweden was substantially more advantageous than the gloomy picture presented by Imhof for Germany. One could assume the changes in Swedish 19th century agriculture to have worsened the situation of women vis-à-vis men. The crop rotation technique was introduced after the enclosure movement. The technique was laborious and led to an increase in the amount of work done by women. The same thing could be said about the rapidly expanding production of potatoes. The great numerical growth of the lower classes—in 1750 crofters, cottagers and day labourers amounted to 27 per cent of the peasant population; in 1860 the ratio had risen to 98 per cent—is likely to have contributed to a further worsening of the situation of women, due to the fact that they were, to a larger extent, forced to seek employment outside their homes.

Figure 2. Sex differential mortality rates for rural Sweden in different age-groups 1751/1760-1901/1910. Female = 100.

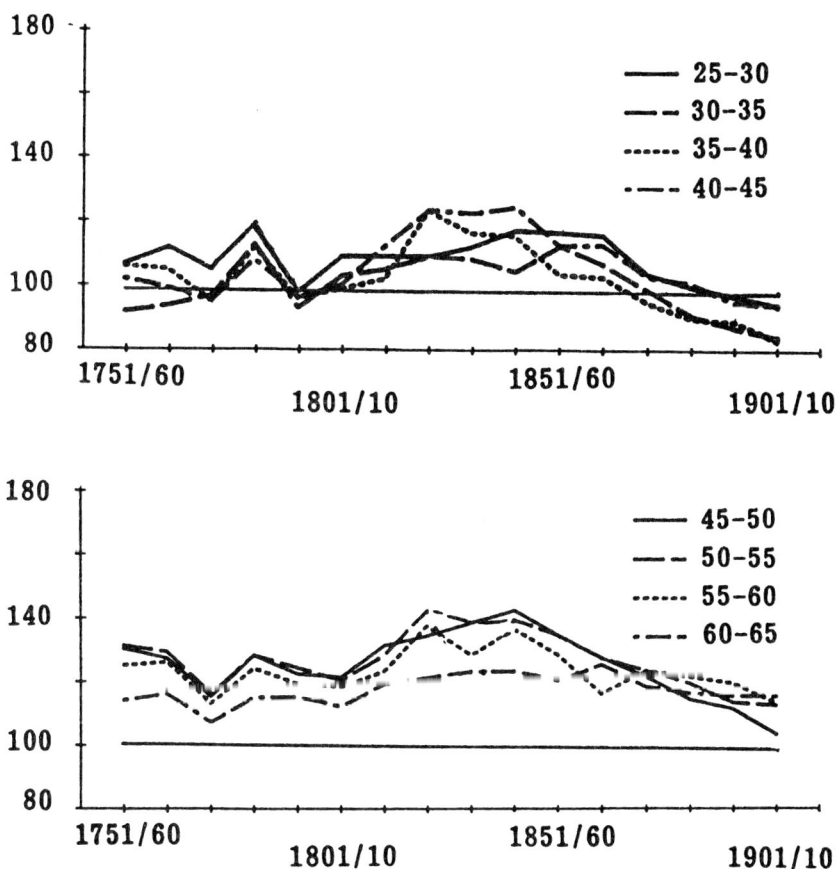

Table 4. Rural Sweden. Age specific sex differential mortality according to civil status. 1821—1830. Index female = 100.

	25/30	30/35	35/40	40/45	45/50
Married	74	87	102	112	137
Unmarried	148	157	186	188	176
Total	113	109	117	123	138

We must remember that Imhof deals with married people, whereas we have been forced to work with aggregates including both married and unmarried people. Swedish statistics do not register mortality according to civil status until 1870.

However, an attempt to reconstruct the mortality according to civil status also for this early period shows a pattern which clearly deviates from the German pattern: in the age groups above 35 there is male excess mortality, although not as apparent as in the total figures (Table 4). We do not know whether the very high excess mortality for unmarried males in all age groups is a specific feature of Sweden since we have no object of comparison.

These observations indicate that the causes of excess male mortality in Sweden ought to be sought primarily in factors affecting the male population. This impression is strengthened by the fact that male mortality was stagnant or rising at the same time as female mortality was declining. [13]

Since we can point to a relatively homogeneous development for the different counties it is reasonable to assume some general factor to have been influential. One such general factor is undoubtedly the enormously large consumption of alcoholic beverages, which from the beginning of the 19th century to the middle of the century was larger than in any other period in Swedish history.

Data on the consumption of alcoholic beverages are inexact and divergent. The number 100 million litres per annum is often suggested for the time about 1830 when the consumption culminated. [14] However, even a cautious estimate of 80 million litres as an average for the period 1825-1830 gives an annual per capita consumption of 30 litres. This should be compared to about 5.4 litres in our day.

We know that alcoholics and large consumers of alcoholic beverages are much more exposed to disease and death than other categories. Today, diseases related to alcohol consumption are considered to be the third most important cause of death in ages below 60. Some experts consider this to be an underestimation. During a period when alcoholic consumption was about 6 times higher than today, the mortality related to alcohol is bound to have been much higher.

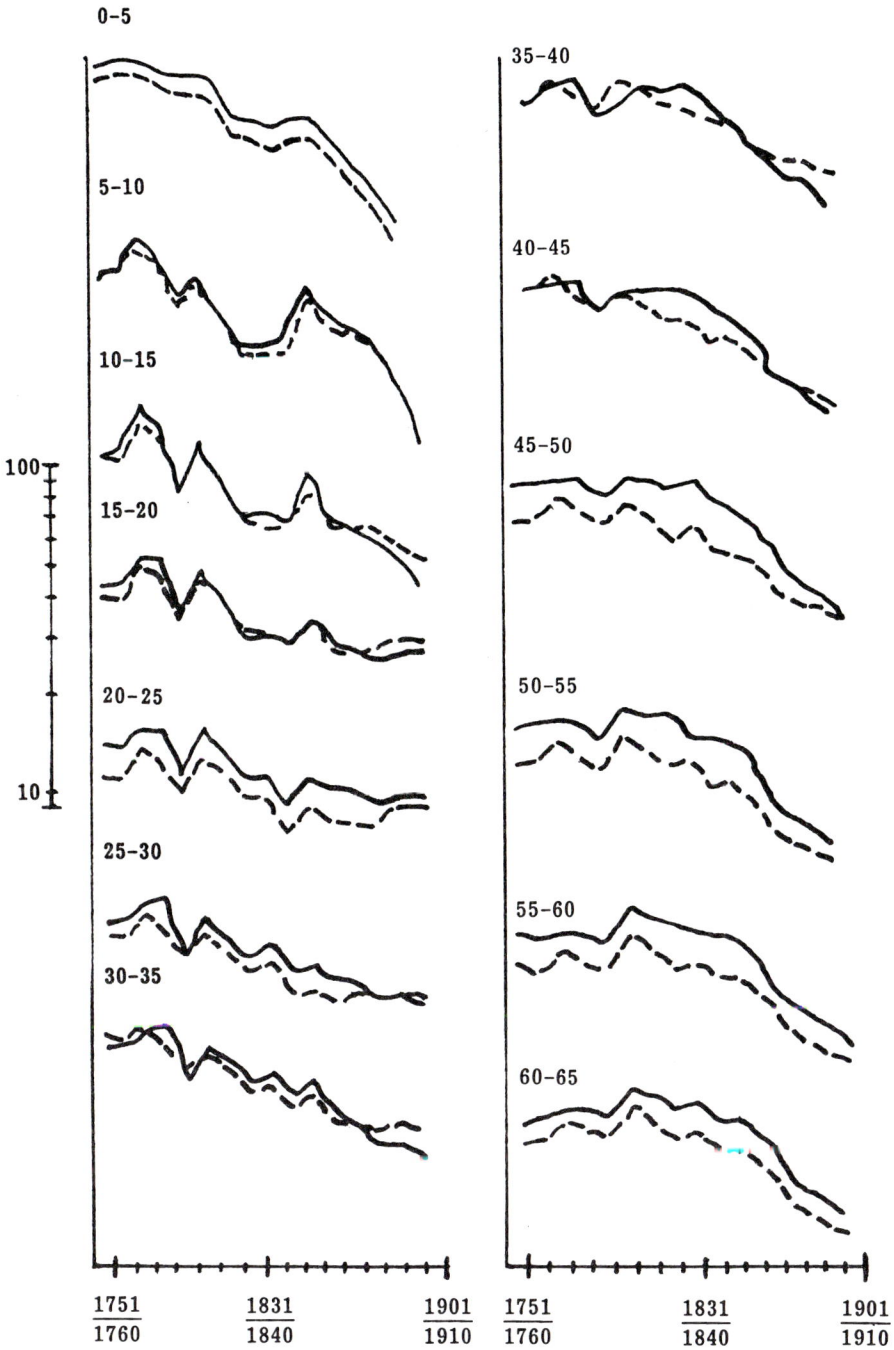

Figure 3. Age- and sex-specific mortality rates for rural Sweden 1751/1760-1901/1910. Male — Female --

The very high excess male mortality in age group 25/50 due to accidents we can see in Table 5 may to a certain extent be related to alcohol; this is also the case with inflammation fevers, especially as excess male mortality is practically insignificant in the age group immediately below. The same is true for the high male excess mortality in violent deaths. On the whole, there are few causes of death for which a relation to alcohol can be excluded.

Table 5. Age specific mortality rates and sex-differentials in mortality 1821—1830. Female = 100. M = Male, F = Female, I = Index

		0-5	5-10	10-25	25-50	>50	Total
Tuberculosis							
Rural	M	1.5	0.4	0.8	2.4	7.4	2.4
Sweden	F	1.5	0.5	1.2	2.2	5.7	2.3
	I	100	67	72	110	132	106
Urban	M	2.3	1.0	1.7	6.6	16.1	5.4
Sweden	F	2.0	1.3	1.6	4.3	10.1	4.1
	I	114	78	106	150	160	131
Stockholm	M	5.9	2.1	3.1	16.2	31.5	11.9
	F	7.8	2.7	2.6	7.0	16.4	7.7
	I	76	77	119	231	192	155
Inflammation fevers							
Rural	M	7.8	1.2	0.9	2.3	7.6	3.4
Sweden	F	6.6	1.0	0.9	1.6	6.0	2.9
	I	118	102	106	144	127	120
Urban	M	5.6	1.4	0.8	2.8	7.0	3.1
Sweden	F	5.7	1.0	0.5	1.6	4.3	2.1
	I	99	144	158	181	163	144
Stockholm	M	8.8	1.5	2.0	6.3	9.0	5.1
	F	8.5	1.8	1.1	1.8	4.6	2.7
	I	104	84	200	350	196	194
Typhoid fevers							
Rural	M	0.9	0.5	0.7	1.2	2.3	1.1
Sweden	F	0.9	0.5	0.8	1.0	1.9	1.0
	I	102	100	87	116	124	108
Urban	M	1.9	1.1	1.3	3.6	5.0	2.7
Sweden	F	1.7	0.9	1.0	1.7	2.7	1.7
	I	112	122	130	211	185	160
Stockholm	M	1.4	0.8	2.1	5.4	7.2	3.9
	F	1.3	0.8	1.1	1.8	3.0	1.8
	I	111	103	191	300	240	225

Dropsy							
Rural	M	0.3	0.3	0.3	0.7	2.6	0.8
Sweden	F	0.3	0.3	0.3	0.9	2.6	0.9
	I	127	100	88	82	100	84
Urban	M	0.9	0.8	0.6	2.0	4.7	1.7
Sweden	F	0.7	0.9	0.5	1.2	2.6	1.5
	I	132	86	131	167	178	114
Stockholm	M	1.1	1.6	1.1	5.1	8.8	3.7
	F	1.2	0.8	0.7	2.8	6.7	2.8
	I	96	188	157	182	131	133
Violent death							
Rural	M	11.4	0.8	0.3	0.8	3.4	2.7
Sweden	F	9.1	0.7	0.3	0.5	2.2	2.0
	I	125	114	117	187	158	137
Urban	M	27.9	1.7	0.6	2.8	7.9	5.5
Sweden	F	23.2	1.7	0.4	0.9	3.4	3.8
	I	120	104	162	330	235	159
Stockholm	M	70.8	2.2	1.0	4.8	15.1	11.3
	F	63.3	2.1	0.8	1.7	7.7	7.9
	I	112	102	125	282	196	141
Accidents							
Rural	M	1.8	0.5	0.9	1.6	1.7	1.3
Sweden	F	1.6	0.2	0.2	0.2	0.3	0.4
	I	118	282	405	889	548	328
Urban	M	1.0	0.9	1.6	3.0	2.7	2.1
Sweden	F	0.5	0.2	0.3	0.3	0.6	0.4
	I	194	409	604	934	486	600
Stockholm	M	0.7	1.2	2.0	4.3	3.7	3.0
	F	0.3	0.3	0.4	0.6	0.6	0.5
	I	194	432	500	717	617	602
Total							
Rural	M	61.7	7.4	5.3	11.5	54.8	23.6
Sweden	F	52.7	7.1	5.1	9.7	47.6	21.2
	I	117	104	104	119	115	111
Urban	M	75.8	12.4	7.8	24.2	69.7	31.0
Sweden	F	66.1	10.2	5.3	12.6	45.1	23.9
	I	115	122	147	193	154	130
Stockholm	M	149.8	14.9	13.7	48.0	103.7	51.7
	F	141.6	12.8	8.3	20.2	60.3	35.2
	I	106	116	165	238	172	147

Note 1: Index is calculated from two decimals.
Note 2: Stockholm is not included in urban Sweden.

The low excess male mortality in tuberculosis is surprising since it is a disease sensitive to alcohol. This was also observed by Gustav Sundbärg, who, however, argued that the consumption of alcoholic beverages among males had an indirect negative impact on female mortality.[15] It is possible that this suggestion might contain a grain of truth. However, it is more likely that women were exposed to tuberculosis due to the fact that they were domestic indoor workers. Thus, this argument is similar to the one proposed as an explanation to excess female childhood mortality. In addition, we know that pregnant women constitute a potential risk group with respect to tuberculosis.[16]

From this, and the reasonable supposition that the consequence of an excess alcohol consumption for mortality may be more serious in the higher age groups in the interval, it follows that we may find a more pronounced excess male mortality in the upper part of the interval compared to the lower parts, where there is a possibility that we may find excess female mortality. This assumption was confirmed by calculations of the mortality rate in tuberculosis for the age groups 20/40 and 40/60, a finding that would harmonize well with our "alcoholic thesis".

The Swedish consumption of alcoholic beverages was not only far in excess of present-day consumption; measured in litres of alcohol per year and inhabitant, it must also have been higher than in modern high-consumption countries such as France and Italy (Table 6). Also, the pattern of consumption in Sweden was different in a sense that made the damaging effects more serious. Firstly, consumption was more concentrated to males, in particular in the age groups between 20 and 70. An assumption that the female share in consumption amounted to 10 per cent gives a per capita consumption for men in these age groups of 107 litres per annum, i.e. 0.3 litres a day. These estimates are for liquor with an alcoholic content of 50 percent. Furthermore, drinking in Sweden—as in the rest of Northern and Eastern Europe—was concentrated to weekends, which was probably more damaging than if the drinking had been distributed over the entire week as in the case of wine consumption in Southern Europe.

Table 6. Litres alcohol per year and inhabitant 1971-1975. Converted to 50 % alcohol.

	Beer	Wine	Spirits	Total
Sweden	2.4	1.4	5.4	9.2
France	1.7	21.4	4.6	27.9
Italy	0.5	22.2	3.8	26.5

The problem of extensive distilling of aquavitae soon became one of the most controversial subjects in early 19th Century Sweden. One witty and malicious radical author most certainly had a point in writing:

> King Oscar in his Palace sits, placid and weary-eyed. Around him his sottish folk, flaccid and bleary eyed.

Of course, it is impossible to determine with precision the extent of excess male mortality that was related to alcohol. However, experience from modern times when it has been possible for physicians to ascertain the close relationship between consumption of alcoholic beverages and mortality, clearly indicates that it could not be wrong to associate excess male mortality in the working ages with the prevailing pattern of alcoholic consumption.

Why did the male mortality hump disappear?

From about 1850, excess male mortality began to vanish. By the end of the century it had even been replaced by excess female mortality in the age groups up to 40/45 (Figure 2). To begin with, this pattern developed during a continuous decline in mortality with a slight lag in female mortality, which was accentuated after around 1880 (Figure 3). For the younger female age groups in the interval, the decline came to a stop, and during the end of the period there was even an absolute increase in the mortality.[17]

We have defended the thesis that an increase in the consumption of alcoholic beverages led to excess male mortality. Thus, a decline in consumption ought to have worked in the reverse direction. Modern research has shown that a decline in consumption quickly results in a decline in the mortality which is related to alcohol. In the beginning of the 1850's, new spirits legislation was passed after lengthy discussions. As an effect, the consumption of alcoholic beverages is likely to have been considerably reduced.

Therefore, it seems reasonable to assume that, to some extent, the slightly faster decline in male mortality in relation to female mortality during the decades after 1850 could be ascribed to the new restrictive policy, in particular as we have found no signs of worsened working conditions for females.

However, the discussion of the change in the sex-differential mortality pattern at the end of the century ought to focus upon the females. During this period, Swedish agriculture changed to a production more specialized on dairy products. There is no reason to doubt that this led to a worsening of working conditions for the woman. She was now much more engaged in occupations such as milking and attendance of animals. She was also allotted the task of cleaning the cow houses—a dirty and fatiguing job. The milking machine was not introduced until after the First World War. This increase in the number of tasks was seldom compensated for by a decrease in the number of traditional tasks. In this situation, the prevalence of tuberculosis exerted an additional negative influence.

So far, the conclusion regarding the negative impact of the transition to dairy production on female mortality seems reasonable. However, a closer investigation seems to call for some modifications. From regional data we do not find the expected correlation between dairy production areas and increasing female mortality; but the latter we also have in non-dairy production regions. In the towns, we also observe a decline, although less pronounced, in excess male mortality. As long as we do not know if these patterns were results of some other negative factor for females in the towns and in the non-dairy producing areas, we cannot assume that the discrimination thesis is valid. It only implies that the patterns are complex.

The truth of this is obvious when studying the causes of death. As can be seen from Table 7, the new sex-differential mortality pattern was the result of an increasing excess female mortality in tuberculosis, while other diseases show no changes.

While the former is in accordance with the discrimination thesis, it seems not to be the case regarding the latter. However, an expected excess female mortality—but not so pronounced—in "other diseases" may be concealed by changes in the traditionally very high excess male mortality from accidents.

Mortality caused by tuberculosis increased, however, rapidly its proportion in the total mortality in the age group 20/40 (Table 7). As a result, the specific sex-differential mortality pattern of tuberculosis might statistically influence the total sex-differential mortality pattern in the interval. But worsening conditions on the female labour market do not explain the increase in mortality due to tuberculosis for both men and women.

Table 7. The mortality in tuberculosis in percent of total mortality in different age groups in rural Sweden (A), urban Sweden (B), and Stockholm (C).

| | Males | | | | | Females | | | |
	20/40	40/60	>60	Total		20/40	40/60	>60	Total
A									
1779-82	19.1	21.1	9.4	8.2		15.8	19.2	7.7	7.4
1821-30	21.4	20.5	10.4	10.2		23.1	22.2	9.8	10.8
1911-14	38.1	15.6	2.4	9.0		48.6	20.7	2.1	11.3
B									
1821-30	32.0	30.3	24.2	20.1		35.8	34.5	17.7	22.8
1881-90	40.2	24.2	11.6	15.3		42.5	27.8	9.6	15.5
1911-14	40.4	17.4	4.1	14.1		51.8	18.8	3.3	14.5
C									
1781-90	27.3	34.7	32.7	19.1		27.4	32.1	24.8	17.3
1821-30	32.4	31.6	32.3	23.0		38.7	31.3	23.7	21.8
1891-00	41.0	24.2	8.9	16.6		42.5	21.6	7.3	13.9
1911-14	44.8	20.0	5.7	17.2		49.2	18.8	1.9	13.5

Thus, we have to calculate with other factors. In analysing the development of mortality in the age group 10/20, we were confronted with a similar phenomenon. In this case, no satisfactory answer could be offered, only a guess as to the epidemiological nature of the disease. This guess may also be valid concerning the age group 20/40. The mortality pattern developed is notable in particular as there is a simultaneous decline in mortality from tuberculosis and all other causes of death in the age group 40/60, and a much faster decline in tuberculosis in the age group above 60.[18]

Earlier, we assumed that worsened working conditions might have affected married women in a particularly negative way. As is shown in Figure 4, this assumption does not hold true in the Swedish case. The lag in total female mortality in the age groups 20/25 refers primarily to a disadvantageous development of mortality for unmarried women.[19] To some extent this is also the case in the age groups 25/30 and 30/35. In 1871-1880, mortality among married women was higher than for unmarried women in all of these age groups. Thirty years later the situation had for the first time in Swedish demographic history reversed.

So far it is difficult to give a satisfactory explanation of this change in the pattern of female mortality. Possibly, the decrease in the mortality for married women in the beginning of the period could be connected with the rapid decrease in mortality due to childbirth and child-bed fever in accordance with Semmelweiss's observations at the end of the 1860's of the importance of hand hygiene in connection with deliveries. The increasing number of midwives might have had similar positive effects.[20]

Table 8. Sex-differential mortality rates in different age gropus in rural Sweden (A), urban Sweden (B) and Stockholm (C). Female = 100.

	Tuberculosis				Others			
	20/40	40/60	>60	Total	20/40	40/60	>60	Total
A								
1779-82	122	141	130	120	97	126	103	107
1821-30	103	126	119	106	114	138	112	109
1911-14	80	81	122	80	122	136	105	103
B								
1821-30	185	176	176	119	219	211	119	142
1881-90	134	137	146	99	150	164	119	121
1911-14	106	151	147	97	168	166	116	113
C								
1781-90	141	141	141	132	141	137	107	117
1821-30	183	243	200	155	241	261	145	155
1891-00	172	224	157	155	183	194	127	125
1911-14	151	221	—	158	184	203	121	120

Note: The figures for Stockholm 1911/14 are based only on 1910.

251

Figure 4. Rural Sweden. Age-specific mortality rates 25/30-45/50 according to sex and civil status 1871/1880-1901/1910.

A = age-groups 25/30, B = 30/35, C = 35/40, D = 40/45, E = 45/50.

— married females, --- unmarried females, - - unmarried males

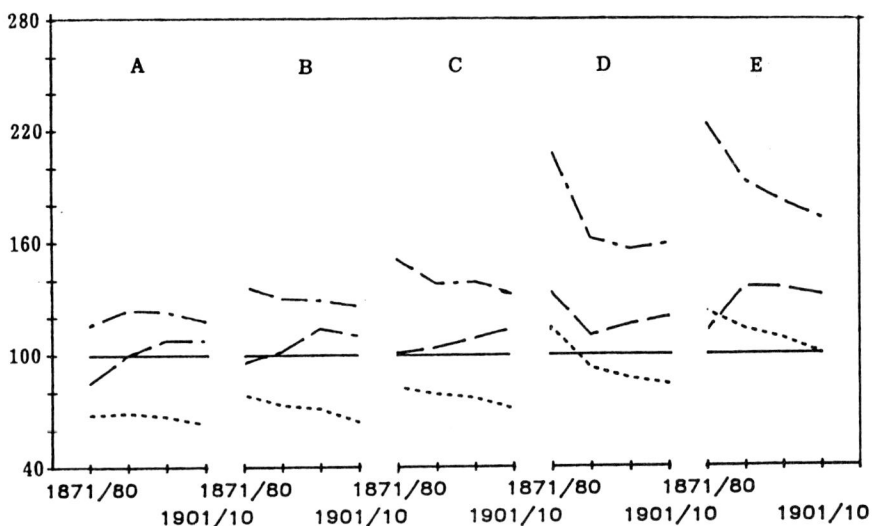

Table 9. Sex-differential mortality rates for married and unmarried in rural Sweden 1871-1880—1901-1910. Female = 100.

Married	20/25	25/30	30/35	35/40	40/45	45/50
1871-80	66	68	79	83	104	123
1881-90	64	69	73	79	92	113
1891-10	60	67	71	77	87	108
1901-10	58	63	64	71	84	100

Unmarried	20/25	25/30	30/35	35/40	40/45	45/50
1871-80	137	136	143	149	156	158
1881-90	124	124	128	136	147	141
1891-10	114	114	113	128	134	135
1901-10	114	109	115	116	133	132

The increase in mortality for unmarried women could, in the same rather uncertain way, be associated with the agrarian transformation; it was the unmarried women in particular who were engaged in dairy production. On the other hand, there were no changes in the relation between married and unmarried men; regardless of age group the mortality for unmarried men was some 80 per cent higher than for married men, which should be compared to the small difference between married and unmarried women. This means that

252

Figure 5. Age-specific mortality rates for rural Sweden according to sex (A) and civil status (B). A: males —, females ---, B: unmarried —, married --, not specified —

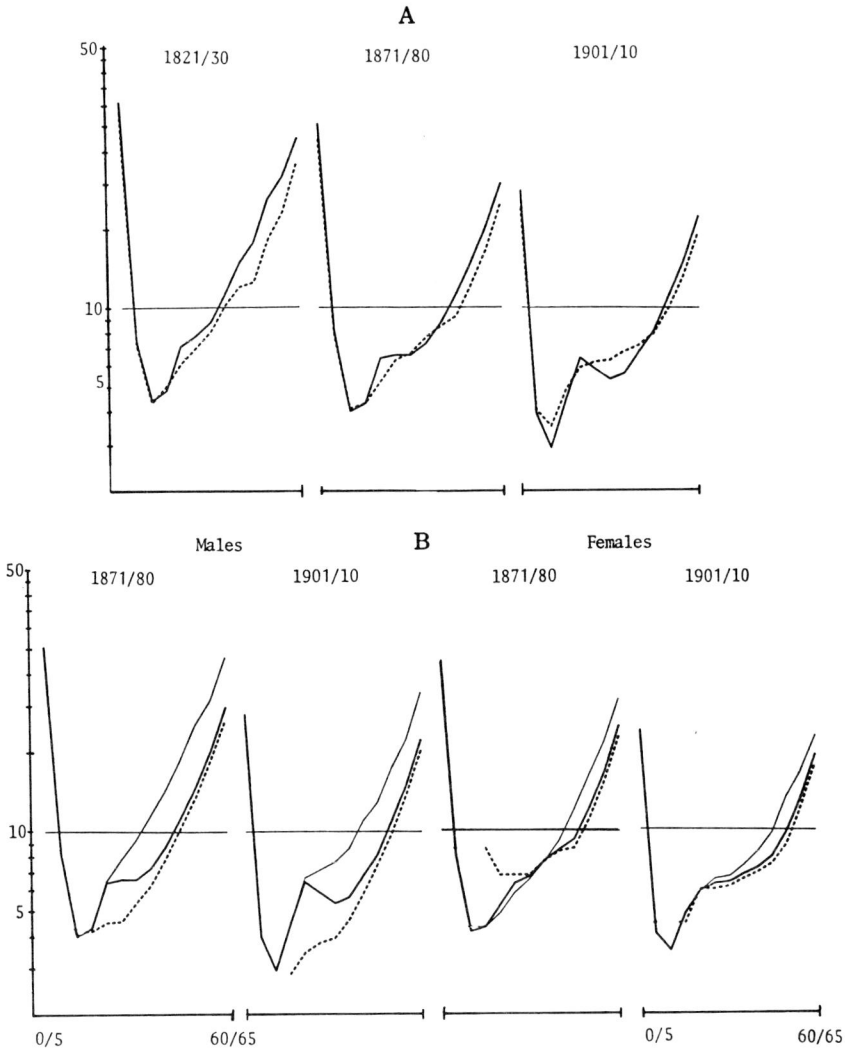

the unmarried men had by far the most disadvantageous position with respect to mortality, followed by the unmarried woman. The married man had the most favourable position up to 40/45 whereupon this position was taken over by the married woman (Figure 4). The causes of this surprisingly great difference between married and unmarried males and, on the whole, the difference in mortality between sex and civil status has not, however, been seriously studied.

The differentiation into sex and civil status also adds new light on the peak in male mortality in the age group 20/25 (Figure 5). This peak is not characteristic for Sweden only; it exists in several other populations and has tempted various interpretations.[21] As this peak is non-existent or only partly present in female mortality it has resulted in a higher excess male mortality in this age group than in the age groups above and below (Appendix).

However, on studying the mortality according to civil status we do not find this male mortality hump, except for the period 1901-1910, a period for which there were tendencies towards peaks in all series regardless of sex and civil status. As the mortality for unmarried males is considerably higher than for married males, and since the unmarried dominate the group 20/25, there ought to be a peak in the series due to statistical reasons if we consider the male mortality unspecified. On the other hand, since the difference in mortality between married and unmarried women is insignificant, we do not find any peak in total female age specific mortality. As the same pattern is likely to prevail in other populations as well, any drastic explanation ought to be rejected as statistical fiction. The mortality peak for both males and females in 1901-1910, regardless of civil status, is likely to reflect the increasing mortality from tuberculosis discussed above.

The huge excess male mortality hump in urban Sweden

What are the reasons behind the enormously large excess male mortality in the working ages in the towns? In 1821-1830 it was between 70 and 125 per cent for urban Sweden and between 100 and 200 per cent for Stockholm alone. This can be compared with between 10 and 42 per cent for the rural areas during the same period (Appendix).

For Stockholm, this mortality hump was due to a marked increase in male mortality at the same time as female mortality remained constant (Figure 7). For the total urban mortality, the only available figures are from 1821-1830 onwards, but we would probably find a similar development (Figure 8).[22]

When explaining the huge male mortality hump in the towns we have to concentrate not only on the excessive consumption of alcoholic beverages, as in the rural areas, but to a larger extent on the conditions of the labour market and the pattern of death causes as well.[23] The combination of these factors was greatly disadvantageous for the men and must have been the main reason for the high excess male mortality in working ages. That the preindustrial labour market was disadvantageous for the males appears to be a general rule. In Stockholm, where poverty seems to have been greater than in most other European cities, this rule seems to have been particularly applicable.[24]

Figure 6. Sex differential mortality rates for Stockholm in different ages - grops 1751/1760-1901/1910. Female = 100.

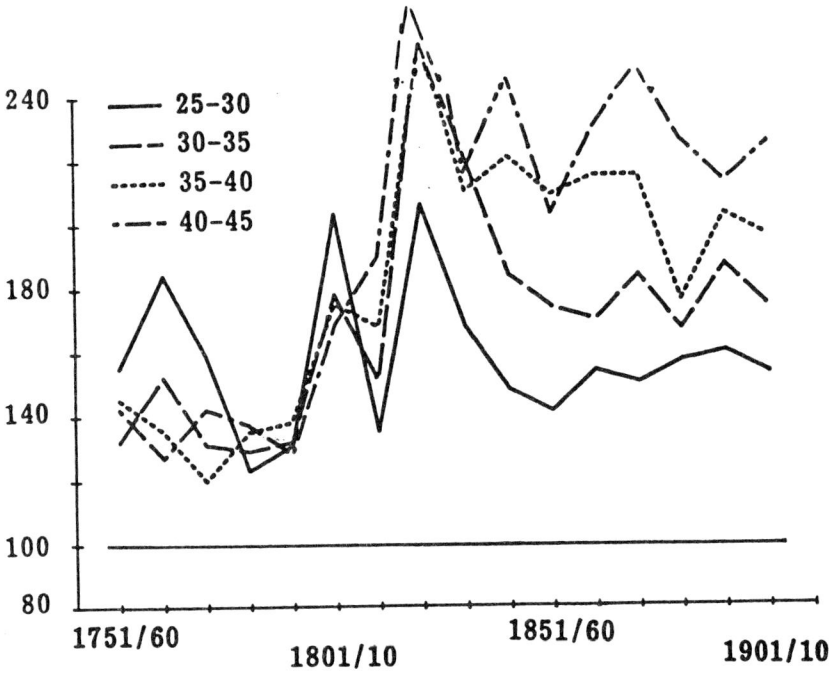

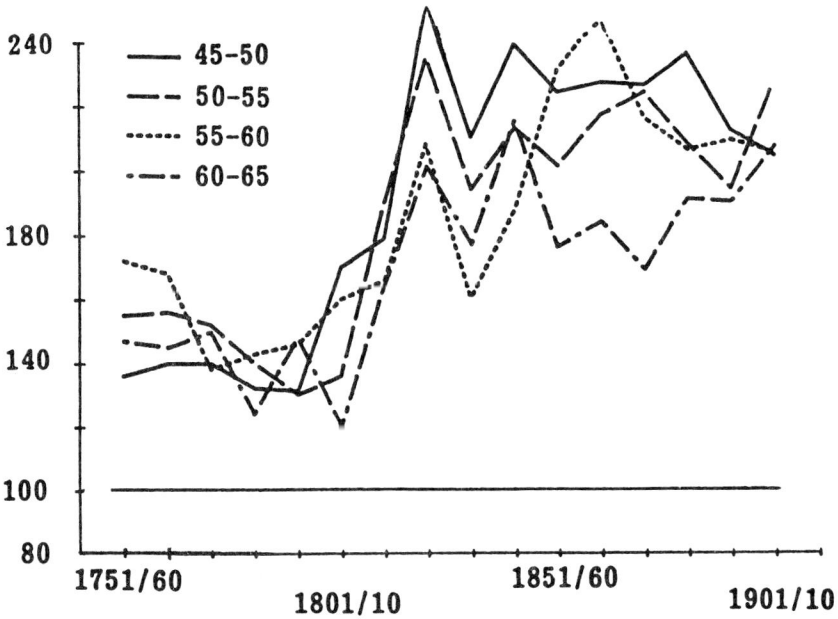

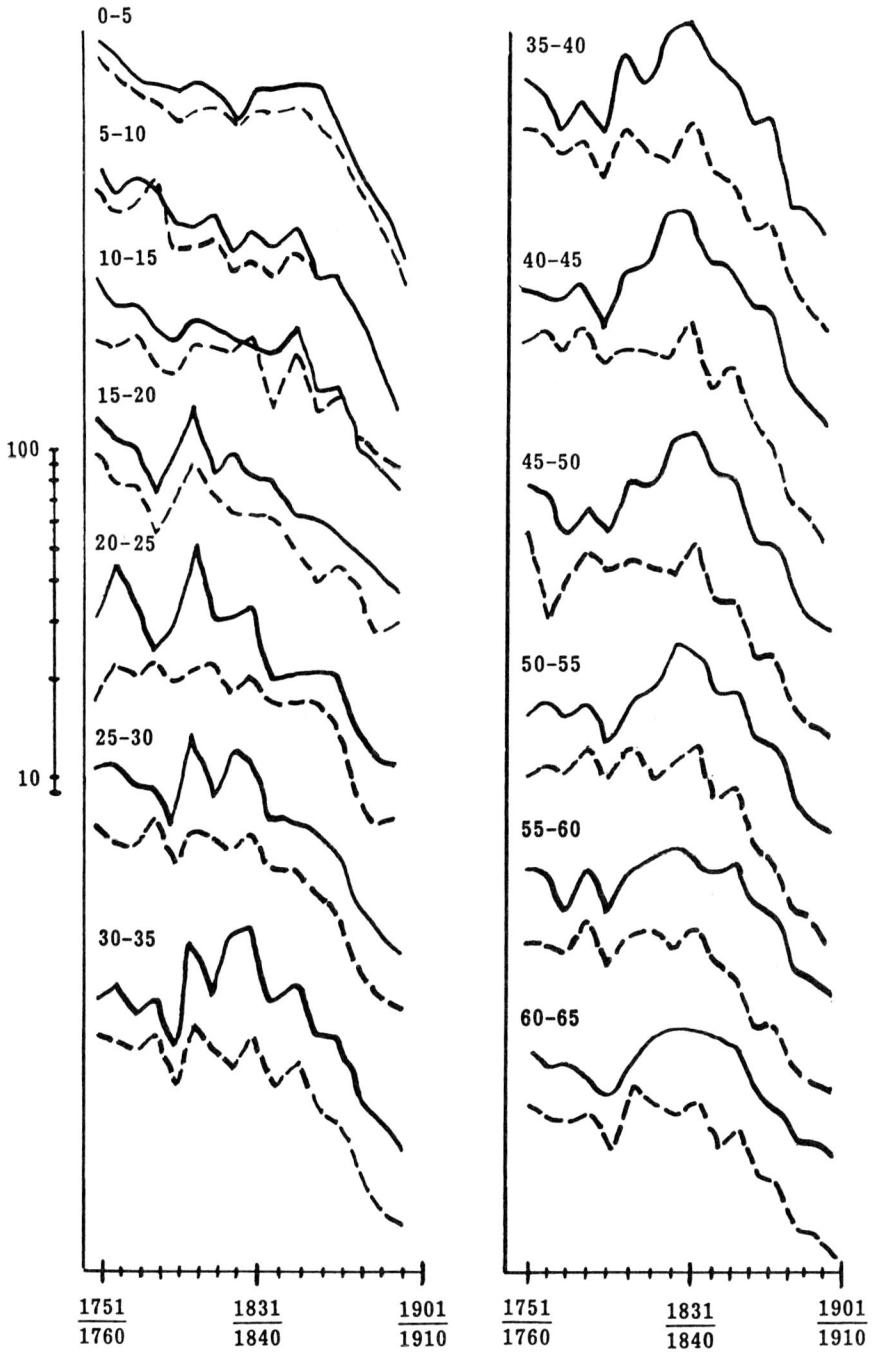

Figure 7. Age- and sex-specific mortality rates for Stockholm 1751/1760-1901/1910. Males — Females ---

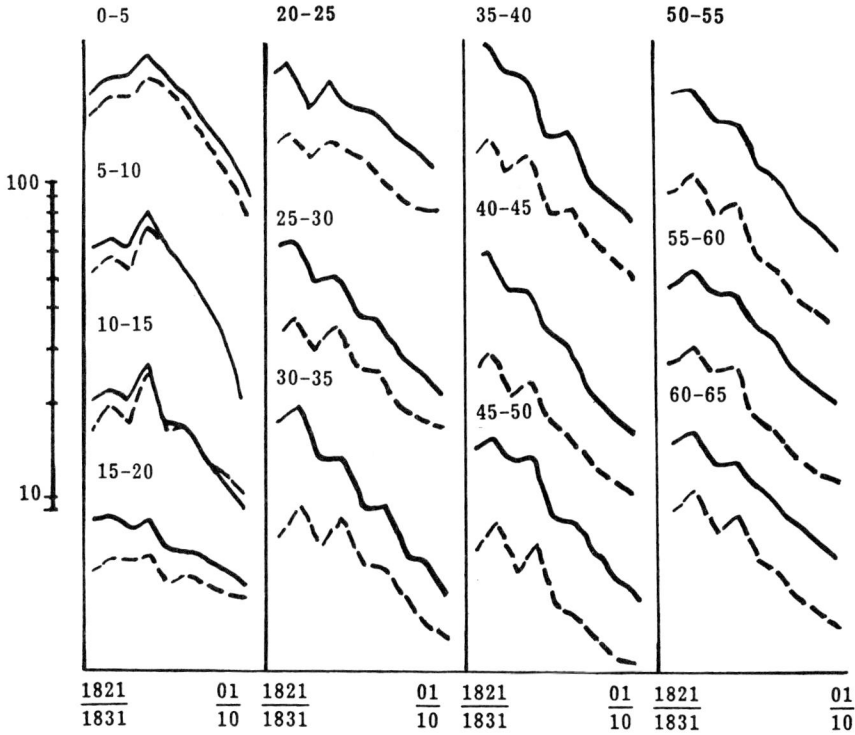

Figure 8. Age- and sex-specific mortality rates for urban Sweden 1751/1760-1901/1910. Male — Female ---

Insecurity with regard to job opportunities, poor housing conditions with several lodgers in one room, and an insufficient diet were factors which left many males in social and economic penury, which is bound to have fostered high mortality rates. Many women, on the other hand, earned their living as maids and were likely to have better living and working conditions than was normal for men. Estimates indicate a lower poverty ratio for women than for men. In the rural areas the situation was the reverse.[25]

In this situation, the prevailing pattern of causes of death is likely to have been disadvantageous for the men. Infectious diseases were the dominant cause of death (Table 5). Tuberculosis was particularly widespread. In 1821 1830 the male mortality from this disease amounted to 35 per cent of total mortality in the age groups 25/50. The male living conditions ought to have increased the risks for the men of being infected with tuberculosis at the same time as their resistance to the disease was reduced.[26] It is symptomatic that the male mortality from tuberculosis until this period increased faster than female mortality which on the whole was constant.

257

When it comes to the consumption of alcoholic beverages, per capita consumption in the towns, not least in Stockholm, was surely far above the national average presented above. Consequently, alcohol was a much more important hazard in the towns.

Alcoholic beverages were more accessible. The taverns in Stockholm were innumerable. Evidence has shown that disease and death due to the consumption of alcohol is directly correlated to access. It has also been shown that an environment which encourages collective gathering is an important incentive to an increased consumption of alcoholic beverages. Jeppe did not drink in the first place because his wife was a bitch but because his companions were drinking as well. Insecure conditions for many workers must have been a further stimulus to drinking. This insecurity however, was not only economic in character. It was also the insecurity felt by the immigrant countryman having to face an entirely new environment. In this environment, self-confidence could be temporarily enhanced by drinking of spirits.[27] This was also true for his relationship to women, the thousands of unmarried maids of Stockholm. Often there were quite practical reasons for drinking. They drank because they froze at their work places or in the cold barracks or lodgings. Sometimes a snaps was the easiest way to take the edge of their hunger. On the whole, drinking was a way of life to an even larger extent than in modern times.

However, drinking is expensive. Although, as we have shown, poverty was widespread in Stockholm at that time, it is likewise obvious that from 1810 onwards there was a gradual improvement in the real wages of workers of Stockholm.[28] In Stockholm and other towns, where unmarried people made up a larger part of the population than in rural areas, it was easier for a man to retain more of an increase in real wages for himself. This improvement occurred at the same time as there was a considerable increase in the supply of liquor due to a liberalization of the legislation (1809), the introduction of potatoes as raw material in the distilleries (1820's), and the establishment of

Table 10. Rates of unmarried of the total population in different age-groups 1870 in urban Sweden and Stockholm.

	25/30	30/35	35/40	40/45	45/50
			Males		
Urban Sweden	67	42	28	21	17
Stockholm	77	53	39	31	27
			Females		
Urban Sweden	65	47	36	32	28
Stockholm	73	56	45	39	37

258

steam distilleries (1830's). These factors combined to lower prices, which in turn worked as a further stimulus to demand. In modern time it is a well-known fact that increasing real wages and stable prices of alcoholic beverages have a stimulating effect on consumption.

There are several indications that the increasing incomes for the lower classes in the beginning were, to a large extent, spent on an increased consumption of spirits. In fact, in the emerging consumer society, the liquor industry became the industrial flagship, and producers and merchants in the liquor trade made quicker profits than others.[29] The correlation between workers' real wages, production of liquor and the excess male mortality in the working ages could hardly be coincidental.

The excess male mortality hump: a slow decrease or stagnation

Why was the decrease in the excess male mortality much slower in urban than in rural areas? In Stockholm there were, on the whole, no changes in the mortality relations between the sexes in the ages over 35.

This pattern developed during a continuous decline in the mortality with a slight lag in female mortality which was accentuated by the end of the century. In this respect, the pattern was similar to that in rural Sweden (Figures 7 and 8). The great difference between the two areas, however, was that the mortality decline was much faster in the urban areas. At the same time, the decline was somewhat faster for Stockholm than for the other towns. This pattern was, however, less developed in the working ages than in the infant and child ages (Figure 9).

The mortality decline in the European towns has often been regarded as an effect of the large-scale improvements in sewage and water supply during this period.[30] The fact that the mortality decline, as regards Sweden, began in the 1840's, i.e. 30 or 40 years before these improvements could have had any substantial positive effect on mortality, indicates that the causal chain is more complex. This conclusion is confirmed by the fact that the decline began simultaneously in the rural areas.

As for rural Sweden, it is reasonable to regard this early decline partly as a result of a cohort-specific mortality improvement and partly as a period-specific improvement; the latter being particularly manifest in the male cohorts. For the rural areas, we assumed that the decrease in the consumption of alcoholic beverages led to a similar improvement in mortality. There is no reason to revise this assumption with regard to the towns.

However, the rapid decline in total mortality after about 1870 ought to be seen in relation to the improvements in sanitation. This is further indicated by the more rapid decline in mortality caused by diseases related to poor water supply or unsatisfactory sewage.[31] Another indication is that the mortality decline for the towns relative to that of the rural areas was faster during this period than during the previous decades. Improvements in sanitation were costly and could be undertaken in densely populated areas only. It is symptomatic that the mortality decline was more accentuated in Stockholm than in the towns in general. When, in the early 20th century, mortality had become lower in the towns than in the rural areas, it was a historically unique phenomenon (Figures 9 and 10). For the first time ever, urban life had become more healthy than rural life seen from the point of view of mortality. It was not until after the Second World War that the pendulum swung back again.[32]

If mortality due to stomach diseases represented one extreme in the total mortality decline, mortality due to tuberculosis represented the other, with a slower decline in age groups 20/40 as well as in age groups 40/60 (females). As the lag was especially manifest for females, the result was a decrease in the excess male mortality (Figure 11). This pattern cannot be observed for any other of the more important diseases. Due to the dominant role of tuberculosis, the total age-specific mortality was influenced. This means that the pattern was similar to that of the rural areas. Therefore, we may raise the question again: How much was a result of worsened working conditions for women and how much could be attributed to a possibly autonomous epidemiological factor of the disease?

Figure 9. Age-specific mortality rates 1821/1830-1901/1910 for males and females in different age-groups for rural Sweden (--), urban Sweden (—) and Stockholm (···)

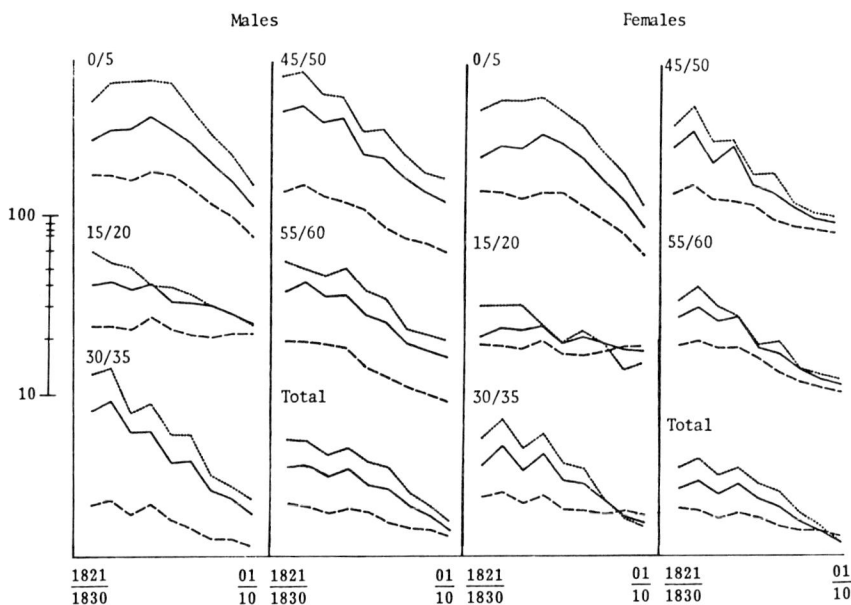

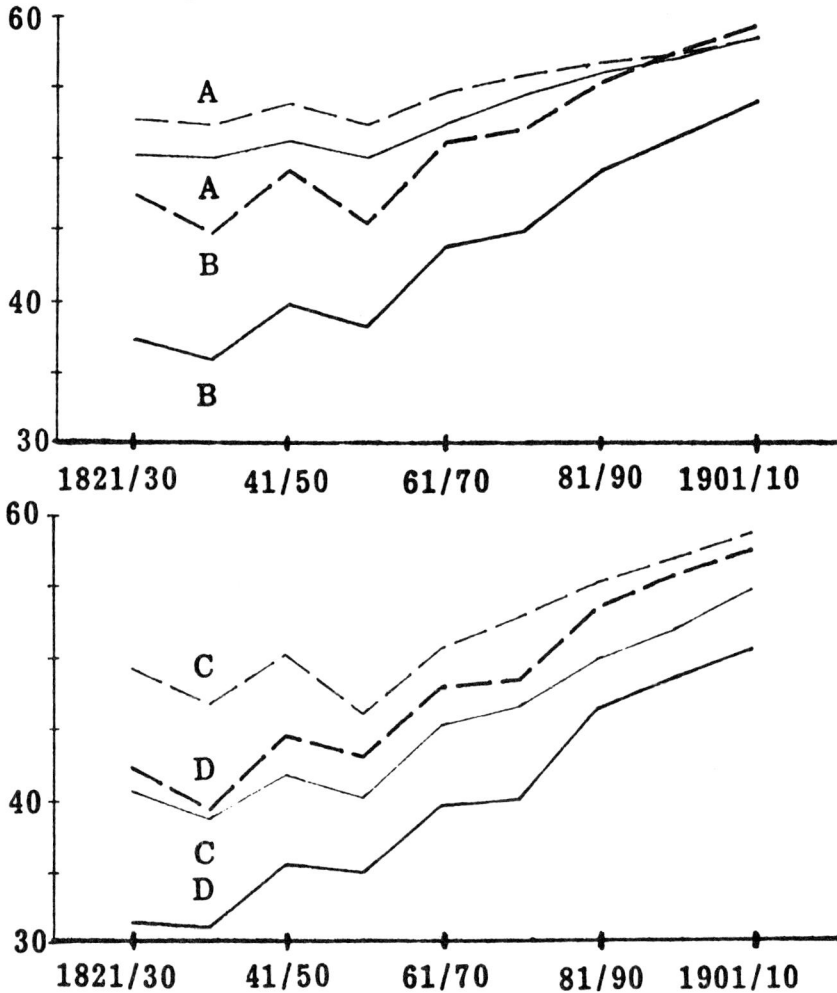

Figure 10. Life expectancy at age five for rural and urban areas 1821/1830-1901/1910. A = Rural Sweden. B = Urban Sweden. C = Urban Sweden excluding Stockholm. D = Stockholm.   Males —   Females ---

A differentiation according to civil status adds some important aspects to the issue. Looking at Stockholm and the age group 20/30, there was excess mortality for married females at the same time as there was a pronounced excess mortality for unmarried men. In higher age groups, the excess mortality among unmarried men becomes more accentuated while the excess mortality among married women disappears. The conventional picture of a significant bad situation for the married women in the early industrial town—as a result of repeated pregnancies under a double work burden—is hardly verified by our data. Her situation was not worse than for an unmarried woman, and much better than that of the married and the unmarried man. This means that, whereas in the rural area the dividing line with regard to mortality goes between married and unmarried people, in the town it goes between the two sexes.

261

Figure 11. Age-specific mortality rates for tuberculosis (B) and other diseases (A) 1875/1880, 1881/1890, 1891/1900 and 1901/1910.
Males —   Females ---

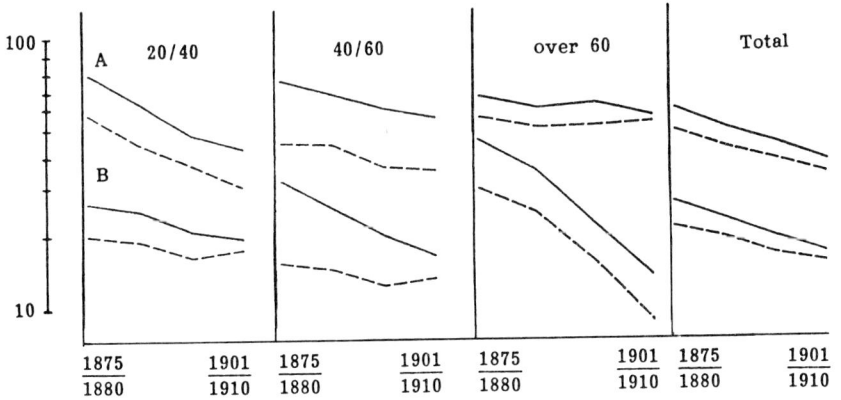

Figure 12. Stockholm. Age-specific mortality rates 25/30-40/45 according to sex and civil status 1871/1880-1901/1910. Index. Married female = 100.
A = age-groups 25/30, B = 30/35, C = 35/40, D = 40/45.

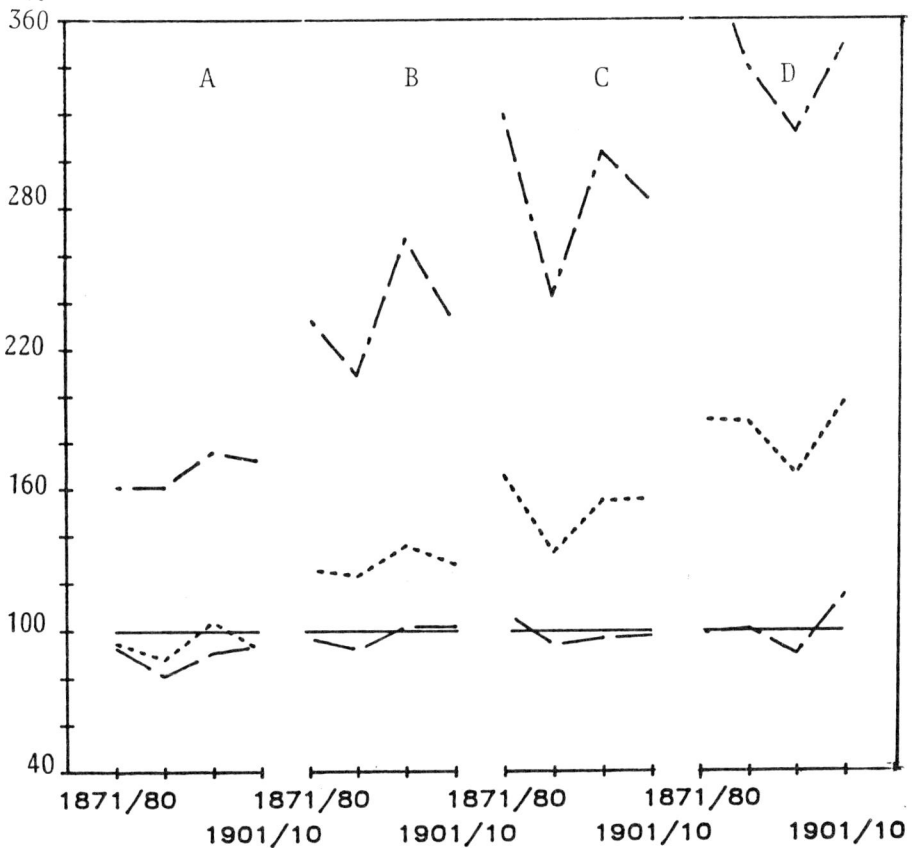

Table 11. Sex-differential mortality rates for married and unmarried in urban Sweden 1871-1880—1901-1910. Female = 100.

Married	20/25	25/30	30/35	35/40	40/45	45/50
1871-80	90	90	110	135	150	184
1881-90	75	90	101	113	147	166
1891-00	79	87	111	122	144	160
1901-10	100	84	107	116	140	156
Unmarried	20/25	25/30	30/35	35/40	40/45	45/50
1871-80	162	176	253	290	371	331
1881-90	167	188	209	244	293	305
1891-00	162	182	233	268	279	287
1901-10	138	162	188	247	249	245

Conclusion

This paper has pointed to the complex causality behind the mortality decline in Sweden during the 19th century. In this we have to consider socio-economic, medical and biological factors. These, as yet little penetrated relations complicate the analysis of the sex differential patterns during the period. However, the homogeneous development in different regions and at different levels of aggregation appears to indicate that it is possible to consider certain general factors in the analysis. The male mortality hump in the working ages during the first half of the century seems to be firmly anchored in an excessive consumption of alcoholic beverages; in the towns this factor was combined with unhealthy working and living conditions. The worsened situation for women at the end of the century, in some cases manifest in an excess female mortality, is more difficult to explain. Possibly, both changes in labour conditions and in the epidemiological climate are important factors. It is difficult to accept that excess female mortality during childhood could be a result of a continuous discrimination of girls. A more fruitful approach would be to concentrate on tuberculosis and the specific conditions for this disease.

Broadly speaking, the change in the sex-differential mortality rates during the first half of the 19th century was to a great extent caused by socio-economic factors; during the second half, on the other hand, biological factors seem to have been involved to a considerably larger extent. Thus, this pattern seems to have been quite the opposite concerning the general mortality decline.[33] A more detailed analysis of this complicated relation is, of course, outside the aim of this paper.[34]

Appendix

Methods and material

For the period 1749-1859, our mortality series are based on figures compiled from the unprinted material of *Tabellverket;* after that from *Bidrag till Sveriges officiella statistik* ser. A and K, (1860-1910) and from *Sveriges officiella statistik* (1911-1914). For every year and region studied, the number of dead people have been compiled according to ages and sex; every fifth year (1749-1774 every third) the whole population also according to sex and ages. In a similar way the number of dead males and females have been compiled according to cause of death up to 1830, when this statistic ended. From 1861 a new cause of death series started (age- and sex-specific) based on doctors' death attests but only for the towns. (1861-1870 every town; 1875-1910 all towns together.) These series have been compiled and computer analyzed. From 1911 the statistics on a national level again gives cause of death series for both country and towns. To a certain extent the material in this paper is taken from a more comprehensive study under preparation "Urban mortality in Sweden 1750 to 1914". In this I also have studied age-, sex- and cause of death-specific mortality in different towns according to size and regional location for the whole period.

On a national level the mortality and population tables of Tabellverket can be used without more serious reservations. For Stockholm the material of the 18th century, especially the population figures for certain years, might be of a lower quality. However, the sex differential mortality series constructed are reliable for our purposes.

The age- and sex-differential mortality rates for rural Sweden 1751-1820 are calculated as Tabellverket only gives mortality figures for Sweden in total during this period. This calculation is an approximation and has its starting point in the relations between the sex-differential mortality rates for rural and total Sweden 1821-1830, with a decreasing rate backwards in time. That the method gives a correct tendency of the mortality development is indicated by the fact that the towns also in the second part of the 18th century show a higher male excess mortality compared with the rural areas; besides, calculating the age- and sex-differential mortality rates for 5 counties with few and small towns (Södermanland, Kristianstad, Kronoberg, Skaraborg and Värmland) 1751-1770 we find a lower excess male mortality than 1821-1830 with the towns excluded. And at least: the age-specific excess male mortality rates for rural Sweden 1821-1850 are higher than for all of Sweden 1751-1810.

The cause of death series of Tabellverket are difficult to deal with from many aspects; especially due to changes in nomenclature and the vagueness and inaccuracy of the diagnoses.

For this paper we only have commented a special problem concerning tuberculosis. For a more comprehensive discussion concerning this topic see B.-I. Puranen, *Tuberkulos. En sjukdoms förekomst och dess orsaker. Sverige*

1750-1980 (Umeå 1984). For the whole country the mortality development of tuberculosis for the period of Tabellverket (1749-1859) are given by G. Sundbärg "Dödligheten i lungtuberkulos i Sverige 1751-1830", *Statistisk Tidskrift* (1905); for the towns 1869-1900 by C. Runeborg and G. Sundbärg, "Dödligheten i lungtuberkulos i Sveriges städer åren 1861-1900", *Statistisk Tidskrift* (1905). For the first period tuberculosis includes "consumptions of the lungs" */lungsot/,* "signs of consumption" */trånsjuka/,* "pine-away diseases" */tvinsot/* and haemotysis */blodhostning/.* Sometimes the causes of death are registered separately, sometimes together. On a national level, the pine-away diseases had about 25 per cent of the total mortality (1776-1800). The distribution over the ages, however, was uneven: (males in per cent) 0/1;84, 1/5;86, 5/10;66, 10/25;27, 25/50;12, 50;20. Concerning Stockholm, the proportion was somewhat lower, 16 per cent of the total mortality in tuberculosis (1781-1790). The age-distribution, however, was the same. Over time, the proportion of pine-away diseases seems on the whole to have been constant. When calculating mortality due to pine-away diseases for the ages 0/25 during the period 1821-1830, when the statistics only register pine-away for the elderly, we have assumed this to be a fact.

In the series of causes of death for the towns from 1861, pine-away diseases are in the beginning also registered as a separate cause of death. Compared with the towns 1821-1830 *(Tabellverket)* the new figures—based on doctors' attests and not on the priests' diagnoses—are higher in total and more concentrated to higher and lower ages. However, in new series from 1875 the pine-away disease as a special cause of death has disappeared, and is possibly included among a new comprehensive cause of death "congenital diseases and defects". Only a very small part may have been included in tuberculosis. This is also the case with the disease in the higher ages, which may possibly be indicated by a slight increase in the mortality due to tuberculosis between 1865-1870—1875-1880.

Runeborg and Sundbärg, calculating mortality due to tuberculosis from 1860, do not, however, include pine-away diseases. Thus, the mortality series due to tuberculosis for the first half of the century include pine-away diseases, but not for the second half.

Possibly, it is less suitable to classify pine-away diseases in the infant and child ages as tuberculosis. This is, for instance, suggested by the new nomenclature in 1875. Another reason is that pulmonary tuberculosis in children has a more acute course and does not have the character of a slow atrophy *(O. Cronberg, 40-points paper in economic history,* Lund 1986). Warrant reasons may possibly also be raised against including pine-away diseases in the higher ages, among tuberculosis. Discussing this problem more in detail is outside the topic of this paper. However, as I am working with series from the end of the 18th century to 1914, and the behaviour of tuberculosis has a central place in my analysis, I have to touch the problem. It is more for practical reasons that I define tuberculosis according to Sundbärg in this paper.

Table 12. Sex differential mortality rates for rural Sweden (A), urban Sweden (B) and Stockholm (C).

A

	0/5	5/10	10/15	15/20	20/25	25/30	30/35	35/40	40/45	45/50	50/55	55/60	60/65	65/70	70/75	Total
1751-60	111	103	103	107	129	106	98	111	101	131	129	128	114	108	103	108
1761-70	111	100	111	111	127	110	97	111	105	128	127	130	114	118	104	108
1771-80	110	106	114	103	118	100	99	100	100	114	114	117	105	112	105	106
1781-90	108	104	109	111	128	116	110	117	114	127	125	127	114	110	106	104
1791-00	107	103	103	102	115	92	90	101	100	126	121	123	114	109	108	106
1801-10	108	104	109	101	123	102	95	104	102	118	117	121	110	112	112	107
1811-20	107	103	104	96	111	101	93	107	114	127	124	125	117	113	111	109
1821-30	117	106	102	98	116	110	110	124	124	134	142	137	121	110	117	111
1831-40	117	107	110	98	115	113	109	117	123	138	136	128	123	117	113	109
1841-50	119	113	102	98	118	110	105	116	125	142	139	136	123	121	126	111
1851-60	121	106	111	104	122	117	113	104	113	134	134	128	120	104	110	109
1861-70	115	107	105	105	127	116	107	103	113	127	127	116	125	115	118	110
1871-80	116	103	96	98	123	104	99	95	103	121	123	123	110	116	115	107
1881-90	114	102	94	94	115	100	91	90	101	114	119	121	115	112	112	104
1891-00	116	98	89	92	108	97	87	89	95	111	113	119	115	112	111	102
1901-10	119	99	85	92	109	94	84	83	94	103	112	113	115	113	110	100

Table 12. Sex differential mortality rates for rural Sweden (A), urban Sweden (B) and Stockholm (C).

B

	0/5	5/10	10/15	15/20	20/25	25/30	30/35	35/40	40/45	45/50	50/55	55/60	60/65	65/70	70/75	Total
1821-30	116	120	125	147	174	198	231	222	225	212	208	176	162	145	134	136
1831-40	116	121	112	138	172	179	206	205	204	186	181	176	154	132	130	127
1841-50	120	117	117	129	147	166	191	208	216	224	200	173	163	154	125	129
1851-60	117	112	107	132	159	144	158	178	194	188	178	167	148	126	127	124
1861-70	110	100	106	130	144	147	152	177	195	194	191	192	167	159	147	122
1871-80	112	101	100	120	153	145	162	176	193	203	195	188	161	160	155	127
1881-90	114	102	99	123	155	145	140	147	175	187	187	176	165	151	139	124
1891-00	117	100	95	122	152	141	155	151	164	181	182	181	162	153	141	122
1901-10	119	102	90	112	138	131	139	149	149	167	179	177	166	152	137	117

*Table 12.*Sex differential mortality rates for rural Sweden(A), urban Sweden (B) and Stockholm (C).
C

	0/5	5/10	10/15	15/20	20/25	25/30	30/35	35/40	40/45	45/50	50/55	55/60	60/65	65/70	70/75	Total
1751-60	114	118	153	126	181	155	132	145	142	136	155	172	147	133	121	126
1761-70	120	116	132	137	207	184	152	135	127	140	156	168	145	172	108	133
1771-80	110	122	124	128	171	159	131	120	142	140	152	136	150	133	124	130
1781-90	112	115	138	158	138	140	136	143	149	144	144	140	121	130	126	120
1791-00	126	110	131	134	150	131	132	138	128	131	130	146	148	132	95	117
1801-10	127	117	118	150	241	203	178	175	169	170	136	160	120	108	117	127
1811-20	113	118	116	116	137	135	151	168	190	179	190	166	164	140	192	125
1821-30	106	116	107	153	172	206	250	259	293	252	235	208	201	163	144	147
1831-40	118	124	108	133	159	168	221	210	216	210	194	160	177	117	128	129
1841-50	120	125	147	125	120	148	184	221	246	239	213	188	215	167	110	132
1851-60	118	118	117	127	125	141	174	200	203	224	201	231	176	154	138	132
1861-70	133	102	115	153	125	154	170	215	230	227	217	240	184	147	139	135
1871-80	115	101	107	122	140	150	184	215	250	220	224	216	160	179	148	138
1881-90	115	98	95	123	154	157	167	178	226	236	268	206	191	168	140	130
1891-00	117	96	94	153	164	160	187	203	213	212	194	209	180	176	155	130
1901-10	120	103	90	128	140	153	174	196	225	204	227	205	177	147	147	128

However, a definition excluding pine- away diseases will not change our main results. From 1821-1830 we will have a somewhat slower decline in total mortality due to tuberculosis; in the higher ages the pattern is similar; in the ages from 10 to about 40 we will have a faster increase (the rural areas) or a more accentuated lag (the towns), and for infant and child ages on the whole an unchanging development instead for a lower decrease. In this connection, we will also point out that dealing with tuberculosis, we are always speaking of pulmonary tuberculosis.

Another problem is how to get homogeneous series according to age-groups and cause of death—tuberculosis—during the whole period for the age-groups over ten years (for the age-groups under 10 years there are no problems) as the classification into age-groups differs. We have chosen to give homogeneous series for the age-groups 10/20, 20/40, 40/60 and over 60. For the period 1821-1830 having only the age-groups 10/25, 25/50 and <50 we have solved this in the following way: Analyzing mortality due to tuberculosis at the end of the 18th century, when causes of death were registered in 5-year intervals, we found a very homogeneous mortality increase. It is reasonable to suppose that in the period 1821-1830, the average 10/25, 25/50 and over 50 concealed a similar pattern. Thus, an interpolation may give rather acceptable figures for the new headings.

Notes

1. See especially S.R. Johansson, 'Deferred Infanticide: Excess Female Mortality During Childhood' G. Hausfater and S.B. Hardy, (Eds.), *Infanticide* (New York 1984). Some general series regarding France, England and Sweden are, however, given in D. Tabutin, 'La surmortalité fémine en Europe avant 1940', *Population*, 1 (1978).

2. See, A.E. Imhof, *The Over-Mortality of Married Women of Child-Bearing Age. An Illustration of the "condition féminine" in the 19th Century.* Paper presented at a conference held by the "Société de Démographie Historique" (Paris 1979). See also A.E. Imhof, 'Women, Family and Death: Excess Mortality of Women in Childbearing Age in Four Communities in Nineteenth-century Germany' J. Evans and W.R. Lee (Eds.), *The German Family* (London 1981). A first version of this paper was presented at the workshop *"Methodological problems in Urban History: Demography and Social Stratification in the Early Phase of Industrialisation, 1750-1850"* (Stockholm 1984). At the same workshop Ulf Jonsson dealt with the issue in his paper 'Mortality Patterns in the 18th and 19th Century Stockholm in a European Perspective'. In her dissertation *Tuberkulos. En sjukdoms förekomst och dess orsaker. Sverige 1750-1980* (Umeå 1984), Britt-Inger Puranen also deals with the problem.

3. Concerning material and methods see Appendix.

4. Tabutin (1978).

5. Johansson (1984).

6. See for instance, P. Bairoch, 'Europe's Gross National Product: 1800-1975', *Journal of European Economic History* (1976); G. Sandberg, 'Banking and Economic Growth in Sweden before World War I', *Journal of Economic History,* 3 (1978).

7. O. Krantz, *Utrikeshandel, ekonomisk tillväxt och strukturförändring efter 1850* (Lund 1986).

8. L. Jörberg, *A History of Prices in Sweden 1732-1914* (Lund 1972).

9. Puranen (1984).

10. Experiences from Malmö, Swedens third largest town, shows that during the 80's about 16 per cent of all in-migrants belonged to the age-group 15/20 years, which can be compared with 20 resp. 18 per cent for the age-groups 20/24 and 25/30. Certainly we have to count on a similar pattern with regard to Stockholm. (G. Fridlizius, 'Agricultural Productivity, Trade and Urban Growth during the Commercialization Phase of the Swedish Economic Development, 1810-70', A. van der Woude, et al (Eds.), *Proceedings from ... Paper for an IUSSP symposium* (Tokyo 1986).

11. See further footnote 21.

12. Imhof (1981).

13. A cohort analysis gives further support to this opinion. The declining child mortality from the end of the 18th century ought to have given these cohorts a possibility to lead a healthier life throughout their entire lifetimes, in spite of the fact that there are no signs of improvements in nutrition, housing, labour market conditions or medicine. For the females, we do find this kind of "natural" development from a cohort point of view. For the males, however, the gains from this favourable start in life could not be reaped when the cohorts entered ages above 30; instead we find a "deformed" cohort manifest in a stagnant age- specific mortality rate. Our analysis is based on cohort tables for Sweden as a whole and Stockholm, and constructed in the

270

following way: First we calculated the average for the sex- and age-specific mortality rates—10 years interval—1751-1780, that are the decades just before the start of the secular decline in mortality in Sweden. The age- and sex-specific mortality rates for the decades 1781-1790—1900-1910 were then related to this average (the age-groups on the Y-axis). Similar values along the same columns would suggest that mortality improvements proceeded in a period-specific way; similar values along the diagonals would suggest that the improvements proceeded in a cohort-specific way. The method is inspired by that used by Preston and van de Walle when analysing the mortality decline in France. S. Preston and E. van de Walle, 'Urban French Mortality in the Nineteenth Century', *Population Studies,* 32, 2 (1978). In another connection this theme will be further developed (Fridlizius, op. cit. forthcoming).

14. See especially T. Larsson, *Reformer i brännvinslagstiftningen 1853-54. Förhistorien.* (Stockholm 1945).

15. G. Sundbärg 'Dödligheten i lungtuberkulos i Sverige 1751-1830', *Statistisk Tidskrift* (1905).

16. Puranen (1984).

17. From a cohort point of view, this process could, in its first phase, be described as new and healthier male cohorts from the 1820's and 1830's reaching working age, which means that the cohorts are becoming less deformed, whereas the position of the females is unchanged.

18. The rapid decline of the mortality in the higher age-groups from a high mortality level was first observed by Sundbärg (1905). Puranen (1984), thinks that this high mortality by the end of the 18th century may be cohort-influenced; it is an effect of a higher mortality due to tuberculosis in the first half of the 18th century. Owing to a lack of material from this time, this thesis cannot be tested. However, we undoubtedly have this pattern as late as 1821-1830, without finding a higher mortality in the decades after 1750, when we have reliable material. Possibly it is more reasonable to suggest that the high mortality due to tuberculosis in the higher ages reflects a society with a generally high infant and child mortality. Children who avoided falling ill—during this period smallpox had a strategic position—went through life with less resistance against other diseases, infectious and non-infectious alike; a particular sensitivity to relapse was one result. The decline in mortality due to tuberculosis from the 1840's in the highest ages, which happened at the same time as a decline in other diseases, is possibly cohort-influenced. The decline can partly be seen as a result of the low infant- and child mortality from the end of the 18th century, which gave these cohorts the chance to go through life with a better immunity against different diseases, not at least tuberculosis. Fewer relapses resulted. The accentuated lag in the mortality due to tuberculosis in the ages around 20 years may mirror the biological structure of the disease.

19. By mistake the age-groups 20/25 is not represented in figure 4.

20. The decline in the long term mortality due to mortality in childbirth and childbed fever in rural Sweden started in the 80's: (per 1000 women in confinement): 1861-1870: 4,8. 1871-1880: 5,1. 1881-1890: 3,8. 1891-1900: 2,8. Examined midwives per 1000 women in confinement: 1861 1870: 359. 1871-1000. 467. 1881-1890: 600. 1891-1895: 700. E.W. Wretlind, 'Döde af barnsängsfeber och barnsbörd i Sverige 1776-1900', *Jordemodern,* 2 (1904).

21. For a review of some of these, see Tabutin (1978), and Preston and van de Walle (1978).

22. Our cohort-mortality interpretation also seems to be valid for Stockholm.

23. U. Jonsson, 'Mortality Patterns in the 18th and 19th Century Stockholm in a European Perspective', *Research Report No. 2 in the project: Stagnating Metropolis: Growth Problems and Social Inequality in Stockholm, 1760-1850.* The Department of Economic History, University of Stockholm (1984), emphasizes the importance of the labour-market for the mortality level. See also J. Söderberg, 'Den stagnerande staden', *Historisk tidskrift,* 2 (1985).

24. J. Söderberg, 'Poverty and Social Structure in Stockholm 1850', *Research Report No. 1 in the project: Stagnating Metropolis* (1982).

25. Söderberg (1982).

26. A detailed discussion concerning these problems is given in Puranen (1984).

27. See also a survey over new drinking research in L. Magnusson, 'Drinking and the Verlag System 1820-1850: The Significance of Taverns and Drink in Eskilstuna before Industrialization', *The Scandinavian Economic History Review,* 1 (1986).

28. J. Söderberg, *Real Wage Trends in Urban Europe, 1730-1850: Stockholm in a Comparative Perspective* (Stockholm 1984).

29. See, for instance, G. Fridlizius, 'Handel och Sjöfart', *Malmö Stads historia,* 3 (1981).

30. See for instance Preston and van de Walle (1978).

31. In urban Sweden during the period 1875-1880—1901-1910 the age-specific mortality due to different stomach diseases, including typhoid, and all other diseases declined in the following way—figures for stomach diseases first. (Index 1875-1880= 100: 0/5: 32, 49. 5/10: 27, 40. 10/20: 32, 67. 20/60: 37, 60. Over 60: 33, 81. Total: 32, 64. Regarding France, Preston and van de Walle are of the opinion, that the mortality decline in the child-ages due to different stomach diseases had a cohort mortality effect; Preston and van de Walle (1978). Possibly we had a similar pattern in Sweden, especially as mortality due to stomach diseases constituted a considerable part of the total mortality in the age group 0/5: in 1875-1880 28,4 per cent (males) and 26,9 (females).

32. The age-specific death probabilities (q), are calculated from age-specific mortality rates (5-years) for ten-year periods (m) according to the formula: $q = \dfrac{5 \cdot m}{1 + \frac{5}{2} \cdot m}$

33. If we accept that the infant- and child mortality decline from the end of the 18th century was primarily the result of a long term change in the relationship between the infectious organism and the human host and that the mortality decline was cohort influenced, the following decline in higher age groups might, to a considerable degree, also have been caused by biological factors. However, at the end of the century, this initial push to a lower mortality was to a large extent caused by socio-economic factors.

34. However, it is obvious that future research in this subject to a larger extent than has often been assumed, must consider a disease synergism, often based on a cohort mode of operation.

Urban Water Supply and Improvement of Health Conditions

Reinhold Castensson, Marianne Löwgren and Jan Sundin

Introduction

Several theories have been launched concerning the decline in mortality in Western Europe during the previous centuries. Thomas McKeown, who discussed a number of those theories, declared that the decline was, without much doubt, caused by improved nutritional conditions. His proof was mainly negative; there were few indications of a dramatic change in the virulence of diseases, and there was no proof that the population had become immune to them. Medical progress was very modest; the only spectacular development was the vaccination against smallpox until penicillin was discovered. By excluding possible alternatives, McKeown thought that he had reason to believe that the improved economy, and thereby the improved nutritional and material standard of living of the people, was to be given most of the credit for the decline in mortality.[1]

Although the results of medical research in poor countries today strongly indicate that nutritional status has great impact upon health, there are many researchers who claim that McKeown overlooked at least one factor which could have contributed to the decline in mortality, namely the preventive work of the medical profession, midwives, local authorities and, at least in Sweden, the Church. Anders Brändström has shown that in some parts of Sweden high levels of infant mortality were caused by the lack of breast-feeding combined with poor hygienic habits. He also showed that infant mortality decreased rapidly when medical doctors and trained midwives managed to convince parents of the benefit of breast-feeding and good hygiene.[2]

Britt-Inger Puranen demonstrated that there were several causes of tuberculosis, for example inferior housing conditions, poor hygiene, and malnutrition. These factors could be changed by the activities of the medical profession and the authorities.[3] Similarly, Jan Sundin and Lars-Göran Tedebrand have shown that health conditions at the Swedish iron foundries seem to have been influenced by the paternalistic system applied there. Infant mortality was lower at the foundries than in the agrarian hinterland, and it decreased earlier at the foundries than in the agrarian surroundings, indicating an open-mindedness towards the improvement of health conditions.[4]

Even if it is evident that economic factors influenced mortality, especially when yearly fluctuations are concerned (as an example see the results of economic historians in Lund)[5], there is still reason to consider whether or not it was possible for authorities and individuals to influence health conditions and to study the attitudes towards the improvement of hygienic conditions. It is known that mortality rates differed between the sexes, between age groups, between social groups, between different geographical regions and between urban and rural areas. It is also known that changes took place during different periods of time for different age groups, social groups and geographical regions. The observed differences make it necessary to be cautious when trying to reduce the number of causes for the decline in mortality to one specific factor.

Some results of studies on mortality rates in the city of Stockholm during the transitional period have been presented by Ulf Jonsson and Johan Söderberg. The results are based mainly on aggregated statistics and a comparison between Stockholm and other European cities, and they show that Stockholm had some specific patterns that may possibly be explained by socio-economic factors.[6] Thus far, however, little is known about the detailed development of mortality in rural areas and even less about what happened in Swedish cities.

Nationwide studies have shown that, as expected, mortality in urban areas was, for a long period of time, higher than in rural areas. The population density was, of course, larger in the urban areas, making hygienic factors more difficult to handle, and exposure to diseases via contacts between different areas more common. However, even this general picture needs to be more closely inspected in order to explain why the urban mortality rate finally reached the levels of the countryside. It is not at all evident that this process was caused by a larger increase in prosperity among the inhabitants of the cities in comparison to their neighbours in the countryside.

The city of Linköping — a case study of mortality decline

The city of Sundsvall, a center of forest industry in northern Sweden, will soon be the object of studies concerning the development of mortality, morbidity and health care during the last two centuries. These studies will further illuminate questions concerning mortality in Swedish cities. In one or two years, another project is planned to be started in which the city of Linköping, situated on the plains in southern Sweden, will be studied. A presentation of the basic development of the decline in mortality in Linköping will illustrate what happened in a relatively typical, middle-sized, Swedish city, and which questions need to be asked in order to go further in understanding this process.

274

Table 1. Social distribution of adult men (above age 15) in the parish of Sankt Lars in 1750 and 1855.

Social group	Year 1750 Number	%	Year 1855 Number	%
"Middle class"	12	4	87	13
Farmers	97	29	60	9
Crofters, other landless	228	67	538	78
Total	337	100	685	100

Source: Tables from the Swedish Table Commission at the Provincial Archives in Vadstena.

Table 2. Social distribution of adult men (above age 15) in the city of Linköping in 1750 and 1855.

Social group	Year 1750 Number	%	Year 1855 Number	%
"Middle class"	97	18	406	24
Craftsmen, masters	100	19	120	9
Apprentices, unskilled workers	332	63	857	67
Total	529	100	1283	100

Source: Tables from the Swedish Table Commission in the Provincial Archives of Vadstena.

Tables 1 and 2 show the socio-economic structure in Linköping and in the adjacent agrarian parish of Sankt Lars in 1750 and 1855. Sankt Lars was by 1750 already a relatively proletarised parish, in which 4 % of the adult men came from the "middle class", 29 % were farmers and 67 % were crofters, soldiers and other members of the landless population. During the following 105 years, the farmers decreased in numbers and percentage, while the landless population and the "middle class" increased in both respects. In the city of Linköping a similar process took place. The number of merchants, factory owners and other members of the upper classes increased, and their share of the population increased from 18 to 24 %. The number of craftsmen with a master's title increased from 100 to 120, but their share of the population decreased from 19 to 9 %. The apprentices, the factory workers and the unskilled labourers increased their share of the population from 63 to 67 %.

Consequently, in both the agrarian parish and the city, a large percentage of the population belonged to the lower classes, and these classes increased their percentage as time progressed. On the other hand, there was also an increase in the "middle class" in both places. In Sankt Lars, however, the figures are partly illusive, since the majority of the "middle class" in 1855 consisted of pupils enrolled at the secondary school in Linköping, but residing in households outside the city limits.

Figures 1 and 2 (Appendix) present the demographic development in Linköping and in the agrarian parish of Sankt Lars. In the latter, the traditional pattern of high mortality, frequently surmounting the fertility rate, prevailed until the end of the eighteenth century. During the first 15 years after 1790 and continually after 1815, the mortality rate dropped and occupied a level far below the fertility rate, thereby creating a natural increase in the population; this increase, however, did not have a full effect due to a negative net migration. Even though there is a fluctuating but clear downward trend in the mortality curve in Figure 2, the dominating features are the two broad peaks of high mortality, one before the end of the eighteenth century and the other during three decades after 1815.

In the city of Linköping, the number of deaths exceeded the number of births until the end of the 1830's. In spite of that, the population increased during two phases: the first phase lasted until about 1780; the second included the entire nineteenth century. This was, of course, the effect of a positive net migration. As in the parish of Sankt Lars, the mortality rate increased during the first decades after 1769, but unlike Sankt Lars, the overall downward trend was much more pronounced after the peak years of 1775—1779. The reason this did not result in a constant excess of births over deaths before 1840, is that after 1845, the birth rate dropped from about 35 per 1000 persons to about 28 per 1000. This drop is at least partially due to the decreasing number of marriages, but thus far, there is no available information as to whether or not it was also caused by family planning.

After 1859, the statistical system in Sweden changed, and each individual parish no longer produced its own tables. The printed statistics do not give detailed reports on ages of death, but do, at least, give the total death rate. It can thus be seen that the general death rate reached a plateau in 1850—1864, a peak in 1865—1869 (caused by cholera and bad harvests) and a steady downward trend again after 1869. Records from census years show that the population in the original city parish grew from 6 138 in 1860 to 14 552 in 1900, a more than twofold increase in 40 years.[7] This increase was, on the average, about the same as for other contemporary Swedish cities. It occurred during a period of falling birth rates; in 1861—1870 the average birth rate in Linköping was 29 per 1000 inhabitants, in 1891—1900 the rate was 23. A certain excess of births over deaths prevailed, especially after 1869, but the main cause of the population increase was net migration.

Now that the general picture of mortality rates has been established for the two areas, attention will be turned to infant mortality in particular (Figure 3 in Appendix). From 1749 until the beginning of the nineteenth century infant mortality was usually lower in the parish of Sankt Lars than in the city of Linköping. While only a modest decline of the infant mortality rate occurred

276

in Sankt Lars, there was a much more pronounced decline in Linköping. After having been frighteningly high until 1794 (between 30 and 45 % and with two high peaks), the infant mortality rate started to fall. The decline took place in distinct "drops", one from a very high level in 1785—1789, a second in 1815—1819 and a third in 1845—1849. This development is quite different from the two peaks of high infant mortality in Sankt Lars.

A curve for infant mortality cannot be produced yet for the period prior to 1859, but fortunately, the city of Linköping was included in a special five-year investigation from 1876 to 1895. The results show that infant mortality dropped again after 1859, and that there was a downward trend during the latter part of the nineteenth century. The infant mortality rate had fallen from 40—45 % in the 1780's to less than 10 percent 100 years later, and the total death rate had become less than half of its original size during the same period!

Figure 4 (Appendix) shows the development of mortality after the age of one in the two areas in 1749—1859. With the exception of the period 1755—1769, when the peak of the agrarian parish had no counterpart in the city, the two curves seem to be shaped by the same, short term factors. Infant mortality was much higher in the city at the beginning of the period, but the level of mortality after the age of one was about the same in both areas before 1785. After that date and up until about 1840, the level decreased in the agrarian parish, while it continued to be high in the city. A downward trend was seen in both areas in the 1830's, but the drop was larger in the city, ending in a "rendez vous" of the two curves around 1840.

Finally, for the city of Linköping, the development of infant mortality will be compared with mortality after the age of one (Figure 5 in Appendix). Short term fluctuations coincided only occasionally. The peak of infant mortality in 1755—1764 had no counterpart in mortality after age 1, and the same situation occurred in 1770—1774 and in 1780—1784. Mortality after age 1 had peaks in 1810—1814 and 1825—1829, but no similar reactions in infant mortality. In general, infant mortality seems to have reacted more negatively during the peak period before 1785, but the decline in infant mortality was also more pronounced after that year. Both curves decline quickly during certain periods, but for infant mortality the declines are steeper downwards during two periods, 1815—1819 and 1845—1849. Although the declines in both curves were quick "drops", there is generally no total correlation in time or speed.

This is roughly what can be extracted from the statistical records. It is, of course, possible to gain a much more detailed understanding of the development by, among other things, dividing mortality into more age groups, by analyzing records of causes of death during peaks and slumps, and reading the comments made by the clergymen about the occurrence of epidemics. A quick look at the records reveals that throughout the period 1749—1859, certain causes of death were more frequently reported by the clergymen. Among these are dysentery, chest pains, fevers and ague (malaria?). In the eighteenth century, prior to the smallpox vaccination campaign, many children died of this disease, and smallpox also occurred sporadically during the nineteenth century. A violent scarlet fever epidemic took place among children in 1846. Other frequent children's disease were, as expected, measles and whooping cough. Adults and older children were stricken by cholera in 1834, 1852, 1855, 1857, 1858 and 1866.[8]

Since this report has a tentative approach, it is anticipated that the rough results presented will be adequate enough to point out some interesting and, as of yet, unanswered questions. Before starting to discuss where the answers to these questions may be found, the picture provided by the presented diagrams will be summarized. First of all, when comparing the city of Linköping to its agrarian neighbour the parish of Sankt Lars, there are both similarities and differences in the development of mortality. Some short term fluctuations coincide in the two areas (considering how some epidemics spread geographically, the opposite would be extremely surprising), and the final trend for mortality rates is downward in both cases.

Many differences, however, also exist. The situation in the city was remarkably gloomy during the eighteenth century and, for mortality after the age of 1, during the first decades of the nineteenth century. The observed deterioration in the mortality situation took place during a period of population increase in the city and can probably be partly explained by that fact. However, what is more striking is the rapid improvement of the conditions during a similar period of population growth after the year of 1800, starting among infants and spreading later to other age groups. Within a few decades, the rates of the city decreased to about the same levels as those of the agrarian parish. Influences of the geographical expansion of the city may also, of course, have been expressed in the neighbouring parish by then, but this does not explain the rapid decline in the mortality rates of the city.

A second observation that can be made, is that the declines of both infant mortality and mortality after age 1, were particularly pronounced during relatively short periods of time. It was not a question of slow, steady declines, but instead of stepwise drops. These periods are, of course, particularly interesting. Finally, it was also observed that there was no obvious common trend in infant mortality and mortality after age 1, and that there is no total temporal correlation between the large drops observed.

The development that took place in Linköping was not unique, it occurred in many Swedish cities during the same period. It is, however, striking that the positive effects were so pronounced despite the initially high level of mortality. In the 1840's, infant mortality in Linköping was almost as low as for the entire country of Sweden, including the rural areas, where mortality was usually lower than in the cities. By 1876—1880, the rates in Linköping were about the same as in the countryside, and well below those of the average Swedish city, and this situation continued throughout the century. This is in sharp contrast to the infant mortality in Linköping in 1751—1860, which was about 75 % higher than in the rest of the country.[9]

What are the reasons for these results? It is of course necessary to find out more about the development of the economic situation in the city. The "mortality wave" in the eighteenth century was probably connected with population growth, deteriorating housing conditions and the growth of a group of economically weak persons and households. The proposition that the economic situation improved during the first half of the nineteenth century cannot be rejected, but it is difficult to be totally content with this explanation alone. Migration to the city was large, people continued to live crowded together in small dwellings and the problems of vagrancy and unemployment were often discussed by the authorities. There was a crisis for traditional crafts and a general increase in the "proletariat" of the city. Did the housing conditions and the nutritional status of the population really improve to such an extent that they could provide an explanation for the decline in mortality? That certainly would have been an astonishing accomplishment.

There are other possibilities which should be considered, even if that will require more than a statistical analysis of time series of mortality and economic fluctuations. At present, the possibility of making estimations about the climate and harvests from historical time series is being investigated with the Linköping University Geographical Information System (LINGIS). Perhaps this system will be able to provide better tools for analysing connections between data concerning mortality and climate.

It is also possible that a qualitative change took place in the health conditions of the inhabitants of Linköping, a change that was connected with child care and hygienic conditions in general. This change, if it did occur, may not be easy to describe, and, if disclosed, it may be difficult to convincingly connect it with the decline in mortality. As a starting point, however, an attempt has to be made to test the hypothesis as thoroughly as possible. First of all, the activities of the agents of health improvement, the medical doctors and the midwives can be studied, in order to find out if their work could have changed the attitudes toward improvement held by the people and the local authorities. Secondly, it can be investigated whether or not the authorities actually reacted, and if so, in what way.[10] The demographic investigation can also be pursued to the level of individuals, households and different areas within the city.

The progressive development of the system for the supply of water and the disposal of sewage could be studied in much greater detail. Primitive systems for these purposes already existed during the first half of the century. In the 1870's the first relatively modern pipelines were installed in Linköping. This development needs to be studied as thoroughly as possible. It is known that water quality and quantity are essential factors affecting health conditions of the populations in developing countries; why should the situation have been different in European cities of the past? Infants suffer severely from bad

279

drinking water, cholera is spread to adults by water, and so on. The quantity of water supplied to each household indicates its level of hygienic standard.

Water supply and waste disposal

Urban water supply in Sweden has long been based on both surface water and ground water sources. Swedish cities are usually located near rivers or streams or are built up close to eskers; these location criteria constitute excellent conditions for sustainable urban water supplies. The disadvantage of being largely dependent on local water resources is the vulnerability to human-induced water pollution. The more densely populated an urban area is, the greater the risk for self-contamination of the water sources. Therefore, in correspondence with urban growth, the water supply systems have to be quantitatively and qualitatively adapted to the development of water needs.

There is some documentary and archaeological evidence of the existence of an 18th century water supply in Linköping; a reconstruction of this is shown in Figure 6. The water supply was dependent on both the extraction of ground water from public and private wells and on the delivery of surface water from the Stångå River. The fact that the city is located on a slope of an esker, made it easy to extract ground water from the upper instream areas.

In 1749, the famous architect Carl Hårleman visited Linköping and made an investigation of water quality. Comparing the river surface water with the ground water from wells, he stated that the best drinking water came from the Stångå River. It tasted and looked good.[11] There were, however, several complaints about bad hygienic conditions during the 18th century. In 1757, the district medical doctor complained about unsatisfactory street cleaning, pigs running loose, and poor drainage and water logging in the lower eastern parts of the city. The eastern church yard was especially affected; since it was located in an undrained, outstream area near the river, it was impossible to use it as a cemetery, because water flooded "half way up in newly dug graves"[12].

Household wastewater from cleaning, cooking or washing was disposed of in the most convenient way, which usually meant simply throwing it into the streets or street gutters. The wastewater, heavily contaminated by human and animal wastes, then soaked into the ground, polluting groundwater which fed wells and the area of the Stångå River used as a drinking water supply. The process is illustrated in Figure 7. A certain filtering effect might have occurred during the infiltration into the ground. But, no doubt, a great deal of the contamination was transported to the wells and then to the river, which was also a recipient for wastes from tanneries and dye works situated upstream the water supply facilities.

Figure 7. The process of self-contamination of ground water in private wells and surface water in the adjacent river. Profile of the town of Linköping and the Stångå river, 1817.

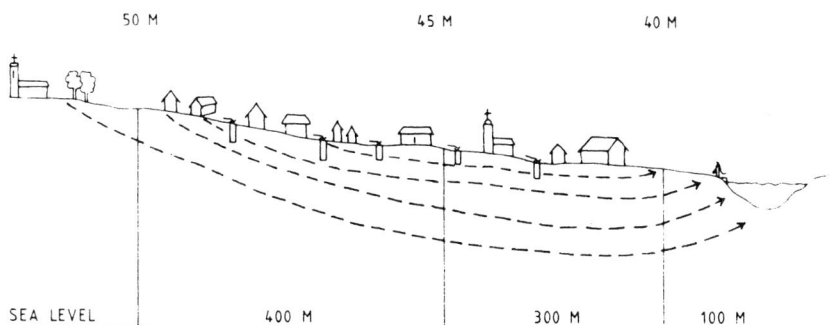

Administrative regulations

Several attempts were made to improve the situation by means of legislation. In 1775, the City Council prohibited the disposal of dirt and manure in the river upstream of the city. At the end of the 18th century, the land owners were obliged to clean the streets twice a week, and later, this was extended to daily street cleaning during the hot summer months. Street cleaning became a heavy burden; in 1799, 27 persons were prosecuted during one week for neglecting their share of the street. Scavengers were hired to take care of the wastes in public areas of the city, however, these services were inefficient and irregular.

The first local Building Act, submitted in 1818, imposed several rules aimed at improving the hygiene of the city. It was prescribed that gutters and ditches should be lined with stones in order to increase the run-off, and annual inspections were stipulated to inform the house owners about their maintenance duties. Similar ordinances were included in the Building Act of 1830.[13]

In general, the efficiency of these types of administrative regulations depended on the willingness of the inhabitants to cooperate with them and on the type of control system used to enforce them. The success of the administrative regulations imposed in Linköping can be partially illustrated by the number of persons punished for disobedience. The lists of fines registered at the two courts in Linköping during the first decades of the nineteenth century, represent a noticeable ambition to keep hygienic standards high. Seven different categories of "uncleanliness" can be discerned in those lists: negligence in cleaning streets or market places; non-participation in the "sanitary guard" (during the cholera epidemic of 1834); transporting manure through the city during forbidden periods (mainly during the hot summer months); negligence in keeping gutters free from ice and other obstacles; washing in the river at forbidden places; bathing in the river at forbidden places; non-notification of the outbreak of an epidemic disease.

The seven categories above are listed in order according to the total number of persons prosecuted for each offense. Out of a total of 218 cases in 1809—1839, 134 belonged to the first category, 31 to the second, 24 to the third. Keeping the streets clean and preventing sick people from other areas from entering the city were evidently the ordinances that concerned the authorities most. The number of prosecutions increased during years of epidemic crisis. The first wave of prosecution appeared in 1812, a year which was characterized by a post-war epidemic and high mortality in the city. Another wave appeared in 1834, when there were, in all, 31 prosecutions of negligent security guards, 5 prosecutions of persons who had not cleaned their parts of the street and 3 prosecutions of persons who had transported manure through the city during forbidden periods. The wave continued at a lower level after the actual cholera epidemic (16 cases in 1835 and 17 cases in 1836), before again decreasing to a few cases per year in 1837—1839. The frequency of prosecutions is illustrated in Figure 8.

In general, however, the prosecution rate was more pronounced during the 1830's than it had been earlier, which indicates the ambitious attempts of the city administration to improve the situation. The threat of cholera was probably one of the reasons for more stringent control, but this, in turn, also had effect on other diseases caused by poor hygienic conditions, especially since the control measured by the number of prosecutions was most active during the hot summer months.

Awareness to the *growing water quality problems* is documented in the records from the City Council. In 1808, the Mayor made a proposal to search for a new surface water source upstream of the old one. A mill barrage had turned part of the river near the city into a sedimentation basin for various wastes from the streets and tanneries along the river banks. After discussing and investigating the problems, it was found that the most inexpensive solution would be to establish a new water supply upstream of the old one; this was carried out in 1817, and pumps were also installed at a later date.[14]

The improvement of water supplies during the beginning of the 19th century was not entirely due to an interest in public health or for the convenience of the urban population. Some cities, especially larger ones, installed simple piping systems to increase access to water in case of fire; the cities were densely covered with wooden buildings, which meant that fires were often disastrous and more ample water supplies were required for fire fighting.

As social changes occur, repercussions are found in the management structure of society. The growth of the Swedish cities during the second part of the nineteenth century was accompanied by an increase in legislation aimed at improving health and order, and the new laws, of course, facilitated the growth of the urban population. Stockholm, by far the largest of the Swedish cities, had to cope with the greatest environmental problems. According to Yvonne Hirdman, the fear of cholera was the reason for establishing a "Health Board" *(Sundhetskommittén)* in Stockholm in 1831. Local health boards were appointed in each parish in order to improve waste collection and food distribution. In spite of this, Stockholm was struck by an epidemic in the summer of 1834, as was mentioned previously. The importance of water and hygiene is further traceable in the Ordinance of Epidemics *(Epidemistadgan)* of 1857, which established permanent health boards in Stockholm. Their tasks were comprised not only of organizing medical care during epidemics, but also of investigating the origins of diseases and working at preventive health care.[15]

In Linköping, a committee was founded to plan preventive measures to divert the threat of cholera in 1831, twenty persons were, however, taken ill in 1834. The committee was turned into a permanent Health Board, working to prevent the risk of epidemics.[16]

The first Ordinance for Local Order *(ordningsstadga)* for all Swedish towns and cities was issued in 1868. Some of the paragraphs were intended to protect surface water and to preempt pollution: cadavers, pigspill and wastes of all kinds were not to be thrown in streams; wastewater and other fluid wastes were allowed to be thrown in gutters, unless they caused major inconveniences; the pollution of common wells, springs or localities of general water supply was forbidden, and the offenders were fined and forced to pay costs and compensate for damage done. In 1874, a Public Health Act and a Building Act were passed. Health boards were set up, with the aim of, among other things, arranging a supply of drinking water of adequate quality.

Figure 8. Number of prosecuted for neglecting sanitary regulations in Linköping 1805-1839.

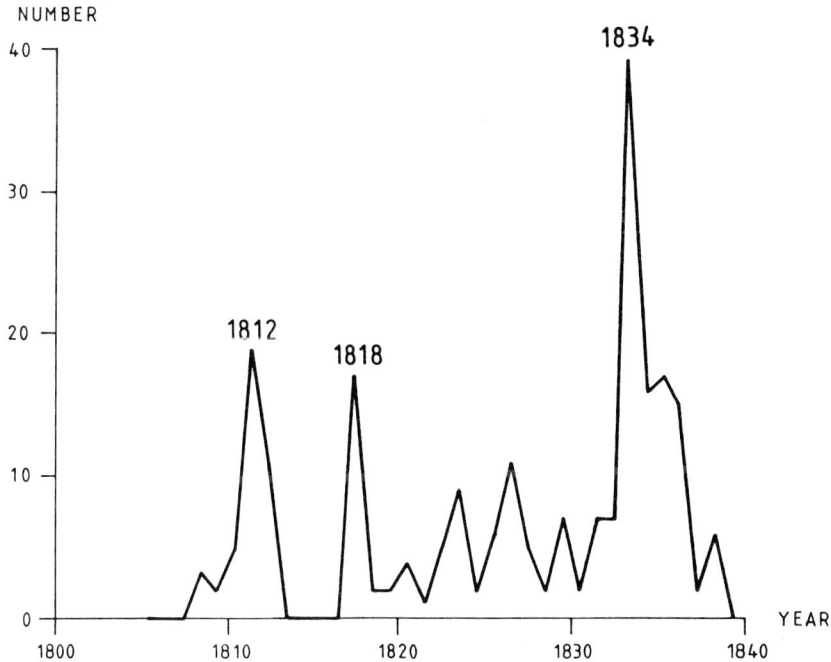

Source: Lists of fines at the Provincial Archive of Vadstena.

Drainage from streets, building lots and market places needed to be led to a common sewage system, and wastewater should be discharged to a suitable recipient, if possible a river, a sea bay or a lake. The Building Act stated that plans putting this into effect had to be made, and without such plans, the construction of new cities or parts of cities was not permitted.[17]

Water-carriage technology

The technology of piped-in water dates back at least to the aqueducts of ancient Rome. In Sweden, a pipe-line system consisting of a net of wooden pipes to various parts of the city of Uppsala was built in 1649, and in 1786, Gothenburg began piping water from a well outside the city to a fountain at the centre of the city. Several examples of this kind could be mentioned, but none of them affected the way of life for the majority of the urban population in Sweden. As is shown in Figure 9, there is, on average, no great lag between the

Figure 9. The construction of piped water supply systems and sewage disposal systems in Swedish towns 1869-1939.

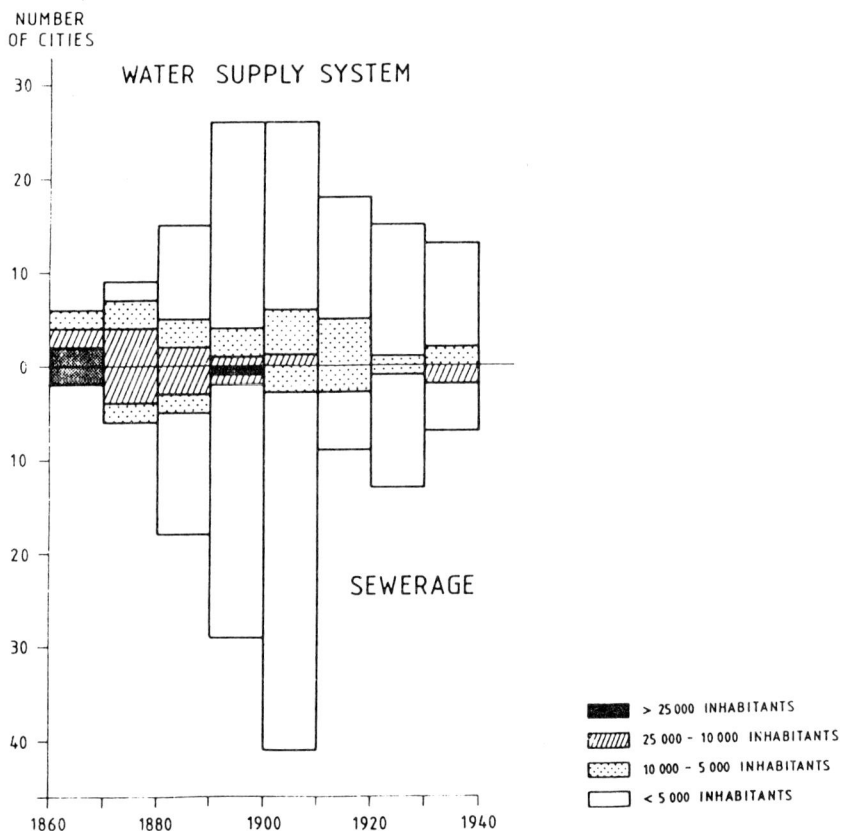

NUMBER
OF CITIES

WATER SUPPLY SYSTEM

SEWERAGE

> 25 000 INHABITANTS
25 000 - 10 000 INHABITANTS
10 000 - 5 000 INHABITANTS
< 5 000 INHABITANTS

Source: SKTF's statistical yearbook 1949.

284

provision of water supplies and the disposal of wastewater. As expected, the larger cities of Sweden (comparatively small from an international point of view) attended to the issue sooner than the smaller ones. In Stockholm, the first common water supply and waste water disposal systems were completed in 1861. The water works of Malmö was constructed in 1866, but wastewater disposal was not effectuated until the 1890's, because Malmö is interspersed by canals. During the 1860's, Gothenburg initiated a sewage system, about five years before new water supplies were constructed.

Annual statistical data from SKTF *(Svenska Kommunal Tekniska Föreningen,* The Swedish Municipal Technology Association), showing the year of construction of water supplies and sewerage, indicate that 13 per cent of the cities established drinking water supplies before constructing sewerage. Twenty-nine per cent of the municipalities provided for wastewater disposal first, but in no less than 41 per cent of the cities, water pipes and sewerage were built simultaneously. For 16 per cent of the urban areas, data concerning years of construction are missing, thus no comparisons can be made.[18]

In Linköping, a private company was founded in 1873 to raise funds for a water supply system. Two years later, water pipes and a sewage system were built. The company established a new water intake 1 kilometer upstream from the two old water supply sites. Water was led by gravity to the new water-works, and from there it was pumped by steam engines to a high reservoir. From the reservoir, mains were laid in the streets for connection to houses and to facilitate public fire prevention. Wastewater was piped straight to the river without treatment.

From 1875 to 1925, the population increased from 8 112 to 29 110 inhabitants. This rapid expansion would probably have been impossible without a feasible technical solution to the water supply problem. The capacity of the privately-owned water-works had become insufficient by the end of the 19th century, and in 1905, it was made public. In 1918, a new water-works was ready for use; the intake was placed at a distance of 2.2 kilometers from town, because the urban sprawl made it necessary to move it further away. A filtering technique to improve water quality was also introduced. The development is summarized in Table 3.

In Linköping, the first water closet was installed in 1882.[19] Although the spread of this innovation was fairly slow, it soon became obvious that wastewater from toilets should not be let out at several places along the river. In 1907, a cut-off sewer was initiated, which collected this wastewater and disposed of it downstream.

The development of the urban water supply system in Linköping is summarized in Figure 10 (Appendix), which illustrates the stages in solving the water supply and the water hygiene problems. Prior to 1870, the main strategy had been to avoid self-contamination, which was accomplished by administrative regulations. As was shown in Figure 1 (Appendix), there was a drop in the death rate up until 1845, which subsequently levelled out.

Table 3. Water delivery distances and water demand for the city of Linköping 1750—1920.

Year	Average water delivery distance (km)	Urban area (sq km)	Population (inh/sq km)	Water demand 1 hd (2)		cbm/yr
1750	< 0.5	0.45	3 970	10	(3)	6 520
1820	0.8	0.61	5 790	15	(3)	19 300
1875	1.8	1.34	6 050	30	(4)	95 300
1920	2.2	1.80	14 995	170	(5)	1 mill

Source: (1) Measurement made from public water source to midpoint of urban area. (2) Household water demand, industrial water demand excluded; lhd = liters per capita and day. (3) Estimates based on investigations of English cities (Caroline Davidson, A woman's Work is Never done, London 1982). (4) Linköping Water-work's Statistics for 1968. (5) SKTF. Annual Statistics for 1920.

Technical solutions, brought about around 1870, are accompanied by a further drop, although this is followed by a remarkable increase of the urban population density. One hypothesis for this is that 5000—6000 inhabitants/km^2 is the maximum population density for a healthy urban water supply, based on local water sources and strict health regulations. After the establishment of well-functioning water supply and wastewater disposal systems, theoretically, there should be no upper limits of population density.

The improvement of water supply techniques is generally considered to be the most important factor in decreasing mortality rates in developing countries today. Carl Lindman ascribed the 1876—1895 drop in infant mortality to hygienic advancements[20], and medical experts of the late 19th century were, with few exceptions, very committed to the idea that improved hygienic conditions meant progress.[21] However, when comparing a series of death rates with dates for the introduction of piped water supply facilities, the latter does not seem to be a very important factor in the reduction of mortality. Figure 11 shows the general mortality of some Swedish cities and the years piped-in water (W) and sewerage (S) were introduced.

As can be seen, there are no changes that are noticeably connected to the year of construction of water pipes (W), to the year of construction of sewerage (S) or to a combination of the two. A cautious hypothesis concerning this may be that the effects of epidemic disease are less pronounced after the introduction of piped-in water and a sewage disposal system. A detailed study of how these innovations have spread is needed. This study should include, among other things, finding out when water was first delivered to the majority of city dwellers, which groups had first access, and the form of distribution. Is water supply more important than sewage disposal, or is it the combination of the two that is essential? There are too many confounding

Figure 11. Crude death rate in some Swedish cities 1860-1910. The dotted line shows the general trend, smoothed by means of a moving averages. W = the year of construction of the first piped-in water supply system S = the corresponding year for a sewage disposal system.

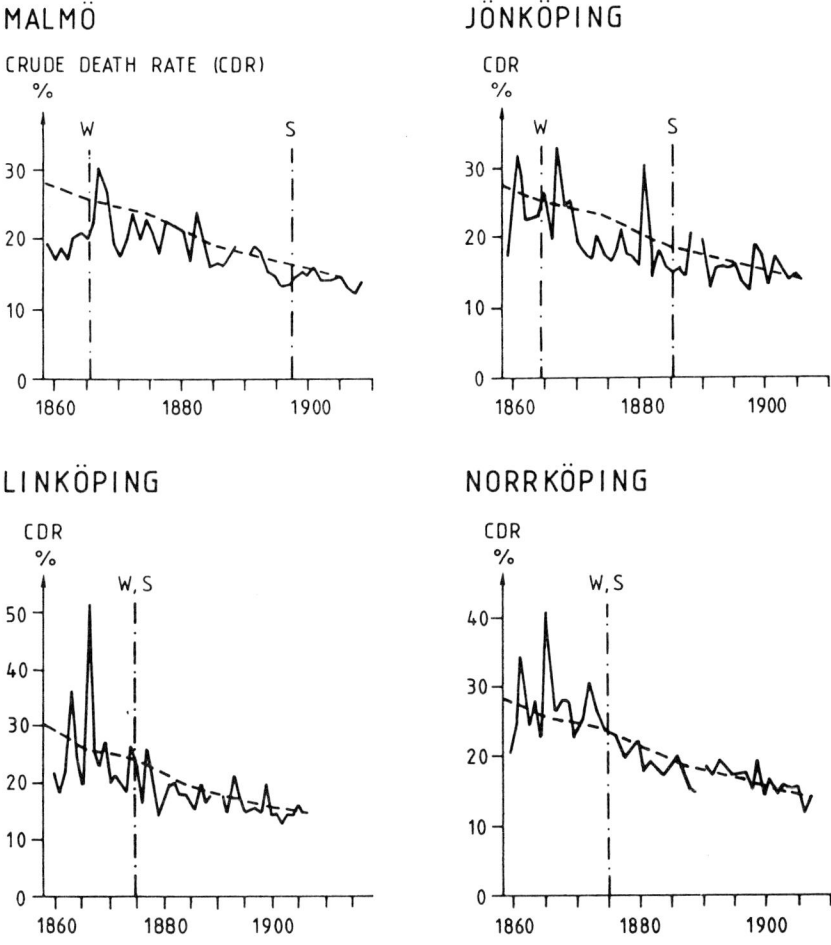

factors that conceal the possible effects of sanitary improvements towards the end of the 19th century.

Conclusion

The development of mortality in a typical, middle-sized Swedish city from 1749 to the end of the nineteenth century has been roughly sketched. What happened there can probably be partly explained by the direct impact of economic change upon the nutrition and health of the population. However, results of recent research in several countries make it necessary to take other factors into consideration.

A few time series do not provide sufficient information for a study of the effects of conscious actions by individuals and local authorities aimed at health improvement. The sources of information that are available were produced by people living during the period of time in question, and they did not anticipate our questions and methods of research. In regard to this, the source situation in Sweden is, in some respects relatively good. This enables an attempt to be made at reconstructing the living conditions of a city. The Demographic Data Base at Umeå University can provide detailed information about individuals, households and neighbourhoods in the city of Linköping. This provides the demographic backbones needed for the proposed investigation. Medical doctors and local authorities have left a large amount of information concerning, among other things, their ideas, their activities, and their control systems. This information can be used to reconstruct other aspects of living conditions in Linköping.

A reconstruction of this type will aid the understanding of some of the underlying factors responsible for the decline in mortality in Linköping. It is always difficult to generalize from one single example, however, much that occurred in Linköping also occurred in other European cities at about the same time. Mortality declined, statutes for better hygienic conditions were issued and followed by a control apparatus, water systems were constructed and the same kind of ideas were spread between medical doctors, between the new group of technical experts in the cities and between literate parts of the population as a whole. The number of local studies in other countries are growing in number each year, and the results of the ongoing "Sundsvall project" will provide larger amounts of valuable comparative knowledge and many hypotheses.

Tentatively, a model of the connection between the decline in mortality and the hygienic improvements in 19th century cities can be proposed:

Figure A.

Demographic transition Characteristics	Urban water supply.
High and constant death rate, often higher than birth rate.	Local water sources; ground- and surface water supply.
Decreasing death rate, equal to or lower than birth rate.	Strengthened administrative regulation of water use and handling of waste. Punishment for disobedience.
Decreasing death rate, lower than birth rate.	Technological solutions: piped urban water supply, and sewers.

This model distinguishes between three stages: a period of high mortality, often above the crude birth rate, in which there was little possibility for city administration to improve the situation (second half of 18th century); a period of declining mortality, caused at least partially by the effects of sanitary regulations and control (beginning of 19th century); a period of continued decline in mortality, to some extent connected with new technical solutions to problems of water supply and waste water disposal (end of 19th century).

Acknowledgements

This study is carried out within the Department of Water in Environment and Society, Linköping University, with financial support from The Bank of Sweden Tercentenary Foundation. The study is part of the ongoing research projects: ''Water and Regional Development — Who and what governs the allocation of water resources in the Motala River Basin?'' and ''Cooperation Conflict Solution and Social Control — Civil and Ecclesiastical Justice in preindustrial Sweden''. The authors are in debt to Lisbeth Samuelsson for redrawing of the figures.

Appendix

Figure 1. Demographic development in the town of Linköping 1749-1904. D = Crude death rates. Five-year averages on 1000 inhabitants. B = Crude birth rates. Five-year averages 1749-1859, ten-year averages 1860-1909 on 1000 inhabitants. G = Population growth during a five-year period on 1000 inhabitants.

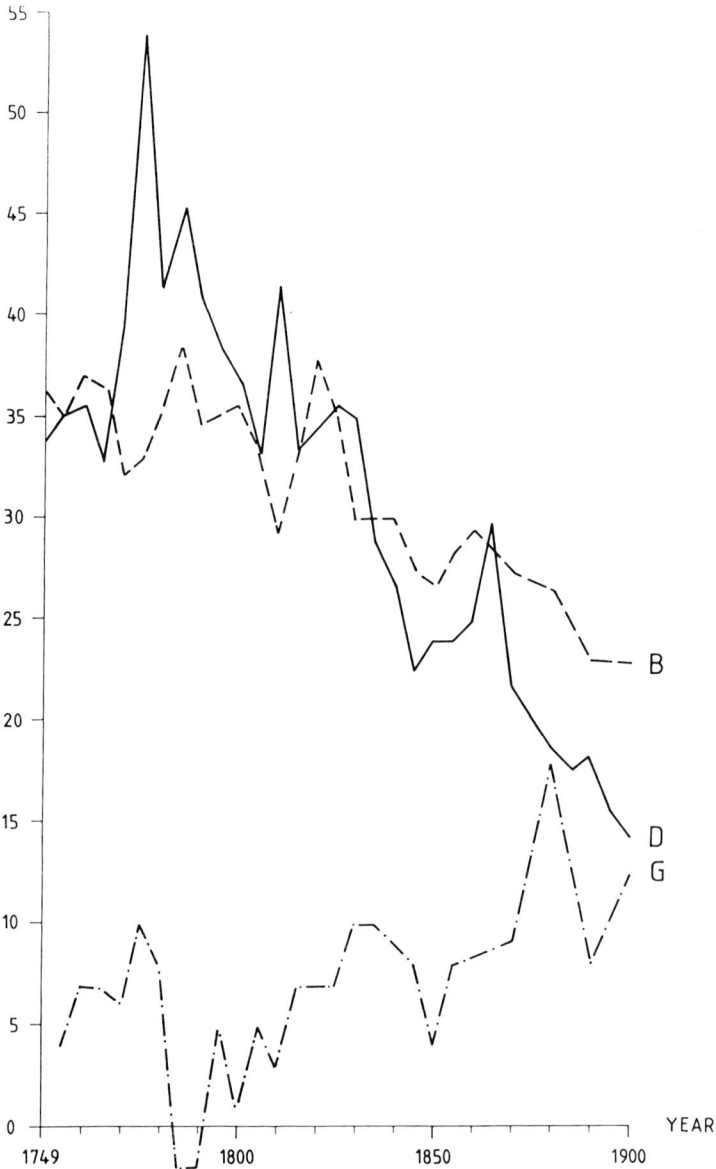

Sources: Statistical tables of the Table Comission at the Provincial Archive of Vadstena. Sven Hellström, 'Befolkning och social struktur' in Linköpings historia. 4. Tiden 1863-1910, Linköping 1978, p. 15.

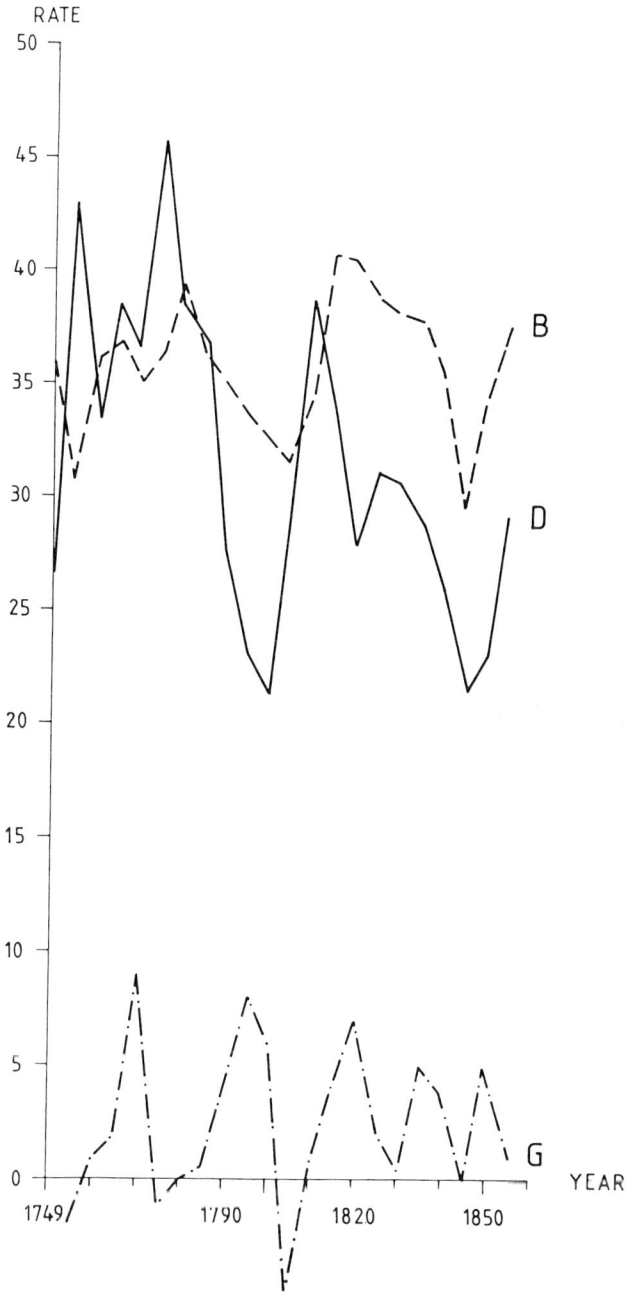

Figure 2. Demographic development in the agrarian parish of Sankt Lars 1749-1859. D = Crude death rates. Five-year averages on 1000 inhabitants. G = Population growth during a five-year period on 100 inhabitants.

Source: Statistical tables of the Table Comission at the Provincial Archive of Vadstena.

Figure 3. Infant mortality in Linköping (L) 1749-1859 and 1876-1894 and in Sankt Lars (S) 1749-1859. Five-year averages on 100 births.

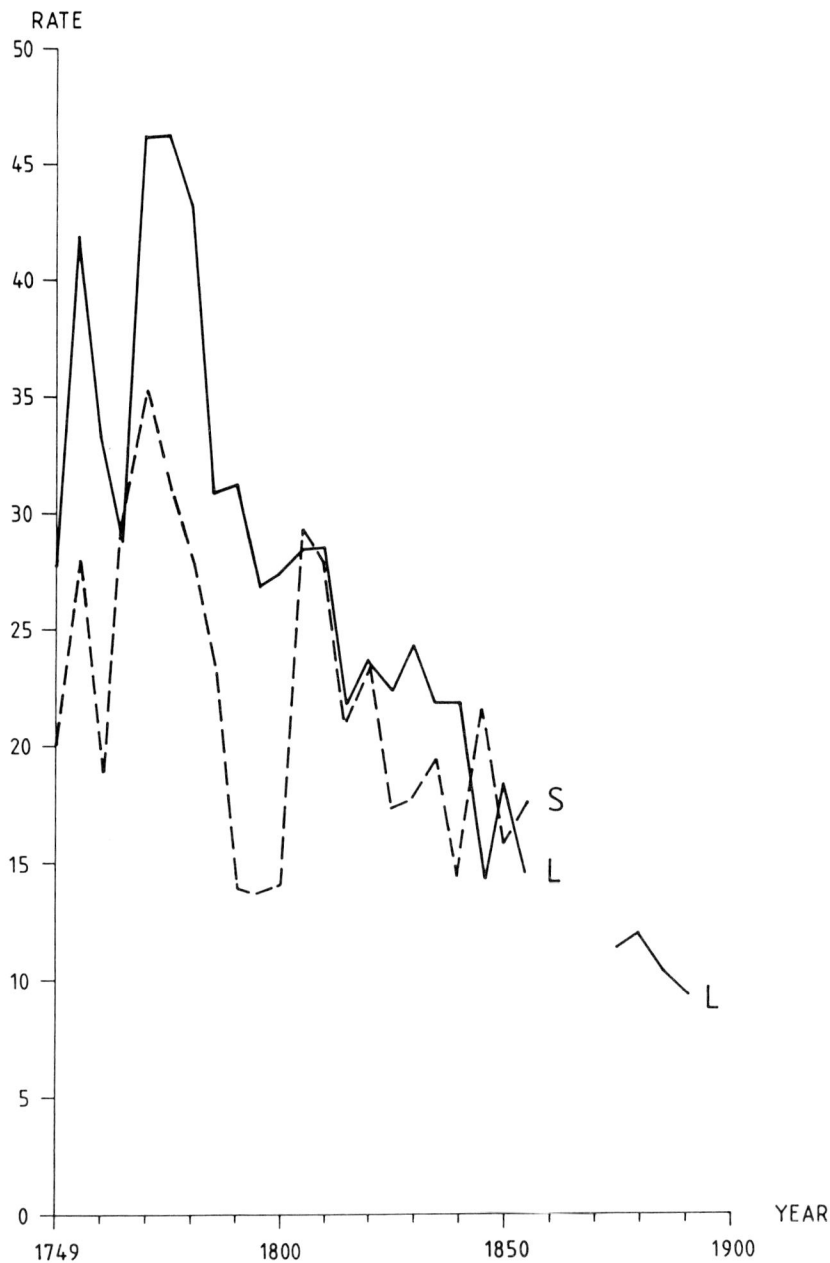

Sources: Statistical tables of the Table Comission at the Provincial Archive of Vadstena. Carl Lindman, Dödligheten i första lefnadsåret i Sveriges tjugo större städer 1876-1895, Stockholm 1898, p. 103.

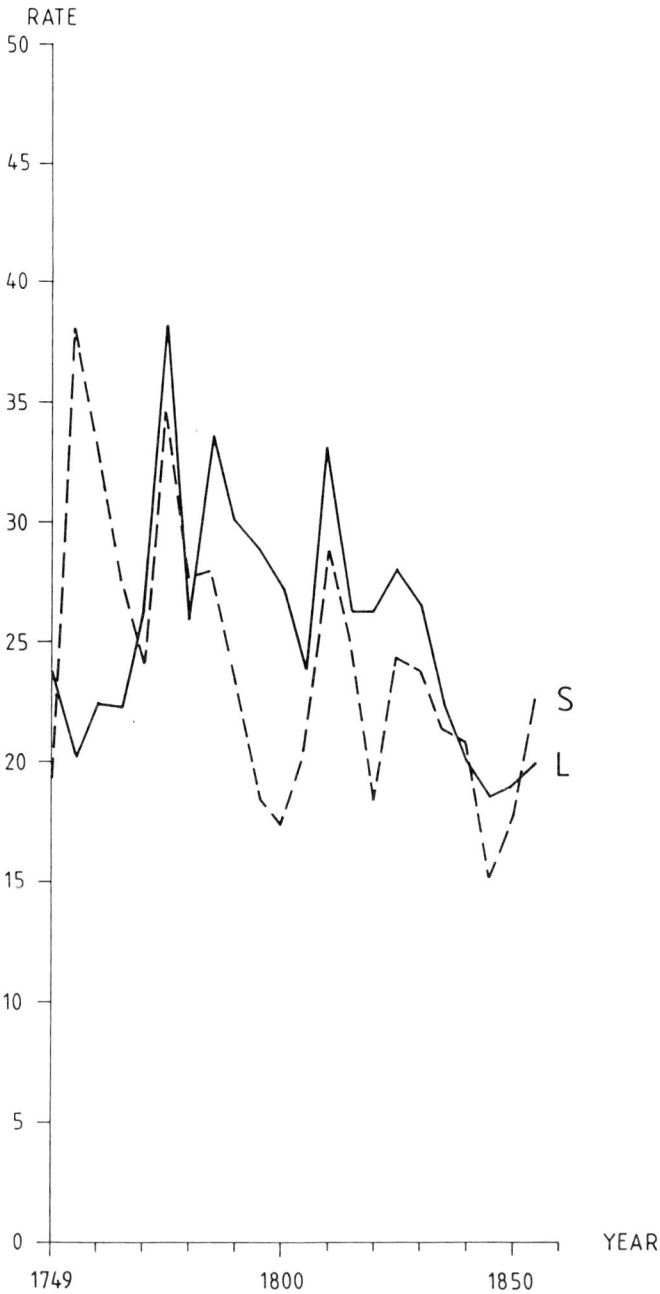

Figure 4. Mortality after one year of age in Linköping (L) and Sankt Lars (S) 1749-1859. Five-year averages on 1000 inhabitants.

Source: Statistical tables of the Table Comission at the Provincial Archive of Vadstena.

Figure 5. Infant mortality (I) on 100 births and mortality after one year of age (A) on 1000 inhabitants in Linköping 1749-1859. Five-year averages.

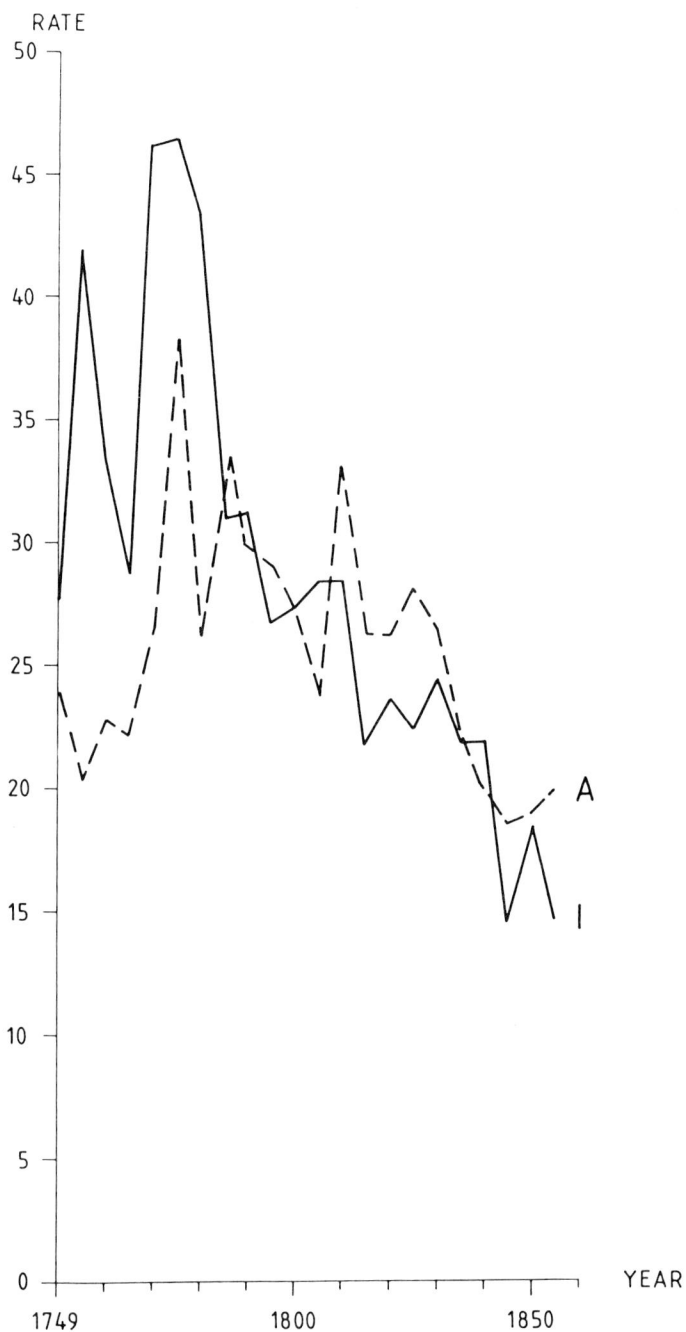

Source: Statistical tables of the Table Comission at the Provincial Archive of Vadstena.

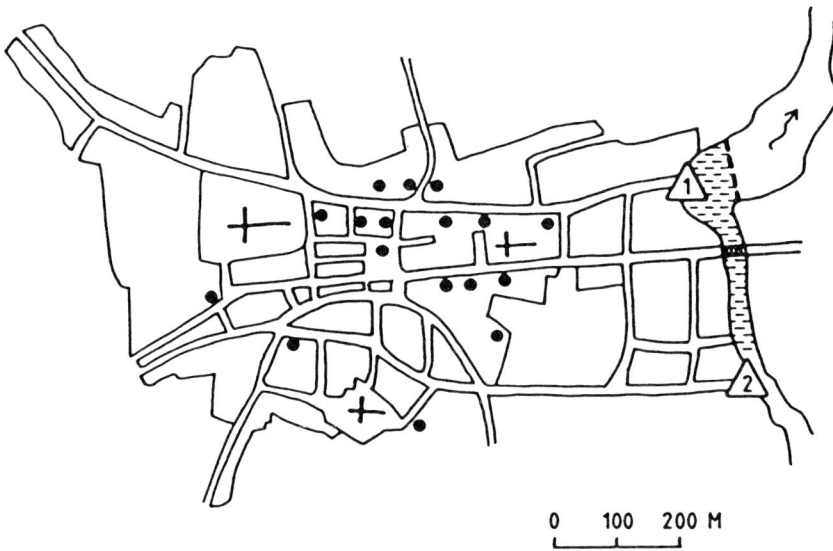

Figure 6. A reconstruction of the urban water supply during the late 18th century in the town of Linköping.

1 ORIGINAL SURFACE WATER SOURCE

2 SINCE 1817 SURFACE WATER SOURCE

● GROUNDWATER SOURCE

– – BARRAGE

AREA OF SELF-CONTAMINATION

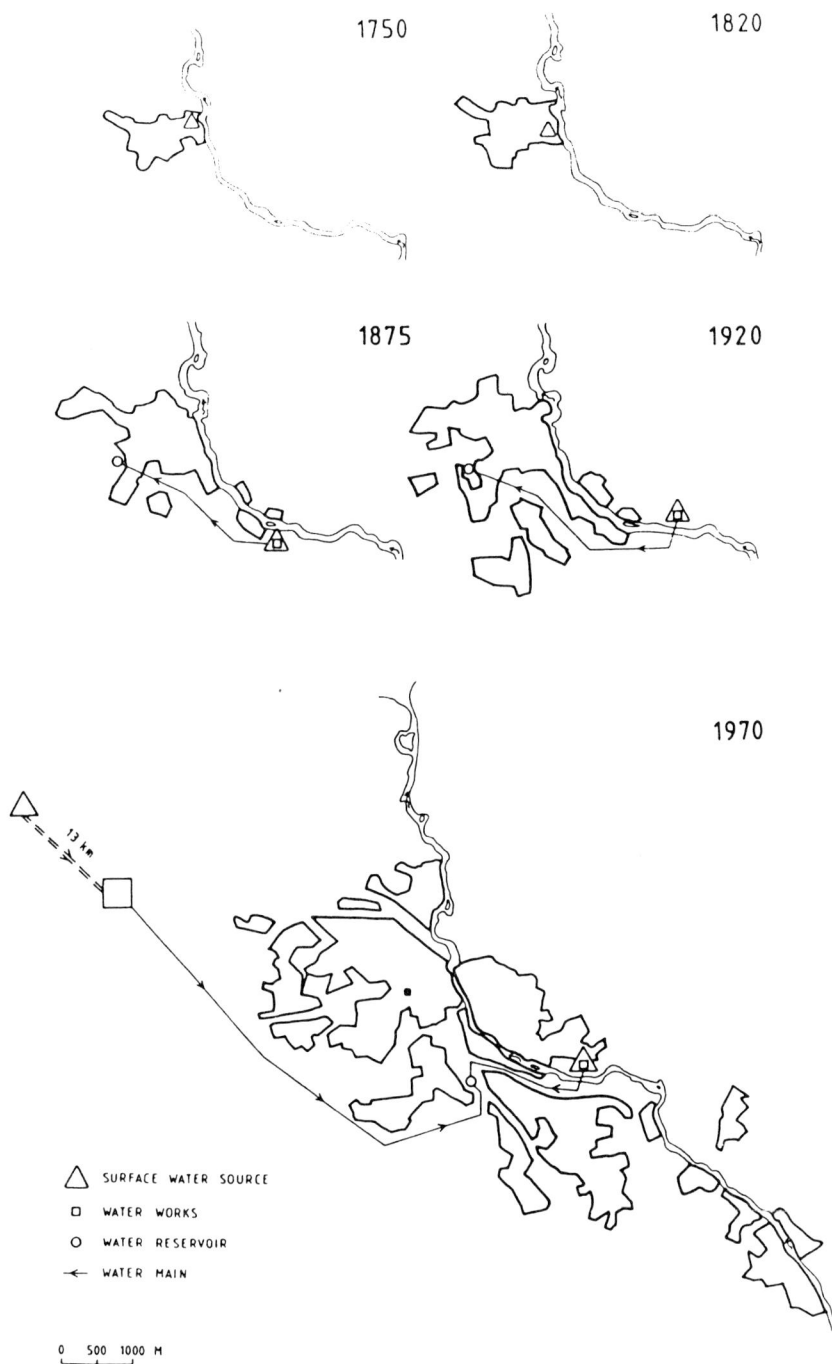

Figure 10. The development of the urban area and the urban water supply systems in the township of Linköping 1750-1970.

SURFACE WATER SOURCE

WATER WORKS

WATER RESERVOIR

WATER MAIN

0   500 1000 M

Notes

1. T. McKeown, *The Modern Rise of Population* (London 1976).

2. A. Brändström, *"De kärlekslösa mödrarna"*. *Spädbarnsdödligheten i Sverige under 1800-talet med särskild hänsyn till Nedertorneå*. With an English Summary (Umeå 1984). On the impact of breast feeding, see also J. Knodel, 'Natural Fertility in Pre-Industrial Germany', *Population Studies*, 32, 3 (1978) and U-B. Lithell, *Breast-feeding and Reproduction. Studies in Marital Fertility and Infant Mortality in 19th Century Finland and Sweden* (Uppsala 1981).

3. B-I. Puranen, *Tuberkulos. En sjukdoms förekomst och dess orsaker. Sverige 1750—1980*. With an English Summary (Umeå 1984).

4. J. Sundin and L-G. Tedebrand, 'Mortality and Morbidity in Swedish Iron Foundries 1750—1875', *Tradition and Transition. Studies in Microdemography and Social Change, Report No. 2 from the Demographic Data Base* (Umeå 1981).

5. See conference reports by T. Bengtsson and others.

6. See conference reports by U. Jonsson and J. Söderberg.

7. S. Hellström, 'Befolkning och social struktur', *Linköpings historia. 4. Tiden 1863—1910* (Linköping 1978), p. 13.

8. Statistical records delivered by the priests to the Swedish Table Commission 1749—1859 at the Provincial Archive of Vadstena.

9. F. Lindberg, *Linköpings historia. 3. 1567—1862. Samhälls- och kulturliv* (Linköping 1976), p. 15; C. Lindman, *Dödligheten i första lefnadsåret i Sveriges tjugo större städer 1876—1895* (Helsingborg 1898), p. 103.

10. Lindberg (1976), pp. 36—40. see also the frequent cases in the city's court against people who did not clean their parts of the streets, who transported manure through the streets at forbidden times or in forbidden ways, etc.

11. Lindberg (1976), p. 37.

12. Lindberg (1976), p. 36.

13. Lindberg (1976), p. 36.

14. Lindberg (1976), p. 38.

15. Y. Hirdman, *Magfrågan. Mat som mål och medel. Stockholm 1870—1920* (Stockholm 1983), p. 143. For French examples of regulations and handling of the water situation see J-P. Goubert, 'Public Hygiene and Mortality Decline in France in the 19th Century', T. Bengtsson, G. Fridlizius and R. Ohlsson (Eds), *Pre-Industrial Population Change. The Mortality Decline and Short-Term Population Movements* (Lund 1984).

16. Lindberg (1976), p. 41.

17. L. Lundgren, *Vattenförorening. Debatten i Sverige 1870—1920* (Lund 1974), p. 28.

18. SKTF's Statistical Yearbook of 1949 (Statistiska uppgifter över vattenverk och avloppsverk, vägar, gator samt renhållningsverk i svenska städer och samhällen för år 1949) (Malmö 1950).

19. S.E. Noreen, 'Bebyggelse', *Linköpings historia,* 4 (1978), p. 41.

20. Lindman (1898), p. 155.

21. Lundgren (1974), p. 200.

Comments on the Session Society and Medicine

Sølvi Sogner

Four very interesting papers have been submitted for this session. Together they straddle five centuries. I don't know if it is by pure accident or by invitation that they do not overlap in chronology. I am all for the long view, and am quite impressed. But in drawing up my commentary I have felt at some loss how to set about it. I settle for a compromise—some remarks for each and some for all. I shall briefly mention common aspects that I will return to in the discussion of the separate papers, which I will then comment on in chronological order.

"Society and medicine"—the session is called. Intriguing title and open to many interpretations. An obvious one is viewing society as the state—and write about how the state shouldered the responsibility of medical care. How taking care of the sick became a public duty, and ceased to be a wholly private concern. This interpretation is all the more obvious in the Scandinavian countries—welfare-states of long standing. And all the papers—three Swedish and one Norwegian—have, to a larger or smaller degree, considered this aspect and adopted this approach.

To view the administration of medical care as a public task, entails viewing it in light of (1) the state economy, and of (2) the public administration. This is all the more important, since we are reviewing half a millennium and the historical context, the specific historic situations will be highly variable.

Øivind Larsen operates with the concept "an ecology of the diseases, an interplay between the diseases and the population they belong to". This concept, I think, conveys the historian's respect for the individualizing of specific epochs, the historic relativity, while the word ecology has a ring to it, reminding us that we are dealing not only with societal matters, but with biological and physical as well.

Ottosson's paper on the battle against the plague drives two theses. The first one claims that the public measures taken were eventually, as they became steadily more effective, the responsible agent for causing plague to disappear in Sweden.

Claiming the decisive importance of quarantine measures in winning the battle of the plague is no novelty. I have great sympathy for this view. I have always found preposterous the importance that has been attached to the scientific proof of the demonstration of micro-organisms that carry disease, and the subsequent underrating of common sense observations that triggered off the scientific research, and in the meantime led to health measures that proved effective.

But it comes as a surprise to meet an advocate of this view here and now. In 1982 Lars Walløe published an article on plague and population in Norway 1350-1750.[1] I see no mention of it in Ottosson's bibliography, and doubt that he can have any knowledge of the article. Otherwise Ottosson would not have written the following passage, "Restricting this problem to the case of Sweden, it is first important to bear in mind that there are no reasons to believe that plague has ever been endemic in the country".

This is exactly the opposite of what the Norwegian scientist thinks. Walløe advances the hypothesis that in between the fairly regular epidemic outbursts of plague in Europe the infectious materia will have been conserved within enzootic reservoirs within Europe itself. He believes that most European countries had this kind of enzootic reservoirs in one or more of their specimens of wild rodents. He mentions a wide variety of rodents that in Siberia in this century have been shown to be carriers of plague—marmot, hare, rabbit, otter, mole, porcupine, and my English fails me: *røyskatt, snømus, ilder, oter, grevling, spissmus, mår*—exactly our own well-known fauna.

In the case of Norway The Eastern and Middle parts were especially hard hit by plague, according to Walløe, and he believes for climatic reasons. This argument is underpinned by the example from Soviet Russia in this century, where it has proved very difficult, in a belt across the whole of the Soviet Union including Asia, to get rid of enzootic plague. This area is very similar to the Norwegian areas just mentioned, and are in the same manner characterized by cold winters with heavy lying snow, and at the same time warm summers and a varied fauna of rodents. Local epidemics in this area of Soviet have been remittent, and repeatedly the health authorities have had to fight them. Walløe says, "It is not an unreasonable thought that this kind of local epidemic occurred in Norway in a similar manner and with greater frequency in the 15th century than in countries further south, and that Norway was enzootically infected with plague for a longer period than e.g. England" (p. 37). He further claims that it is reasonable to think that the same was true of Sweden, being comparable to Norway as to the conditions mentioned.

Walløe does not, however, forward any explication for the disappearance of plague—he contents himself with saying that plague has on three occasions in historical time spread from its enzootic native grounds in Siberia and ravaged the world in short time—in the 6th century, in the 14th century, and then in 1894: "Medical science can give no reasonable explanation for why such sudden bursts of epidemic disease happen, and why the disease after a while looses foothold. The problem is the same for several kinds of disease, not only plague". It is, however, evident from his line of reasoning that he attributes no decisive importance to human measures concerning the disappearance of plague in Scandinavia around 1700.

We are thus confronted with two seemingly irreconcilable views, based on fresh research, neither of which can be proved or disproved with our present state of knowledge.—I am glad to say that Ottoson tells us that the study of the history of plague in Sweden has not more than begun. The same can be said for Norway!—There is therefore, as we have seen, reason to believe that plague may have struck Scandinavia in two ways—from within and from without.

As far as the plague coming from without is concerned, Ottoson has very carefully argued the case of ever improving official measures being taken against it, eventually crowned with success. His case is all the better represented for showing all the counter arguments. And we can offer at least one Norwegian example to back him up: The plague epidemic of 1710/11 came indubitably from the continent and Norwegian public authorities were all aware of it in time to take precautions. A strict quarantine was upheld. Any Swede crossing the border was to be shot dead immediately and the corpse buried without touch of hand. And Norway went free of plague. The last plague occurred in 1654.

Ottoson's second thesis concerns society's shouldering of responsibility for fighting disease. Fighting the plague was analogous to military defence, and hence naturally included among main traditional public duties. By extension to other epidemics, the battle of the plague thus became of importance for developing public responsibility in general in the area of medicine.

He sees this as a natural extension of military defence, for several reasons—by direct analogy: defence against intruding alien elements, as well as through its being fought partly by already existing military means. Stimulating this development was the contagion theory of spreading disease. It is an interesting observation that the theory of miasmatic spreading of disease—stressing factors in the environment—could not in this period make great advances—the administrative and technological apparatus for this not yet having been created. Custom administration and military forces, able to control and uphold quarantines and lay cordon sanitaires, were however already in existence and lent themselves readily to the purpose, once this line of action was decided upon. It was a line of public medical action tailor-made to what the state was capable of at the time.

Ottoson draws attention to the fact that economic considerations naturally weighed heavily when public authorities issued orders about quarantine for chips for the 40 days required, isolation, cordon sanitaire, closing or postponing of markets. He offers several telling examples. These economic considerations take into account, as far as I can tell, the problems that will arise for the little people just as well as for the authorities.

This brings us to the paper by Johannisson. Johannisson in her paper sets out to discuss "The public rationale of the community's care of the sick". An historian of ideas, she feels free to concentrate upon the ideology of the theoreticians and the policymakers. It is her right. Still, the pedestrian historian misses a more detailed and explicit exposition of the factual historical situation and the concrete measures,—practice linked to the philosophy. E.g. I feel bewildered by the last paragraph, where "a bed in hospital, a clean shirt, hot food and access to doctors' is taken to represent the community's new offer to the sick, and this is opposed to what people otherwise would have had to resort to in case of sickness, "a dirty straw mattress in a hovel in the slum". This description does not ring true to me. I do not think that neither the 18th century hospitals nor the domestic dwellings of the average Swede at the time are given accurate representations in these sweeping statements. As general statements, I think hospitals are presented too favourably, private dwellings too unfavourably. And in any case, how many clean hospital beds all told were there to go around, and what chances did actual slum-dwellers have of admittance in case of need? This rhetorical question I found the answer to, when I came to Umeå, in Anders Brändström's paper: Not very many! 650 beds in 1800!

The introduction to the paper states quite clearly what the paper is about. A question is asked, in general terms: Why cure the sick? It is a catchy phrase and awakes our interest immediately. The author is quite right in feeling confident that her contemporary readers—all of them welfare state patients at one point or other in their career—can hardly be expected to come up with any interesting answers to that question. But she has one in store for us. It is pointed out that from the community's point of view, curing the sick is done for economic reasons. Of course it is for economic reasons, but not altogether, and what of it if it were.

I am not sure whether the author generalizes the problem or is treating it as a historical category, changeable over time. To judge by her own words, I suspect she is generalizing: "To illustrate the question I have chosen a particular historical period and a particular social ideology, namely mercantilism". Is it really the intention to show that communities, then and now, cure the sick for economic state-egoistic reasons? Does she expect her thesis to hold for the present situation? Does the 18th century only serve as an illustration of a point she is making in general concerning society and medicine? I leave this question pending. Since the discussion in the paper is wholly concerned with the 18th century, I will comment on it as if the thesis was limited to this more restricted period.

I feel the case which is presented to us suffers from a too one-sided treatment. The counter-arguments are lacking. How can Johannisson be so sure of her conclusion, "The authorities had begun to see the sick, even if the reason was hardly their concern for the suffering individual but rather their wish to return potential manpower capital to its place in the production machine in order to work, pay taxes and produce children for the nation". Johannisson implies that there is a lack of the true welfare attitude on the part of the 18th century government officials and policy-makers.

And what is more, she holds it against them. The latter attitude, I think, is moralizing and out of place. Examples: "Nothing was too private, too intimate, too sensitive for inclusion in the national welfare (that is actually the word used?!) program". "The individual had to be sacrificed for the prosperity of the nation, his freedom and rights and his own personal prosperity limited. The most naked expression of this view came when a cash value was placed on the individual". "The reasoning (of the mercantilists)—dizzying in its unabashed rationalism". "Thus the mercantilist view was pursued to its logical conclusion, where human worth seemed to be synonymous with capital value".

As for the welfare motive, she says: "Welfare for all was only a theoretical goal". The policy-makers did have in mind then, after all, the welfare for all? I feel we have not been treated to a full discussion of what mercantilistic policy was all about. To quote Charles Wilson, "the ends it sought varied; they ranged from the immediate profit of individuals and the pockets of princes to the power of the state and the welfare of great communities of people".[2] Johannisson says, and I subscribe to her statement, that "State power had to come first, and the individual had to subordinate his private needs and hopes to its claim for priority". What I disagree with is the interpretation that the fact that state interests would have to come first, also meant that common welfare was not also intended. How could welfare for all otherwise be attained ultimately, one may ask? It was too early to afford such a luxury, as we understand it today.

The Swedish brand of mercantilism can off hand be expected to be more digestible to modern stomachs than most. Why otherwise should that country in later years have attained, ahead of all others, the renown of forerunner among welfare-states? Some time, somewhere we must be able to uncover the frail beginnings. Others have held opinions differing from Johannisson's. To quote Eli Heckscher, giant among students of mercantilism and whose name I miss in the bibliography, Swedish mercantilism was distinguished by its close affiliation with an interest in natural science and technology.[3] According to him, Sweden was practically uninfluenced by contemporaneous German economic thinking, known as Cameralistics, and which, according to Heckscher, in its most pronounced form intended to "make all of economic life into the servant of the state or the prince and above all make it serve the interest of state finances". According to Heckscher such ideas were not acceptable in Sweden, because of the form of government in the Freedom era, the political traditions such as they were and the national character which had been developed through the past. Heckscher is not necessarily right, but if he is not, I would like to see him refuted.

We note in passing that the German cameralistics was the dominant influence in Denmark in the period, when it came to economic thinking. And the Danish brand does not seem very offensive. Danish 18th century pamphleteers agree that consideration be taken to the common weal, the welfare of the whole community. The interest of the individual must give in to the collective. But it is the common welfare and security of the inhabitants of the realm that is the ultimate aim and the duty of the government, the state to provide. In order to provide this, the economy of the society must function in the best of ways. How this was to be brought about was the theme of endless discussions as it was no easy matter to decide. Hence profit maximizing allusions abound in the pamphlets. The words used and the sheer volume of the economic argumentation should not preclude the fact that this was striving for the betterment of all the people, though of course not in the sense that we would understand it today.[4]

For just as in the case of Sweden, as Johannisson ably points out, the second half of the 18th century is a breakthrough in Denmark for new ways of thinking in several areas, not least the field of medicine with which we are concerned. It is this budding new public concern within a new field that is interesting. Argumentation will always make use of the most persuasive phrases. In the 18th century economics was "in". That the new ideas are formulated in—to our modern minds—shockingly crude phrases, should not mislead us into taking them at face value. Of course there is good economy in saving the lives of prospective industrious citizens. But even if there was genuine economic concern behind the new initiatives, even if it was mainly economic concern, I cannot see that it need reflect negatively upon the new initiatives. What is important is that they in addition to, for the period, sophisticated new economic reasoning *also* embraced a new humanitarian aspect, a new public humanitarian thinking and a new concern on the part of the authorities.

Brändström's very interesting paper supplies information on how this new humanitarian spirit finds material expression. His is a sketch of the new hospitals—where the sick are the protagonists. We have been kept so busy here that I have not been able to do justice to his paper, which I first received in Umeå. However, I have made a note of the very interesting comparison with English and American hospitals regarding venereal diseases. Swedish hospitals—and Norwegian, I may add—were "mainly designed to treat patients with such complaints", whereas in other countries they were preferably not admitted! "The strongest argument for the financing of hospitals was the fear of uncontrolled spread of syphilis", "... the whole nation would be infected unless something was done". Are we here confronting something crucial in attitudes, representing differences between Scandinavian and other countries? I pose the question.

Anyway there is a concern here for the common welfare. Brändström makes a point of the difference between the public Swedish hospitals and the voluntary hospitals abroad, a point that could have been enlarged upon. Papers on this theme from outside of Scandinavia are missed, although the author himself makes some very interesting comparisons with foreign research.

The tables on the very high percentages "cured" are intriguing. "Cured", "improved", "incurable" and "dead" are the four possible outcomes of a stay in hospital. A very convincing case, however, is presented that hospitals were not the death-traps that they have been made out to be, nor that they were only used by the destitute. Myth-dispelling and innovative are epithets that come to mind, when describing the paper.

Øivind Larsen's and Fritz Hodne's concern is the establishment of the medical profession over the last two centuries. During the period that the two previous papers dealt with, doctors were few and far between. Around 1800, for instance, there were 100 doctors in Norway, and even that number was an enormous increase on the situation 200 years earlier. 200 years later, in 1986, there are 11.600—a hundred-fold increase, whereas the population had only quadrupled. Larsen-Hodne draw our attention to how well correlated the increase of the number of doctors and the decline of mortality have been—the more of the former, the less of the latter. Carefully—I think maybe too carefully—they will not draw causal links from one phenomenon to the other. They underline that the treating capacity of each doctor was limited, but still there was a rising demand for more doctors. They prefer to see the two developments—more doctors and declining mortality—as part of the same process.

What process? I find them a bit less explicit on this point than I would like. They introduce the concept "an ecology of the diseases, an interplay between the diseases and the population they belong to". And in the last paragraph they claim that the "development of the medical profession is a part of the ecological system to which the diseases belong". I take it that this alludes to the change of the disease pattern that has taken place during these two last centuries,—"how morbidity, mortality and the causes of disease totally alter during the years of transition"—the now well-known shift from the preponderance of epidemic diseases to cancer and cardio-vascular diseases. I find the choice of words mystifying, and still they are undoubtedly the natural scientist's respectful attitude toward phenomena that are not easily put on an explicatory formula. I would have been more blunt and given praise where praise seemed due. The battle put up by the medical profession against epidemic disease has seemed victorious. But of course there will be future wars to fight and maybe in different ways and with different warriors—health and therapeutic personnel in general rather than doctors. History never repeats itself, and the circumstances always differ. Each period has its own imprint and its particular problems and differ in the ways of tackling them. To call it an ecological system has a ring of determinism to it, reminiscent of the disappearance of endemic plague, if such there was.

Larsen-Hodne claim that people's attitudes toward medicine are decisive for what happens in the medical field. Medicine does not develop autonomously, divorced from a social and economic reality. Very successfully this idea has inspired the structure of the book, Doctors and Society[5], which was published this summer, and which Larsen-Hodne have co-authored together with a political scientist. The development of the medical profession is here seen as an integral part of the economic and social history of the nation during the same period. This is a rare approach for this kind of history writing, professional associations congratulating themselves upon some anniversary—in the present case it is the Norwegian Medical Association celebrating the first hundred years. Usually the subgroup under scrutiny is studied as a butterfly on a pin and the reader must himself supply the general historical context—if he is able to.

Probably the approach chosen is more feasible for medicine than for most other sectors, for several reasons. One reason is the considerable part of the national resources that are being allocated to health services in our society today—absolutely as well as compared to what was the case 200 years ago. Another reason is the peculiar semi-official position of the medical profession. As Larsen-Hodne point out, after some delay when the education of lawyers, priests and officers were receiving more public attention in consideration of their importance to the government in the task of running the country, a shift is discernible round the middle of last century. A turning point is 1860, the year when district physicians became public servants in a hitherto unknown manner, by heading the new local health boards. The growth of hospitals set up for public money is another important factor in this development.

The national economic growth during those 200 years explain how this development was possible. And is also the background against which changes of attitude to medical policy must be seen. Larsen-Hodne distinguish a turning point in attitude around 1890. Before that time bad health had seemed "for a long period to be accepted as a toll, perhaps as a price which had to be paid for the expanding economy". But as conditions improve, people's demands change—"health and absence of sickness gain in weight and importance" as "cure and relief of disabling and discomforting ailments" became steadily more available. After World War II a new shift of attitude is discernible, which they define thus: "Attitudes towards health problems, public economy and social equality had shifted the needs into a quest for absence of pain and distress, a quest for comfort and welfare".

People get what they ask for, to say it crudely. And as time changes they ask for different things, and different people ask. We recall the bishop Lurentius Paulinus Gothus and what he asked for in 1623—penance by the people, and from the authorities food-supply and rigorous measures against transmission of the contagion of plague, at the pain of capital punishment. From each government according to capacity...

And the capacity has differed. In the 18th century the principle for the government in Denmark-Norway for raising the necessary funds to introduce new public works was to let the taxpayers locally contribute toward the novelties. If they wanted them badly enough, they would pay up. Today we are reaching the limit of what the taxpayers are able to pay for the public medical system that we have eventually acquired. Private measures are now called for. Are we coming full circle? Society's attitude toward medicine and the State's attitude toward medicine is no longer necessarily the same. Larsen-Hodne do not in their paper sketch the possible future development, after all we are doing history of the past not of the future. Still I believe these questions are raised in the recent book, and I believe it would be fruitful for the discussion if they would let us in on some of their thoughts and ideas on this line of development, as seen in light of the historical development with which they are so well acquainted.

Notes

1. L. Walløe, 'Pest og folketall 1350-1750', *Historisk tidskrift,* 3 (1982), p. 1-45.

2. C. Wilson, 'Mercantilism', *The Historical Association, General Series,* Pamphlet No. 37 (London 1958), p. 26.

3. E. Heckscher, *Svenskt arbete och liv* (Stockholm 1976), p. 224.

4. E. Oxenbøll, *Dansk økonomisk taenkning 1700-1770* (Copenhagen 1977), p. 58-88.

5. Ø. Larsen, O. Berg and F. Hodne, *Legene og samfunnet* (Oslo 1986).

Fighting the Plague in 17th- and 18th-Century Sweden: A Survey

Per-Gunnar Ottosson

Introduction

The study of the demographic transition cannot be confined to the decades during which it occurred. The question must also be raised whether it was an effect of a development which began centuries earlier. In the context of the present conference *Society, Health, and Population during the Demographic Transition,* the purpose of this paper will be to focus some problems concerning the long-term effects of plague.

Since the 18th century Western Europe has been free from the factor which, according to M.W. Flinn "probably exercised the single most effective check on the growth of population: plague"[1] He further maintained that "without plague, the kind of uninterrupted population growth that has characterised and transformed Western Europe since the eighteenth century would have begun several centuries earlier". The latter assertion cannot be either confirmed or denied. It leads to unanswerable questions, such as whether the nutrition resources would have allowed an earlier expansion of population, and what role other epidemic diseases would have played in that case. It has also been shown in several local studies that populations stricken by the plague had remarkable powers of recovery.[2] After the Middle Ages the population crises caused by plague appear to have been only temporary. The long-term effects of plague are to be sought in other areas. First, while it is a fact that Western Europe was free from plague after the 1720's, its presence in North Africa, the Levant, and Russia still constituted a threat in the 19th century.[3] If these epidemics had reached Western Europe they would have led to at least temporary halts in population growth.

But how was this avoided? Was it due to good fortune or good management? This is the first question I would like to raise on the basis of Swedish sources. The second, and I am convinced, the most important question concerns the role of plague in the development of public health. I will argue that the long-term effects of plague are to be sought primarily within that area.

The study of the history of plague in Sweden has only just begun. There is only a small number of local studies of plague, of which the most important concern the plague in Stockholm 1710-1711 by O.T. Hult (1916) and L. Preinitz (1972).[4] This essay must be regarded as only a preliminary report on my project which is concerned primarily with the social, religious, and medical response to plague in Sweden (the project is financially supported by the Swedish Council for Research in the Humanities and Social Sciences).

On the disappearance of plague

The question of the disappearance of plague from Western Europe is a very much discussed issue, and it is not possible to take all the arguments into account here. Basically the arguments concern two kinds of explanation: (1) biological or ecological factors, not the outcome of conscious, human manipulation; (2) human measures, such as isolation and quarantine.

Restricting this problem to the case of Sweden, it is first important to bear in mind that there is no reason to believe that plague has ever been endemic in this country. There was and is no ecological niche for the microbe *Yersinia pestis*. Its natural environment is among partially resistant ground squirrels, where there can exist a balance between the *Y. pestis* and its host. Epidemics of plague arise when the microbe is, by means of flea-vectors, transferred from wild rodents to domestic rodents, such as the black rat *(Rattus rattus)*, which has a very low resistance to plague. When the rats die, their infected fleas may instead transfer themselves to human beings. Subsequently, interhuman transmission is also possible by means of the human flea *(Pulex irritans)*. Even if *P. irritans* is a less effective vector than the rat fleas *(Xenopsylla cheopis* and *Nosopsyllus fasciatus)*, this could be compensated for by its greater numbers in areas of poor hygienic conditions, where people wore a great deal of clothes.[5] Since rats and fleas do not travel long distances within a short period of time, the spread of plague is dependent on human transportation. Particularly shipments of grain and textiles are apt to transport and conceal infected rats and fleas.

The disappearance of plague has sometimes been attributed to a change in the rat species dominant in Europe. During the 18th century *Rattus rattus* was gradually replaced by *Rattus norvegicus*. While the latter does not nest so close to human beings as the former, its fleas are considered less likely to infect human beings. This hypothesis can, however, be rejected for the simple reason that the decline of *R. rattus* began long after the disappearance of plague in Western Europe. It is certainly not a factor which can explain the disappearance of plague in Sweden. *R. rattus* did not begin to decline until the beginning of the 19th century in the south, and remained in Central Sweden throughout the century. It was still existing in the Stockholm area around 1900.[6] However this does not explain the decline of plague, it rather makes it even more puzzling that the disease did not reappear after the 1710's. On the other hand, it is a factor which makes it less likely that plague might return now.

310

A.P. Appleby has instead argued that the effect of the recurrent waves of plague was that the rats became immune or developed a high degree of resistance.[7] This is, however, biologically doubtful. If rats had developed a partial resistance the result would have been that they would have provided permanent reservoirs of the microbe. Plague would have become permanent as an endemic disease, although the epidemic outbreaks would have become fewer. The notion that such a species as susceptible as *R. rattus* would have developed total immunity to plague, lasting for generations, must be refuted until it has been proved experimentally. However, the usual intervals between plague epidemics might be attributed to short-term immunity among rats (and people).

The effectiveness of isolation and quarantine has been disputed on a number of grounds. The medical theories of *miasma* and *contagion* on which the measures against plague were founded did not take into account the roles of rats and fleas; the attention was focused on people and goods. Since rats and fleas would not have spread without the aid of human transport, these theories might still have led to the development of effective measures. It is very easy to demonstrate how deficient the barriers against the import of plague-infected fleas and rats were. The disappearance of plague was, however, a prolonged and irregular development. If biological factors had been determinative for the end of plague we would expect a much more uniform development. It is more likely, as P. Slack has argued, that "only the irregular adoption and incomplete success of the anti-plague measures can account for that".[8] J.-N. Biraben has, in his monumental study of plague, called attention to the fact that the development of measures against plague went from a local to a national or international level. Local measures had varying amounts of success and this might account for the irregular spread of the disease. In the course of time lessons were learned which finally made it possible to exclude plague from larger areas.[9]

The development of public measures against plague in Sweden

The general pattern of development from local measures against plague to more general and better organized ones also applies to the development in Sweden.

The Black Death and the subsequent plagues during the Middle Ages in Sweden did not result in a development of an organized public health as in Southern Europe. The first half of the 16th century appears to have been a period when Sweden was largely free from plague or other severe epidemic diseases. The expansion of settlements which occurred at this time must have been a consequence of a marked increase in population.[10] From 1547 to 1552 there are a number of references to epidemics which might have been plague in the present sense of the term. In November 1548 King Gustavus Vasa warned against a plague which was thought to have been introduced into

Stockholm by means of shipments of merchandise.[11] For this reason the great fair at Uppsala was cancelled. There is no evidence that any more general measures were taken. The royal letters express only concern about the shortage of soldiers. Sporadic sources suggest a slow diffusion of the pestilence with local variations.

Even if the years 1565-1566 are known as the time of the great plague in one medical tract,[12] King Eric XIV appears to have worried only about the loss of soldiers.[13] From the time of King John III efforts were made to implement more general measures against the spread of plague. The first Royal Ordinance of the plague year 1572 was, however, concerned only with the protection of the royal court.[14] The first decree regarding the quarantining of ships from plague-infected areas was issued on the 24th of July 1577, owing to the fact that plague was raging in Denmark and the German coastal towns.[15] John III ordered that, since experience had shown that the disease was contagious and could spread by means of merchandise, no ship from places suspected of being infected by the plague was to be permitted to enter any of the chief Swedish seaports (Öregrund, Norrköping, Söderköping, Västervik, and Kalmar), but should be required to lie at anchor in the roadsteads until it became clear whether or not there was any disease on board. Interestingly enough the same Ordinance warns against the import of heretical books from Germany, which was thus put on a pair with the plague. This general decree regarding quarantine did not, however, involve any sanctions, and did not apply to all ports. It was without effect, and there was nothing to stop plague from spreading during the following years. Later Royal Ordinances were not proclaimed until after the calamity was a fact. Neither were any general measures taken during the epidemics of 1588-1589 and 1602-1603.

During the first decades of the 17th century Sweden remained, like its neighbours, free from plague. The country was subsequently struck by a period of plagues beginning with the disastrous one of 1622-1624, and followed by the epidemics of 1629-1630, 1638-1640, and 1653-1657.[16]

The sources for the dimensions of the plague problem in 17th-century Sweden are, however, very scanty. One of the oldest series of parish registers is from Västerås.[17] Due to its situation on Lake Mälaren, Västerås was exposed to all the epidemics which struck Stockholm. The adjoining diagram shows the effects plague could have. The first epidemic for twenty years, in 1623, had severe consequences, while those that followed were comparatively mild, due to congenital or acquired immunity in the remaining population. It may also be noted that, apart from the years of crisis, there was an excess of births over deaths in Västerås.

At this time any administrative preparedness to meet plague with the kind of measures generally taken in Europe was still absent in Sweden. The authors of vernacular plague-tracts insisted, however, that the authorities should take more responsibility for the prevention of plague. The usual argument implied that just as it was a function of the "armed estate" to protect the country from

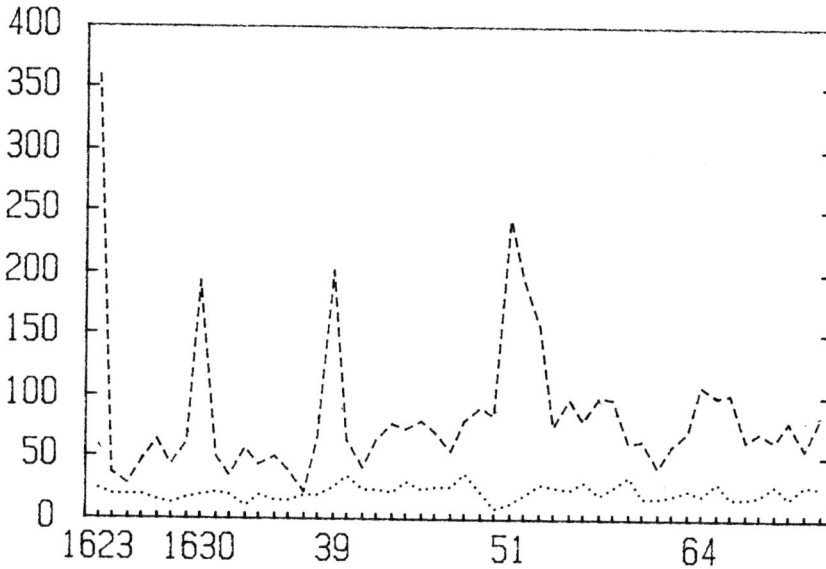

invading hostile armies, it was also their function to protect the people from invading contagious diseases. As early as 1620, when plague had begun to rage in the neighbouring countries, one Laurentius Carolstadius published a tract directed primarily at the authorities urging them to take actions against the threat of plague.[18] Throughout this tract a clear parallel is drawn between military defence and protection against plague. Bishop Laurentius Paulinus Gothus was still more clear-cut in his exhortations to the different estates to fulfill their various duties during times of plague.[19] Supporting his arguments with a host of Biblical quotations he insisted that the authorities must not abandon their duties in such times. First they must exhort their subjects to penitence. Then steps must be taken concerning their physical well-being. The food-supply must be ensured, since it was generally thought that there was a connection between starvation and plague. Furthermore rigorous measures against transmission of the contagion should be taken. The bishop maintained that spreading the plague should be equated with murder, and capital punishment imposed. These notions had also the full support of Martin Luther in his plague-tract, *Ob man vor dem Sterben fliehen möge*, which after the catechism was his most frequently printed tract in Swedish during this period.

In monolithically Lutheran Sweden there were no religious obstacles to an active policy for the control of plague. The Lutheran doctrines and ethos rather provided support for the notion that practical measures should be taken in addition to repentance and prayer. There was no expressed opposition to natural precautions, such as that of the Puritan movements in England.[21]

With the notifications of plague in neighbouring countries a Royal Ordinance was issued on the 20th of March 1620, containing a ban on all navigation between Swedish seaports and suspected places under the threat that the ships defying the ban would be confiscated.[22] There was, however, no special effort to ensure that the ban was respected when the threat was imminent. It was left to the local authorities to take action, but they could not do much, and in the summer of 1622 plague began to spread over the country. On the 17th of October, two months after it was known that the plague had arrived, King Gustavus Adolphus decreed that all markets should be postponed to the winter.[23] This was the only general measure taken. The king then only issued more detailed rules for the City of Stockholm concerning the isolation of the sick, but this did not occur until after the plague had been raging there for some time.[24] The epidemic continued throughout 1623 without interruption. The provincial governors of the country depicted in their reports to the Royal Chancellery the calamities the plague had brought about. They called attention above all to the problems of tax enforcement and the conscription of soldiers.[25] It was not until the end of this plague period in December 1624, that there was a marked tightening up of the statutes, when the burghers of Gothenburg were prohibited from leaving the infected town by a penalty of death. This was the first time the death penalty was imposed in connection with plague.[26]

The most ambitious ordinances against the spread of plague were issued by Christina, the queen mother, within the duchy she so autocratically ruled. Her decrees contained detailed instructions both to her town of Nyköping and the surrounding countryside, concerning the nursing and isolation of the sick, public decontamination and the burning of aromatic substances according to the medical theories of the time.[27] However, in defiance of the royal decree she permitted markets to take place, the only proviso being that they should not be visited by persons from infected areas. The reason was explicitly economic, but it was also given a religious justification.[28]

It is obvious for the whole period that the application of effective measures against plague was in conflict with economic interests. For the country people the markets provided their only possibility of turning their products into cash or exchanging them for other goods. The imposed isolation of towns meant economic disaster for the burghers. The state, which was rearming, demanded large resources in revenue and men. For the individual it must have meant the constant weighing of the risk of starvation against that of plague. For the government the risk of plague had to be weighed against the needs of the armed forces. The result was a hazy policy with several compromises. When finally steps were taken they became more and more strict and well-organized during the following decades. From 1638 the first printed Royal Ordinance imposed the death penalty for breaking the rules of isolation.[29] During the 1650's the quarantine system developed, but it was only during the final phase of the last epidemic of the 17th century that the protection against suspected vessels had found a reasonably effective form.

During the 1660's several European countries experienced their last plague epidemics. Of Swedish territory only the island of Gotland was struck by plague, in 1662, whereupon no ships from there were allowed to call at mainland ports.[30] In view of this it is reasonable to assume that susceptibility to plague was still low after the recent epidemic. In 1664 a new Royal Ordinance was published forbidding any traveller from Holland or any other plague infected area to land in Sweden on penalty of death.[31] At this time the only risk lay in long-distance shipments from Holland and England which were fairly easy to control thanks to the improvements in customs administration. This remains the only instance where there is some reason to believe that the imposed measures were successful.

During the plague-free decades at the end of the 17th century medicine became more established with the formation of the *Collegium medicum* in 1663, which more and more developed from a body of physicians into a public agency with special duties in preventing epidemic disease. A system of district medical officers was also developed. Around 1710 nine provincial towns had physicians who could advise the local authorities concerning the prevention of disease, and who could diagnose suspected cases.[32]

As soon as the notifications of plague in neighbouring countries in 1709 became known to the government an ordinance of general quarantine was issued, and Sweden was not affected by plague that year.[33] Quarantine is, however, only effective as long as the risk of infection is restricted to ships from a limited number of countries, and as long as there is a reasonable administrative system for its control. This was not the case in the following year. Sweden was a country in crisis after the catastrophe at Poltava. The harvests had failed and mass starvation had followed. After the defeat on the eastern frontier hosts of refugees came from the plague infected Baltic provinces. There was no possibility for the authorities to control the spread of plague. Furthermore the authorities were very irresolute, and hesitated until the very last moment before taking action.

At the end of August and the beginning of September 1710, the Royal Senate and the *Collegium medicum* officially tried to suppress the rumours of plague, while at the same time preparing for the worst. Cases of suspected plague was examined by the physicians and discussed in the Royal Senate.[34] Even if there was no doubt that there was plague in Stockholm, it was stated officially that it was only a kind of fever. In order to calm the citizens a deliberately misleading article appeared in the weekly magazine on the 24th of August which denied that the disease was the plague.[35] This occurred a week after the first cases of plague in Stockholm had been diagnosed. In the Ordinance of the 2nd of September it was forbidden on penalty of death to receive travellers from plague-infected areas. However, only plague in the provinces and on islands was mentioned, not the plague in Stockholm, which had already taken 300 lives.[36] The only action taken in time to prepare the people for the plague was that the *Collegium medicum* was ordered to publish a plague tract with medical advice for ordinary people.[37] From the records of the Royal Senate it is apparent that they were calculating with the remote possibility of limiting the plague to one district of Stockholm. They knew that as soon as news of the plague was officially made public it would involve the total closure of the city, and substantial food supply problems would result. As late as the 10th of September it was ordered that it should be noted in the passports of travelling merchants that the air was sound in Stockholm.[38] The same day letters were sent to the Pomeranian government, and the provincial governors, that their subjects could without any danger of contagious disease trade with the capital.[39]

It was not until the 20th of September that the Magistrate published a tract for the citizens of Stockholm concerning how they should behave in order to prevent the spread of plague.[40] That week 584 plague victims were counted. It took even longer before an ordinance was promulgated for the whole country. This occurred on the 8th of November. By that time the Royal Senate had fled to Arboga, and large areas of the country were affected by plague. The decree included strict regulations concerning the isolation of plague-infected areas. The most provocative paragraph concerned the burial of plague victims. It was decreed that they should be buried immediately, without ceremony, outside the towns, on the nearest hill.[42] This was, of course, founded on the medical notion that *miasma* from plague victims might poison the air. The *Collegium medicum* had, however, only insisted that special churchyards should be arranged, and that the bodies should be covered with lime. This statute provoked determined opposition among the people. The authorities were apparently not aware of how much a proper Christian burial meant to ordinary men. Exclusion from the churchyards put the plague victims in the same category as impenitent criminals and witches. The bishops did what they could to induce the clergy to emphasize in their sermons how little such ceremonies meant, but with little apparent effect. In some places there were riots, people kept cases of plague secret in their homes, and they buried their dead secretly in the churchyards.[43] The result was that the authorities totally lost control of the spread of plague. It also means that the demographic historian cannot rely on the parish registers of that time.

An assessment of the fight against plague during the 16th and 17th centuries and the early 18th century cannot lead to any other conclusion than that the steps taken were generally inoperative. Sweden was hit by plague whenever the neighbouring countries were. The failure of the measures against plague did not lead to a questioning of their effectiveness in principle; the failure was blamed on the ignorance and disobedience of the people. The notion remained that it was a function of government to protect the country against contagious disease. The Lutheran mentality left no room for defeatism. The belief that plague was a consequence of sin meant that it should be combated as something evil both by means of penitence and by natural means. These ideas were further supported by the mercantilistic ideology of the 18th century, which encouraged a greater interest in the problem of how to increase the population.

In the course of the 17th century medicine became more firmly established within society. The leading physicians were all concerned with promoting public health. The medical theories of epidemic disease were still based on the ancient ideas of *miasma* and *contagion*, although these concepts had received more detailed chemical interpretations. In Sweden there were no important conflicts between these ideas; it was only a question of emphasis. The idea of miasma led to a stress on factors in the environment, and the call for public sanitation. In a number of speeches at the Royal Academy of Science physicians demanded action against the insanitary environments in towns.[44] A special government commission on health took steps in that direction around the middle of the 18th century.[45] There were, however, no lasting results. Public hygiene was a matter for local authorities, which did not have the necessary administrative or technological capability until the 19th century. The ideas concerning contagion, which led to an emphasis on isolation and quarantine, were more likely to be accepted by the authorities. Although infant mortality and endemic diseases received more attention, plague was still what was most feared. The fight against foreign contagious diseases could also be carried out using means which were natural for a central government: customs administration and military defence. Defending the country from foreign disease became equated with defending the country from foreign armies.

The military character of the quarantine legislation during the 18th century in Sweden as well as in other European countries is obvious. The last Western European plague, in Provence, began in the summer of 1720. The reaction in Sweden was, however, slow. It was not until December that the *Collegium medicum* discussed the problem.[46] In 1721 a committee was appointed to suggest appropriate measures.[47] A Royal Ordinance was issued in December 1721, containing very rigorous regulations, by which ships could be confiscated, and the crews executed for breaking the quarantine rules.[48]

New quarantine ordinances were subsequently issued as soon as rumours of plague, usually in North Africa and the Levant, reached the government (1738, 1733, 1739, 1743, 1744, 1768, 1770). Since similar measures were taken by all European maritime countries, ships from plague-infected areas must have had very few opportunities to call at European harbours; to get through all the way to Scandinavia would have been practically impossible. It was rather the case that plague threatened Scandinavia from another direction, since earlier epidemics had usually come from the other side of the Baltic.

Plague was still endemic in the Ottoman Empire in the 19th century, where there were several epidemic outbreaks. It was primarily the Austrian territories that were threatened, and in order to prevent the advance of plague the Austrian government established a military sanitary cordon along the more than one thousand miles of frontier with the Ottoman Empire.[49] Even if its usefulness has been disputed, the fact remains that the plague no longer penetrated into Western and Central Europe, and that this development coincided with the consolidation of this cordon.[50] Plague could, however, spread from the Ottoman Empire to Russia, and it was thus a threat also to Scandinavia.

During the summer of 1770 plague reached Poland, and the Swedish government accordingly reinforced the quarantine regulations.[51] In order to prevent the plague from penetrating, General Ehrensvärd, who was still responsible for the defence of Finland, was ordered to establish a sanitary cordon along the eastern frontier.[52]

The general posted sentries from the Savolaks Regiment on all roads and paths crossing the eastern border. When winter came, and the danger was thought to be over, the sentries were withdrawn. During the following spring, when plague began to rage in Russia, frontier guards were posted again, and army guard ships patrolled the archipelago. In 1772 the threat came still closer. In February General Ehrensvärd received a report that the disease had advanced to the Ladoga-Novogorod area, and was approaching St. Petersburg. He again demanded permission to reinforce the guard, and to maintain a *cordon sanitaire* by force. This was officially permitted by a Royal Ordinance and a circular letter to the governors of Finland in March 1772.[53] Moreover in February a committee consisting of medical and military experts was appointed to take the steps necessary for the protection of the country from plague.[54]

According to reports sent to the committee a close watch was kept along all the busiest parts of the border. The only point where crossing was permitted was at Aborrfors, where a quarantine-station had been established. The period of quarantine for travellers from Russia was fixed at forty-two days, in accordance with the instructions of the *Collegium medicum*. An expedition was also sent from Stockholm in order to determine the efficiency of the *cordon*.

It is, however, difficult to make a retrospective assessment of the use and efficiency of the measures taken on the basis of official records. A total closure of the border was neither possible, nor necessary. The danger lay in the busy trade between Finnish farmers and Russian towns. There was a clear risk that cartloads of produce might conceal plague-infected rats or fleas. There was also reason to stop this trade in order to resolve the supply problems in Finnish towns. The abolition of the trade with Russia soon proved to have this result. The *cordon* was, however, opposed by the *Mössorna* party, which supported the principle of free trade.[55]

It is also difficult to judge how serious the threat from Russia really was. The sources are ambiguous, and dependent on their authors general view of quarantine measures. There was never any epidemic in the St. Petersburg area comparable with that of the Moscow area. There was a high death rate in the Novogorod gubernia during 1771, but it is not certain to what extent it was due to plague.[56] Cold winters might also have helped to stop the spread of the disease.

Conclusion

The disappearance of plague was basically due to the character of plague as an invasive disease. There was no ecological niche in Western Europe for the microbe. It was thus possible to exclude the disease by means of measures, such as isolation, quarantine, and *cordon sanitaire*. In the course of the 18th century this had developed into a reasonably cohesive system in Western Europe, where Sweden played an important role by defending the northern flank.

The long-term effect of plague is to be found in its role in the development of public health. During the periods of plague public authorities gradually became convinced that it was one of their functions to protect the citizens from epidemic disease. This was to a great extent due to the fact that the defence against contagion was associated with military defence, and the steps to be taken accorded with the traditional functions of central government.

When plague ceased to be an actual threat, attention could be directed to other health problems in society. The quarantine system did not prove to be effective against other diseases, such as cholera, and liberals opposed it for economic reasons. The sanitary movements introduced new methods in the fight against epidemic diseases. However, the notion persisted that it was a function of the state to protect its citizens from wasting diseases. This remains the heritage of plague in history.

Notes

1. M.W. Flinn, 'Plague in Europe and the Mediterranean Countries', *Journal of European Economic History*, 8 (1979), pp. 131-148.

2. See e.g. L. Bradley, 'The Most Famous of All English Plagues: A Detailed Analysis of the Plague at Eyam, 1665-1666', *The Plague Reconsidered: A New Look at its Origins and Effects in 16th and 17th Century England. A Local Population Studies Supplement* (Matlock 1977), pp. 63-94; M. Mattmüller, 'Die Pest in Liestal: Notizen zu den demographischen Implikationen der frühneuzeitlichen Epidemien', *Gesnerus*, 40 (1983), pp. 119-128; A. Perrenoud, 'Les mecanismes de recauperation d'une population frappée par la peste. L'epidemie de 1636-1640 à Geneve', *Schweizerische Zeitschrift für Geschichte*, 28 (1978), pp. 265-288.

3. See the survey in J.-N. Biraben, *Les hommes et la peste en France et dans les pays européens et méditerranéens*, Vol. 1 (Paris 1975), Annexe IV.

4. O.T. Hult, *Pesten i Sverige 1710* (Stockholm 1916); L. Preinitz, *Studier rörande pesten i Stockholm 1710-1711*, Department of History, Uppsala (Unpublished licentiate-thesis 1972).

5. Concerning the epidemiology of plague, see e.g. R. Pollitzer, 'Plague', *WHO, Monographs Series*, 22 (Geneva 1954); R.E. Blount, 'Plague', *A Manual of Tropical Medicine*, 5 ed. (Philadelphia 1976), pp. 224-233; Biraben (1975), Vol. 1, pp. 7-21; Bradley (1977), pp. 11-23. The thesis that plague in Scandinavia was diffused primarily by interhuman transmission is maintained in L. Walløe, 'Pest og folketall 1350-1750', *Historisk Tidskrift*, 1 (Oslo 1982), pp. 1-45. It is there further argued that plague had a permanent enzootic reservoir in Europe, see esp. p. 34.

6. S. Ekman, *Djurvärldens utbredningshistoria på skandinaviska halvön* (Stockholm 1922), p. 90.

7. A.B. Appleby, 'The Disappearance of Plague: A Continuing Puzzle', *The Economic History Review*, 33 (1980), pp. 161-173.

8. P. Slack, 'The Disappearance of Plague: An Alternative View', *The Economic History Review*, 34 (1981), pp. 469-476, on p. 473.

9. Biraben (1976), vol 2, pp. 182-185.

10. L.-O. Larsson, 'Kolonisation och befolkningsutveckling i det svenska agrar-samhället 1500-1640', *Bibliotheca Historica Lundensis*, 27 (Lund 1972).

11. Konung Gustav den förstes registratur, Vol. 19, pp. 341 f.

12. S. Berchelt, *Om Pestilentzien och hennes Orsaker ...* (Stockholm 1589), fol. 6r.

13. C.M. Stenbock (Ed.), 'Erik XIV:s almanacksanteckningar ...', *Skrifter utgifna af Personhistoriska samfundet*, 6 (Stockholm 1912), pp. 27, 33, 38.

14. Stockholm: Riksarkivet (RA: The National Archives), Riks-registratur (RR) 1572-1-16, fol. 16r.

15. RR 1577-7-24, fol. 166r.

16. The identification of these epidemics with bubonic plague is based primarily on my analysis of contemporary medical tracts: P.G. Ottosson, *Den svenska pestlitteraturen* (1572-1711) (Linköping 1986).

17. Uppsala: Landsarkivet (The provincial archives), Västerås Domkyrkoförsamling C 1.

18. L. Carolstadius, *Een kort Mening/Om en Troghen och Försichtigh öfwerheetz Kall och Embete vthi Pestilentie Tijdher/sitt Land och Rijke från then Smittesamme Kranck-heetz Pestis/Fiendtlighe infall och Tyranij at frija/ frelsa och förswara. Korteligen och hastelighen författat aff Laurentius Carolstadio—Psal. 41. Eccles. 7 Bene illi qui prudenter, aegros tractat. Nam quo tempore ipse aliquid aduersi patietur, Dominus vicissim ei auxiliabitur* (Uppsala 1620).

20. L. P. Gothus: *Loimoscopia Eller Pestilentz Speghel. Thet är: Andeligh och Naturligh Vnderwijsning/Om Pestilentzies Beskriffwelse/Orsaker/Praeservatijff/Läkedomar och Befrijelser: Stält och Sammanfattadt Så wäl allom Christrognom vthi Gemeen/Som i Synderhz Läre- Wärie- och Näre-Stånden/til Nödtorfftigh Vnderrättelse /Sampt Timmeligha Wälfärdz och Ewigha Salighetz Befordring. Widh Ändan är tilsadt/D.D. Mart. Lutheri Grundrijke Vnderwijsning/om Pestilentziske Förwaringar.* (Strängnäs: O. Olofzson, Enaeus, 1623).

21. Cf. P. Slack, *The Impact of Plague in Tudor and Stuart England* (London 1985), Ch. 9.

22. RR 1621-1-14, fol. 78v-79r.

23. RR 1622-10-17, fol. 326.

24. RR 1623-2-8, fol. 41v-42v.

25. RA: Kammarkollegium, Kansliet, E IIa:2,7.

26. RR 1624-12-30, fol. 474v-475v.

27. RA: Kungl. Arkiv, Drottning Christinas d.ä. Registratur, 1623-7-15, fol. 188v-193r; 1623-8-25, fol. 220r-223v.

28. Ibid., 1623-9-10, fol. 241r-242v.

29. Kungl. Placat 1638-11-17.

30. *Handlingar rörande Skandinaviens historia.* Vol. 31 (Stockholm 1850), p. 155.

31. Kungl. Placat 1664-9-7.

32. O.E.A. Hjelt, *Svenska och finska medicinalverkets historia 1663-1812* (Helsinki 1892), vol 2, p. 3.

33. Kungl. Placat 1709-8-25.

34. RA: Collegium medicum protokoll (CMP) 1710-8-18, pp. 290-293; Svenska riksrådets protokoll (SRP) 1710-8-19, p. 766-769.

35. *Stockholmiske Post-Tidender* 30, 1710-8-30.

36. Hult (1916), p. 23.

37. RR 1710-8-4, fol. 239. The tract *Kort underrättelse/Huru man sig förhålla skal/när Gud Land och Rike med en grymm Pestilentialisk Fahrsoot straffa täckes. Uppå Höga öfwerhetens Nådigas Befallning Upsatt af Kongl. Collegio Medico I Stockholm Åhr 1710* (Stockholm: H. Werner) was published during the first week of September, CMP 1710-9-8, p. 318.

38. SRP 1710-9-10, p. 938.

39. Ibid., and RR 1710-9-10, fol. 419r-421r.

40. *Förordning/Angående Åtskilige Måhl/som böra i acht tagas wid den nu påstående Fahrsoten* (Stockholm: S. Werner).

41. Kungl. Placat 1710-11-8.

42. Ibid., paragraph 17.

43. See e.g. the discussions in SRP 103a, 1711, fol. 25v-27r, 34v, 220, 780r-783v, 437v-438r, 504r-505r.

44. E.g. A. Bäck, 'Tal om farsoter, som mäst härja bland Rikets Allmoge', *Kungliga Vetenskaps Akademien, Praesidii tal* (Stockholm 1765); N. Dalberg, 'Tal om luftens beskaffenhet i stora och folkrika städer...', *Kungliga Vetenskaps Akademien, Praesidii tal* (Stockholm, 1784); J. Leche, *Tal om luftens beskaffenhet i Åbo, samt huru politien, i samråd med medicin bör förekomma sjukdomar...* (Stockholm 1761); J.L. Odhelius, 'Dödligheten i Stockholm', *Kungliga Vetenskaps Akademien, Praesidii tal* (Stockholm, 1785); cf. S. Lindroth, *Svensk lärdomshistoria: Frihetstiden* (Stockholm 1978), pp. 460-462.

45. O. Hjelt, *Svenska och finska medicinalverkets historia 1663-1812* (Helsinki 1891), vol 1, pp. 339-350.

46. Hjelt (1891), Vol. 2, p. 200.

47. RA: Äldre Kommittéer (ÄK) 674.

48. R.G. Modée, *Utdrag utur all ifrån den 7 decemb. 1718 utkomne Publique Handlingar...* (Stockholm 1742), vol 1, pp. 307-310.

49. E. Lesky, 'Die österreichische Pestfront an der k.k. Militärgrenze', *Saeculum*, 8 (1957), pp. 82-106.

50. G.E. Rothenberg, 'The Austrian Sanitary Cordon and the Control of the Bubonic Plague: 1710-1871', *Journal of the History of Medicine and Allied Sciences*, 28 (1973), pp. 15-23.

51. Modée (1742), Vol. 9, pp. 449-452.

52. O. Nikula, *Augustin Ehrensvärd* (Helsinki 1960), pp. 492ff.

53. Modée (1742), Vol. 9, pp. 828-829; RR, Inrikes civilexp. 410r-411v.

54. RA: ÄK 677.

55. O.E.A. Hjelt, *Johan Haartmans verksamhet vid universitetet i Åbo under åren 1754-1787* (Helsinki 1911), p. 93.

56. J.T. Alexander, *Bubonic Plague in Early Modern Russia: Public Health and Urban Disaster* (Baltimore and London 1980), pp. 229-254.

Why Cure the Sick? Population Policy and Health Programs within 18th-Century Swedish Mercantilism[1]

Karin Johannisson

The intense interest of the European mercantilists in population policy is well-known. The primary goal of mercantilism, which dominated the economic debate between about 1650-1750, was to obtain more power for the state. In essence this goal meant a favourable balance of trade in a rapidly expanding colonial world. A major emphasis was placed on developing natural resources, of which population was considered the most important. The stimulation of population growth began, therefore, to be seen as a fundamental responsibility of government.

In Sweden, mercantilism became the central ideology after the great political defeat around 1720. The country was deprived of manpower and capital; reduced from a great power to a small estate on the outskirts of Europe. An acute need for a rapid recovery became apparent. On all political levels, within public debate and scientific institutions, a program for progress, based on exploring and developing natural resources, was emphasized. Productive workers were the key to the realization of this program.

From the 1730s onwards the axiom "a plentitude of poor people is a country's greatest wealth", formulated by one of the leading mercantilists, Anders Nordencrantz, was elevated into a national credo. The matter could be put into still clearer terms: "A population of proper size is a country's finest possession; for low enforcement, chastisement and thrift make the people manageable and industrious". For greater religious legitimacy the Book of Proverbs was quoted time after time: "In the multitude of people is the King's honour: but in the want of people is the destruction of the prince" (Proverbs 14:28).

The basic idea was that a surplus of people also created a surplus of demand, which in turn inspired initiative, tillage of the land and industry. Thus an abundance of people, kept just above subsistence level, would automatically stimulate business, increasing the power and wealth of the nation.

How, then, to achieve the desired increase in population? There seemed to be two main ways: to encourage immigration and to stimulate nativity. (A third, to make the existing population survive through better health conditions and health services, was not yet advanced.) For ideas on the former point, Swedish mercantilists had only to look to England. There William Petty, founder of the new science of political arithmetic, had presented a series of radical proposals at the end of the seventeenth century. These included the prohibition of all emigration, the recall of colonists from America and the settlement of the entire populations of northern Scotland and Ireland (1.8 million people!) on more fertile English land.[2]

Similarly, a widespread interest in colonization projects of all kinds, population settlement and population-stimulating measures flourished in Sweden. The suggestions are in some case astonishing. The ideal of colonization found its most grandiose expression in the many schemes for the development of Lapland, "our Swedish India". In the same spirit, others wanted to send people to Finland (then part of Sweden), or toyed with the notion of transporting criminals to colonize less attractive areas. Anders Berch, one of the mercantilist ideologists, quotes with approval the example of ten life-prisoners and ten women from the workhouse who "after drawing lots were paired off and ... sent to Greenland."

Any method of encouraging foreigners to come to Sweden was acceptable. Berch particularly had in mind the people of Silesia and Meissen (good potters!), "who would suit us well". Others complained that Sweden had made little effort to attract groups who had suffered religious or political persecution, in particular the 30,000 Protestants of Salzburg, who had been banished from their native land by an edict of 1731. They could, for example, have been placed in the sparsely-populated, northerly province of Västerbotten. Further proposals were made regarding the movement of population between the different Swedish provinces. Either the population should be distributed more evenly over the full area of the country, or it should be concentrated in a few (the most fertile) provinces. It was thought that in the latter case the densely-populated areas would expand "organically" as a result of natural population growth.

There was great optimism about the rate at which the population might increase. A doubling in the space of twenty years would be no impossibility, many believed. Over the long term, the population of Sweden ought to be able to grow to ten, twenty, even thirty million people. (The true population, in the mid-eighteenth century, although not made known at the time, was just over two million.)

Such optimistic calculations were not mere eccentricities, outside the mainstream of public discussion. They were to be heard from most of the leading mercantilists and even in the reports which the Office of Tables (founded in 1749 and the predecessor of the Central Bureau of Statistics) submitted to Parliament.

How could they come up with such fantastic figures? In this case the optimism was based on exaggerated hopes for Sweden's natural resources. These hopes had been inherited from a national romantic tradition of the preceding century. Sweden had been depicted in those days as the chosen land, where the sons of Noah had decided to settle for its natural riches.

This romantic tradition now merged interestingly with the seemingly cold rationalism of the mercantilists. Sweden was bulging with dormant resources. "To keep any kind of land unused and unfruitful, now and in the future, dare no man who has seen the new ideas that can spring from human ingenuity, when spurred by need, in a populous country", asserted the Director of the Land Survey Board, E.O. Runeberg. Sweden, above all others, is the country in which the good Lord "has let abundance fall from his footsteps", agreed Johan Kraftman, professor of economics, in even more exalted tones.

Moreover, the Nordic climate was unusually favourable, a number of writers maintained. The cold protected the people from infectious diseases and made them "merry, lively and manly". The snow on the ground prevented nutritious substances from evaporating and, when it melted, transformed the rotting leaves and needles into rich humus. The woods were teeming with useful game— "if anyone seriously tried to domesticate our moose, they might well become our camels" —and lakes and rivers were swarming with salmon and other splendid fish, pearl-filled molluscs, oysters and lobsters. The people could also rejoice over what the Swedish climate spared them from. They were spared from the burning sun of hotter countries "where the people, drained by the heat, for much of the year must splash around all day in their water barrels". They could walk in the forests without fear of tigers, lions, leopards and apes and they could fish in lakes and rivers without being frightened by dreadful hippopotamuses and bloodthirsty crocodiles. Given persevering application, all this splendour would show a wonderful capacity to multiply. "When wildernesses and wastes are cultivated, a whole new land will be created, much more fruitful than this, milder in climate, pleasanter in every way, rich and able to support and feed many million people more than now."

This faith in the future was proclaimed exuberantly, in language imbued with the biblical legend of paradise, in sweet harmony with the Gothic vision of Sweden as a great power. It was an extravagant and rather absurd optimism, perhaps without parallel in the history of Swedish society. As the natural resources were already present, the real need entailed increasing the number of productive labourers. One way in which to achieve this goal has already been mentioned (to encourage immigration and prohibit emigration). The other way—and in a long term perspective the more profitable one—was to stimulate nativity. Many drastic suggestions were put forward, interesting for their apparent disregard for cultural and religious tradition. William Petty had struck the keynote in England. To stimulate nativity, for example, he had advocated a rationalization of sexual morality, in the form of various types of contractual marriage, more liberal attitudes to the incest taboo, tax penalties on any woman between 18-44 not bearing child during the year and prohibition for all women older than 44 "to make claim to a man". To increase the work output of the existing population he had also suggested that seven-year-olds should be put to work and that workers should work more and eat less (e.g. by cutting down their lunch-breaks and/or fasting on Fridays).

In Sweden there was great ingenuity in the suggestions both for increasing the population and for extracting as much work as possible from the people that Sweden already had. Unnecessary holidays ("when the workers only get drunk") could be done away with; thralls could be imported; emigration could be made a crime; prisoners of war, beggars and criminals could be put in the workhouse and small children could begin doing simple work at the age of four.

Procreation was to be encouraged by all possible means, but only among the working classes, not among the "consuming" sections of the population. The Office of Tables devoted much attention to this question in the 1750s and 1760s. In which month were most children conceived: in spring, when the light returned: in summer, at harvest time: in the autumn, when the pantries were full, or around Christmas? Tables of the monthly numbers of births were drawn up, showing that most children were conceived in December. However, the figures permitted no conclusions more significant than that "Christmas games make hearts light and cradles heavy". As a matter of fact October turned out to be the worst month for conception, although it was a month of many weddings ("which shows that the new love devours more than it brings forth").

In this way the mercantilists discussed every aspect of the subject. Nothing seemed too private for inclusion in the national welfare programme. Their population policies were notable for their mixture of rationalism and unbounded optimism. In their social implications they were progressive: they recommended tax exemptions and bounties for the newly wed, a new policy on crime and more orphanages and workhouses. However, hospitals were not included in the programme, a point to which I shall return.

The mercantilistic ideology was mechanistic and depersonalized. People were the means of power. In a long term perspective the welfare of the state was certainly supposed to be accorded also to each of its members. But state power had to come first and the individual had to subordinate his private needs and rights to its claim for priority. His material wants were seen as limited to the most primary needs: food, clothing, accommodation. His wages had to cover these—but nothing more. This view found its most naked expression when a cash value was placed on the individual (labourer).

Once again, inspiration was to be drawn from William Petty, who had assigned a fixed capital value to each member of the population, about £ 70, an approximate mean between a year-old baby (£ 4) and a 20-year-old (£ 140), or between the daily rates for slaves and mercenary soldiers). Similar calculations were performed in Sweden. The highest value was set on a married workman (2,391:99 dalers), followed by an unmarried workman, then "a person in general", by which was meant an average for the total population (612 dalers). A woman was assigned a capital value three-quarters of that of a man. Finally came the children, divided by age group down to the infants, whose worth was negligible, as they required on average "one-fifth of a person in care and tending" and thus had to be reckoned as a minus item equal to one-fifth of the full value of an adult. This reasoning can be illustrated as follows: "If we assume that by his eighteenth year a youth is equivalent to a full adult workman, and that a child of the common people does not begin to be of use until his ninth year, and that not until his eighteenth year has he atoned for all the discommodity and damage that he caused before his ninth year, then a youth can be seen as non-deductible capital, increased by the accrual of compound interest, which only begins to yield an annual return through simple interest after his eighteenth year. So if a youth is given a political value of 1,195 dalers in his eighteenth year, he must be valued at 998.8 in his fifteenth, 746.3 in his tenth, 557.6 in his fifth and 416.7 dalers in the cradle."[3] Thus the mercantilist view was pursued to a point where human worth seemed to become synonymous with capital value.

At the same time this scheme was, however, contradicted by reality. The most valuable unit according to this system would indeed be the healthy labourer who sired many children. The average life expectancy was, however, about 33 years and one child in three died before the age of ten; epidemics and illness claimed tens of thousands of lives every year.

At first the mercantilists did not really want to see the problem. The high child mortality rate was certainly remarked upon, but it was treated mainly as an abstract, economic problem. Thus it could be stated that "whoever can make farmers' children live longer enriches the community at once by 416.7 and eventually by 2,391 dalers". The problem of disease was similarly treated in tables and financial calculations. Yet again, English mercantilism supplied the model. Nehemiah Grew, the renowned English doctor, secretary of the Royal Society, had boldly pointed out that from a purely economic point of view dead subjects were preferable to sick subjects, who were only an unnecessary drain on capital and a public or private encumbrance.[4] William Petty calculated more optimistically on the basis of England's current population at the time: "Suppose that by the advancement of the art of Medicine a quarter part more may be borne and a quarter part fewer dye. Then the King will gain and save 200,000 subjects per annum, which valued at £20 per head, the lowest price of slaves, will make 4 million per annum benefit to the Commonwealth".[5] On these assumptions the task of medicine was to achieve what it could in the form of profitable results, i.e. direct capital growth.

In the mid-1750s the Swedish Parliament began to notice the medical predicament of the country. The situation was wretched. Doctors were extremely few and far between and not likely to concern themselves with the poor. Those in acute need of treatment had to obtain what help they could from barbersurgeons, bonesetters and wise old women; the chronic cases ended up—if there was room—in the hospital.

The eighteenth century hospital was, as is well known, a complex institution. It offered very little indeed in the way of medical care. It contained outcasts of every category: the aged, the incurable, the deranged, the handicapped and the down-and-out of all kinds. The criterion was that they had to be unfit for work. The state's task was to make sure that none but those wholly incapable of work were admitted to hospital, as one of the mercantilists stated. However, the total inadequacy of the hospitals was already apparent from the first figures produced by the Office of Tables in 1749. They showed only 1,679 inmates, but a further 28,991 people who were also considered in need of admission. In addition there were 1,571 labelled "mad" and 1,581 "ill with the falling sickness".

The new statistics provided an entirely new instrument for the consideration of Sweden's human resources. The figures for mortality and causes of death were at first treated optimistically. When in 1752 Parliament asked the College of Physicians to comment on the figures for 1749, the reply radiated on optimism and an assurance that were as typical of the time as was the precision of the figures. For example, it was said (note that the figures do not cover all mortality in Sweden in the year concerned) that of the 7,191 people who had died of smallpox and measles, the College considered that "at least 6,000 could have been preserved by sensible care and appropriate medicine"; of the 4,054 dying of fevers, 3,000 people "could have been saved"; of the 3,112 who succumbed to dysentery, 2,000 could have been restored to health; of the 1,704 victims of ague at least 1,000 could surely have been saved if midwives had been available; 2,816 people had died of whooping cough and of them 2,000 could probably have regained their health, and so on.[6]

The percentage of potential cures is nearly 75 %! Nils Rosén von Rosenstein, Professor of Medicine at Uppsala, was equally optimistic: mortality could be reduced by half "and thus 30,000 lives be spared".

The reports of the College of Physicians to Parliament are of interest, in that they regard as a matter of course that population-policy was the obvious purpose of medical care. In 1756, for example, there is a comment on the Office of Tables' statistics to the effect that at least 17,000 of the 50,000 who died each year could be cured if there were more doctors and more medicaments. How many children would these 17,000 not produce and how much tax would they not pay to the Swedish Exchequer!

On the whole the situation was portrayed in an optimistic tone that can hardly have been in keeping with the capabilities of medicine in the mid-eighteenth century. As here, for example:

"In the autumn of 1753 smallpox was common in Enköping, and most deadly, so that 18 or 20 children had to be buried, and that in a small town, every week. The spots always ran together, with diarrhoea throughout their sickness, which meant that they never came quite to a head and the afflicted died with pitiful convulsions and mortification on the eleventh or fourteenth day. But then a doctor was appointed to come to the assistance of the suffering and medicine was dispensed without charge: which, praise be to God, so succeeded that the sickness was halted."

"In 1754, towards autumn, St. Anthony's Fire (ergotism) broke out in the County of Kronoberg. It was like the falling sickness, with convulsions and fits of violent jerking or spasms, which occurred from time to time and began either with vomiting or diarrhoea, and ended in fever and terrible delirium. The sickness was slow, often fatal, and spread before anything could be done, across the counties of Kronoberg, Kalmar and Blekinge. The College sent forthwith a complete description of the cure and prevention of this disease to the affected places. Which with God's gracious blessing led to the sickness declining and eventually quite disappearing."[7]

In fact improvements came slowly and decades were to pass before mortality began to fall extensively. By then the number of district medical officers had greatly increased and the first hospitals, wholly dedicated to the sick, had been opened (the first in 1752; by 1780 there were already seventeen).

To what extent then, did the arguments put forward within mercantilistic ideology, i.e. economic arguments, influence these improvements? Can it be said that public authorities decided to invest in health services, primarily because of their wish to return potential manpower capital to its place in the production machine in order to work, pay taxes and produce children for the nation?

Moreover, were the mercantilistic arguments the only ones presented for an improved health programme?

There is, for example, the remarkable speech, "The epidemics which most afflict the country people of the nation", delivered at the Royal Swedish Academy of Sciences in 1764, by Abraham Bäck, the patriarch of Swedish doctors. He, too, considered the situation wretched. He, too, as a good mercantilist, emphasized economic motives, pointing out that the future of Sweden was threatened by devastating diseases, depriving the country of much productive labour. However, he combines this perspective with the idea that the severe epidemics affect the lower strata of the population most heavily because of their poverty, which in various ways makes them especially susceptible to disease. Therefore, the working people should not be kept at a level of mere subsistence, rather their social conditions and lives in general should be considerably improved. In this way, Bäck concludes, "many productive members could be snatched away from the jaws of death".[8] On the whole, his reform programme is characterized by a striking socio-political clearsightedness.

So whose voices did the authorities listen to? Of course, there is no simple answer, only a complex one.

What can be stated is that mercantilistic arguments—in their naked cost-and-benefit reasoning—dominated the Swedish debate during the decades around 1750, when public health services became more and more a responsibility of government. Sick and prematurely deceased workers were not profitable workers. In the long run, therefore, organized health and medical services would benefit society.

These arguments were stressed in the important reports sent in to Parliament by the Office of Tables, as well as by the College of Physicians. Economic arguments were certainly effective in bringing about change; this is true for the 18th century as for our own time. Behind these arguments there may, of course, be motives of, for example, a humanitarian nature.

My purpose has been to present the mercantilistic arguments for health care, to show their pragmatism and apparent disregard for cultural and religious traditions. From the point of view of results, i.e. more hospitals and expanding health services, the arguments used to bring about this change, may, of course, seem secondary. For the sick individual, a bed in hospital and access to rest, hot food and medical care certainly increased his chance of recovery.

Notes

1. This article is based on K. Johannisson, *Society in Numbers: Statistics and Utopias in Eighteenth century Europe* (forthcoming); idem, *'The Interchangeable Man: Individual, Disease and Society in a Historical Perspective'* (preliminary version). An interesting article discussing economic motives for health care in a historical perspective is R. Fein, 'On Measuring Economic Benefits of Health Programmes', G. McLachlan and Th. McKeown (Eds.), *Medical History and Medical Care* (London, 1971). Generally on mercantilism see E. Heckscher, *Merkantilismen,* vol. 1-2 (1931, rev. ed. Stockholm 1953).

2. On Petty see E. Fitzmaurice, *The Life of Sir William Petty* (London, 1895); E. Strauss, *Sir William Petty* (London 1954); W. Letwin, *The Origins of Scientific Economics: English Economic Thought 1660-1776* (London 1963), chap. 5; H. Westergaard, *Contributions to the History of Statistics* (London 1932), pp. 28-37; E.S. Pearson (Ed.), *The History of Statistics in the 17th and 18th Centuries ... Lectures by Karl Pearson ... 1921-33* (London 1978), pp. 49-72; P. Buck, 'Seventeenth-Century Political Arithmetic', *Isis,* 68 (1977); ibid, 'People Who Counted: Political Arithmetic in the Eighteenth Century', *Isis,* 73 (1982).

Petty's works reprinted in Ch. H. Hull (Ed.), *The Economic Writings of Sir William Petty,* I-II (Cambridge 1899); *The Petty Papers: Some Unpublished Writings of Sir William Petty Edited From the Bowood Papers by the Marquis of Lansdowne,* I-II (London 1927).

3. E.O. Runeberg, 'Försök til en politisk värdering på land och folk i anledning af Laihela Socken', *Kungl. Vetenskapsakademiens Handlingar* (Stockholm 1759), p. 194.

4. N. Grew, 'The Heanes of a Most Ample Increase of the Wealth and Strength of England in a Few Years' (1707), referred to in E.A. Johnson, *Predecessors of Adam Smith: The Growth of British Economic Thought* (New York 1937), pp. 117-38.

5. W. Petty, 'Anatomy lecture', in The Petty Papers (London 1927), II, p. 176.

6. A. Hjelt, *Svenska medicinalverkets historia 1663-1812* (Helsingfors 1892), I, pp. 155-56.

7. *Berättelse om Kongl. Collegii Medici föremål och författningar til sjukdomars botande och förekommande i Riket ...* (Stockholm 1756), pp. 6-7.

Health Conditions, Population and Physicians in Norway 1814-1986. Notes on the Development of a Profession

Øivind Larsen and Fritz Hodne

Demography, public attitudes, and the development of a medical profession

The aim of the present article is a modest one: to offer some notes on the rise of the medical profession in Norway during the last century or so, and report some findings on the role of the medical profession in the modern health revolution. These findings are more fully reported in a work that appeared in June 1986 as part of the centenary of the Norwegian Medical Association.[1] Here we review, in the form of summary statements, findings concerning three of the themes discussed in the book, viz. (1) the demographic transition, (2) popular attitudes towards disease during the latter half of the 19th century, and (3) the development of the medical profession. A detailed documentation is omitted here. Interested readers should consult the book *Legene og samfunnet* (Physicians and society) itself.

Medicine in the demographic transition

By now the timing and pattern of the modern health revolution is well established, together with the main changes in the population.

Three main stages are well documented in the recent demographic history of Norway. Prior to 1815 both the birth rates and the mortality figures fluctuated around traditional and high levels. Just after 1815 and the end of the Napoleonic wars there occurred a sharp drop in the mortality rate (25% by 1826). The new, lower mortality rates proved to be permanent, while the birth rate remained unchanged at its traditional level until the very end of the nineteenth century. The resulting gap between births and deaths led to a rapid population growth. In two hundred years, from the end of the eighteenth century and until now, the Norwegian population quintupled, up from some 900 000 to 4.2 million. Due to brisk emigration to America, however, mainly 1860-1930, the population growth in mainland Norway was somewhat muted. Next, beginning in the 1890s, there occurred a drop also in the birth rate, the urban areas in the lead. In a third stage, evident from the 1930s, mortality and natality rates, having diverged for more than a century, now met again and resumed parallel courses, but at much lower levels. This new situation, apart from the post World War II-baby boom, has remained relatively stable, in Norway as in other high-income countries in the post-industrial phase. By the 1980s their populations have become just about stationary, in some cases even declining. To sum up: All the tendencies implied in the term the demographic transition have been observed in the recent demographic history of Norway.

Going from description to explanation, we find that the Norwegian statistics confirm the current view that the modern health revolution, documented in terms of mortality as sketched above, came about mainly through the gradual elimination of traditional epidemic diseases, among them cholera, typhoid fevers, tuberculosis, whooping cough, scarlet fever, diphteria, and measles. This salutary process, which above all benefited infants and children, has to a large extent coincided with the rise of the medical profession in Norway. Hence the question, what has been the role of physicians in the recent health revolution?

As background we have provided a summary of the international debate on this issue in the work referred to above, including the views of the McKeown school with its insistence upon the primary role of improved nutrition and the subsequent findings by scholars that have undermined the nutrition argument.

An original contribution to the ongoing research consisted in running a regression analysis 1865-1929 of central government health expenditures and mortality. The idea was to uncover statistically significant relationships between medicine and health and thus obtain a measure of the contribution of medicine to the outcome. Specifically, as a proxy for medicine we used central government health expenditures in fixed 1910-prices, and as a proxy for health we used infant mortality rates (0-1 years) and average mortality rates.

The results were statistically significant; but for that reason, they might just as well reflect underlying common factors, such as material progress, expressed as gains in annual per capita income. The suspicion was amply confirmed as we ran regression tests on the health and income data for the same period, lagging the health data five years to allow for imputed effects of income changes. Again, the scores obtained turned out to be statistically significant, though less so when the time span 1865-1929 was divided up into separate subperiods. The statistical relationship turned out to be weakest for the latest period 1920-1929. This result was obtained also when we regressed health data against public outlays on health, which suggested decreasing marginal returns.

Though inconclusive, our statistical tests clearly tended to reduce the assumed role of medicine in the rise of the modern health situation and underscore the role of economic factors, including nutritional factors. This interpretation, however, would seem to be immature, which became evident as we considered other relevant data, bearing on the issue. On a very high level of aggregation scholars, inspecting these and similar results, have in fact been induced to speak of an ecology of human disease, in which the development of the medical profession could be viewed as just one element in a larger system of societal development, interacting with other factors, including social, scientific and economic changes.

In the following sections we will have more to say on the possible contribution of medicine to the modern health situation, and begin with a summary of a study of attitudes towards disease:

Shifts in popular attitudes towards disease

Consider first our previous study on the public attitudes towards epidemic disease during the period 1868-1900.[2] This study examined the degrees of acceptance of epidemics and endemic infections by the local health authorities, and sought to identify possible changes in acceptance levels during the period. The underlying assumption was that the tolerance levels could be regarded as a reliable measure, not only of the public's confidence in the curative powers of medicine and its practitioners, but also of any real scientific progress in medicine. Moreover, the demand and supply side for medical services could be assumed to interact in such a way that a lowering of the public acceptance of epidemic disease reflected both increased public confidence and increased curative skills on the part of medical practitioners.

The study was based mainly on the annual medical reports on health conditions in Norway, given by the local medical officers and edited at county level before they were summarized, commented upon and published by the central health authorities. The general idea of the study was to obtain a systematic comparison of the reported morbidity and mortality figures with the judgment implied in the accompanying verbal descriptions of the same health conditions.

A special set of tables had to be constructed to reveal the longitudinal trends in morbidity and mortality. They showed remarkable changes, among them a striking increase in urban areas in both morbidity and mortality rates until the 1890s. The verbal descriptions were scaled by means of a numerical score system. Thus the ordering was checked against the numerical description of the epidemiological situation as found in the tables. In this manner an index was constructed that indicated any variation in the degree of acceptance of or concern about disease.

One interesting result of the study was that above all in the capital, where contagious disease was rampant, especially in the crowded working class quarters, a marked change in tolerance levels could be observed from the 1890s, that is, the decade when the national birth rate began to fall. Disease and poor health, it seemed, long regarded as inevitable elements in the natural order, now increasingly came to be conceived as avoidable nuisances. At the same time the notion of health began to acquire its modern meaning as the absence of sickness.

A reasonable interpretation of these findings would be that, granted the above assumptions, contemporary opinion in Norway in the 1890s at any rate assigned medicine a major role in combating epidemics and ameliorating health conditions, since it appears unlikely that acceptance levels could change unless accompanied by increased public confidence in medicine and in medical practitioners. In other words, it seems inconceivable that medicine could have retained its reputation in the face of repeated failures in curing and preventing illness, environmental and individual. Equally, it appeared unlikely that increased public confidence in the doctors could emerge unless the doctors really had something new to offer. This applies both to the county governors and to expert medical officers in charge of the preparation and publication of the official health reports. Finally, it must be added that many of the innovations introduced by the medical community in the last decades of the nineteenth century belonged to the area of public hygiene, where needs were urgent and initial results spectacular.

The physician and his self image

Old and recent studies that analyze Norwegian doctors as members of a profession, also shed light, albeit indirectly, on their role in the modern health revolution.[3] These studies offer a variety of information on doctors, including their social background, their incomes, their career patterns, and less explicitly, they tell us about the doctors' attitudes towards themselves and the medical profession. The main source for our own studies has been different editions of the biographical handbook *Norges leger* (Physicians in Norway), the first of which dating back to 1873. This series of handbooks has since acquired status as a calendar of "who is who" in Norwegian medicine. While the first edition contained biographies of 875 doctors, of whom 421 were alive in 1871, the latest, 1986 edition, produced by a team under the direction of Øivind Larsen and published by the Norwegian Medical Association, provides information on approximately 11 600 living physicians, active or retired.

In our book *Legene og samfunnet* the main results of a study of a ten per cent sample of the Norwegian physicians in 1984 are published. A questionnaire was circulated, wherein they were asked for additional information beyond what had been collected for the biographical work *Norges leger*. They were also asked for personal views, including a judgment on their own function and role in society. To supplement this evidence a small group of doctors, carefully chosen with reference to age group, type of work and living place in Norway was selected for in-depth interviews. The idea of these interviews was to bring out their career aims, values, expectations, and reflections on the changing role of their profession. One interesting result that emerged from these interviews, was that the younger generation of physicians, who had graduated in the 1970s, differed markedly from the older generations over the entire gamut of issues, for instance the function of medicine and the social role of physicians. The change in part undoubtedly reflects the emergence of new values, competing with the older, dominant career goals. Such a shift is of special interest, because Norwegian physicians are a young population group; half of them being born after World War II.

Two important conclusions of this study were:

1) The majority of the somewhat older doctors still tended to define their job comprehensively, that is, they felt that their responsibility not only included therapy and cure of individual patients, but also efforts to remove elements in the environment detrimental to popular health. This comprehensive approach is a direct continuation of the policy and practice upheld by the medical community for over a century. A common keyword is public hygiene. Looking back, it may well be that it has been in the area of public health that the Norwegian Medical Association has had its greatest impact on health. Indeed, the hygiene movement from its inception in the nineteenth century has been commanded by doctors who entertained a very broad view of the tasks of the medical profession. But while highlighting the achievements of medicine — the eradication of important contagious diseases — the hygiene movement also suggests the difficulties in summarizing in a simple manner the role of medicine as distinct from social and economic progress in the modern health revolution; since, depending on the level of analysis, the doctors would appear to be both the agents of and the effects of that revolution. Hence the summary nature of the next sections of this paper, dealing with the formation of the medical profession in Norway.

2) The rise of specialization in medicine, increasingly formalized in hospital medicine, notably after World War II, has led to the gradual disappearance of the old generalists and even the disappearance of jobs requiring such abilities. Accordingly, the new physicians have come to define their jobs more and more narrowly, as indicated by the testimony of the younger physicians.

Increased demand for medical services

As described by Laache, a national, medical profession developed in Norway in the course of the nineteenth century.[4] When Norway achieved its political independence from Denmark in 1814, albeit in a union with Sweden, the country was still suffering from the repercussions of the Napoleonic wars. A series of nation-building tasks lay ahead; the medical problems being only part of them. Lindbekk has shown how the education of lawyers, teachers, ministers, officers and other civil servants for the central and local administration dominated for a long time.[5]

At the start in 1814 the small group of doctors had received their training outside Norway. As the surgical and the medical education had just recently been united into one curriculum at most universities and medical academies, the doctors in Norway at the time had gone through different types of medical training programmes, some rather incomplete and all rapidly becoming obsolete. This group gradually disappeared as the training capacity of the new, Norwegian university, established 1811 in the capital Christiania (from 1925: Oslo), increased.

In general, outpatient practice was the typical work for a physician in Norway throughout the nineteenth century and even up till the late 1940s. As most patients were treated in their homes, the home call was the hallmark of the Norwegian doctor. The scattered location of the population, the long distances, the poor communications and transportation meant that the typical Norwegian doctor also experienced a remarkably itinerant life, including all the inherent perils of travel.

The nature of this ambulatory, general practice of the first generations of national, Norwegian doctors offers important inputs to the discussion as to the possible effects of the medical profession on public health. The curative capacity of each doctor was limited. In addition, the medical remedies and techniques available to the doctor for a long time were rather ineffective. These facts pose the question why—despite the professional handicaps—the demand for doctors could survive and even increase. The answer is in large measure found in the changed attitudes towards health and sickness. Increasingly, the comfort and reassurance rendered by the visiting physician outweighed the public and private expenditures involved in their provision.

The masters of public health

Life as a doctor in the nineteenth century was not easy. In a population still in the process of adjusting to a monetary economy, offering medical services for a cash return was difficult. Therapeutic results, even if successful, seldom softened this reality. Nevertheless the emerging medical profession experienced a growing esteem. The esteem was based on competence rather than on wealth or social rank. If doubts lingered, the medical legislation adopted by the country's parliament, for a century settled the position of the doctor, above all the law passed in 1860, setting up the municipal health boards. Henceforth the district physician, designated by law to act as chairman of the health boards, became an important civil servant with authority to intervene in public life in efforts to prevent disease and social misery. Not least in the period when epidemics ravaged and the mechanisms involved in the transfer of contagious disease remained unsolved, the district doctors played an important part in the general preventive health care, which in turn helped bring down morbidity and mortality rates.

Hospitals, specialists and science

In the wake of the nineteenth century a new medicine appeared, more rigorously based on science and scientific experiments. The bigger hospitals in turn accelerated the process of moving the care of the sick out of the homes. New scientific results in medicine stimulated this development and new public programmes of social security made it possible. Gradually, more doctors found employment in hospitals, where some of them combined work as public doctors and in some cases private medical practice with scientific interests, perhaps inspired by study tours abroad.

This is no place to detail how medicine leaped forward in the beginning of the 20th century, nor should it be doubted that a substantial part of the efforts to conquer morbidity and mortality had its background in economic and social rather than medical developments. However, the medical achievements not only enabled the members of the medical profession to save lives; successful cure of and relief from disabling and discomforting ailments gradually gave medicine and physicians an important place in the national idea of welfare and living standards. Dentists around the same time felt themselves enveloped by similar sentiments.

In the first half of the twentieth century, the typical Norwegian doctor still worked in his outpatient practice as a generalist. In the years after World War I, however, a small but growing number educated themselves as specialists. A technical innovation at this time revolutionized medical practice: The introduction of the automobile vastly increased the physicians' capacity for home calls. In combination with a new public system for doctors' salaries and fees, Norwegian medicine in the inter-war period came to be ranked as the most attractive among the academic professions. Wage statistics underscore the contemporary attraction exerted by medicine in these years. To be a doctor could mean a top income and top social status, without destroying the notion of a calling or a social service. At any rate recruitment to medicine reached till then unknown levels in the 1930s. The large number of new students made entrance regulation necessary. School marks were chosen as criteria, which meant that the most clever students were selected for medical education. How this regulation, inaugurated from 1940, and practiced at varying degrees ever since, influenced the development of the profession in the subsequent decades, remains to be studied in detail, but it is probable that the entrance regulations caused a shift in medical interests and orientation.

The fulfilment of welfare standards

The number of doctors in Norway around 1814 was about one hundred. One hundred years later this number had increased tenfold (1910:1266), and in 1986 there are approximately 11 600 Norwegian physicians, which represent another tenfold increase. From time to time warnings have been voiced that the profession would outgrow its market and undercut the employment situation of its members. Such tendencies in the past, however, have been followed by periods of resurging demand for doctors, which suggests that the demand for health services is highly elastic.

After World War II the demographic transition, as noted earlier, came full circle in Norway. That is, both mortality rates and birth rates settled on stable, low levels; moreover, in most groups the frequency of child-bearing reached the rates which were to become typical for the post-industrial societies. The epidemiological transition became history too; that is, cardiovascular diseases and cancer climbed to the top of the list of causes of death. By contrast, life threatening infections, the former major cause of death, had largely been eliminated through preventive medicine and new medical technology.

Preventive medicine has resulted in new, hygienic standards of behaviour. Hygienic behaviour thus constitutes a third, independent factor in the disease prevention. Rather being part of culture than of medicine, norms for cleanliness, social contact etc. add substantially to the effects of preventive and curative medicine. Still, our post-epidemic society has not eliminated the threat from microorganisms, in so far as they may be spread through socially accepted behaviour. New norms for sexual behaviour provide current examples.

Paradoxically, it was in the post-World War II-period that the demand for health services exploded. Since the 1950s hospitals were built at an unprecedented rate. The call for more doctor's services was strong, especially from the rural districts. The physicians working there usually faced all the work they could overcome. The paradox dissolves, however, when it is recalled that the costs for health services were gradually transferred from the individual patients to the public sector, notably the central government. That holds both for investment and current account expenditures. Socialized medicine thus removed the private budget constraints; accordingly, demand for medical services, offered free or almost free, became unlimited.

Omitting the documentation here, it might be suggested that the motives for seeking doctors' help now underwent a complete change. The change reflected new attitudes towards health problems, towards payment for health services, and towards social equality. The need was not so much a quest for the absence of pain and distress as a quest for comfort, welfare and equality. And in a system of socialized medicine the doctors and their services were at hand. The demand for the extension and the multiplication of health services became a political issue, which in a system of free elections could hardly be rejected. Hence, from the 1960s, came the massive expansion of health expenditures for medical and social purposes.

The limits of the health economy

The so-called health crisis of the 1970s and the 1980s will not be described here, beyond noting that the demand for social and medical welfare continued to grow unabatedly, while costs reached unacceptable levels. Budget restraints were felt as cutbacks in welfare. The failure of the system sparked a public debate which, despite its intensity and political character, so far has left no

338

doubt that the populace feels entitled to good health as part of a new standard of public welfare. The medical profession, traditionally identified with the health services, naturally has become the prime target for public criticism, although the doctors by now mainly have been reduced to actors with limited influence on decisions.

The subsistence of a subgroup

Ties and isolation

Demographic data and career patterns of the members of the medical profession depict a group strongly governed by its internalized set of rules. Supported by a strong corporation, The Norwegian Medical Association, these rules make up the central criteria that define a profession. The independent general practitioners of the past have gradually been replaced by the hospital employees as the typical doctors. However, the strongly regulated hospital careers merely strengthened the professional ties. There is some evidence suggesting that the enforced occupational mobility among hospital doctors, who frequently move between the different hospitals, can lead to a degree of social isolation for the group as a whole. How would a subgroup with strong internal ties react to demands for change which easily could be felt as a threat? In our book, referred to above, this topic has been discussed, in part based on questionnaires returned by the ten per cent sample of the physicians. Suffice it to say that the answers provide no simple interpretations and that the internalized rules for the members of the profession now face a thorough revision in order to fit the realities.

To study professions

To the present authors, looking at professions as demographic subgroups has proved useful. Surprisingly, in the case of the medical profession the linkage between the objectives of the individual members and the development of the profession itself, seems far less close than could be expected. Economic and social goals of the members apparently differ from those of their profession; the difference extends even to the proper definition of disease, hence, the basic tasks of the profession.

In our work on the sociology of the profession, reported in some detail in the book mentioned, we have, moreover, come to the conclusion that in the development of a close-knit social system such as the medical profession, the expectations and identifications of its members play a role that so far has been underestimated. Expectations and identifications serve as common intermediate factors. Products of an exclusive training and work experience, these intermediate factors have helped foster a specific professional ethic and outlook. We assume that the satisfaction of basic needs forms an important factor in all occupations; indeed, the strive for such satisfaction may be considered a controlling force in their development. The medical profession provides interesting testimony; the profession has until quite recently amply met the members' desire for financial rewards and social recognition, and compensated for the unpleasant aspects of the career, including frequent moves and the oppressive hierarchy of hospital medicine.

The medical profession and the recent changes in health conditions

The recent years have witnessed far reaching changes in health conditions, and in the work of doctors, both of which have led to a critical debate among doctors as to their role and future prospects. Lately historians and economists have joined the debate. At a time when socialized medicine has reduced the independent practitioner to an employee, paid a negotiated salary, the questions are raised again, in regard to the possible role of medicine in the demographic transition 1815-1930.

The popular view that medicine had minimal impact on the health situation, compared to the weight of improved social and economic conditions, is too simple. According to that view, the development of a medical profession, e.g. in Norway, should be secondary to the growth of welfare, which by its nature has its origins in economic growth.

Nevertheless, the study of the medical profession, summarily sketched above, reveals that at least in the popular imagination the physicians have retained a sort of indispensability. The physician is still considered indispensable in some three albeit "stereotypical" roles: (1) the life-saving hero, mainly assisting in emergencies, (2) the provider of comfort, well-being, and safety, and (3) the medical officer, as an extension of the medical and social service system. Within the medical profession itself an additional role is cherished, viz. the scientist, the provider of new medical knowledge. In our considered opinion, these popular stereotypes represent pitfalls in a valid assessment of the historical contribution of medicine to the modern health revolution. Admittedly, these stereotypes have persisted for a long time; and this fact should be recalled also when the role of physicians have been assessed in earlier times.

Additionally, one has to take into account the doctor's own perennial dilemma. They have always, at least in Norway, been positioned between the market and the bureaucracy. Occasionally, that position involve the impossibility of reconciling mutually exclusive goals: Providing services according to public demands normally excludes the role of social conscience.

Further studies of the health professions with demographic and sociological methods will hopefully yield a better understanding of historical trends and provide guidelines for medical policies in the future.

340

Notes

1. Ø. Larsen, O. Berg and F. Hodne, *Legene og samfunnet* (Oslo 1986). Øivind Larsen was educated as a physician and holds a chair in medical history at the University of Oslo. Ole Berg, a political scientist, is a member of the Department of political science at the University of Oslo, and Fritz Hodne, an economist, is professor in Economic History at the Norwegian School of Economics and Business Administration in Bergen.

Specifically, Øivind Larsen analysed the individual physician, his social background over the last century, his education, his work and the changing perception of his role as a member of a profession. Ole Berg described the rise and development of the Norwegian Medical Association itself, with underpinnings in current sociological theories of the nature and role of professions, including their role as interest organizations. Fritz Hodne, on a still higher level of aggregation, summarized recent findings by Norwegian scholars on the demographic, social, and economic changes that accompanied the modern health revolution in Norway and set the results against current international research and debate in these areas.

The present paper mainly deals with topics covered by Hodne and Larsen and references for further reading are given in the reading lists accompanying their chapters.

2. Ø. Larsen, H. Haugtomt and W. Platou, *Sykdomsoppfatning og epidemiologi 1860-1900. Epidemiske sykdommer i Norge og helsemyndighetenes vurdering av folkehelsen — presentasjon av data* (Oslo 1980).

3. H. Palmstrøm, 'Om en befolkningsgruppes utvikling gjennom de siste 100 år'. *Statsøkonomisk tidskrift,* 49 (1935) pp. 161-370; T. Lindbekk, *Mobilitets og stillingsstrukturen innenfor tre akademiske profesjoner 1910-1963* (Oslo 1967); U. Torgersen, *Profesjonssosiologi* (Oslo-Bergen-Tromsø 1972).

4. S.B. Laache, *Norsk medicin i hundrede aar* (Kristiania 1911).

5. Lindbekk (1967).

The Silent Sick. Life-Histories
of 19th Century Swedish Hospital Patients

Anders Brändström

Jacques Revel and Jean-Pierre Peter have critically analyzed studies about the history of diseases. Scholars have, they argue, studied in great detail almost every disease, its origin, its spreading, and its effects on mankind. The results have been published in the form of morbidity and mortality rates. Doctors, and their ceaseless lasting struggle against suffering and poor health have been carefully assessed. The therapeutic regimen, the medical instruments, and the clinical apparatus have all been given a history of their own, but the patient, the sick and suffering, have remained anonymous [1].

The history of a disease should, quite naturally one would think, be centred around the people afflicted by it. Who were they? How did they feel about their situation? What became of them? Questions quite natural to the social historian, but difficult to find in the vast literature on the history of medicine. According to Revel and Peter disease has been awarded its own history, together with the crusaders of medical science campaigning against them. The sick patient has only existed in a footnote, or as an often bizarre example: as a monster from the operating theater. The patient has only been worth mentioning because of his role as some sort of a medium for an interesting disease [2].

Whether this holds true for the majority of literature on the history of medicine is a matter of opinion. One thing is, however clear, it certainly holds true for most studies dealing with the history of hospitals.

There are numerous hospital histories that manage, almost with clinical perfection, to avoid even mentioning that there actually were sick people in the wards. Instead we get detailed analyses of the architecture of the hospital, the design of separate wards, the system of sewage, when the hospital changed from wooden to iron beds, and whether the walls were white-washed or not. The staff of the hospital always seems to be of the utmost interest. Famous surgeons and doctors are presented: we get to know of their education, how they struggled against disease and ignorance, what scientific achievements they made, etc. The nurses, the apothecary, the clerks, the maids, and the guardians of the insane are presented to the reader. The patients are, however, seldom mentioned. Sometimes even the word patient is avoided; in some studies "number of beds" seems to be used as an equivalent. Typically, the most detailed historical analysis of Swedish hospitals is an architectural history [3]. I do not even consider the numerous histories written in memory of hospitals as being particularly analytical or historical in their approach.

Because of this we know much more about the hospital as a monument of the art of constructing pompous buildings. Their function as some sort of experimental laboratory for skilled scientists, and as a playground for philanthropists and/or politicians is well-known. But the patients have remained silent and anonymous.

During recent years there has been a trend toward a new kind of history of medicine, which emphasizes the social interaction between medicine and society. Scholars like Henry Sigerist, Charles Rosen, and Erwin Ackerknecht have of course always had a social dimension to their research. Studies made by authors from the social sciences and the humanities have, however, increased dramatically. New questions have been asked, and old ones analyzed in a different perspective [4]. Since sickness and health are two of the most fundamental aspects of human life and therefore have great cultural and social impact on society, it is quite natural that the effort to understand disease is of the greatest interdisciplinary interest. This has altered the course, not only of the history of medicine in general, but also of the history of hospitals.

One way of writing a new hospital history is to put more emphasis on the history of the patients by using the often excellent records of admissions and dismissals. By using these sources we get a detailed and clear-cut picture of who the eighteenth- and nineteenth-century patients were, why they visited the hospital, how they were treated, and what happened to them during their stay. In the Scandinavian countries Øivind Larsen has used hospital records for patients in his study of the Navy Hospital in Copenhagen and the Kongsberg hospital in Norway. In her investigation into the political and social motives behind the foundation of hospitals in Denmark, Signhild Vallgårda studied the patients admitted to Fredriks Hospital and Kommunehospitalet in Copenhagen, and Praestø Amts Sygehus in Naesved. There is no study in Sweden where full use has been made of patients records. Most of them are written in the above mentioned fashion, though there are some exceptions [5]. Arthur E Imhof has used patients' records from the Charite-Hospital in Berlin in order to describe the sick [6]. In England , E M Sigsworth, John Woodward and Steven Cherry have made important contributions by using the same type of material. In the USA, William H Williams and Guenter B Risse have also directed much more interest toward the patient. Guenter B Risse has recently published a book about the Royal Infirmary of Edinburgh, where he makes extensive use of patients' records, prescription bills, case-books, and students' notebooks. Risse can thereby give a detailed picture of the diseases of the patients, their social background and medical treatment and its effect [7]. In these studies we can, for the first time, say that the patients begin to emerge upon the arena, and that they are given their own history.

The first hospitals

Swedens first hospital, the Serafimer Hospital in Stockholm, was founded in 1752. Earlier attempts at founding a hospital—the so-called *Nosokomium*—had failed due to the lack of capital and interest. The Serafimer Hospital in Stockholm opened with a capacity of eight beds, and with the intention of curing pauper sick people from the whole country. The hospital was financed mainly by taxes and contributions from each of Swedens counties. It did not, of course, take long before people realized that the Serafimer Hospital was too small and it was used only by the citizens of Stockholm. In 1765 Swedish Parliament therefore gave permission for the foundation of county-hospitals. The Swedish Government contributed to the finances from a fund *(Medicinalfonden)* designed especially for this purpose. The contributions were, however, very modest and the county hospitals had to be financed also by the the local authorities through taxes, Church collections, and private donations.

It is important to remember how Swedish hospitals were financed. Because of the large proportion of money from public means, and the fact that they were to be governed by State authorities, on both a local and central level, they never assumed the character of a Voluntary hospital, so common in England, Scotland, and the United States. This, in turn, as we shall see, had an effect upon admission policy, and also upon the reliability of some of the information in the patients' records.

The Swedish county hospitals were rather small in comparison with those in England and Scotland, and extremely small compared with hospitals such as the Massachusetts General, or Hôtel Dieu in Paris with more than 1400 beds. Paris alone had more than 30 hospitals with a total number of more than 20 000 beds [8], which is the same as the total number of hospitals in Sweden in the year 1800. The Swedish hospitals could not offer more than approximately 650 beds at that time. The average size of a county hospital was 16 beds, with an average of 80 admissions per year [9]. The largest hospital at the turn of the eighteenth century was the Serafimer hospital in Stockholm with 140 beds.

The modest size of Swedish eighteenth- and nineteenth-century hospitals is a drawback when making comparisons with the development of institutional care in other European countries. On one hand, one could argue that because they were so small, they were scientifically backward. The hospital physicians lacked perhaps both medical knowledge and the right equipment in order to be successful in their work. Swedish hospital mortality rates would be higher because of primitive therapy. On the other hand, one could argue that Swedish hospitals were fortunate, in that their modest size protected them from the horrors of overcrowding. The latter was frequently reported from Hotel Dieu in Paris, where evidently at times up to four persons were obliged to share the same bed. Thomas McKeown, quoting Florence Nightingale, pictures nineteenth century hospitals as overcrowded and filthy hellholes [10]. The much feared "hospital disease", which made it almost impossible for English physicians to admit persons suffering from infectious diseases, should therefore not have caused any problems in Swedish hospitals.

The conclusion we can draw from this argument is that Swedish county hospitals should have had patients with a totally different disease panorama and with much lower mortality rates. A third possibility would be that the negative effects of primitive therapy and the positive effects of modest size evened things out, thereby creating a seemingly similar situation in comparison with large European hospitals. Thus, by not being larger than a single ward at the Royal Infirmary of Edinburgh, their possible contribution to the history of hospitals in Europe would be more as something picturesque and exotic. With this in mind we turn our attention to the county hospital in Härnösand.

The County Hospital of Härnösand

In 1776 a "hospital" was founded in the town of Sundsvall, the first in the county of Västernorrland: a rented room with two beds. The doctor in charge was the provincial physician. There is no evidence that this "hospital" ever admitted any patients, since no records were kept. When Johan Sahlberg, the physician in charge, moved to Härnösand the hospital was closed, and all the equipment was transferred to Härnösand. In 1788 the first real hospital opened with nine beds available for the treatment of sick people. Six of the beds were to be reserved for the sick poor, and three for those who could afford to pay the modest sum of 4 Skillingar per day. During the first decades the hospital gave shelter and medical care to about 20 patients each year. The hospital served a triple function; as an ordinary hospital for curable sick; as an asylum; and as a *"Kurhus"* for patients suffering from venereal diseases, mainly syphilis. There was only one physician in charge of the hospital, the "Kurhus" and the home for the insane. However, when surgery had to be performed, the surgeon employed by the town of Härnösand was called in.

The three different functions of the hospital were in practice separated only by administrative procedures. Records of admissions and dismissals were kept separately, and each function also had separate account books. In practice, however, the insane could still enter the records of the hospital and the boundaries between the "Kurhus" and the hospital were often fictitious. The "Kurhus" and the ordinary hospital also benefited from the same public taxes, while the home for the insane received its own funding from 1828 onwards.

346

Map 1. Sweden and the county of Västernorrland

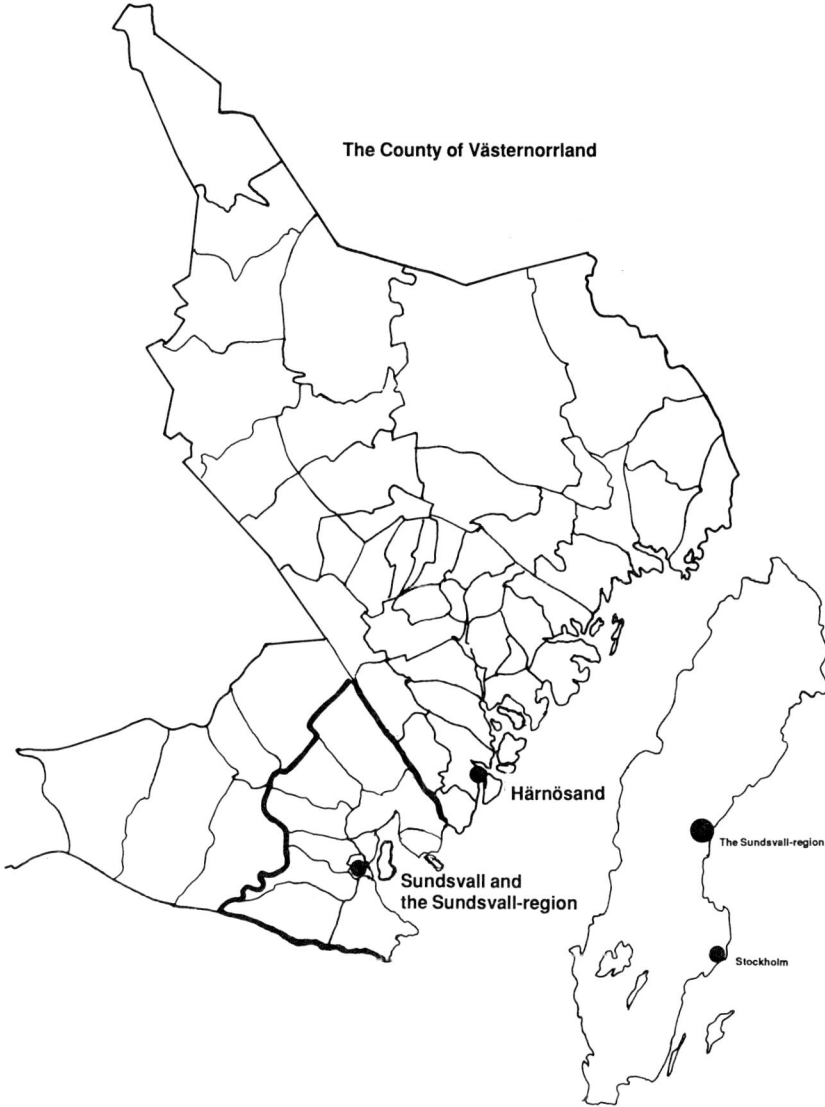

The County of Västernorrland

Härnösand

Sundsvall and
the Sundsvall-region

The Sundsvall-region

Stockholm

This article will deal with the patients' records from the hospital and the "Kurhus" during the fifty years between 1814 and 1864. In Figure 1 we can see the total number of patients admitted to the hospital each year. In 1820 the insane were moved to a separate building, whereby the number of beds could be increased to 30. The hospital now admitted around 100 patients each year. The hospital expanded in 1845 and 1853, and with approximately 60 beds now available, over 250 patients were admitted each year. Between the years 1814-1864 a total of 6837 admissions were entered into the records.

The majority of the sick, nearly 90 per cent, came from the county of Västernorrland. 20 per cent of them were living in the town of Härnösand, and 10 per cent came from parishes close to Härnösand. The hospital did certainly function as a county hospital, but this did not mean that patients from other regions were excluded. On the contrary, the hospital physician A A Lenström cured sailors from Denmark, Norway, and Germany. He admitted seasonally employed workers and handicrafts from Finland, and in late September 1863 he even had a patient from New York: 26 year old Frans Crocked, who was treated in the hospital for 7 days, suffering from *Erysipelas* or "the rose" and cured.

As in the case of the Serafimer hospital in Stockholm, the majority of patients came from the town and the surrounding countryside. This fact has also been confirmed from studies of the County Hospital in Umeå [11]. The purpose of the hospital was to help the needing sick in the local region, but in practice the physicians, or rather the County Governor who had the final say, always admitted those who got sick or injured while they were passing through. The hospital was located by the coast and in an area where the shipping of goods was an important part of the economy. Trade contacts with other countries were frequent, and this explains the rather large proportion of foreigners in the hospital: mostly sailors. In Table 1 we can see the occupational structure of the hospital's patients.

A majority of the patients admitted to the hospital originated from the lower social classes. The largest group was unskilled workers from the sawmill industry and agricultural workers. A large category was patients with unspecified occupational titles such as "the girl" or "the widow", titles usually equivalent to a very low position on the social scale. The majority of sailors, with the exception of those who came on foreign ships, were enrolled in the Swedish war-fleet. The category "Lower middle class" included civil servants, such as clerks and postofficeworkers. Included in this group were also sea captains and officers from the Navy and the Army.

What is striking in Table 1 is the rather large proportion of patients with a relatively high social position in society. Every fifth patient belonged to the lower middle class, the peasantry, or the crafts. It is of course true that a majority of patients came from the lower social ranks, but the County Hospital of Härnösand was certainly not occupied only by the "industrious poor"; those unfortunates who by no means could care for and support themselves

Figure 1. Total number of admissions each year. Härnösand 1814-1864.

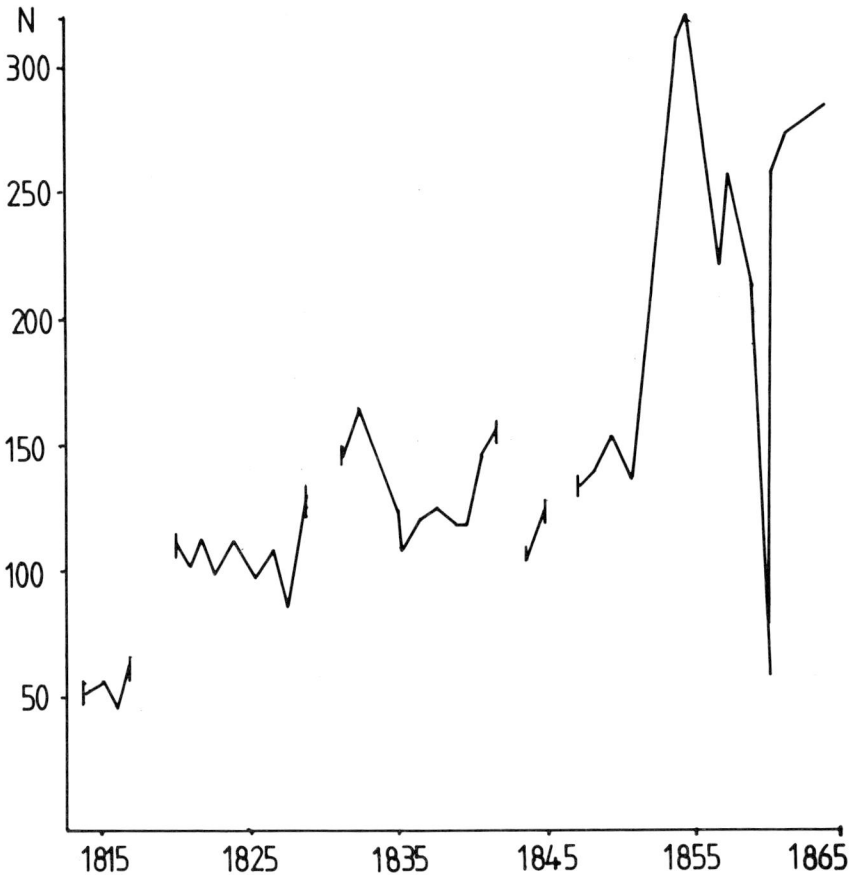

Figure 1. Total number of admissions each year. Härnösand 1814-1864.

during their illness. It is also incorrect to say that the lower classes were over-represented at the hospital. It is probably more correct to argue that the occupational structure of the patients actually represented the social structure of contemporary Härnösand. This is an interesting finding, since it contradicts the popular belief that eighteenth- and early nineteenth-century hospitals were nothing more than almshouses—used by an unfortunate minority, and avoided by the majority [12]. In fact, one is tempted to say that anyone who was struck by a disease which popular medicine at home could not heal, went to the hospital. However, there is so far insufficient evidence to support such a hypothesis.

The hospital was not full of the aged and infirm, either. The sick admitted were men and women in their prime of life. In Table 2 we can see that more than 50 per cent of the patients were between 20 and 39 years of age. Only 14 per cent were more than 50 years old. The physician also admitted more than

Table 1. Occupational structure of admitted patients. Härnösand 1800-1864.

Occupation	N	Percent
Lower middle class	238	3.5
Farmers	614	9.0
Handicrafts	518	7.5
Crofters	573	8.4
Soldiers and sailors	682	10.0
Workers in industry and agriculture	2133	31.2
Unspecified	1343	19.6
No occupation given	736	10.8
Total	6837	100.0

Table 2. Age structure of the patients. Härnösand 1814—1864.

Age	N	Percent
under 1 year	32	0.5
1—9	303	4.4
10—19	924	13.5
20—29	2273	33.2
30—39	1213	17.7
40—49	785	11.5
50—59	533	7.8
60—69	331	4.8
70—	97	1.4
No information	346	5.1

300 children under the age of 10, which was a very extraordinary procedure. Young children were usually considered as unsuitable patients because of their "sensible nature", and the fact that they often suffered from infectious diseases. For the same reason pregnant women were usually not admitted [13].

The disease panorama

During this conference we have had the opportunity to discuss the difficulties in interpreting the nomenclature for the causes of death during the eighteenth- and nineteenth centuries. It is a well-known fact that medical science of that time had a totally different concept of the functions of the human body, and the specific nature of disease. Eighteenth and nineteenth-century medical philosophers also based their concepts of disease and causes of death on a confusing mixture of symptoms and purely theoretical assumptions. Because of this, the great nosologies written by Linnaeus (1763), or by

Boissier de Sauvage (1768) presented problems of interpretation even to physicians of that time [14]. It was therefore common that many of the great clinicians in Europe, William Cullen in Edinburgh for instance, often wrote their own simplified nosologies to be used in their teaching wards [15]. If, therefore, we try to understand names of diseases or causes of death according to the concepts of our own times, we will meet with severe difficulties [16].

Guenter B Risse has discussed the problem of interpreting the disease panorama in the late eighteenth century when studying the Royal Infirmary of Edinburgh. In his opinion it is essential for our understanding of hospital care to try to retain the framework that originally formed the disease concepts at the Infirmary. I quote: "Instead of trying to match the archaic labels with specific modern medical terms, the general scheme retained the eighteenth-century nosological terminology but redistributed disease entities to their presumed contemporary nature and affected body system". He, therefore, placed a disease that the Edinburgh physicians named "Chlorosis", which is possibly an irondeficiency anemia, but in William Cullen's nosology was a genus among the adynamic neuroses—under diseases affecting the sexual organs—because Cullen considered it a form of amenorrhea [17].

It was common for Swedish physicians to study medicine abroad. Linnaeus was, for instance, one of Boerhaave's pupils in Leyden [18]. At the turn of the eighteenth century the University of Edinburgh, with William Cullen, the Professor of Medicine, was the centre of medical education in Europe. It is not clear whether contemporary Swedish physicians visited Edinburgh, but Cullen's influence on Swedish medicine is noticeable. His nosology was evidently used at several hospitals, as was his Farmacopoeia Pauperum. The names of the diseases in the County Hospital of Härnösand therefore bear great similarities to those of the patients at the Royal Infirmary of Edinburgh. It is therefore possible to use Risse's classification system on Swedish material, which opens up interesting comparative perspectives between the hospitals.

Risse has categorized the diseases into 17 classes, depending on the organ and the part of the body that was considered to be affected. The same system has been applied on patients' records from Härnösand in, however, a slightly simplified form. The results are displayed in Table 3.

"Diseases affecting the sexual organs" were usually syphilis, but also included phymosis, amenorrhea, and menorrhagia. "Surgical infections" include abcesses, bone caries, fistulas, sores, gangrene, and ulcers. "Infectious diseases" were different types of fever; intermittent fever, hectic fever, and nervous fever; but also smallpox, and typhus. "Respiratory diseases" cover asthma, breast pain, cynache, dyspnea, phtisis, consumption, pleurisy, pneumonia, and tuberculosis. "Tumors and cancers" meant that the patients suffered from scrofulas, cancers, tumors, metastases, and the like. The physicians made a distinction between cancerous sores and ordinary sores depending on the structure of the surface.

Table 3. Disease panorama among patients. Härnösand 1814—1864.

Disease	N	Percent
Disease affecting sexual organs	1918	28.1
Surgical infections	703	10.3
Infectious diseases	681	10.0
Respiratory diseases	652	9.5
Traumatic conditions	442	6.5
Tumors and cancers	372	5.4
Diseases affecting the digestive system	307	4.5
Circulatory disorders	280	4.1
Neurological diseases	262	3.8
Mental diseases	254	3.7
Musculoskeletal disorders	241	3.5
Others, no information	226	3.3
Diseases of the skin	180	2.6
Urinary tract diseases	105	1.5
Eye problems	100	1.5
Surgical procedures	86	1.3
Inflammations of unspec origin	28	0.4
All diseases	6837	100.0

"Traumatic conditions" include all the different types of wounds caused, for instance, by accidents such as burns, dislocations, fractures, luxations, congelations, shot wounds, and the like. "Diseases of the digestive system" include vomiting, worms, cholera, colic, gastric complaints, dyspepsia, enteritis, icterus, dysentery, and diarrhea. The term "Neurological diseases" cover epilepsy, headache, hemiplegia, paralysis, phrenitis, atrophia, and apoplexia. "Mental diseases" on the other hand were diseases such as mania, hysteria, melancholy, nymphomania, nostalgia, stupidity, and madness.

"Circulatory disorders" were a kind of disease difficult to diagnose, since physicians lacked our modern clinical equipment. The diseases that belonged to this group were usually called hydrops, anaemia, anasarca, ascites, and dropsy. Under the heading "Musculo-skeletal disorders" we find most of the ailments caused by many years of long hard labour and draughty dwellings: back pain, ischias, rheumatism, and pain in the limbs. "Diseases of the skin" were likewise often due to harsh living conditions, and lack of personal hygiene. Here we find complaints such as itches, scurvy, tinea capitis, eruptions of the skin, and leprosy. It is worth mentioning that the term leprosy had changed its meaning during the eighteenth century. It no longer meant the disease that seriously disfigured the sick. Eighteenth century physicians were well aware of this fact, and instead they often used the term "black scurvy" for the "earlier" form of leprosy [19].

Then we have the category "Eye problems" where we find such ailments as amaurosis, and opthalmia. Finally, under the heading "Others" we find miscellaneous diseases affecting the urinary tract, pains of unspecified origin, minor surgical conditions etc.

As we can see from Table 3 the most common disease category among the patients at the county hospital of Härnösand was diseases affecting the sexual organs. Nearly all of these patients suffered from syphilis in various stages. In this respect Scandinavian hospitals were different from most other European and American hospitals in their admission policy [20]. In England voluntary hospitals refused to admit people suffering from venereal diseases, mostly due to moral judgments. Venereal diseases were considered the worst form of punishment for the sins of the flesh, and therefore very improper for admission [21]. In the United States many hospital physicians refused to admit venereal sick even after the turn of the nineteenth century [22]. One should not forget that hospitals were also expected to serve an "educational" purpose, i.e. to improve the Christian moral of the pauper classes, and venereal patients were thought to have a bad influence on other sick souls. The Royal Infirmary of Edinburgh did, however, admit venereal patients at an early stage, but it was mostly due to the fact that they had a contract with the Royal Navy to admit sick sailors, who frequently suffered from this disease [23]. In Sweden it was exactly the other way around. The strongest argument for the financing of hospitals was the fear of an uncontrolled spreading of syphilis. During the first half of the eighteenth century, governmental commissions estimated that within a few decades the whole nation could be infected unless something was done to stop the disease [24].

Confinement in hospitals was also the only effective way to control the disease. The only known method for curing syphilis was by giving the patients large doses of mercury, until they began to show acute symptoms of poisoning. The patients started to drivel—the method was called the *salivation cure*—whereby the substance which caused the disease was considered to be expelled. The method was extremely dangerous and time-consuming. The patients had to be monitored daily by the physician, and therefore confinement in hospital was necessary. Hospitals naturally also served as a quarantine.

Because of the relative importance of the venereal patients, hospitals actually received far more financial support from the Government for this purpose, than they ever received for the treatment of ordinary sick people. This was the case almost throughout the whole of the nineteenth century. Hospitals which served the double function as both general hospitals and as "Kurhus" could, however, use the financial surplus, if there ever was any, from the treatment of venereal patients.

The venereal patients had the longest duration of stay of all sick at the hospital in Härnösand. In some extreme cases they had to remain there for nearly two years, but the average time of confinement was approximately 70 days (Appendix A). The average for all patients, regardless of what ailment they suffered from, was 54.9 days. It is also interesting to notice that of these patients who came to the hospital from outside the county of Västernorrland, nearly 50 per cent suffered from syphilis.

Surgical infections came second with 10.3 per cent of the patients. Those suffering from sores and fistulas had to stay in the hospital for quite a time— an average of 64.9 days. This was probably due to the fact that most of them came to the hospital with wounds in a very bad condition. It was natural for people to try to heal, for instance, severe cuts at home before they went to the hospital. Because of the unfamiliarity with hygiene the sores often got seriously infected and gangrenous. Only when all popular cures had failed did they seek hospital admission. There are examples where patients had suffered from wounds for months and even years, before they finally went to see a doctor [25].

Infectious diseases, mainly fevers, came in third place in the disease panorama at the hospital. 10 per cent were admitted with this symptom. Fevers were one of the most important classes in the nosologies of the eighteenth century, since they seemed to affect not only a single organ, but the whole body. More than twelve different types of fevers were specified, and each one of them could in turn have subgroups. It is, however, not my intention to go into detail about this complex "disease" in this paper. I can merely point to some other studies that deal with the problem more extensively [26]. Because of the nature of fever—you either get well fairly quickly, or you die—the average stay at the hospital for fever patients was very short, 30.9 days. This also meant that a majority of the patients suffering from infectious diseases came from short distances. Every fourth patient from Härnösand suffered from fever, but only 1.4 per cent of the patients from outside the county of Västernorrland belonged to this category.

The same can be said of respiratory diseases. In most cases the chance of survival was limited. It was often meaningless to even consider a long journey to the hospital. Patients belonging to this category either got well quickly, were dismissed as incurable or were faced with a certain death. Because of this the average stay was only 34.4 days, and a majority of the patients came from nearby.

There is little to say about the rest of the disease panorama at the County Hospital of Härnösand. Patients suffering from other diseases than the above-mentioned came in equal numbers, whether they lived nearby or at a far distance. The shortest duration of stay was experienced by patients suffering from diseases of the digestive system. They remained in the hospital for only 25.9 days.

On the whole the patients in Härnösand remained in hospital much longer than patients at the Royal Infirmary of Edinburgh, where the average length of stay was only 29.1 days [27]. Whether this was due to more efficient treatment, or merely to economic reasons, it is hard to say. The patients at the County Hospital of Härnösand suffered, however, from roughly the same type of diseases. At the Royal Infirmary of Edinburgh, there were, of course, fewer patients with venereal complaints, 19 per cent, and infectious diseases were more common, 15,6 per cent (Appendix B). The patients in Härnösand suffered, on the other hand, more often from neurological and mental diseases, and cancers. But on the whole the proportions were pretty much the same.

Before we leave the disease panorama among the hospital patients, we shall try to answer one more question. Were there "social diseases" i.e. did certain social categories of patients suffer from a particular disease? If we take a look at the hospital records, we find that there is only one disease that had a distinct social pattern: disease of the sexual organs. 17.4 per cent of the lower middle class patients suffered from this complaint; 18.6 per cent of the farmers; 18.2 per cent of the soldiers and sailors; 24.1 of the crofters; 23.8 per cent of the handicrafts; and finally, 31.4 per cent of the industrial and agricultural workers.

It is obvious that syphilis was more common among the lower classes admitted to hospital care. Surprisingly enough, soldiers and sailors had a low percentage. In the medical debate of the time contemporary physicians frequently attacked sailors for being the primary source of syphilis. Several doctors demanded that there should be an obligatory close examination of every sailor when he returned after a voyage. Naturally if promiscuity was common among sailors a relatively small number of them could spread syphilis. But such promiscuity should also have worked the other way around and infected sailors, so perhaps their reputation was exaggerated, or alternatively, which remains to be checked, Naval seamen were treated elsewhere.

Gateways to death?

The contribution of the early modern hospitals to public health and population growth is under frequent debate. Were hospital physicians, with their simple remedies, and, in our view, rather obscure therapeutic regimen, successful or not? Were patients healed, or simply put to eternal rest by a physician with medical knowledge rooted in medieval thinking? Did, on the the other hand, some of the herbal remedies, other than cinchona bark, really have a noticeable effect on disease? And what about the surgeons? Were they simply butchers, who stood with blood up to their ankles and amputated legs from tormented patients? Or were they, despite the lack of anesthetics and proper knowledge of antiseptics, skilled surgeons who in most cases did their patient good?

There seem to be two different opinions among historians. One is represented by Thomas McKeown, who in his books and articles pictures the eighteenth- and nineteenth-century hospitals as being nothing more than gateways to death. Entering a hospital meant, according to McKeown, that the chance of recovery for a pauper sick was reduced to practically nothing. Already weakened by disease, he underwent severe bleeding, received strong purgatives and was forced to share his bed with a couple of other unfortunates. In the filthy and overcrowded wards infectious diseases spread like a prairie-fire. The chance of surviving an amputation of one of the limbs was less than 50 percent. Hospital physicians had practically no knowledge of effective remedies. They also selected their patients carefully, and refused to admit anyone who they might fail to cure. Thomas McKeown's conclusion is therefore that hospitals in no way contributed to public health and population growth. They more likely contributed to the spreading of disease [28].

There are, however, quite opposite views on the role of early modern hospitals. E M Sigsworth, Steven Cherry, and John Woodward, present a far less rigid picture. Woodward carefully examines the statements made by McKeown, and argues that he actually has no evidence at all to support his standpoint. Woodward claims that McKeown has misinterpreted the whole picture, simply by selecting information uncritically [29]. By using patients' records, Sigsworth, Cherry, and Woodward picture the hospitals as quite successful in curing the sick. The problems of overcrowding and filth did exist, according to Steven Cherry. They were, however, not a constant problem. Only during the second half of the nineteenth century, when population pressure on the hospitals became a problem, did mortality rise [30]. Cherry also claims that physicians admitted patients with diseases that without hospital treatment frequently would have led to death [31].

English hospital records do, however, present several source critical problems, especially in the use of the term "cured". The Voluntary hospitals were to a high extent dependent upon donations for their existence and it was therefore of great value to be able to present as favourable statistics as possible. Because of this, there is a risk that many patients were dismissed just before death. English hospitals also had a system of "out-patients", i.e. sick treated in their own homes by visiting hospital physicians. These patients evidently entered the records as "in-patients" in times when it was necessary to show good statistics for the total number of patients treated.

In the following we will examine how successful the hospital physicians in Härnösand were. We will, however, not limit our investigation to the patients' records. In order to be able to answer the question of whether patients were dismissed to cover up for unfavorable statistics, or simply because the physicians imagined that they had cured their patients, we will follow a small cohort of patients in the church records until their time of death. It will then be possible to calculate the time between dismissal and death. We will also compare the diseases that they suffered from during their stay at the hospital with their causes of death.

Results of treatment

I have no intention to analyze early nineteenth-century therapeutic regimen in this article. To be able to fully understand how and why the physicians acted as they did we would have to take our point of departure from Galenic medical theory dating back to the year 200 A.D. Let us just say that the Swedish physicians, through frequent travels abroad, an internationally recognized university in Uppsala, and a well-functioning system of medical journals, were well aware of the medical findings and theories in Europe. At the hospitals a fairly new and updated pharmacopoeia was in use, the Swedish Pharmacopoea svecica (1775). It was also translated into German and used in their hospitals. In return Swedish hospitals frequently consulted the "Pharmacopoea pauperum" printed in Hamburg, and Cullen's "Pharmacopoeia Pauperum" [32]. We have, therefore, no reason to believe that Swedish hospital physicians were less well-trained, or lacked contemporary medical knowledge in comparison with their European colleagues.

The physicians used mainly four classifications when patients were dismissed from the hospital. Patients were either considered "cured", or their physical state had "improved". Some were dismissed as "incurable", and the rest left the hospital in coffins. In some rare cases patients became tired of seemingly everlasting therapy, and simply "escaped" from the hospital.

74.3 per cent of all patients admitted to the County Hospital of Härnösand were dismissed as cured. 11.5 per cent had recovered enough to be dismissed as improved, 3 per cent were incurable, and 8 per cent died. The percentage of cured patients was approximately the same at the Royal Infirmary of Edinburgh: 70.7. 10.4 per cent were dismissed as relieved, 0.1 as incurable, and 4.1 died. The larger proportion of patients leaving the County Hospital as incurable could perhaps be explained by the great number of neurological and mental patients. Swedish hospital physicians were also more generous in admitting patients with diseases difficult to cure, since they were financed otherwise. The physicians at the Royal Infirmary of Edinburgh considered as many as 3.8 per cent of all patients as "improper". This could also explain the high mortality rate in the County Hospital of Härnösand—twice as high as in the Edinburgh hospital.

According to Risse, the mortality rate in the Royal Infirmary of Edinburgh should have been somewhat higher. The custom of discharging moribund patients was not only a scheme to improve hospital statistics but a response to the demands of relatives and patients themselves to die in their own homes. Mortality was also increasing at a steady rate in the Infirmary, and was reported to be 6.4% in 1810 [33].

The total number of patients cured or dead is one thing. The real differences appear when we look at single disease categories. From Table 4 we can see that the physicians were successful in curing the patients whom the hospital had originally been designed for. Patients suffering from diseases affecting the sexual organs, the majority of all admissions, were cured in over 90 per cent of all cases. Patients dying or considered incurable were rather few in number. Most of the patients suffering from syphilis entered the hospital at an early stage. Their disease was considered to be in its "primitive stage". There were, however, also patients with syphilis in its third and last stage. With their brains attacked, madness followed and finally inevitable death.

Table 4. The result of treatment at the county hospital of Härnösand 1814—1864.

Disease	Cured	Improved	Incurable	Dead	Other
Sexual organs	90.6	4.2	0.8	2.7	1.7
Surgical infections	77.8	12.4	1.4	5.0	3.4
Infectious diseases	89.1	1.2	0.1	9.0	0.6
Respiratory diseases	57.2	20.1	1.7	16.6	4.4
Traumatic conditions	82.6	7.7	0.7	5.4	3.6
Tumors and cancers	59.4	11.3	8.6	12.6	8.1
Digestive diseases	70.4	15.0	0.7	11.4	2.5
Circulatory disorder	42.1	21.4	2.5	31.1	2.9
Neurological	49.6	29.4	6.9	9.5	4.6
Mental	32.7	25.6	29.1	6.3	6.3
Musculoskeletal	64.7	22.4	4.6	5.0	3.3
Others, and unspec	94.0	2.8	—	2.8	0.4
Diseases of the skin	71.7	17.8	4.4	3.9	2.2
Urinary tract disease	45.7	26.7	3.8	16.2	7.6
Eye problems	68.0	22.0	6.0	3.0	1.0
Surgical conditions	73.3	9.3	4.7	10.5	2.2
Unspec. inflammations	57.1	14.3	3.6	17.9	7.1
All diseases	74.3	11.5	3.0	8.0	3.2

The high rate of cured patients with venereal diseases is, however, not that easy to interpret. Syphilis is characterized by spontaneous and long periods of rest. This probably made the physicians believe that their patients had been cured. The patient could then appear at the hospital once again, not infected a second time, but suffering from the same syphilis. The therapy with mercury did have some effect though, and many patients evidently were healed [34]. We shall, however, return to this problem.

Low percentages of cured were found among patients suffering from diseases of the respiratory organs, circulatory disorders and neurological and mental diseases. It is quite natural that a nineteenth-century physician could not cure, for instance, epilepsy. Patients with mental diseases were often transferred to asylums if they did not respond positively to purgatives and bleeding, and clearly, these diseases are not cured even today. Patients with circulatory disorders and diseases of the respiratory organs also had the highest mortality rates. The chance of survival when suffering from dropsy, aneurysm, or hydrops was only two out of three. Every fifth patient suffering from respiratory diseases, mainly tuberculosis, survived. Many of these patients "improved" during their stay in the hospital, probably due to the fact that they received rest, warmth, and regular meals.

We can draw the same conclusion from the patients suffering from musculo-skeletal disorders. Patients with rheumatism felt much better when they received shelter inside the hospital and were treated with hot baths, massage and medicine containing alcohol. They were not cured, many of them were chronically ill, but they felt much better. The dividing line between health and sickness is not absolute. Today we often tend to look upon health as a state of complete physical and psychological well-being, forgetting that our nineteenth-century ancestors probably had a much different view [35]. To be cured could simply just mean that the patient was fit enough to contribute to his family's provision.

Some former patients came back to the hospital later in life. This group of readmitted patients is of the utmost interest, since it might shed light on the meaning of the term cured. If patients were frequently readmitted and suffering from the same complaint as they had been treated for earlier, it might indicate that they had never really been cured in the first place.

6837 admissions were recorded at the hospital between the years 1814 and 1864. By using the patients' name, age, occupation, and residence it has been possible, with a fairly high degree of accuracy, to manually link them together within the sources. Thus we can calculate that 599 patients returned to the hospital at least once. 98 of them came back twice, 21 returned three times and 4 patients were readmitted four times. One man, a syphilitic farmer called Jon Olsson from Norby in the parish of Njurunda, was readmitted to the hospital five times between 1821 and 1826. During his first four visits he was dismissed as cured, but after the fifth he only left the hospital as "relieved". The readmissions sum up to a total of 1322 cases in the patients' records, which means that 5515, or 80.7 per cent, were admitted for treatment only once.

It seems to be typical that it was the patients suffering from syphilis who were the ones to return most frequently to the hospital. Since the physicians lacked modern laboratory equipment it was impossible for them to tell for certain whether a patient definitely was cured or not. When syphilis has its first periods of "rest" all symptoms and signs, such as rashes and ulcers, disappear. It was only after the disease had started to disfigure the body that the doctors could tell for sure that syphilis was still present. In Table 5 the total number of readmissions is presented for each disease category, but only for those patients who each time left the hospital as cured.

The dominant role played by syphilis for the readmission of formerly "cured" patients is obvious. 99 patients, nearly 6 per cent, returned to the hospital, although they had been considered as cured by the physician. 88 of them left as cured, but 10 of were readmitted a second time. Eight left the hospital as "cured" for the third time, but still one of the poor souls came back for his fourth stay at the County Hospital. He was finally dismissed as "cured"! The only two groups of patients equivalent to those suffering from syphilis, as regards percentage of readmissions, were those with circulatory disorders: 7 out of 118 patients came back, and those with tumors and cancers, 11 out of 221 were readmitted. For the other disease categories the percentage of readmitted patients varied between one and four per cent, the lowest for those suffering from traumatic conditions, infectious diseases and diseases of the skin. Patients cured from mental diseases were never readmitted.

Table 5. Readmissions to the County hospital of Härnösand 1814—1864

Disease	Cured	Number of readmissions		
		1	2	3
Sexual organs	1737	99	10	1
Infectious diseases	607	10	—	—
Surgical infections	547	13	1	—
Respiratory diseases	373	12	—	—
Traumatic conditions	365	3	—	—
Tumors and cancers	221	11	1	—
Digestive diseases	216	6	—	—
Musculoskeletal	156	3	1	—
Neurological diseases	130	5	1	—
Diseases of the skin	129	1	—	—
Circulatory disorders	118	7	—	—
Eye problems	68	1	—	—

It is possible, of course, that many of them really did leave the hospital in a healthy state, and that they then contracted a similar disease. Many readmissions could probably be explained in this way, and the only way to check for this would be to study each individual case history. Time has, however, not permitted such an inquiry in this article. On the other hand, when we are dealing with diseases that we know were hard to diagnose and cure, it is more likely that the doctors were sometimes bound to draw hasty conclusions. This must certainly have been true in the cases of patients suffering from syphilis, because of the extraordinary characteristics of this disease.

The disease first shows its nature after an incubation period of between 10 days to 10 weeks, usually in the form of small, hard and painless swellings on the sexual organs. The disease is therefore hard to detect in this first stage, especially in women. The swellings will disappear, even without treatment, in about eight weeks. The infecting organism, the spirochete Treponema pallidium, continues to move through the body into the lymph nodes. After a period of 2-4 months skin lesions in the form of an eruptive rash or ulcerating sores begin to appear. This marks what is called the second stage of the disease. The rash or the sores may heal in 2-6 weeks, but they might well be visible for a couple of months. The second stage may last for 2-4 years, during which the ulcerating sores can reappear several times. After this stage the untreated disease moves into a latent period, where, in fact according to statistics, 25 percent of those who have contracted the disease are healed spontaneously. The latent period may last for 15-25 years when finally the nervous system is damaged. In this third and last stage, with their brains attacked, the sick are finally faced with certain death. It has been calculated that third stage syphilis accounted for as many as 10 per cent of admissions to insane asylums [36].

We can summarize from Table 4, by saying that early modern hospital physicians actually were capable of curing, at least in their own judgment. This picture becomes, however, somewhat modified in the light of the results in Table 5. Between one and six per cent of the originally cured patients were readmitted to hospital suffering from what could have been the same ailment. Whether these figures are to be considered high or not is more a matter of opinion. In the case of syphilis, especially if we take the exceptional characteristics of the disease into consideration, we must, however, be more skeptical as to the high figure of "cured" in Table 4. Patients with venereal diseases had the highest rate of readmission, and if we also bear in mind the average numbers of days that were necessary for the treatment, 69.5 days (See Appendix A), we might reason that there is a connection with the spontaneous healing periods of the second stage. It is, in this respect, safe to argue that a majority of the venereal patients suffered from second stage syphilis. It is highly unlikely that people went to see a doctor or that social control forced them into institutional care, just because of some small hard swellings.

Despite all this the early nineteenth century hospital still deserves a much better reputation than it has received from, for instance, Thomas McKeown. More than 4,000 patients left the hospital as cured, and they never returned. Whether this was due to the therapeutic regimen, or simply to the healing powers of nature, it is more difficult to say. The fact that patients received a warm bed, regular meals, and lots of rest, naturally did a lot of good.

Explicit problems of treatment were mainly posed by patients suffering from internal diseases, i.e. affecting organs that the physician could not see or touch. All they had were theoretical assumptions on how the human body functioned. It is no surprise then that they often failed with these cases.

The cohort-investigation

In order to better understand the meaning of the term cured, we shall turn our attention to a small cohort of 325 patients dismissed from the hospital [37]. Using the information about residence in the patients' records they have been traced to their home parishes after their dismissal. By scanning through the death and burial registers, death-dates were found for all of them. The death- and burial registers also give the cause of death in some cases, according to the priest's judgment [38]. The time span between dismissal and death has then been calculated and cross-tabulated with the categories of dismissal. The results are presented in Table 6.

104 out of 224 patients dismissed as cured were still alive more than 10 years after their stay at the hospital. Only ten of them died within the first year after dismissal, and they were actually patients who were over 60 years of age. A majority of those dismissed as "improved" also lived for at least more than a year. Only patients who left the hospital as incurable had a really low life expectancy. In Table 6 we can also see that only two of the 325 patients were

dismissed and died on the very same day that they left the hospital. Since one was incurable and the other only improved, we can conclude that the cohort investigation, even if it is limited, does not support the assumption that patients were dismissed from the hospital to make up for unfavorable statistics.

The only former patients who actually died of the same diseases as they had been treated for at the hospital, were those who had suffered from circulatory disorders and tumours. 4 out of 12 patients who had been treated for dropsy later died from it. Two of them had even been considered as cured. Out of 16 patients treated for tumours, 6 eventually died from cancer, but only one had been dismissed as cured.

The venereal patients should be mentioned once more. 161 of the 325 patients in the cohort suffered from syphilis. 3 of them died in hospital, 5 died during the first year, 6 during the next 3 years, 13 lived up to nine years, and 134 lived more than 10 years after dismissal. None of them were re-admitted to the hospital. Only two of the 161 patients' cause of death could be connected with venereal disease, and only one of them was dismissed as cured. Indeed many lived long enough to die of "old age".

If we combine these results with the readmissions in Table 5 we have a large proportion of venereal patients who were dismissed as cured, never returned and did not die of causes connected with the disease. 1737 venereal patients left as cured, 99 were readmitted, some of them several times, and roughly 20 percent died within 10 years after dismissal. If we make the assumption that these patients died directly or indirectly because of their disease, we still have more than 1300 patients who seem to really have been cured. This would mean that over 70 per cent must have been cured out of the 1918 admitted venereal patients.

Table 6. Time span between dismissal and death among patients at the county hospital of Härnösand, 1814—1864.

| | Time Span | | | | | | |
| | Days | | | Years | | | |
Result	0	1—29	30—364	1—4	5—9	10—	Total
Cured	—	1	9	15	15	184	224
Improved	1	1	5	13	3	22	45
Incurable	1	2	5	2	4	13	27
Dead	18	—	—	—	—	—	18
Other	—	1	3	1	1	5	11
Total	20	5	22	31	23	224	325
Per cent	6.2	1.5	6.8	9.5	7.1	68.9	100.0

Now, the problem is a bit more complicated than this. We know that third stage syphilis might take as long as 15-25 years to appear (we find no traces of it in the causes of death for the cohort, though), and some of the patients could have later been admitted to the County Hospital in Sundsvall (founded in 1844) [39]. Some patients might also have arranged some sort of private care. It still seems unlikely, however, that this should account for all of the 1300 patients. Naturally, we need more research in this field before we can say anything definite.

Conclusions

In this paper we have examined the patients at the County Hospital of Härnösand between 1814 and 1864. During this time 6837 admissions were recorded at the hospital. The patients came from various social backgrounds. Almost every fifth patient in fact came from social groups among the population that were relatively well-off. One could say that the social structure of the hospitals' patients clearly reflected the social composition of contemporary Härnösand. Most patients were in their prime of life, and the conclusion must be that people did not consider the hospital such a horrifying institution that it should be avoided at all costs.

The most common complaint among the patients was venereal disease, mainly syphilis. Nearly every third patient suffered from a disease affecting the sexual organs, and it was especially common among patients who came to the hospital from long distance. In second and third place came surgical infections and infectious diseases. In comparison with the Royal Infirmary of Edinburgh the disease panorama at the County Hospital was approximately the same, although the Swedish hospital had a larger proportion of venereal patients. This was probably due to the fact that Scandinavian hospitals were mainly designed to treat patients with such complaints, while in other countries they were considered "improper" for admission.

Patients admitted to the County Hospital stayed there for a long period of time. The average stay was almost 55 days. The longest duration of stay was recorded for the venereal patients, and those suffering from mental diseases. The former group had to undertake salivation-cures, i.e. treatment with mercury, which was a dangerous and time consuming method.

A majority of the patients, 74.3 per cent, were dismissed from the hospital as cured. The best chance of recovery was among the venereal patients, those suffering from infectious diseases and traumatic conditions. Patients with mental diseases, circulatory disorders, or respiratory diseases had a far lesser chance of being dismissed as cured. Of the patients suffering from circulatory disorders, over 30 per cent died in hospital. The investigation has, however, shown that nineteenth century Swedish hospital patients were in fact cured, not killed.

Even if we take into consideration what happened to the patients after they were dismissed, our positive impression of the hospitals is not altered. Only in very few cases were patients dismissed shortly before they died. Most patients lived for more than 10 years after their dismissal and very few died of the same disease as they had been treated for.

The number of readmissions to the hospital of formerly cured patients does, however, slightly modify this positive picture. It was especially common for venereal patients to be released as cured, only to return a couple of years later with the same ailment. It is likely that the physicians had difficulty in determining whether this disease was cured or not since syphilis is characterized by long periods of "rest", when all symptoms and signs disappear. In order to fully determine whether the readmissions were due to a generous use of the term "cured" by the physicians we will have to study individual case histories more systematically. This will also be done in the near future.

This paper has also pointed to the fact that there are more similarities than differences between small Swedish county hospitals and large European hospitals. They shared the same disease panorama, with the exception of venereal patients, they were equally successful in their treatment of their patients, and their physicians probably applied the same therapeutic methods[40]. Since Sweden has excellent source material, where it is possible to trace patients, both before and after their stay in hospital, further and deeper studies of Swedish county hospitals could make an important contribution to the international discussion on the role of the early modern hospitals. Life-histories for patients would not only answer questions about the possible connections between public care and population growth, but also, and much more important, become a real history of the hospitals, i.e. a history as if told by the patients.

Table A. Average stay in days at the county hospital of Härnösand 1814—1864

Disease	Number of days
Disease affecting sexual organs	69.5
Infectious diseases	30.9
Surgical infections	64.9
Respiratory diseases	34.4
Diseases of digestive system	25.9
Musculosketal disorders	58.9
Neurological diseases	54.8
Mental diseases	88.4
Traumatic conditions	57.3
Diseases of the skin	55.5
Circulatory disorders	45.7
Tumors and cancers	49.0
Eye problems	53.9
Mucus of unspec origin	69.8
Total average	54.9

Table B. Diseases at the Royal Infirmary of Edinburgh.

Disease	N	Percent
Diseases affecting sexual organs	578	19.0
Infectious diseases	476	15.6
Surgical infections	347	11.4
Respiratory diseases	340	11.2
Diseases of the digestive system	197	6.5
Musculosketal disorders	181	5.9
Neurological and mental diseases	162	5.3
Traumatic conditions	149	4.8
Diseases of the skin	125	4.1
Circulatory disorders	79	2.6
Tumors and cancers	75	2.5
Eye problems	61	2.0
Other	277	9.1
Total	3047	100.0

Source: Risse (1986), p. 124

Notes

1. J. Revel and J-P. Peter, 'Kroppen. Den sjuka människan och hennes historia', J. Le Goff and P. Nova (Eds), *Att skriva historia* (Stockholm 1978), p 267.

2. Revel and Peter (1978), p 272. See also, M. Foucault, *The Birth of the Clinic* [La naissance de la clinique] (London 1973), p 97.

3. A. Åman, *Om den offentliga vården. Byggnader och verksamheter vid svenska vårdinstitutioner under 1800- och 1900-talen* [Public Care. Buildings and Activities in Swedish Institutions for Social and Public Care, During the Nineteenth and Twentieth Centuries] (Uddevalla 1976).

4. See discussion about the 'new medical history' in, for instance R. Porter (Ed), *Patients and Practitioners. Lay Perceptions of Medicine in Pre-industrial Society* (Cambridge 1985), pp. 1; R. McGrew, *Encyclopedia of Medical History* (London 1985), pp. 177.

5. Ø. Larsen, '''Söe-Quaest-Huuset''—Das Marinespital zu Kopenhagen und seine Funktion 1788-1791' *Medizinhistorisches Journal* (1970);—'Skykehusets funksjon i bergstaden Kongsberg i arene 1769-1772 [The Role of the Hospital in Kongsberg, 1769-1772] *Medicinhistorisk årsbok* (1969);—'Das Krankenhauswesen in Norwegen im 19. Jahrhundert', H. Schadewaldt (Ed), *Studien zur Krankenhausgeschichte im 19. Jahrhundert im Hinblick auf die Entwicklung in Deutschland* (Göttingen 1976); S. Vallgårda, *Sjukhus och fattigpolitik. Ett bidrag till de danska sjukhusens historia 1750-1880* [Hospitals and Poor Relief. A Contribution to the History of Danish Hospitals 1750-1880] (Odense 1985), Chapter V. Å. Boman has written an interesting study of the Västerås hospital 1786-1893, based on patient records. He has, however, concentrated his analysis only to the disease panorama. Å. Boman, Sjukvården vid Västerås lasarett 1786-1893 [Care and Treatment at the Västerås Hospital 1786-1893] *Nordisk Medicinhistorisk Årsbok,* Supplementum XII (1986).

6. A. E. Imhof, 'The Hospital in the Eighteenth Century: For Whom?', P. Branca (Ed.), *The Medicine Show* (New York 1977).

7. E.M. Sigsworth, 'Gateways to Death?. Medicine, Hospitals and Mortality, 1700-1850', P. Mathias (Ed.), *Science and Society 1600-1900* (Cambridge 1972); J. Woodward, *To Do the Sick No Harm. A Study of the British Voluntary Hospital System to 1875* (London 1974); S. Cherry, 'The Role of a Provincial Hospital. The Norfolk and Norwich Hospital, 1771-1880', *Population studies,* 26, 2 (1972);—'The Hospitals and Population Growth: The Voluntary General Hospitals, Mortality and Local Populations in the English Provinces in the Eighteenth and Nineteenth Centuries', *Population Studies,* 34, 1-2 (1980); W. H. Williams, *America's First Hospital: The Pennsylvania Hospital, 1751-1841* (Wayne, Penn 1976); G. B. Risse, *Hospital Life in Enlightenment Scotland. Care and Teaching at the Royal Infirmary of Edinburgh* (Cambridge 1986).

8. E. Falkum, and Ø. Larsen, *Helseomsorgens vilkår. Linjer i medisinsk sosialhistorie* [The Conditions for Public Health Care] (Oslo 1981), p.85. See also, G. Ljunquist, *Om sjukdomsbot och mediciner* [Therapy and Remedies] (Uddevalla 1965).

9. R. Wawrinsky, *Svenskt lasarettsväsende förr och nu* [Swedish Hospitals, Past and Present] (Stockholm 1906).

10. T. McKeown, 'A Sociological Approach to the History of Medicine', *Medical History,* 14, 4 (1970).

11. A. Brändström, 'Umeå lasarett och de första patienterna' [The County Hospital in Umeå and its First Patients], *Västerbotten,* 3/4 (1985).

12. See for instance Foucault (1973), p.42, and . J. V. Vogel, *The Invention of the Modern Hospital: Boston, 1870-1930* (Chicago 1980).

13. Woodward (1974), p.45.

14. L. S. King, *The Medical World of the Eighteenth Century* (Chicago 1958), pp. 212.

15. Risse (1986), p.189.

16. Risse (1986), p.121. See also, B-I. Puranen, *Tuberkulos. En sjukdoms förekomst och dess orsaker. Sverige 1750-1980* [Tuberculosis. The Occurrence and Causes in Sweden 1750-1980](Umeå 1984), pp 102.

17. Risse (1986), p.121.

18. B. M. Bergvall, Svenska medicinares och kirurgers utländska studieresor under 1700-talet [Studies Abroad Made by Swedish Physicians and Surgeons During the Eighteenth Century] *Unpublished paper* (Uppsala 1961).

19. Risse (1986), p.162.

20. Vallgårda (1985), p.41.

21. Woodward (1974), p.49.

22. Vogel (1980), pp.70.

23. Risse (1986), pp.101.

24. I. Lönnberg, 'Översikt över sjukhusväsendets utveckling i Sverige' [The Development of Hospitals in Sweden], *SOU* 1922:43.

25. Brändström (1984), p.162.

26. See for instance King (1958), pp.128. O. Temkin, *Galenism. Rise and Decline of a Medical Philosophy* (London 1973), p 165. Foucault (1973), pp. 180.

27. Risse (1986), p.173.

28. McKeown (1970), p.351.

29. Woodward (1974), passim.

30. Cherry (1970), Part 1, p.71.

31. Cherry (1980), Part 2, p.260.

32. Ljungqvist (1965), p.144.

33. Risse (1986), p.234.

34. U. Högberg, *Svagårens barn* (1983), p 165.

35. Falkum and Larsen (1981) have an interesting presentation of the concept of health, pp.18.

36. McGrew (1985), pp. 229; M. Bergmark, *Från pest till polio. Hur farsoter gripit in i människors öden* [From Plague to Poliomyelitis] (Stockholm 1983), pp 87.

37. Time has not permitted a larger cohort investigation at this stage, since the cohort had to be constructed manually. This article is, however, part of a larger project about the county hospitals in Härnösand and Sundsvall. The cohort investigation will be taken much further and, with the help of computer-registered church records, some 21 000 case histories.

38. Puranen (1984), pp.35.

39. The patient records for the county hospital of Sundsvall are at present being computer-registered. The material will cover the period between 1844-1900, and some 21,000 recorded admissions.

40. When we compare therapeutics and success of treatment between Härnösand and the Royal Infirmary of Edinburgh, we do, however, have to remember that Risses' investigation covers a somewhat earlier time period, 1770-1800. There could be differences because of this, but they should not be exaggerated. The real breakthroughs in medicine did not happen until during the last decades of the nineteenth century.

Nutrition and the Decline in Mortality since 1700: Some Additional Preliminary Findings

Robert W. Fogel

The issues

Between c. 1700 and 1980 there was a decline of about 35 points in the standardized American death rate (see Table 1).[1] Between the same years, the British rate declined by about 21 points. About 70 percent of the American decline and about 50 percent of the British decline took place before 1911.

The causes of this remarkable decline remain a puzzle. Until the mid 1950s it was widely attributed to improvements in medical technology. During the past three decades Thomas McKeown vigorously disputed that view in a series of highly influential papers and books. McKeown agreed that there had been a considerable expansion of hospital services and important advances in medical knowledge during the eighteenth and nineteenth centuries but he argued that such advances had little effect on the decline in death rates until the twentieth century. An epidemiologist, McKeown gained prominence for biomedical research, including his studies of the relationship between birth weight and perinatal mortality rates in Birmingham after World War II, before turning his attention to long-term changes in medical practices and demographic rates.[2]

The nutritional contribution: The English experience

McKeown's explanation for the decline in mortality rates after 1700 is most fully set forth in his book on *The Modern Rise of Population* (1976) and he subsequently restated and cogently summarized his argument in 1978 and 1983. In the place of medical technology, McKeown substituted improvement in nutrition as the principal factor affecting the decline in mortality. He does

This is an abridged version of professor Fogels paper. The whole paper has been published in *Long-Term Factors in American Growth* (National Bureau of Economic Research, 1986). The abridgement has been made by permission of the author and the University of Chicago Press.

not make his case for nutrition directly but largely through a residual argument in which he rejects the other principal explanations. The alternatives to nutrition are advances in medical technology; reductions in the virulence of pathogens; human acquisition of immunity through natural selection, genetic drift, or acquired immunities; personal hygiene; and public sanitation.

Table 1. The probable decline in standardized death rates between 1700 and 1980 in the United States and Great Britain.

Part A. Standardized Death Rates (per thousand)

Approximate Date		*United States*	*Great Britain*
1.	1700	40	28
2.	1850	23	24
3.	1910	15	17
4.	1980	5	7

Part B. Percentage of the total decline which occurred between c. 1700 and the specified date

Approximate Date		*United States*	*Great Britain*
5.	1850	49	19
6.	1910	71	52
7.	1980	100	100

Sources: United States: The age distribution is standardized on the weights computed from persons alive in 1700 in the pilot sample of genealogies that is described in the next section of this paper. *Line 1.* Fogel, *et al,*'The Economics of Mortality in North America, 1650—1910: A Decription of a Research Project', *Hist. Meth.,* 11 (1978), p. 76, with New England and Chesapeake rates weighted by the New England and Southern populations for 1700 as given in U.S. Bur. Cen. 1975, p. 1168. *Line 2.* Unpublished mortality tables for whites in 1850, cited in M.R. Haines, 'The Use of Model Life Tables to Estimate Mortality for the United States in the Late Nineteenth Century', *Demography,* 16 (1979). *Line 3.* S.H. Preston, N. Keyfitz, and R. Schoen, *Causes of Death: Life Tables For National Populations* (New York 1972), pp. 728, 730. *Line 4.* U.S. Nat. Cent. Health Stat. (1983), p. 12. Great Britain: The age distribution is standardized on the weights given in E.A. Wrigley and R. Schofield, *The Population History of England, 1541—1871: A Reconstruction* (Cambridge 1981), p. 529 for 1701—1705; male and female death rates were equally weighted. *Line 1. Ibid. Lines 2 and 3.* R.A.M. Case, *Chester Beatty Research Institute Abridged Serial Life Tables, England and Wales 1841—1960,* I (London 1962), pp. 41, 53, 65, 76. *Line 4.* G.B. Cent. Stat. Off. (1983), p. 43.

McKeown's analysis turns on a careful consideration of the British pattern of decline in death rates due to specific infectious diseases between c. 1850 and 1971. During this period the standardized death rate attributable to infectious diseases declined from 13.0 per thousand to 0.7 per thousand. About 54 percent of the decline was associated with airborne diseases, 28 percent with water- and food-borne diseases, and 18 percent with diseases spread by other means.[3] This simple classification permits McKeown to assess the probable impact of public health measures and personal sanitation. Cleaning up the public water supply and improving sewage systems, he argues, would have had little effect on the airborne diseases. Moreover, as long as water supplies were polluted, individuals could not protect themselves against such water-borne diseases as typhoid and cholera by washing regularly. Under such circumstances "the washing of hands is about as effective as the wringing of hands".[4] In his view public health measures did not become effective until the very end of the nineteenth century. The sharp declines in food- and water-borne diseases (which he dates in England and Wales with the start of the eighth decade) were not only due to better water and sewage systems but to improvements in food hygiene, especially pasteurization. He attributes the rapid decline of infant mortality between 1900 and 1931 mainly to the development of a "safe milk supply".[5] McKeown argues that improvements in personal or public hygiene would not have reduced deaths from airborne diseases unless they reduced crowding, and crowding generally increased during the nineteenth century.

McKeown's skepticism about the efficacy of early medical measures is based on his study of the temporal pattern of decline in the death rates of the most lethal diseases of the nineteenth century. Tuberculosis, the leading killer in England and America during much of the nineteenth century, is a case in point. During 1848-1854 tuberculosis causes nearly one out of every six English deaths from all causes, and one out of every four due to infectious diseases. It was not until 1882 that the tubercle bacillus was identified and an effective chemotherapy for this disease was not developed until 1947. Nevertheless, the death rate of respiratory tuberculosis declined to just 43 percent of its 1848-1854 level, by 1900 and to just 10 percent of that level before the introduction of streptomycin in 1947. Similarly, the major decline in the death rates from bronchitis and pneumonia, whooping cough, measles, scarlet fever, and typhoid all preceded the development of effective chemotherapies. McKeown also doubts the efficacy of the lying-in hospitals which were established during the eighteenth and nineteenth centuries, noting that well into the third quarter of the last century "hospital death rates were many times greater than those for related home deliveries".[6]

McKeown is skeptical of the contention that the decline in mortality rates was due to a decline in the virulence of pathogens. He notes that scarlet fever and influenza have fluctuated in their severity in short periods of time and acknowledges that these fluctuations were due to changes in the character of these diseases. He lists typhus as another disease that might have declined due to changes in the pathogens. However, the fraction of the total decline attributable to these three diseases is small. On a more general plane he notes that infectious diseases that are now relatively benign in developed nations are still quite virulent in less developed countries and argues that it is quite unlikely that pathogens would have lost their virulence only in developed countries. McKeown also minimizes the impact of natural selection, arguing that in the case of tuberculosis too much of the population had been exposed to the bacillus for too long a period before the decline, and the decline itself was too rapid, to be consistent with natural selection.

McKeown's arguments in favor of a nutritional explanation fall into two categories. First, he cites evidence that per capita food supplies in England increased sporadically during the late eighteenth and early nineteenth centuries and then regularly in the late nineteenth and in the twentieth centuries. Second, he emphasizes findings of medical researchers currently working in the developing countries who have concluded that there is a synergistic relationship between malnutrition and infection, and that malnutrition significantly increases the likelihood that a victim will succumb to an infection. In this connection he cites a report of the World Health Organization which concluded that malnutrition was an associated cause in 57 to 67 percent of the deaths of children under age 5 in Latin America.[7]

The nutritional contribution: The American experience

McKeown's argument has been extended to the American experience by Meeker and by Higgs.[8] According to Meeker, the period from 1880 to 1910 witnessed both a substantial rise in per capita income and a decline in mortality rates. In cross-sectional regressions for 1890 to 1900, city mortality rates are significantly related to housing density variables and state mortality rates are significantly related to income. In his 1973 paper Higgs estimated the decline in rural mortality rates for the period from 1870 to World War I. Despite the absence of direct observations on rural mortality, Higgs was able to infer a series by making use of three other series (the aggregate crude death rate, the urban crude death rate, and the share of the population that was urban) and an identity that related the rural crude death rate to these series. This procedure produced a rural crude mortality series which declined at approximately the same rate as the urban mortality series, the total decline over 50 years amounting to between 30 and 40 percent. Higgs argues that whatever role public sanitation and medical care might have played in the urban context, they were of minor consequence in rural areas which were undersupplied with physicians, and which continued to draw water mainly from wells, springs, and cisterns, continued to rely on privies, and continued to consume unpasteurized milk. Like McKeown, Higgs concluded that "the great bulk of the decline in rural mortality before 1920 is probably attributable to rising levels of living among the rural population".[9]

372

Objections to the nutritional argument

Virtually all those who are attempting to explain the secular decline in mortality rates in Europe and America agree that improvements in nutrition made a contribution. But some scholars believe that McKeown and others have greatly exaggerated the case.[10] The doubts arise partly because of major gaps in the evidence. Razzell, for example, doubts McKeown's claim that the food supply in England grew more rapidly than the population before 1840. He argues that at least for the eighteenth century the evidence is "much more consistent with a reversed hypothesis — that the standard of the diet was a function of population change".[11] Even more basic is the absence of adequate evidence on mortality rates. Before 1837 in Great Britain and before 1900 in the United States information on death rates is so sparse that historical demographers are at odds not only on the levels of mortality but even on the direction of change.[12]

In the American case, for example, fragments of evidence led Thompson and Whelpton to believe that mortality rates declined fairly steadily from the middle of the eighteenth century to 1900.[13] On the other hand, Yasuba's examination of available urban death registrations and some scattered registrations from rural communities led him to conclude that mortality rates increased between 1800 and 1860.[14] More recently, a study of Deerfield, which has vital records that extend back to the early eighteenth century, revealed that mortality was low and stable within this rural town of western Massachusetts until the turn of the nineteenth century. Between 1795-1799 and 1840-1844, however, mortality rates nearly doubled.[15]

It is not merely the evidential gaps in the argument of McKeown and others that aroused the concern of critics. Certain facts seemed to contradict the case for nutrition. The absence of a significant gap between the mortality rates of the peerage and the laboring classes in England before 1725 was particularly vexing. "If the food supply was the critical variable", Razzell argued, mortality reductions should have been "concentrated almost exclusively amongst the poorer" classes and the mortality rates of the aristocracy should have been "unaffected".[16] Yet as Table 2 shows, between the fourth quarter of the sixteenth century and the beginning of the second quarter of the eighteenth century, the mortality rates of the aristocracy were about as high as those of the general population. Both the high mortality rates of the nobility before 1725 and the rapid fall in these rates thereafter, although there was no apparent change in the diet of the peerage, predisposed Razzell "to look at the food supply hypothesis very critically."[17]

Efforts to relate both short- and long-term variations in the mortality rates to variations in bread or wheat prices have also undermined the nutritional explanation. Appleby's regressions, which related London deaths from specific diseases to bread prices over the period from 1550 to 1750, led him to conclude that there was no correlation between the supply of food and deaths due to plague, smallpox, or tuberculosis and only slight correlations between bread prices and deaths due to typhus and "ague and fever"[18]. More sophisticated analysis by Lee revealed statistically significant but weak relationships between short-term variations in death rates and in wheat prices.[19] According to Schofield short-run variations in English mortality were "overwhelmingly determined" by factors other than the food supply and the long-run trend in mortality was unaffected by the trend in food prices.[20]

Lindert's examination of the work of Lee, Wrigley, and Schofield confirmed their conclusions on the absence of a notable relationship between food prices and mortality rates. Nevertheless, he was discontented with results that implied that living standards "left little or no mark on mortality". The puzzle, he acknowledged, extended to his own work with Williamson, since they have not yet been able to "find a firm casual link behind the obvious correlation between income and life expectancy after 1820". He suggested that the resolution to "the mystery of independent mortality" trends might require more complex attacks on the issue. That would be the case if the "life-extending" effect of income "was hidden behind the shift toward earlier death in the growing unhealthy cities." He also suggested that diets may "have improved in ways unmeasured by income".[21]

Table 2. Cohort Life Expectation (e_0^0) in the English peerage and in the English population as a whole.

Birth cohort (century and quarter)		Peerage (both sexes)	England and Wales (both sexes)
16th	III	38.0	35.6
	IV	37.2	38.0
17th	I	34.7	37.3
	II	33.0	35.5
	III	31.9	34.2
	IV	34.2	33.5
18th	I	36.2	35.1
	II	38.1	33.8
	III	40.2	36.3
	IV	48.1	37.0
19th	I	50.6	
	II	55.3	41.5
	III	58.6	44.6
	IV	60.2	
20th	I	65.0	

Sources: Column 1: T.H. Hollingsworth, 'Mortality in the British Peerage Families Since 1600', *Population,* numéro spécial (1977), Table 3. *Column 2:* The observations for 16-III through 18-IV are from Wrigley and Schofield (1981), p. 530; the observations for 19-II and 19-III are computed from the cohort life tables in Case, *et al.* (1962), pp. 1-28, which were derived from registration data.

Other investigators have found evidence which suggests that McKeown underestimated the impact of public health measures on the decline in mortality during the nineteenth century: Estimates of the cause of mortality rates in the three largest urban areas of France during the nineteenth century by Preston and van de Walle led them to the conclusion that water and sewage improvements played a major role in the urban mortality decline.[22] Not only were the declines concentrated in the waterborne diseases but the rate of decline was much more rapid in the two cities that introduced vigorous sewage and pure water programs than in the one that did not. On the other hand, deaths due to tuberculosis did not decline in Paris over a 33 year period, although deaths due to other airborne diseases showed small declines. Even these declines could have been due to the clean up of the water supply. Preston and van de Walle stress that diarrhea and other waterborne diseases have important nutritional consequences because they "reduce appetite, reduce the absorption of essential nutrients, increase metabolic demands and often lead to dietary restrictions".[23] Thus, cleaning up the water systems not only reduced deaths caused by waterborne diseases but also contributed to the reduction in deaths due to airborne diseases because the reduction in waterborne diseases improved the nutritional status of the population, especially of infants and young children.

The concepts of "nutritional status" and "nutritional adequacy"

The last point calls attention to a terminological issue that has confused the debate over the contribution of improvements in nutrition to the decline in mortality. Although some investigators have equated the term *nutritional status* with the amount of food that is consumed, epidemiologists and nutritionists use the term in a different way. To them *nutritional status* denotes the balance between the intake of nutrients and the claims against it. It follows that adequate levels of nutrition are not determined solely by the level of nutrient intake but vary with the circumstances of an individual. Whether the diet of a particular individual is nutritionally adequate depends on such matters as his level of physical activity, the climate of the region in which he lives, and the extent of his exposure to various diseases. As Nevin S. Scrimshaw put it, the adequacy of a given level of iron consumption depends critically on whether or not an individual has hookworm.[24] Thus, it is possible that the nutritional status of a population may decline even though that population's consumption of nutrients is rising if the extent of exposure to infection or the degree of physical activity is rising more rapidly. It follows that the assessment of the contribution of nutrition to the decline in mortality not only requires measures of food consumption but of the balance between food consumption and the claims on that consumption. To avoid confusion, in the remainder of this paper I will use the terms "diet" and "gross nutrition" to designate nutrient intake only. All other references to nutrition, such as "nutritional status", "net nutrition", "nutrition", "malnutrition", and "undernutrition" will designate the balance between nutrient intake and the claims on that intake.

Conclusion

The decline in mortality rates since 1700 is one of the greatest events of human history.[25] I was inclined to say "one of the greatest achievements of humankind," but the fact remains that we still do not know how much of that achievement was due to causes beyond human control. The paper published by McKeown and Brown in 1955 marked a turning point in the effort to provide a warranted explanation of the decline in mortality.[26] Bridging the worlds of social scientists and of medical specialists, they brought into the discussion most of the range of issues that have been under debate for the past three decades. That debate not only defined the issues more clearly than previously, but also revealed that the critical differences were quantitative rather than qualitative. Nearly all the specialists agree on the range of factors that were responsible for the decline in mortality but they have had quite different views about the relative importance of each of the factors.

The unresolved issue, therefore, is not really whether a particular factor was involved in the decline, but how much each of the various factors contributed to the decline. Resolution of the issue is essentially an accounting exercise of a particularly complicated nature, which involves not only measuring the direct effect of particular factors but also their indirect effects and their interactions with other factors. Our preliminary investigations indicate that the construction of data sets rich enough to permit such a complex accounting is critical to the successful outcome of the exercise. What is needed is a data set that can cope with the changes in the cause-of-death structure which, as Preston indicated, has varied significantly over time and place.[27] To identify the locus of influences of each of the principal factors that contributed to the decline we need not only disease-specific but age-specific, and generation-specific information, because the influence of both risk-increasing and risk-averting factors appear to vary markedly both over lifetimes and over generations.

The findings on the extent and the locus of the nutritional contribution presented in this paper are preliminary in two respects. First, we anticipate that more complete data will lead to revisions in the estimates we have presented. Second, nutritional status is only the first of numerous other factors which contributed to the mortality decline in America since 1700 that we hope to measure. Our preliminary results indicate that the contribution of improvements in nutritional status was neither inconsequential nor overwhelming; although it made a substantial contribution, the factors which contributed to the majority of the decline are still unmeasured. Moreover, although our preliminary estimates indicate that improvements in nutritional

376

status may have accounted for about four tenths of the mortality decline, this contribution was confined largely to the reduction in infant deaths, particularly to late fetal and neonatal deaths and to deaths during weaning. The concentration of the impact of improved nutrition in these age categories raises the possibility that increases in diarrhea and other diseases which diverted ingested nutrients from growth both before and after birth, rather than a decline in food intake, was the main cause of the decline in nutritional status and the rise in mortality during the middle decades of the nineteenth century.

Several important issues have been obfuscated by the confusion between diet (the gross intake of nutrients) and nutritional status (the balance between nutrient intake and the claims on that intake). The blurring of these concepts has diverted attention from the ingestion of harmful substances, which are not only devoid of nutritional value but which prevent the body from assimilating nutrients at critical ages, especially in utero and in early childhood. Alcohol may have been the most devastating of these substances because it was long and so widely consumed by pregnant women. But the administration of opiates to infants also appears to have been widespread for some stretches of time and may have been as widespread among the upper classes as it was among the lower ones. Even salt, in the quantities in which it was consumed prior to the development of refrigeration, was a toxic substance that may have taken a heavy toll at late ages. We are just beginning to become aware of the full range of ingested toxic substances and their role in the high mortality rates of the early modern and early industrial eras. More attention needs to be paid to the role of a variety of contaminants, including lead, arsenic, snakeroot, and mold poisoning.[28]

Preoccupation with diet, especially the excessive focus on adult diets, has diverted attention from an array of intrauterine occurrences that undermined nutritional status and raised mortality rates during infancy and early childhood. Overwork of pregnant mothers and bacterial infections of minor consequence to mothers could have caused serious retardation of fetal development, especially when the insult occurred during the first trimester.[29] Intrauterine infections not only contributed to the large proportion of low-weight births, but increased the incidence of birth anomalies that severely affected the respiratory, circulatory, renal, skeletal, immune, and neurological systems and thus undermined physical development throughout the first year, and often well into the second year and beyond.[30] Whether caused by a poor diet, by toxic substances, by overwork, or by intrauterine infections, low birth weight not only increased perinatal death rates but also late infant and early childhood death rates. Recent studies suggest that the incidence of arteriosclerotic diseases at middle and late ages may be promoted by adverse intrauterine and infant environments.[31]

The preliminary results not only indicate that the factors contributing to the unanticipated cycles in heights and mortality were concentrated at particular ages but that the routes of influences might have been quite round about. These findings point to new issues in the standard-of-living controversy. It may turn out that the difficulties created by improved transportation and rapidly growing cities carried over into the rural regions surrounding the cities, so that urban disamenities imposed costs on the rural populations that have not yet been measured.[32] In the American case it is difficult to believe that per capita food consumption was declining during the last two-thirds of the nineteenth century since there is so much evidence pointing in the opposite direction.[33] Yet there could have been more unequal distribution of food products, especially of meat, which adversely affected the nutritional status of the poor. This appears to have been the case with blacks whose nutritional intake apparently declined, and whose mortality increased, between 1860 and 1880.[34] A more subtle and possibly more pervasive effect on the living standards of laborers and their families, both in the cities and the countryside, may have come from increased exposure to risks (not captured or only partially captured by current measures of real wages) that more than offset the rises in consumption. This possibility does not invalidate indexes of real wages which were designed to cope with a specific set of issues. Rather it raises new issues which require new measures, measures that will supplement the information obtained from the older ones.

The new findings suggest that much more attention needs to be given to the way that population pressures, urbanization, and other economic factors affected not just those of working age but the very young. It may well be that the main damage to the standard of living of workers occurred at exceedingly young ages, in ways that no one at the time fully appreciated, and in a manner that does not conform well to current scenarios regarding the factors and individuals responsible for the hardships of working-class life during the nineteenth century. Nutritional and other health insults delivered in utero or early life not only appear to have affected adult health and longevity, but significantly reduced the later productivity of those who recovered from early insults.[35]

The search for data sources capable of dealing with both the new and the old issues on the interrelationship between demographic and socioeconomic variables has gained considerable force in recent years. Scholars have pushed in many different directions, and nearly all of the work has borne fruit. Careful examination of published data on disease-specific causes of death in U.S. cities have revealed that expenditures on sewers and waterworks had a relatively small effect on the decline in urban mortality before the beginning of the twentieth century,[36] that the main diseases in which rural death rates were consistently lower than urban death rates in 1890 and 1900 were those which are nutritionally sensitive, and that the urban-rural differential was greater for infants and young children than for older persons.[37] These findings, although consistent with the nutritional hypothesis, raise questions about the role of exposure to disease, a variable that could not be measured

378

in these studies. The weak relationship between public health expenditures and mortality rates could reflect the propensity of cities with the most virulent environments to make the heaviest expenditures. Similarly, urban-rural differences in disease-specific mortality rates might be more a matter of differences in exposure rates than in nutritional status. Such issues have led to a search for data sources that make it possible to measure exposure rates.

In this connection, there is much to be gleaned from a reexamination of published data in both state and local sources which can now be more effectively exploited than previously because of computers. Close examination of such published sources have revealed subtle aspects of the mortality structures[38] and of influences upon them that were not adequately appreciated in the past. Condran and Cheney , for example, have found that in Philadelphia during 1870-1930, medical intervention was effective, despite the absence of "high-tech" chemotherapy, because of the role of medical personnel in spreading knowledge about the environmental sources of diseases and in isolating carriers of diseases.[39] Among the more suggestive findings of these recent studies of published data was the discovery by Higgs[40] of marked cycles, around a declining trend, in the mortality rates of 18 large American cities between 1871 and 1900 that are strongly associated with variations in the rate of immigration.[41]

Work on the manuscript sources is still at an early stage, but as the studies by Wrigley and Schofield (1983), Preston and van de Walle (1978), Haines (1983), and Preston and Haines (1983)[42] have already indicated, these sources will not only permit us to push the empirical analysis of the causes of the decline in mortality further back in time but also to shed light on factors that are not apparent in published data. Linked micro data sets will make it possible to disentangle factors that are intricately convoluted in aggregate data. The ability to measure the separate and joint effects of nutritional status, disease exposure rates, medical practices, public sanitation, and intergenerational transmission of behavioral patterns will not only illuminate the past but will directly contribute to a better understanding of important issues in current economic and social policies.

Notes

1. This paper is a progress report on two projects jointly sponsored by the National Bureau of Economic Research and by the Center for Population Economics of the University of Chicago. Aspects of the research reported here were supported by grants from National Science Foundation; the Social Science Research Council, London; the British Academy; the Exxon Educational Foundation; the Walgreen Foundation; Brigham Young University; the University of California at Berkeley; Harvard University; Ohio State University; the University of Pennsylvania; Princeton University; the University of Rochester; and Stanford University. I have drawn on the work of fellow collaborators in the two projects including S.L. Engerman, R. Floud, G. Friedman, C.D. Goldin, R.A. Margo, C. Pope, K. Sokoloff, R.H. Steckel, T.J. Trussel, G. Villaflor, K.W. Wachter, and L. Wimmer. J. Bourne, C. Ford, M. Fishman, J. Moen, and J. Walker have been effective research assistants. C. Miterko efficiently typed and corrected the various drafts. A.M. John has generously made material from her study of Trinidad available to me, and D. Levy permitted me to cite some of the results of his study of life expectation in colonial Maryland. I am especially indebted to J.M. Tanner for his encouragement and advice since the beginning of both projects and to P.H. Lindert for insightful comments and criticism and for the correction of several errors in the draft presented at the Williamsburg conference.

An earlier version of this paper was commissioned by Gunter Steinmann and other organizers of the "Conference on Economic Consequences of Population Change in Industrialized Countries", which was held in Paderborn, West Germany during June, 1983. Successive versions of the paper were presented to seminars at Caltech, the London School of Economics, the Graduate Institute of International Studies (Geneva), Harvard, Chicago, Birkbeck College, Minnesota, Northwestern, Pennsylvania, Princeton, Toronto, Rochester, and Indiana. Numerous revisions were made as a consequence of points raised during these sessions. I have also benefitted from comments and criticisms by M.J. Bailey, R.K. Chandra, M.G. Coopersmith, E. Crimmins, J. Cropsey, P.A. David, L.E. Davis, N. Davis, G.R. Elton, A. Fishlow, R.A. Easterlin, F. Furet, D. Galenson, R.E. Gallman, H. Goldstein, M.R. Haines, R. Hellie, J.A. Henretta, S. Horton, T.A. Huertas, H.C. Johansen, D.G. Johnson, W. Kruskal, P. Laslett, E.P. Lazear, S.E. Lehmberg, M. Livi-Bacci, T. McKeown, W.H. McNeill, L. Neal, D.C. North, G.H. Pelto, S. Peltzman, S.H. Preston, M.G. Reid, J.C. Riley, A. Sen, W.C. Sanderson, R.S. Schofield, T.W. Schultz, N.S. Scrimshaw, S.G. Scrikantia, J.L. Simon, S. Stigler, C.E. Taylor, B. Thomas, R.H. Tilly, E. van de Walle, S.C. Watkins, S.B. Webb, E.A. Wrigley, and W. Zelinsky.

The findings presented in this article are tentative and subject to change. They do not necessarily reflect the views of the NBER or any other cooperating institutions or funding agencies.

2. J.R. Gibson and T. McKeown, 'Observations on All Births (23,970) in Birmingham, 1947. I: Duration of Gestation. III. Survival', *Brit. J. Soc. Med.,* 4 (1950), pp. 221-233; 5 (1951), pp. 177-183; Gibson and McKeown (1951), II: Birth Weight, pp. 98-112.

3. T. McKeown, *The Modern Rise of Population* (New York 1976a).

4. T. McKeown, 'Fertility, Mortality and Cause of Death: an Examination of Issues Related to the Modern Rise of Population', *Population Studies,* 32 (1978), pp. 535-542, p. 540.

5. McKeown (1976a), p. 122; McKeown (1978), p. 540.

6. McKeown (1976a), p. 105.

7. McKeown (1976a), p. 136.

380

8. E. Meeker, 'The Improving Health of the United States, 1850-1915', *Explor. Econ. Hist,* 9 (1972), pp. 353-373; R. Higgs, 'Mortality in Rural America, 1870-1920: Estimates and Conjectures, *Explor. Econ. Hist.,* 10 (1973), pp. 177-195; R. Higgs, 'Cycles and Trends of Mortality in 18 Large American Cities, 1871-1900', *Explor. Econ. Hist.,* 16 (1979, pp. 381-408.

9. Higgs (1973), p. 189.

10. M. Livi-Bacci, 'The Nutrition-mortality Link in Past Times: A Comment', *Journal of Interdisciplinary History,* 14 (1983), pp. 293-298.

11. P.E. Razzell, 'An Interpretation of the Modern Rise of Population in Europe: A Critique', *Population Studies, 28* (1973), pp. 5-170, p. 8.

12. P.H. Lindert, 'English Living Standards, Population Growth, and Wrigley-Schofield', *Explor. Econ. Hist,* 20 (1983), pp. 131-155; R.A. Easterlin, 'Population Issues in American Economic History: a Survey and Critique', *Res. Econ. Hist.,* 1, Supplement (1977), pp. 131-158; M.A. Vinovskis, 'Mortality Rates and Trends in Massachusetts before 1860', *J. Econ. Hist.,* 32 (1972), pp. 184-213.

13. W.S. Thompson and P.K. Whelpton, *Population Trends in the United States* (New York 1933).

14. Y. Yasuba, *Birth Rates of the White Population in the United States 1800-1860* (1962).

15. R.S. Meindl, and A.C. Swedlund, 'Secular Trends in Mortality in the Connecticut Valley', *Hum. Bio.,* 49 (1977), pp.389-414. p. 398.

16. Razzell (1973), pp. 6-7.

17. Richard Hellie has called my attention to "the coincidence of the lowest life expectation (in Table 2 above) with the Maunder Minimum (the Little Ice Age)," and notes that "the declining life expectations of the English peerage parallels the worsening of the enserfment process in Russia, with the nadir of life expectations coinciding with the completion of the enserfment process." He suggests "that low yields and the generally unhealthier-than-usual climatic conditions" may have "played a role in driving both processes." From a letter to R.W. Fogel dated July 17, 1984.

18. A.B. Appleby, 'Nutrition and Disease: the Case of London, 1550-1750', *J. Interdiscip. Hist.,* 6 (1975), pp. 1-22.

19. R. Lee, 'Short-Term Variation: Vital Rates, Prices and Weather', E.A. Wrigley and R.S. Schofield (Eds.), *The Population History of England, 1541-1871: A Reconstruction* (Cambridge, Mass. 1981), pp. 356-401.

20. R. Schofield, 'The Impact of Scarcity and Plenty on Population Change in England, 1541-1871', *J. Interdiscip. Hist.,* 14 (1983), pp. 265-291. p. 282.

21. Lindert (1983), pp. 147-148.

22. S.H. Preston and E. van de Walle, 'Urban French Mortality in the Nineteenth Century', *Population Studies,* 32 (1978), pp. 275-297.

23. Preston and van de Walle (1978), p. 218.

24. From comments made at the Bellagio Conference on Hunger and History, June, 1982.

25. The decline in the mortality rates of low-income countries since 1950 is even more remarkable than the mortality decline in the industrialized nations between 1700 and

1980. The less developed nations have accomplished in three decades what took two centuries or more in the industrialized nations. A significant part of this acceleration is due to the transfer of medical and economic technology from the industrialized nations to the less developed nations (cf. S.H. Preston, *Mortality Patterns in National Populations: With Special References to Recorded Causes of Death* (New York 1976); S.H. Preston, 'Causes and Consequences of Mortality Declines in Less Developed Countries During the Twentieth Century', R.A. Easterlin (Ed), *Population and Economic Change in Developing Countries* (Chicago 1980); S.H. Preston, *Resources, Knowledge, and Child Mortality: a Comparison of the U.S. in the Late Nineteenth Century and Developing Countries Today.* Paper presented at International Population Conference, Florence; June 1985.

26. T. McKeown and R.G. Brown, 'Medical Evidence Related to English Population Changes in the Eighteenth Century', *Population Studies,* 9 (1955), pp. 119-141.

27. Preston (1976).

28. E.H. Ackerknecht, 'Diseases in the Middle West', *Essays in the History of Medicine in Honor of David J. Davis* (Illinois 1952); N.S. Scrimshaw, 'Functional Consequences of Malnutrition for Human Populations: a Comment', *J. Interdiscip. Hist.,* 14 (1983), pp. 409-411; M.K. Matossian, 'Mold Poisoning and Population Growth in England and France, 1750-1850', *J. Econ. Hist.,* 44 (1984), pp. 669-686.

29. W.M.O. Moore, 'Prenatal Factors Influencing Intrauterine Growth: Clinical Implications', R. Boyd and F.C. Battaglia (Eds), *Perinatal Medicine* (London 1983); A.A. Kielmann, C. De Sweemer, D. Chernichovsky, I.S. Uberoi, N. Masih, C.E. Taylor, R.L. Parker, W.A. Reinke, D.N. Kakar and R.S.S. Sarma, *Child and Maternal Health Services in Rural India: The Narangwal Experiment. Vol. 1: Integrated Nutrition and Health* (Baltimore 1983); L.S. Hurley, *Developmental Nutrition* (Englewood Cliffs, N.J. 1980); R.H. Steckel, *The Health and Mortality of Slave Children Reconsidered: Were the Abolitionists Right?* mimeo, Ohio State Univ (1985).

30. P.M. Fitzhardinge and E.M. Steven, 'The Small-for-date-infant. I. Later growth patterns', *Pediatr.,* 49 (1972a), pp. 671-681; P.M. Fitzhardinge and E.M. Steven, 'The Small-for-date-infant. II. Neurological and intellectual sequelae', *Pediatr.,* 50 (1972b), pp. 50-57; I. Bjerre, 'Neurological Investigation of 5-year-old Children with Low Birth Weight', *Act. Paediatr. Scand.,* 64 (1975), pp. 33-43; H. McFarlane, 'Nutrition and Immunity' *Nutrition Reviews: Present Knowledge in Nutrition,* 4th ed (New York 1976); S. Shapiro, M.C. McCormick, B.H. Starfield, J.P. Krischer and D. Bross, 'Relevance of Correlates of Infant Deaths for Significant Morbidity at 1 Year of Age, *Am. J. Obstet. Gynecol.,* 136 (1980), pp. 363-373; R.E. Christianson, B.J. Van den Berg, L. Milkovich and F.W. Oechsli, 'Incidence of Congenital Anomalies among White and Black Live Births with Long-term Follow-up', *Am. J. Pub. H.,* 71 (1981), pp. 1333-1341; M.C. McCormick, 'The Contribution of Low Birth Weight to Infant Mortality and Childhood Morbidity. New England', *J. Med.,* 312 (1985), pp. 82-89.

31. A. Forsdahl, 'The Poor Living Conditions in Childhood and Adolescence: An Important Risk Factor for Arteriosclerotic Heart Disease?', *Brit. J. Soc. Med.,* 31 (1977), pp. 91-95; M.G. Marmot, M.J. Shipley and G. Rose, 'Inequalities in Death-specific Explanations of a General Pattern', *The Lancet,* 1 (1984), pp. 1003-1006.

32. Cf. J.G. Williamson, 'Urban Disamenities, Dark Satanic Mills, and the British Standard of Living Debate', *J. Econ. Hist.,* 41 (1981a), pp. 75-83; J.G. Williamson, 'Some Myths Die Hard—Urban Disamenities One More Time: A Reply', *J. Econ. Hist.,* 41 (1981b), pp. 905-907; J.G. Williamson, 'Was the Industrial Revolution Worth it? Disamenities and Death in 19th Century British Towns', *Explor. Econ. Hist.,* 19

(1982), pp. 221-245; S. Pollard, 'Sheffield and Sweet Auburn—Amenities and Living Standards in the British Industrial Revolution: A Comment', *J. Econ. Hist.,* 41 (1981), pp. 902-904.

33. M.W. Towne and W.D. Rasmussen, 'Farm Gross Product and Gross Investment in the Nineteenth Century', *Trends in the American Economy in the Nineteenth Century, Conference on Research in Income and Wealth vol. 255-315* (Princeton, N.J. 1960); R.E. Gallman, 'Commodity Output, 1839-1899', *Trends in the American Economy in the Nineteenth Century, Confer. on Research in Income and Wealth vol. 245* (Princeton, N.J. 1960),pp. 13-71; M.K. Bennett and R.H. Pierce, 'Changes in the American National Diet, 1879-1959', *Food Res. Instit. Stud.,* 2 (1961), pp. 95-119.

34. E. Meeker, 'Mortality Trends of Southern Blacks, 1850-1910: Some Preliminary Findings', *Explor. Econ. Hist.,* 13 (1976), pp. 13-42; R.W. Fogel and S.L. Engerman, *Time on the Cross* (Boston 1974); W.O. Atwater and C.D. Woods, 'Dietary Studies with Reference to the Food of the Negro in Alabama in 1895 and 1896', *U.S.D.A. Off. Exp. Stat. Bull.,* 38 (1897), p. 3-69; H.B. Frissell and I. Bevier, 'Dietary Studies of Negroes in Eastern Virginia in 1897 and 1898', *U.S.D.A. Off. Exp. Stat. Bull.,* 71 (1899); U.S. Dept. Lab., 'Conditions of Negroes in Various Cities', *Bull. No. 10* (1897).

35. Cf. R.W. Fogel, S.L. Engerman, R. Floud, R.A. Margo, K. Sokoloff, R.H. Steckel, J. Trussell, G.C. Villaflor and K.W. Wachter, 'Secular Changes in American and British Stature and Nutrition', *J. Interdiscip. Hist.,* 14 (1983), pp. 445-481.

36. G.A. Condran and E. Crimmins-Gardner, 'Public Health Measures and Mortality in U.S. Cities in the Late Nineteenth Century', *Hum. Ecol.,* 6 (1978), pp. 27-54.

37. G.A. Condran and E. Crimmins, 'Mortality Differentials Between Rural and Urban Areas of States in the Northeastern United States 1890-1900', *J. Hist. Geog.,* 6 (1980), pp. 179-202.

38. Preston (1976).

39. G.A. Condran and R.A. Cheney, 'Mortality Trends in Philadelphia: Age- and Cause-specific Death Rates 1870-1930', *Demography,* 19 (1982), pp. 97-123.

40. Higgs (1979).

41. The fact that the debate launched in the mid-1950s still continues should not distract attention from the considerable advances in knowledge that have occurred because of the debate. Investigators have probed increasingly into aspects of issues that were obscure at the outset. The point is well illustrated by the evolution of research on the pathways of airborne diseases. McKeown (1976a) stressed direct exposure; Preston and van de Walle (1978) called attention to the risk-increasing effects of the lowering of resistance to airborne pathogens brought about by infections caused by water-born pathogens. Thus, in the course of the debate the concept of nutritional status has been refined and the factors which affect it have been elaborated. Similarly, Condran and Cheney (1982) have provided evidence that medical intervention became increasingly effective before the dramatic chemical breakthroughs that became apparent during and after World War II. However, the extent of mortality reduction due to these less dramatic contributions has yet to be measured.

42. E.A. Wrigley and R.S. Schofield, 'English Population History from Family Reconstitution: Summary Results 1600-1799', *Population Studies,* 37 (1983), pp. 157-184; Preston and van de Walle (1978), pp. 275-297; M.R. Haines, *Inequality and Child Mortality: a Comparison of England and Wales, 1911 and the United States, 1900,* mimeo, Wayne State Univ (1983); S.H. Preston and M.R. Haines, *New Estimates of Child Mortality in the United States at the Turn of the Century,* mimeo, Univ. of Pennsylvania (1983).

383

Hospitalization, Birth Weight and Nutrition in Montreal and Vienna 1850-1930

W. Peter Ward

We still know very little about the benefits which social welfare institutions conferred upon the poor in the days before the welfare state. In fact we often seem to think that they provided no benefits at all. From our present vantage point the Victorian poor house, the orphanage and the asylum seem very bleak places indeed.[1] Yet the basis for this assessment is not wholly clear and it often seems to rest on rather slender evidence. The hungry Oliver Twist's famous cry for gruel — "please Sir, I want some more" — is as damning an indictment of institutional care as any in nineteenth century literature but it is the product of a literary imagination, not a social enquiry. The politics of early twentieth century reform often rested on the Dickensian view. The assumption that the poor got little benefit from agencies formed to assist them justified the move toward state welfare programs and the growth of the helping professions which they spawned. But was this assumption correct? Were the charities of former times as ineffectual as they sometimes seem in retrospect? This paper brings new evidence to bear on this question.

The evidence comes from the patient registers of two lyingin hospitals, the little-known Montreal Maternity (between 1851 and 1905) and the celebrated Geburtskliniken of the Allgemeines Krankenhaus in Vienna (between 1872 and 1930).[2] At the outset it must be admitted that, in one important respect, the premodern maternity justified pessimistic assessments about nineteenth century philanthropies. Before the development of antibacterial drugs, lying-in hospitals were dangerous places for patients. Intermittent cycles of high maternal mortality plagued most of these institutions, in part because they normally cared for an impoverished and unhealthy clientele, in part because they provided congenial places for the spread of puerperal septicemia. During the first half of the nineteenth century the Geburtskliniken in Vienna were notorious for recurrent outbreaks of childbed fever, events which led Ignaz Semmelweis to his well known contributions to an evolving theory of disease transmission.[3] But mortality rates are not the only test of an institution's contributions to well-being, and when we look beyond them to other measures we can see the lying-in hospital in a somewhat different light.

In this instance the weight of children born in these hospitals provides us with another yardstick. Weight at birth is one of the most common indices of infant well-being employed by the health professions today. Throughout the developed and much of the developing world, babies are routinely weighed within moments of their delivery. The optimum weight of a newborn child lies between 3000 and 4500 grams. Infants weighing either less or more are exposed to greater risks of illness and death than those whose weight is optimal. The more birth weight falls below this lower limit, in particular, the more the risk increases. For many years common therapeutic practice in western hospitals has been to designate newborns weighing less than 2500 grams as low birth weight infants and to provide them with intensive care. At present many hospitals also give special treatment to babies between 2500 and 3000 grams. Because of its close association with higher levels of morbidity and mortality, low birth weight is a primary health problem in the developed and the developing world today. In most western nations low birth weight is largely the result of premature birth, the causes of which are complex and not fully understood. In most non-western nations, where the problem is far more widespread, it is largely the result of malnutrition.

But nutrition is not the sole determinant of neonatal weight. Three sets of factors combine to influence the weight of a child at birth: genetic, medical and socioeconomic. A mother's genetic legacy to her infant (and to a slight extent a father's too) has an important bearing on the birth weight of her baby. Her health before and during the pregnancy, and the health of her unborn child, also affect the course of fetal development and its outcome. Among socio-economic factors (which include income, education and social class), nutrition is particularly important. One recent analysis indicates that between 40 % and 50 % of the variance in birth weight at the end of normal pregnancies within a homogeneous social group may be due to nutritional factors.[4] For this reason, when used with care, birth weight data may help us understand the nutritional condition of past populations. The patients of these two hospitals offer two cases in point.

At the outset the social composition and functions of each institution must be identified. These two hospitals, like virtually all public maternities in Western Europe and North America before the twentieth century, served poor women who needed charitable aid in childbirth. The Montreal hospital fulfilled this function throughout the period considered here.[5] Most of its patients were British immigrants for, in the manner of that city, a similar Roman Catholic institution existed for poor French Canadian women. Between 2 % and 3 % of civic births occurred at the Montreal Maternity annually. The Allgemeines Krankenhaus Geburtskliniken were probably the largest maternity clinics in the western world at this time. Between 8000 and 12,000 deliveries took place in them annually during the 60 years of this study. These constituted just under 20 % of all Viennese births before 1910, the proportion rising to about 40 % by 1930. Like the Montreal Maternity the Geburtskliniken served a poor and largely unmarried clientele until the early twentieth century. But thereafter the growing sophistication of obstetric practice and the rising popularity of hospital delivery attracted an increasing number of patients from more advantaged social classes. Thus, as the hospital assumed a more a modern role, it lost some — but by no means all — of its charitable functions. In 1930 its patients remained predominantly working class.

In addition to providing medical aid to women in childbirth birth hospitals also sheltered some patients for extended periods before their children were born. Then, as now, a majority gave birth soon after their admission but in both institutions a significant minority arrived more than a week in advance. In Vienna one patient in five was hospitalized for eight days or more, and one in ten stayed at least three weeks. The proportions in Montreal were even higher, two in five and three in ten respectively.[6] As a result, because patients received institutional care for varying lengths of time in the prenatal period it is possible to examine the relationship between hospitalization and weight at birth.

The duration of institutional care before delivery is particularly important because, while the rate of fetal weight gain is greatest during the third trimester, it diminishes toward the end of the normal gestational period. The fetus of a woman who spent less than a week in hospital before her due date would not likely be greatly affected by the hospital environment. In part this would be because the period itself was short, in part because the rate of weight gain would have slowed by this time. The longer a woman remained under hospital care, however, the longer she was exposed to institutional influences and the greater the exposure during that period when the rate of fetal weight gain was more rapid. A woman who spent upwards of three weeks in hospital before delivery would experience its effects for a significant part of the time in which her unborn child was growing most quickly.

The two population samples examined here were constituted in the following way. The Montreal clinic records list all patients who attended the hospital between 1851 and 1905. All live, single born infants delivered at full term (280 days plus or minus 14) were selected for analysis.[7] In Vienna, because the annual number of births was far greater, 200 cases were chosen randomly from the patient records of Clinic 1 for all years but one between 1872 and 1930. (The exception was 1882, in which weights were not recorded for one three month period and therefore only 150 were noted.) From this population all live born singleton infants were selected. In the absence of reliable information on gestational age all infants weighing less than 1500 grams were then excluded from the sample, thus removing the most obviously premature from the analysis. This eliminates the exaggerated biases created by the intermittent presence of extremely low values but it does not discard all premature infants as was done in the analysis of the Montreal data.

In both hospitals the longer women remained in hospital care before their children were born the heavier their infants were on average (see Table 1)

Table 1. Weight at birth by length of hospitalization before delivery.

Days	Montreal Weight (g)	Std. Dvn. (g)	N	Vienna Weight (g)	Std. Dvn (g)	N
0—7	3453	545	1876	3108	487	7360
8—21	3468	541	409	3197	470	1037
22+	3539	533	911	3241	447	1003

In Montreal, women who came to the maternity two or three weeks before delivery bore children 15 grams heavier than those who remained a week or less. The difference is relatively slight and is probably not significant. Patients who stayed more than three weeks delivered infants 85 grams heavier than those of short term cases and in this instance the difference is considerable. The differences for comparable periods of care in Vienna were somewhat greater still — 89 grams for intermediate term and 133 grams for long term patients respectively.[8] Graphs 1 and 2 indicate the trends over time.

Here the data have been further aggregated and slightly smoothed because of the small size of some cells. Each graph reveals the high consistency with which the infants of long staying mothers outweighed those of short staying patients.

Figure 1. Vienna: Mean birth weight by duration of hospital stay. Three year running average.

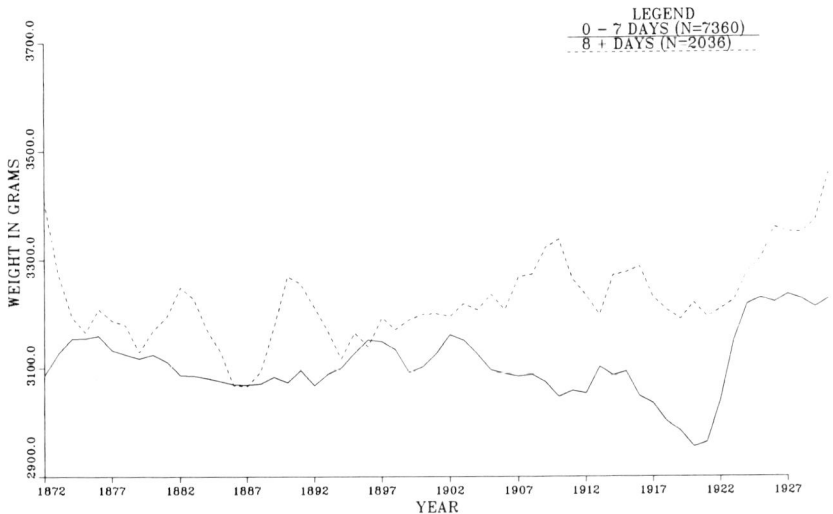

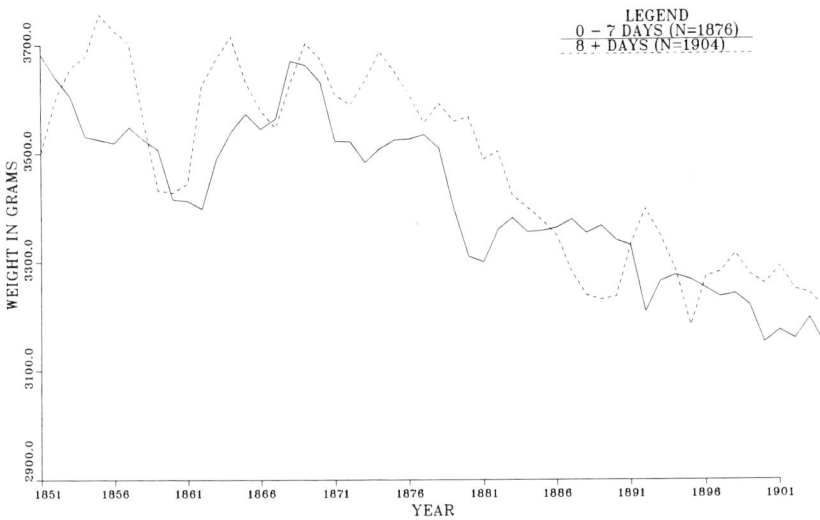

Figure 2. Montreal: Mean birth weight by duration of hospital stay. Three year running average.

The clinical records of each hospital offer no indication that the patients who came to the maternity well before delivery did so for medical reasons.[9] Among Viennese patients place of residence, marital status and occupation were most strongly correlated with length of hospitalization. Women who lived in Vienna were hospitalized slightly more than four days before delivery on average while those from outside the city remained three times as long.[10] Younger patients stayed a day longer than older ones and the unmarried remained twice as long as the married.[11] Domestic servants and the unemployed stayed twice as long as other occupational categories.[12] The special needs of unmarried and unemployed pregnant women are largely self evident. Nor are those of domestics particularly obscure. In Vienna as elsewhere pregnant servants commonly were dismissed when unsympathetic employers discovered their condition. Thus the internal evidence indicates that the women who came to Geburtsklinik 1 long before their babies were due did so because they lived far away or because they needed charitable aid.

The Montreal records list neither occupation nor place of residence and therefore are somewhat less informative. Nevertheless they support the conclusions just reached. On average patients came to the hospital two days earlier during the cold months of the year than the warm ones, a reflection of Montreal's notoriously harsh climate.[13] As in Vienna, younger patients remained longer than older, in this case by five days; the unmarried outstayed the married by nine days.[14] But two other facts emerge from this data which are less easy to explain. Protestants were hospitalized five days longer than Catholics and the Canadian born five days longer than immigrants.[15] This suggests the existence of a more effective, informal system of mutual aid among Catholics and newcomers than among Protestants and the native born in nineteenth century Quebec. Perhaps this was true but, if so, this is the first sign we have seen of the fact.

If the explanation for longer hospital sojourns is not medical, and if no evident differences exist between patients with short and extended sojourns except those which were rooted in place of residence and economic vulnerability, then the higher birth weights of infants who came early to hospital must almost certainly have been due to the care they received while there. The care itself was simple. In essence it consisted of rest and regular meals. Most women in these hospitals were used to hard physical work. The great majority of unmarried Viennese patients were domestic servants and unskilled or semiskilled labourers. Married women laboured hard at home unpaid. Although we have no occupational information on the Montreal patients there is no reason to suspect that they were fundamentally different. By relieving these women from the burden of work, hospitalization reduced their nutritional requirements. At the same time the patients received regular meals, freeing at least the destitute from the haphazard diets which must otherwise have been their lot. The ultimate effect for patients was to increase their average net nutritional intake.[16]

Graph 1 offers further support for this conclusion. Between 1915 and 1922 the Austrian economy progressively collapsed under the cumulative burdens of warfare and post-war imperial dismemberment. Food shortages were serious throughout this period, especially during the hyperinflation of the early 1920's. The mean birth weight of infants in the Vienna sample dropped continuously at this time, reaching a low of 2977 grams in 1921. As Graph 1 reveals, however, the women who delivered soon after their arrival absorbed virtually all of the decline. On average those with extended institutional care bore children with weights slightly below those of their pre-war counterparts but without the sharp decline revealed in the infants of short stay mothers. Hospitalization shielded longer residents from the worst effects of the crisis.

The French physician Adolphe Pinard, a pioneer in the movement to promote antenatal care for pregnant women, was the first to detect a relationship between institutional care before delivery and elevated birth weight levels. In 1895 he published a study of 1500 Parisian mothers, 500 who had worked until just before delivery and 1000 who had spent at least 10 days in one of two refuges before giving birth. Those from the refuges bore children 140 to 180 grams heavier than those without extended institutional care.[17] Pinard also offered evidence that women who worked were more likely to deliver prematurely. As a result he emphasized the importance of rest during the later stages of pregnancy to maternal well-being and fetal development, and he called on the state to intervene in the interests of both, not to say the nation and the species.

> Au point de vue de l'humanité, au point de vue de l'augmentation de la
> population, au point de vue de l'évolution de la race francaise, il est

390

nécessaire, il est urgent que les pouvoirs publiques interviennent pour protéger la femme enceinte, pendant les trois derniers mois de sa grossesse, et le foetus pendant les trois derniers mois de sa vie intra-uterine.[18]

In subsequent years other European studies confirmed Pinard's major findings and also demonstrated a relationship between arduous work and lower birth weight levels.[19] The German Doctor Karl Fuchs provided evidence contradicting the argument that women with strenuous occupations delivered lighter babies than those without. But he too noted the beneficial effects of hospitalization: "Geregelte Lebensweise, Ruhe, gute Kost".[20] By the early twentieth century the importance of rest in the later months of pregnancy had gained wide acceptance in the medical profession.[21]

The Austrian physician Sigismund Peller examined the influence of hospital care upon birth weight more carefully than did any other investigator during this period. Through a series of studies between 1913 and 1924, on patients from a separate Geburtsklinik in the Vienna Allgemeines Krankenhaus, he "confirmed the dependence of foetal development upon maternal nutrition and maternal physical rest".[22] In later life Peller claimed to have challenged established erroneous opinion on the subject but in fact he did little more than place greater emphasis on the importance of nutrition to birth weight than his predecessors had done. After Peller, however, interest in this facet of research on fetal growth lapsed. The influence of hospital care upon birth weight is not a factor considered in recent research, nor has it been since the 1920's.

Despite its limitations the work of Pinard, Peller and others supports the argument set forth in this paper. Most early investigators employed small cross-sectional samples from a single point in time, and all of them neglected long term trends. In an age when knowledge of the energy value of foods was still rudimentary most concluded that rest, which could readily be observed, caused the higher birth weights yielded by mothers with extended institutional prenatal care. Only Peller attempted to assess the independent role of nutrition and he failed to recognize the close relationship between increased rest and improvements in net nutrition. But the two were opposite sides of a single coin. Thus the benefits obtained from increased rest were fundamentally those of improved nutritional welfare.

The long term trends examined here derived from two maternity hospitals with broadly similar medical and social functions, but strikingly different cultural, socio-economic and national contexts. In the face of such great differences in setting the similar relationships between extended hospital care and higher birth weight levels are all the more striking. By themselves these bits of evidence do not call for a wholesale re-evaluation of nineteenth century voluntarist philanthropy. But they do suggest that common assumptions about the inadequacy of social welfare institutions in the past are simplistic and rather too negative. There can be little doubt that the women who took refuge in these institutions for prolonged stays fared much better than if they had not come, and better as well than those who did not enjoy the same advantages. For the former hospitalization brought significant and measurable, if short term, benefit. For their children the result was a better start in life.

Acknowledgements

I wish to thank Elizabeth Mancke, Virginia Green and Frank Flynn for their advice and assistance. This project is funded by the Hannah Institute for the History of Medicine, a division of Associated Medical Services, Toronto, Canada.

Notes

1. For example see M.W. Flinn, 'Medical Services under the New Poor Law', D. Frazer (Ed) *The New Poor Law in the Nineteenth Century,* (London 1976) in which Flinn describes the care of the sick in workhouse infirmaries as "a standing reproach to a nation which thought of itself as civilized." p. 55.

2. The Montreal Maternity Hospital patient records are deposited at the McGill University Archives, Montreal. The Allgemeines Krankenhaus records are housed at the Wiener Stadt) und Landsarchiv in Vienna.

3. E. Lesky, *The Vienna Medical School of the 19th Century* (Baltimore 1976), pp. 181-91.

4. J. Metcoff, 'Maternal Nutrition and Fetal Development', *Early Human Development,* 4, 2 (1980), p. 101.

5. R.R. Kenneally *'The Montreal Maternity, 1843-1926'*, M.A. thesis, McGill University (1983).

6. In Vienna the proportion staying eight days or more was 21.7 %, twentytwo days or more, 10.6 %. In Montreal the proportions were 41.3 % and 28.5 %.

7. W.P. Ward and P.C. Ward, 'Infant Birth Weight and Nutrition in Industrializing Montreal', *American Historical Review,* 89 (1984), pp. 329-30.

8. Some categories of births in these hospitals were not evenly distributed between short and long term stays; in Montreal and Vienna the birth order of the child and, in Montreal, gestational age were distributed slightly unevenly. As both of these factors influence weight at birth their distributional patterns might possibly affect the mean weights when considered by length of stay. In all instances, however, the distributional differences were small and tended to offset one another. Women bearing their first child were slightly overrepresented among long staying patients but this influence was counteracted by the slight overrepresentation of multiparous women who were short staying patients. In the Montreal data the proportion of premature children was slightly higher among short than long staying patients. Because premature births were excluded from the Montreal analysis these births had no effect on the weight means analyzed here. But in consequence the presence of a slight surplus of premature births among short term patients in Vienna may be suspected and, if this were true, it would tend to inflate the influence of hospitalization on birth weight.

9. S. Peller, *Quantitative Research in Human Biology and Medicine* (Bristol 1967), p. 133.

10. The mean length of stay for women from working class districts was 4.1 days, for those from better districts 4.6 days and from neighboring Lower Austria 12.2 days.

11. The mean length of stay for women 25 and under was 6.9 days, for women 26 and older 5.8 days. The unmarried stayed 6.7 days on average, the married 3.1 days.

12. Domestics stayed 7.0 days, the unemployed 7.1 days and all other occupational categories between 2 and 4 days.

13. During October to March the mean stay was 18.4 days while from April to September it was 16.4 days.

14. Women 25 and under stayed 19.0 days on average while those older stayed 14.0 days. The unmarried remained in hospital 19.7 days while the married stayed only 10.6 days.

15. The mean duration of stay in each instance was: Protestants — 19.5 days, Catholics — 14.8 days, Canadian born — 20.5 days, immigrants — 15.0 days.

16. Net nutrition is nutrition "after the claims of work and of the disease environment have been met". J. Komlos, 'Patterns of Children's Growth in East-central Europe in the Eighteenth Century', *Annals of Human Biology,* 13, 1 (1986), p. 43.

17. A. Pinard, 'Note pour servir a l'histoire de la puericulture intrauterine', *Bulletin de l'academie de medecine,* 3 serie, 34 (1895), pp. 593-97.

18. A. Pinard *Clinique Obstétricale* (Paris 1899), p. 60.

19. G. Pechin, *Contributions a l'étude de la puériculture avant la naissance. Etude statistique du poids des enfants nés a la clinique Baudelocque de 1890 a 1907,* M. D. These, Faculté de Médecine de Paris (1908); E. Grenier, *Quelques documents concernant la durée de la gestation et le poids de l'enfant a terme.* (Statistique de la Clinique obstétricale de Bordeaux, 1898-1912), (Bordeaux 1913); H.T. Ashby, *Infant Mortality* (Cambridge 1915), p. 62.

20. K. Fuchs, *Die Abhängigkeit des Geburtsgewichtes des Neugeboren vom Stand und der Beschäftigung der Mutter,* M. D. Dissertation, medizinischen Fakultät, Friedrichs-Universität Halle-Wittenberg (1879), p. 46.

21. For example the prominent Scottish doctor W.L. Mackenzie observed in 1906, "It is probable that the poorer child suffers from long before birth because the mother is not permitted to rest during pregnancy". Mackenzie, *The Health of the School Child* (London 1906), p. 38.

22. Peller (1967), pp. 131-38.

Mortality: Trends, Fluctuations and their Socio-Cultural Background

Gösta Carlsson

History and the epidemiology of death

Explaining demographic events in the past may be made a little easier by reflection on the lessons to be drawn from the study of more recent problems. Even if the conclusions sometimes turn out to be negative they are nonetheless relevant. Forewarned is forearmed, and our difficulties with the contemporary situation will serve as a caution not to expect rapid progress with historical aspects, nor be unduly discouraged by the absence of clear-cut results.

Also, we should not be too hasty in blaming our uncertainties on the remoteness of the phenomena, and on the paucity of data. Differential mortality can be a hard nut to crack even when modern research technology is applied to something occurring before our eyes. As an example, Finnish middle-aged men suffered from phenomenally high death rates, and this as late as the 1970's. This placed them more or less outside the range of variation among developed countries, an indisputable fact and surely a striking one. The writer is not aware that a satisfactory explanation has yet been found. As a more remote problem one could mention the disappearance (for practical purposes) of plague from Western Europe after the great London outbreak in 1665. Various explanations have been put forward but do not seem adequate, either taken singly or in combination, despite the existence of excellent covering laws on parasite, hosts and vectors.[1]

For more constructive hints the story of cancer research may be consulted. If the causal role of cigarette smoking for lung cancer can be regarded as firmly established this is largely because the epidemiological evidence is unusually clear and consistent.[2] Cross-sectional and time-series analyses of national populations point in this direction, and so do individual-level risk studies of smokers versus non-smokers. Whatever doubts may have remained are dispelled by the obvious relation to a classical carcinogen, tar. One conclusion, then, is that a broad spectrum of methods and theorizing need to be applied, here ranging from the population to the molecular level (the genetics and chemistry of carcinogenesis). On the other hand, given this convergence, quite unsophisticated methods of analysis have sometimes proved sufficient, with respect to time and trend analyses little more than visual inspection of time paths. For other locations of cancer equally strong differentials and trends exist, e.g. for cancer of the stomach, yet no explanation has been found.

Turning to the secular decline of mortality in Sweden and Western Europe, its early onset in relation to advances in clinical medicine has long been accepted as evidence against curative medicine as the main cause, say before 1900. Much of the international writing is unavoidably coloured by the English experience, which is the experience of a markedly urbanized society in which progress in sanitation and preventive medicine could have strong effects, especially on water-borne infection. For Swedish demographic history this factor would seem of limited importance as the country long remained rural, though some of the great improvement in the Stockholm rates might be ascribed to the advent of piped drinking water and sewage disposal in the later decades of the 19th century.

For a time the view of McKeown prevailed, that the main forces behind the decline were advances in material conditions, especially nutrition and possibly housing standards.[3] It is well-known that this theory has come under attack, for instance in a recent volume on population change with emphasis on Swedish problems[4] and also in an earlier one on the European experience.[5] Before we proceed to examine some of the empirical evidence and the pro's and con's in the matter, thought has to be given to the alternatives initially open to the historians, demographers and sociologists trying to get a clearer understanding of that supremely important fact, the great mortality decline.

Mortality and the bounds of the possible

It is tempting to follow a method of exclusion when one is dealing with a phenomenon like mortality and its variation over time and space. If certain factors can be successively ruled out, or relegated to a secondary role, the field is narrowed down and we may feel almost compelled to accept what remains. The use of this principle among writers was discernible when existing theories of health and survival were examined some years ago in connection with a study of health in a population perspective.[6] At the time McKeown's solution, improved living conditions behind the mortality decline, seemed reasonable enough. Other possibilities like curative medicine, sanitation, or changes in the virulence of pathogens and resistance of the human hosts, appeared less plausible or too speculative. Yet the dangers of the method were plain; certain alternatives might be dismissed too quickly, and the final one not handled critically enough. In fact, having been critical for a while we might end by grasping at straws. One difficulty was then noticeable with regard to the nutrition (and housing) answer, the very limited advantage privileged groups, like the ruling houses or the aristocracy, seemed to enjoy. The historical record was consulted very imperfectly and there may well exist cases of a greater demonstrated advantage in longevity among the rich and powerful. Still, this does not appear to be a dependable fact.

It should be added immediately that the issue is a complex one. Thus, the single major experimental study known to the author, the Minnesota starvation study, failed to reveal any clear relation between undernourishment and infection, with the significant exception of tuberculosis of the lungs.[7]

What now seems the most glaring weakness in the line of reasoning described above (also followed by the author in his earlier writing on the subject) lies in the omission of yet another factor beside sanitary reforms, host-parasite ecology (including climate) and nutrition. The missing complex is of a behavioral-cultural nature and includes several elements with a corresponding range of possible labels, e.g. health-related behaviors, life-styles, folk-medicine, or self-care practices. No claim is made that the idea is entirely new or that the role of such behavioral facts has been entirely neglected in the literature. Breast-feeding belongs to this category and has been extensively studied as it affects infant mortality;[8] we may here leave on one side its bearing on fecundability and fertility. The cultural dimension has been explicitly recognized with regard to breast-feeding and child care.[9] With respect to adult mortality there is less to build on, and it is understandable if researchers should find such a mixed bag of hypothetical influences uninviting; there is certainly a risk of ending up with all too many intangibles. Yet there is nothing mystical or far-fetched in the notion. An extreme case of protection through a cultural factor is cited by McNeill; a group of nomad hunters successfully evaded the dangers of infection from the rodents they hunted though these provided a reservoir of infection for *Pasteurella pestis*.[10] A set of rules had evolved that served admirably to minimize the danger. For these rules, however, only magical reasons could be given by the actors. Even if we cannot expect demonstration cases of this order in the 19th or even 18th century setting of Sweden behavioral-cultural hypotheses deserve more attention.

Death rates in a 200-year perspective

It will be helpful to compare different age-groups and their mortality response over longer stretches of time with an eye to finding more, or less sensitive ages and thereby clues to causal agents. The plan is less easy to carry out than might be surmised for difficulties are met at the most elementary level What is the larger, or the smaller change with rates at different levels, as for young people versus the ages above 40 or 50? A little of the same difficulty makes itself felt when male and female rates are compared. In the absence of a true model or theory of mortality (in a general sense) our choice of descriptive parameters will be a highly intuitive affair with consequent weaknesses in the interpretation of numerical results.

As a rough solution the total amount of change between the second half of the 18th century and our own time, for any given age category and separately for men and women, will be taken as the unit. The highly variable magnitude of this change in terms of the number of deaths per thousand, e.g. for early middle life versus old age, is neglected. The total shift could be thought of as the gap between "traditional" and "modern" mortality, or even as a measure of "preventible" death, though both characterizations are misleading to some extent. There is clearly no such thing as a fully stable, traditional level, nor can we safely assume that the rates of the 1970's and early 1980's will remain stationary though they change little over a decade. And modern mortality still contains "preventible" death, notably vascular disease and cancer among the middle-aged and older which might be avoided or postponed through dietary and environmental reforms. Equally, violent death (mainly suicide and accidents) plays a role among young people which cannot be regarded as a fixed, biological condition.

For any given five-year the mean rate 1751-1800 (D_1) serves as indicator of "traditional" mortality while the 1976-1980 rate (D_4) is used for "modern" mortality. Two intermediate values are formed from the 1851-1855 (D_2) and 1896-1900 (D_3) rates. Early change (E) is defined as the difference D_1-D_2, middle change (M) as the difference D_2-D_3, and late change (L) as the difference D_3-D_4, where all these differences are divided by total change D_1-D_4. By necessity, then, the sum $E+M+L$ equals 1 and as mentioned above no judgement can be passed on the magnitude of total change for one age-group versus another, a price paid for the solution. The results are shown in Figure 1. They are, of course, in general predictable from the known facts of the secular decline but are nonetheless striking and worth some comment.

Figure 1. Distribution between Early (E), Middle (M), and Late (L) change in Mortality.
E Change from traditional to 1851-1855 level
M Change from 1851-1855 to 1896-1900 level
L Change from 1896-1900 to modern level.
For explanations, see text. First observation infant mortality.

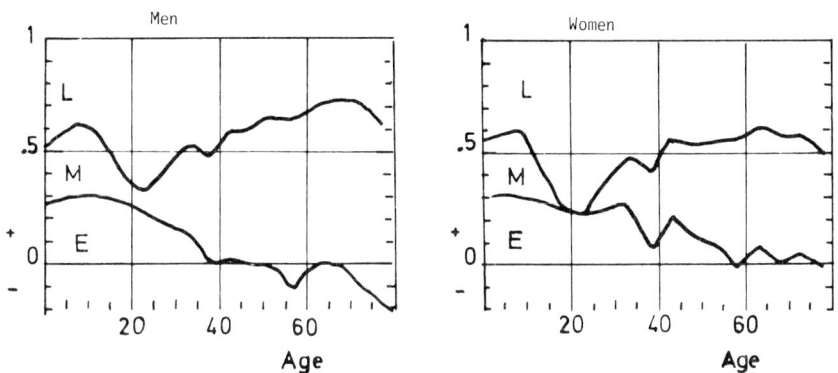

It is immediately apparent that three broader age-categories can be distinguished though the boundaries are not absolutely sharp. There is first infancy and childhood, with the total decline relatively well distributed between the three sub-periods. There is some change in the early 19th century (and indeed earlier) but there is further and continuous decline into this century. Next we have adolescence and early adulthood, roughly between 15 and 25 or 30. Here there is still early change, some of it perhaps a "spill-over" from the childhood effects, whether for medical or socio-cultural reasons. On the other hand, the latter part of the 19th century is something of a lost half-century. The rates decline very little, especially among women. Much of the historical change in this age-span takes place in the 20th century.

For the ages over 30 or 35 the picture again looks different. There is little or no early change (though too much should not be made of the reversals, the negative change visible in the graph). To that extent, and seen entirely in the light of trends, a nutrition and economic-growth explanation of declining death rates faces less difficulty for the population over 35. After 1850 there is a very marked fall in death rates for these ages. In fact, much of total, traditional to modern change for the middle-aged and older is an event of the second half of the 19th century. Late change (after 1900) contributes relatively little among men, somewhat more for women.

At this point some words of caution are in order. Dependence on a single five-year time period, 1851-1855, with the wobbly rates then prevailing, introduces some uncertainty. In further work it will be desirable to start from smoothed data (later rates present much less of this problem as noted earlier). As a check the 1846-1850 rates were used instead, these are generally a little lower and raise the bottom curves, the E-M boundary, somewhat. It can be reported, however, that the results are not affected in essentials, the same typology appears with much the same strength.

A second remark is that the constraint of the method needs to be remembered, i.e. the imposition of a forced unity sum of the terms E, M and L. Thus, the dominance of M among men past their youth (and to a somewhat lesser degree among women) could point to medical or social stagnation in the 20th century, a failure of further death prevention, as well as to rapid progress 1850-1900.

It still remains to find the causes behind these differences and distributions, be they social, medical or of some other origin. There is a reasonable suspicion that falling alcohol consumption was an important factor in the progress of the 1850-1900 period among middle-aged and older men. This, presumably, affected women less. If one looks at the original rates these improved more for men than for women. Age-group for age-group, women still enjoyed lower rates around 1900 but the distance to the male rates had shrunk. There is nonetheless a basic similarity between the male and the female rates in their general course which argues against a heavy stress on explanations built exclusively on the situation of men.

The aberrant case of adolescents and young adults would seem to lead to tuberculosis and its causes as a part of the answer. The age- and sex-incidence of tuberculosis in this century is in agreement with this interpretation.[11] The sustained and more evenly distributed change for children, with an early onset, requires a different explanation again, in the direction of child-care practices mentioned earlier, perhaps even a more fundamental change of attitudes toward children and the value of young lives.

Mortality fluctuations

The manifestations of change we have to contend with are further illustrated in Figure 2 by the curves for infant mortality and mortality in the age span 30-59. The latter, built on rates for five-year age intervals and standardized by the 1880 Swedish age-distribution could be expected to respond to environmental and life-style changes among adults, and is sometimes applied to modern data for this reason. It is certainly desirable to separate infant (and early childhood) rates from these pertaining to adults, but the first impression is one of close agreement in trends between the two. The accidents of scale are partly responsible for this impression, but there is also agreement in some of the early peaks and troughs; for the middle and late 19th century the impression fades. As with other demographic series, notably fertility and nuptiality, one is struck by the gradual dampening of the marked oscillations

Figure 2. Death rates and wage index. 5-year values.

A Mortality 30-59, per 1000
B Infant mortality, per 100
C Wage index.

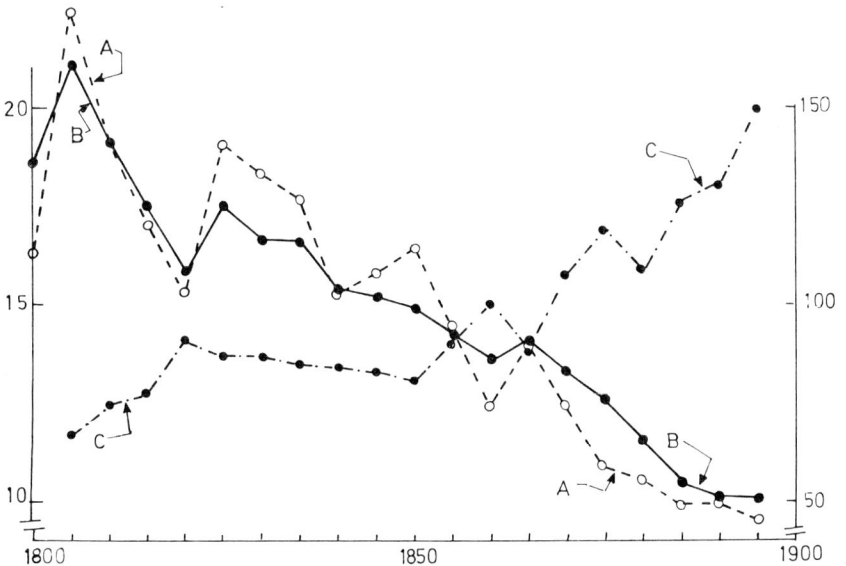

characteristic of the early 19th century, the series gradually become "all trend". From the technical point of view this introduces a worrisome lack of stationarity in variance.

As the series in Figure 2 are composed of five-year averages they are not suitable for a study of short-run fluctuations, from year to year; to these we will return in a moment. Meanwhile it may be noted that the third curve appearing in Figure 2, which stands for a wage index deflated by cost of living brings out one difficulty with the classical income and nutrition theory.[12] There is little sign of a sustained improvement before the 1850's as far as this indicator can tell us though death rates had then fallen appreciably. This weakness has been more fully discussed by Fridlizius, who finds little evidence for rising standards before the middle of the century.[13]

It is out of the question to attempt any kind of review of the rapidly growing body of time-series analysis on annual data. Caution dictates a judgment of conflicting results (or interpretations) and the absence of a clear consensus on the ties between short-run economic fluctuation and short-run mortality changes. Within the present study the relationship between deflated agricultural wages and mortality series was probed. The period is 1820-1865, to avoid the disturbances of the earliest part of the century and of the late 1860's. The results can best be described as indecisive though not without signs of the expected negative correlation. For adult mortality (30-59) first differences were used, for infant mortality both first differences and residuals from the linear trend, which could be fitted with some success in this case. The adult rate shows only a weak relationship with correlations below -.20 and with no evidence of improvement through the inclusion of a lagged value of wages. For infant mortality first differences give a correlation -.451 (R^2 = .204) with the index of wages, again on the basis of first differences. The outcome is acceptable by the Watson-Durbin criterion (d = 2.52). If one combines the last with the preceding first difference for wages the relationship weakens. The latter method produces stronger relations with nuptiality and fertility, and these can be cited to give a standard of comparison. Here we have an R^2 equal to .423 for the fertility series (overall measure of marital fertility 20-45) and .517 for the marriage rate. Again residuals show acceptable low autocorrelations.

While the outcome cannot be called entirely negative it gives no firm support to a nutrition-based model; it may well be that weather conditions, as has been suggested in the literature, are acting independently on harvest and infection risks. Fridlizius and Ohlsson found the pattern of mortality variations and economic conditions a complex matter, with quite modest statistical effects, varying from one phase of the transition to the next.[14] Like other authors they also point to the lack of a dependable connection between the two facts when one looks at different regions. It remains to discuss variability in space as an analogue to variation over time, this will form the subject of the next section.

Two remarks should be added to the discussion of mortality and nutrition (or other similar variables). First the implications of a weak or non-existent relationship for the interpretation of fertility variations. As is well known there were large annual fluctuations in marital fertility in Sweden before the turning point of the late 1870's or the 1880's. They were certainly too large to be explained by short-turn fluctuations in the number of new marriages in combination with a fixed duration schedule of fertility.[15] If they tended to follow food prices and incomes, as the results mentioned above suggest, two explanations seem possible. Either there was an element of deliberate family planning influenced by the economic outlook, or we have an impact of nutritional (and weather) factors on conception probabilities and pregnancy wastage. The effects of harvests, food prices, wages, or perhaps climatic conditions on health assume importance also in this regard.

The second remark concerns the nature of negative or inconclusive evidence. The question is what chances there are for a causal system to become visible enough in the data. The importance of response lags is obvious and often recognized; presumably the dominance of infectious disease, usually of short duration and leading to death or full recovery, lessens the problem. Tuberculosis, however, needs to be remembered here. Also, there may exist non-linear response characteristics, as illustrated in Figure 4, while the standard methodology of data scanning is linear. These and similar considerations underline the virtue of using more than one approach to the problem in terms of data, periods and statistical manipulations.

Variability through space

More than one writer on the subject of death rates has remarked on the absence of a dependable relation between measures of economic development or prosperity, and mortality in regional data, e.g. Lee[16] with respect to German and Fridlizius[17] to Swedish figures. In these cases data for regions were combined with an over-time perspective; the question is then raised if geographical sub-divisions are replications of a common process. More frequent is the use of momentary or short-period values for such divisions within a socioeconomic framework, in the sociological tradition often referred to as the ecological approach.

The use of data for spatial units is beset with technical problems fully as troublesome (and analogous) to those of time-series methods. As they are rather less well known a few further words of comment will be in order before we turn to Swedish data on mortality by county in a mixed cross-sectional and longitudinal perspective. On such data operate the effects of serial or autocorrelation, here between units close in space, with the added complication of two dimensions instead of one as for time. This means the loss of independence among units, a consequence historically known as Galton's problem. A methodology has been developed to overcome some of these difficulties[18]; through its computational requirements and unfamiliarity it is exacting and will be followed only very partially here. One important point is the shape of the "spatial correlogram", how quickly or slowly the degree of similarity between units decays with increasing distance. There may exist an overall gradient, say a north-south gradient analogous to a long-term trend. As for secular trends it will be capable of almost an infinity of explanations. A more limited degree of dependence, analogous to modest autocorrelations in a time series quickly vanishing with increasing lags, would seem comparatively benign.

For Swedish counties, excluding the ambiguously located insular county of Gotland, we have 24 units and 47 "joins", cases of a common border between two counties. An index (I), expressing the degree of co-variation within these pairs, a parallel to the auto-(serial)correlation of lag 1, can be formed with results as follows:[19]

	I.
Infant mortality, 1861	.187
Mortality for ages 30-59, 1861	.367

A feeling for the magnitude of these values may be obtained by citing the ordinary correlation coefficients, resulting from the identical data: .363 (infant mortality) and .578 (mortality 30-59).

The results do not seem to reveal a strong gradient but are nevertheless a warning not to treat county data as we ordinarily handle unit data. An important question is the substantive overlap or identity between the forces acting on infant versus adult mortality. In the preceding section the long-run and short-run agreement in the time course of the two rates was discussed, now the spatial cross-correlation may similarly be used, ultimately both procedures should throw light on the identity question mentioned above. To avoid the danger of working with autocorrelated variables it might be advisable to use the spatial analogue to first differences, here differences between counties having a join. Thus we form the difference with respect to infant mortality between adjoining counties A and B, and similarly for adult mortality (30-59 years of age). For the 1861 rates it can be reported that the ordinary correlation coefficient between the differences is +.617, a substantial level of agreement, presumably unaffected by any major graphical gradient. Again, all these results ought to be regarded as preliminary until a more thorough analysis has been carried out.

As a further step in this exploration the correlations appearing below were computed. They are based on 24 counties, this time the city of Stockholm was left out as having all through the period rates placing it outside the normal range. In Figure 3, then, are shown coefficients indicating stability through time on the one hand, and cross-correlations indicating overlap between infant and adult mortality on the other. In the discussion of the results it will be advantageous to look back to the time series data reported earlier.

Figure 3. Correlations for 24 counties. Double-headed arrows denote correlations.

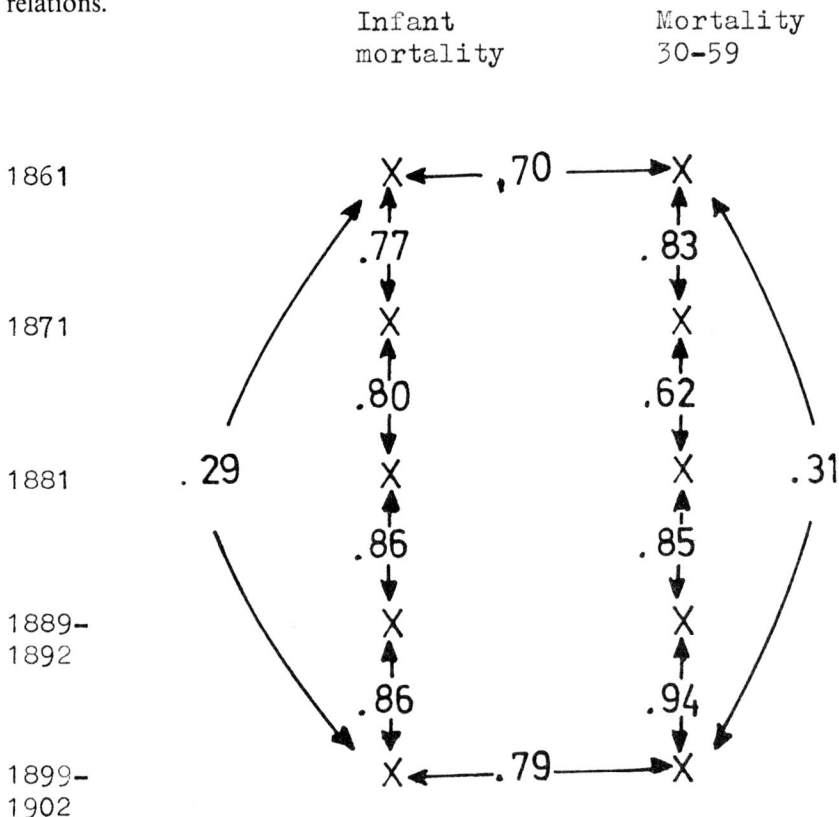

	Infant mortality	Mortality 30-59
1861	X ←— ,70 —→ X	
	.77	. 83
1871	X	X
	.80	.62
1881 . 29	X	X .31
	.86	. 85
1889–1892	X	X
	.86	.94
1899–1902	X ←—.79—→ X	

The evidence from continuity and change

By and large the spatial pattern of variation and co-variation argues for substantial overlap between infant and adult mortality with regard to underlying factors. In 1861 as well as 1899-1902 a high correlation is observed between the two rates on the basis of county data. The effort to check this result for the 1860 data by means of the spatial analogue to first-difference analysis did not lead to a different conclusion.

The 40 years intervening between the initial and terminal data brought considerable change in the relative position of counties. It is especially noticeable that those of northern Sweden lost their initially favourable ranks, here mortality remained stationary or even tended to rise while it fell in other parts. Again this is true of both adult and infant mortality. A manifestation of this mobility of counties in relative position is the weakening of stability correlations with time. Over a decade ranks change little, whether for infant or adult mortality, but over 40 years the correlations are quite weak, yet leaving the high synchronic correlation between the two rates intact.

On general grounds one would expect geographical differences, such as those reported above, to be sensitive to economic, cultural-behavioral or general environmental factors, less to disturbances having their origin in specific epidemics. The latter would presumably affect all or at least many counties about the same time and leave their relative positions less affected. The high short-term (10 years) stability rather supports this view. This still leaves a broad spectrum of influences, including nutrition, sanitary and medical standards, and health-related folkways. No clear correlation is observable between an index of economic level and mortality rates around 1860 though the index used, wages deflated by the price of rye on a county basis, may be inadequate for the purpose.[20] In any event only weak correlations appeared for either rate, around or under $+.20$.

It would have been an interesting finding if the infant-adult correlation in mortality rates is weaker for short-run variations through time as compared with the variations over space so far discussed. This would argue for separate disease spectra as far as epidemic disease is concerned, and might provide a point of departure for further theorizing (or speculation) on causal backgrounds. However, the data do not look obliging on this point. The impression from different time series, and different approaches to the series, is somewhat mixed, and it would be unwise at this point to place too much stress on the distinctiveness of the spatial differences as contrasted to the temporal variation. Though there are indications of weaker relationships between infant and adult mortality for fluctuation in the relatively short run in the five-year mortality series 1801-1900, ($r = +.216$) a stronger correlation is apparent for the annual series 1875-1909 if residuals from linear trends are used ($r = +.631, d = 1.67$). With first differences instead the relationship weakens ($r = +.301$). Finally, the annual series 1820-1865 produce quite a substantial measure of agreement with $r = +.694$ for first differences.

The upshot of this is that we are still left with a wide array of possible causal factors, as mentioned earlier a common predicament among epidemiologists. The gradual transformation of the pre-existing structure of county differentials points to gradual change, or gradual response to more sudden change, but leaves open the question where to locate the change to medical, environmental or cultural-behavioral factors.

The study of death rates makes one realize the danger of being over-specific in causal attribution. Special reasons can be found for the decline of infant and child mortality, such as improved child care practices, and most particularly a change to breast-feeding. That still leaves unexplained the parallel fall of adult rates, and the pronounced short-term and short distance co-variation between the two. It may also be noted (without disparagement of the valuable work done by historians and others in this area) that trends and the precise extent of breast-feeding seem difficult to establish in the Swedish case.

Epidemics and weather conditions may be responsible for simultaneous up's and down's in death rates for different ages but are of less help with geographical variation and co-variation as described earlier. If the nutritional factor is found insufficient, as many writers have suggested and as the county data would seem to indicate, the difficulty becomes more acute.

With this one is brought to the well-known formula of multi-factorial causality. About this it can be said that it sounds eminently reasonable, but also that it leads to a kind of impasse. The history of fertility, and no less fertility research offers an instructive parallel, with a constant use of a "modernization" complex to explain the secular decline, and on occasion a shorter period or renewed change, as in the 1960's. Considering the grab-all character of the explanation one is perhaps not likely to miss a crucial factor, for it includes a wide array such as industrialization, urbanization, growth of the profane and decline of the sacred, compulsory schooling, women's liberation and paid employment, and advances in contraceptive technology. At the same time the lack of precision is obvious. There are similar drawbacks to accepting a "modernization" super-factor in the case of mortality trends, including both dietary improvement, medical advances, a more rigorous application of preventive medicine, new lay practices, and in addition perhaps a change in the virulence of pathogens.

Whether disaggregation, ultimately down to individual-level data, will be more productive is debatable. Again fertility research offers an example. The reproductive behavior of couples today can and has been investigated in survey and interview studies, and the results evaluated by highly competent specialists. Despite all these efforts no straightforward answer to questions of long-term change or recent fluctuations has emerged. One of the leading practitioners of survey methodology within this area has lately expressed his doubts about the use of individual data when population-level results are needed.[21] Returning to mortality it should be noted that studies of exposure or life-styles, e.g. by mean of occupational mortality, typically leave us in doubt about the direction of causality; poor health can be expected to be associated with downward mobility. The intrinsically large stochastic element, cited in the case of fertility outcomes, is also a feature of death and survival.

Cultural change and mortality

The possibility of a behavioral or cultural component in the battery of forces behind mortality trends was introduced in an opening section, but requires some additional comment and classification. As then pointed out the idea is far from new, and it fits easily into the multi-factorial mode of thinking toward which researchers lean anyway. It is important, however, that "cultural-behavioral" is not understood too narrowly, or as referring necessarily to "ideology", or perhaps deep currents in the "collective unconscious". In fact no strictly unitary concept is assumed, and the labels suggested earlier ("folk-medicine", "health-related behaviours", "life-styles", etc) point to a variety of phenomena with a common basis in social learning and socio-cultural transmission. The most promising policy will be to stay with elements like concrete behaviors, skills, and beliefs.

As life and health are permanent concerns in practically every cultural setting, much change can be located in the sphere of the instrumental, in knowledge and practices bearing on health. The possible influence of organized medicine and the medical profession needs to be assessed, and here is one direction further research could take. It is striking that the goals and operating rules of that system were quite modern in their conception, and this already at the beginning of the 19th century or even earlier.[22] Instructions to the local medical officers (*"provinsialläkare"*) laid emphasis on preventive medicine, the importance of educating the lay public on the matter of health risks and their elimination, and on knowing the local population and the "medical topography" of the district, i.e. the epidemiological map.

Admittedly the stock of soundly established experience and rules of conduct was limited, and the skeptic may wonder how much useful knowledge there was to impart. On two points, at least, medical writers were insistent, eloquent and essentially correct in their judgment: on the importance of breast-feeding for the health of the child, and on the adverse effect on adult health of heavy drinking.[23] To what extent they were listened to is another question, not easily settled, especially not for the period before *circa* 1850. The precise extent of breast-feeding is difficult to establish. For the latter part of the 19th century a falling trend in alcohol consumption can be observed, but data are lacking before 1855.[24] The problem has received some attention within the context of mortality trends.[25]

As usual the concepts become a little blurred at the edges, and there is some overlap between professional medicine, especially in its preventive aspects, and the cultural-behavioral complex now discussed. With regard to breast-feeding the propaganda *for* breast-feeding and *against* artificial feeding from doctors and licensed midwives is part of a more general pattern. It is noteworthy that the late 18th and early 19th centuries saw the emergence of a literature in the vernacular on the treatment and prevention of illness aimed at a larger audience than medical personnel[26]; apparently this was a general European phenomenon.[27] The examples given do not exhaust the influences from the medical profession. Nor do they prove that change had to come through this channel at all. Home-care and self-care skills could develop in more than one way. The principle of contagion seems to have been well established internationally (and over-generously applied), as witnessed by Defoe's *Journal of the Plague Year* (1722). It suffered a temporary eclipse among specialists in the 19th century as a result of wrongly interpreted data but may have played a role in building up certain elementary defenses.[28] Dietary improvements of a qualitative kind belong to this area and may not at all, or only dimly, be reflected in customary statistical series.

There is a fundamental question of social theory involved in the behavioral-cultural hypothesis as expounded here, and several consequences of some weight. There is an underlying assumption of a "structurally open" situation, the possibility of changes in beliefs, attitudes and behaviour as an independent (complex) factor, not deterministically governed by basic economic-structural features. It is particularly worth observing that such change cannot be ruled out because there is no good theory leading us to expect it. The brief introductory survey of unexplained trends should be warning enough against this fallacy. Speaking of behavioral trends in general the plain fact is that most of them lack convincing explanation even when their existence is beyond doubt. That existence, the reality of the change, has to be established, but the absence of convincing reasons for the emergence of change is not a strong argument against believing in it.

The hypothesis here advocated makes death, in a sense, more of a behavioral (and cognitive) phenomenon, and to that extent brings it closer to fertility. Accordingly, fertility changes from the 1870's and onwards provide us with examples of behavioral trends of some interest in the present context. Already the late 19th-century shifts show a remarkable simultaneity in onset and course between a number of populations in Western Europe, despite rather great differences in levels of economic development and urbanization, say between Sweden and England. The decline of fertility in the 1960's is no less striking in the nearly identical time of onset among a number of high-income populations. Though more homogeneous in structural terms than a hundred years earlier they could not be called structural copies of one another. It makes good sense to combine general knowledge of such change with the historical at hand, here on mortality in countries, regions or parishes.

One has to be careful, however, and not accept too much as known. There is a tendency to reject behavioral change as explanation because no clear lags or socio-demographic gradients can be discovered, but the basis for this appears quite shaky.[29] It would seem reasonable to expect the entire process to be a gradual and time-consuming one, the overall change being a composite fact with many subsidiary changes or adjustments. From this does not follow that lags of a national, regional or social nature should be apparent. Single innovations could spread at an astounding rate, as shown by the international diffusion of smallpox vaccination (not a major factor in the Swedish decline).

A final remark touches on the place of the behavioral hypothesis within a two- or multifactor model. The presence of behavioral-attitudinal change does not preclude an impact of such facts as poor harvests, cold weather, or new epidemics. If we visualize the behavioral shift as one between two discrete states, a variable fraction of the population having moved from "traditional" to "modern" behavior at any given time, a three-variable problem can be represented as in Figure 4. Here the abscissa denotes some economic factor like harvest or grain price, while the ordinate stands for mortality considered as response. Were the entire population "traditionalists" in conduct and outlook the curve T would depict the exposure-response relation, with all "modern" the curve M would similarly show the impact of harvest or price fluctuations on mortality. For a considerable period we have, then, a mix between the two, gradually shifting in the direction of M. The exact shapes of the curves are not meant to be taken as realistic but the flatter shape of M would produce precisely the dampening and eventual disappearance of short-term fluctuations which is such a conspicuous feature of the 19th-century development. It is also clear that time-series analysis which stresses year-to-year changes (residuals from trends, first differences) might give a different answer from a study of trends.

Further probing and testing of behavioral-cultural hypotheses (there will be many, not one) will require data from more than one customary field: the medical sociology of pre-industrial and early industrial society, and the medical anthropology of these populations, and their nutrition. Also needed will be an application of communication theories to an environment different from the mass-media world of today. And these populations proved quite capable of behavioral change, and less tradition- and custom-bound than is often assumed.

Figure 4. Model with three variables. (See text)

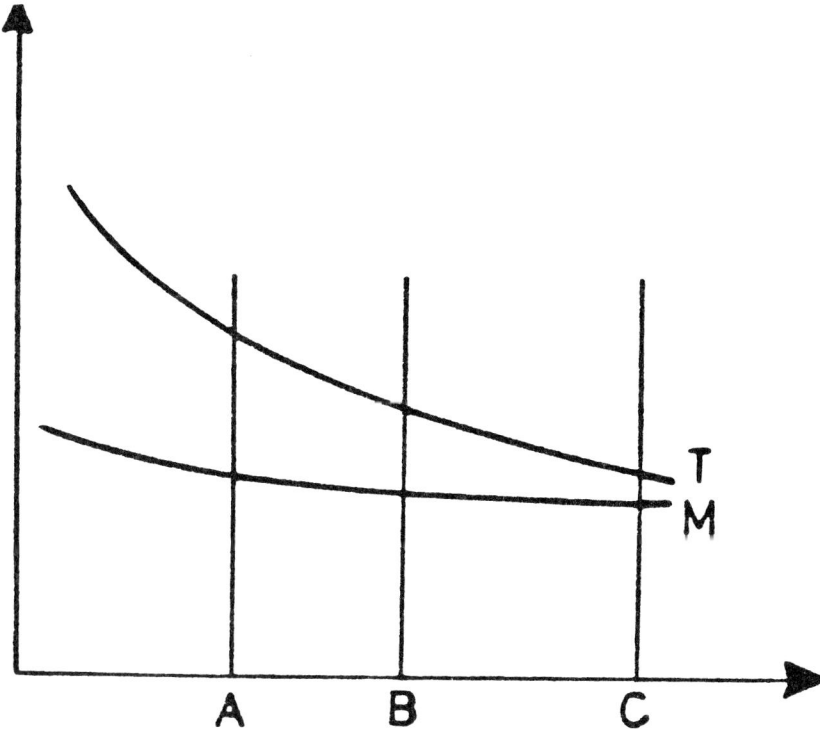

Notes

1. A.H. Gale, *Epidemic Diseases* (London 1959).

2. J. Cairns, *Cancer: Science and Society* (San Francisco 1978), pp. 42-46.

3. T. McKeown, *The Modern Rise of Population* (London 1976).

4. T. Bengtsson, G. Fridlizius, and R. Ohlsson (Eds.), *Pre-Industrial Population Change* (Stockholm 1984).

5. W.R. Lee, 'Introduction', and 'Germany', W.R. Lee (Ed.), *European Demography and Economic Growth* (London 1979), pp. 10-26 and 144-195.

6. G. Carlsson, O. Arvidsson, L.O. Bygren, and L. Werkö, *Liv och hälsa* (Stockholm 1979), chap. 1.

7. A. Keys, et al., *The Biology of Human Starvation* (Minnesota 1950), chaps. 46-47.

8. U.-B. Lithell, *Breast-Feeding and Reproduction* (Uppsala 1981); A. Brändström, *"De kärlekslösa mödrarna". Spädbarnsdödligheten i Sverige under 1800-talet med särskild hänsyn till Nedertorneå* (Umeå 1984).

9. J.-P. Goubert, 'Public Hygiene and Mortality Decline in France in the 19th Century', Bengtsson, Fridlizius and Ohlsson (Eds.) (1984), pp. 151-159.; C. Corsini, 'Structural Modifications in Infant Mortality in Tuscany between the 17th and the 18th Centuries', Bengtsson, Fridlizius and Ohlsson (Eds.) (1984), pp. 127-150.

10. W.H. McNeill, *Plagues and Peoples* (Oxford 1976), chap. 4.

11. B.-I. Puranen, *Tuberkulos. En sjukdoms förekomst och dess orsaker. Sverige 1750-1980* (Umeå 1984), p. 135.

12. L. Jörberg, *A History of Prices in Sweden 1732-1914* (Lund 1972), vol 2, p. 350.

13. G. Fridlizius, 'The Mortality Decline in the First Phase of the Demographic Transition: Swedish Experiences', Bengtsson, Fridlizius and Ohlsson (Eds.) (1984), pp. 71-114.

14. G. Fridlizius and R. Ohlsson, 'Mortality Patterns in Sweden 1751-1802: A Regional Analysis', Bengtsson, Fridlizius and Ohlsson (Eds.) (1984), pp. 329-355.

15. G. Carlsson, 'Nineteenth-Century Fertility Oscillations', *Population Studies,* 24 (1970), pp. 413-422.

16. Lee (1979).

17. Fridlizius (1984).

18. A.D. Cliff and J.K. Ord, *Spatial Processes* (London 1981).

19. Cliff and Ord (1981), chap. 1.

20. Jörberg (1972).

21. N.B. Ryder, 'Where Do Babies Come from?', H.M. Blalock Jr (Ed.), *Sociological Theory and Research* (New York 1980), pp. 182-202.

22. H. Bergstrand, 'Läkarkåren och provinsialläkarväsendet', W. Kock (Ed.), *Medicinalväsendets historia i Sverige 1813-1962* (Stockholm 1963), pp. 121-124.

23. G. Lundquist, 'Alkoholfrågan', Kock (Ed.) (1963), pp. 536-544.

24. P. Frånberg, *'Den svenska supen'*, K. Bruun and P. Frånberg (Eds.), Den svenska supen (Stockholm 1985), chap. 1.

25. Fridlizius (1984). *See also Fridlizius' article in this volume (Editors notice).*

26. Puranen (1984), pp. 54-64.

27. Goubert (1984).

28. McNeill (1976), pp. 265-266.

29. A. Perrenoud, 'The Mortality Decline in a Long-Term Perspective', Bengtsson, Fridlizius and Ohlsson (Eds.) (1984), p. 65; Fridlizius (1984), p. 99.

Height, Health and Nutrition
in Early Modern Sweden

Sune Åkerman, Ulf Högberg and Mats Danielsson

Introduction

When we have been studying the social and economic development of the 19th century it has been natural to concentrate on the effects of the industrialization process. This is quite natural. The industrialization undoubtedly created drastically new conditions for the majority of people and thorough reconstruction of most western societies. This, however, does not imply that the period before the onset of industrialization can be labelled a stable one. On the contrary it was a most dynamic period as regards social, economic, demographic, and political conditions. Although this is a rather well-known fact the first half of the 19th century still tends to be looked upon as a pre-industrial period characterized by a comparatively stable rural sector. It was during this early modern period however that several preconditions for the new production system were born.

Against this background there are good reasons to study more thoroughly the changes of the standard of living of common people both in the urban settings and in the countryside. Compared to England the Scandinavian countries have not a long tradition as regards this type of studies. But recently some scholarly work has been devoted to the problem of improvement or deterioration in the living conditions. From that point of view it is most important to get some sort of measurements linked to the individuals which can disclose better than GNP per capita what really happened to people in general. It is also a crucial problem for us to find out the health situation within different quarters of these hierarchical societies. As we will see this is not quite impossible.

There are various indicators of health which reveal the changes of nutrition of man through history as well as various standards of living of present day societies. Thus mean birth weight in developing countries is about 500 gram less than in developed counterparts of the world. Furthermore, the percentage of low weight of individuals—2.500 gram or less—is only about 5 % in our part of the world while in developing countries this percentage is as high as 20 to 30.

Illustration 1. The intriguing causative relationships of health improvement and height increase.

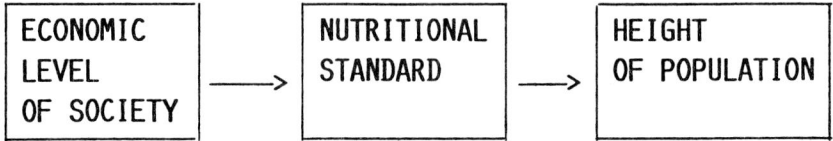

```
┌─────────────┐        ┌─────────────┐        ┌─────────────┐
│ ECONOMIC    │        │ NUTRITIONAL │        │ HEIGHT      │
│ LEVEL       │ ────>  │ STANDARD    │ ────>  │ OF POPULATION│
│ OF SOCIETY  │        │             │        │             │
└─────────────┘        └─────────────┘        └─────────────┘
```

In the General Lying-in hospital of Stockholm the mean birth weight increased with 419 gram between the years 1850/60 and 1935/45. Age of menarche, the beginning of the menstrual function and age of menopause, the time of natural cessation of menstruation are also dependent of nutritional factors during childhood. In Norway for example the age of menarche has decreased from 16.2 to 12.5 years between 1844 and today. Likewise the age of menopause has increased from 46.5 to 51.5 years.

However, the most consistent indicator of maternal and childhood nutrition standard seems to be height. This indicator can be studied through the history of man. It can be used for very early time periods by archaeologists, historians and anthropologists. In fact, height is the only parameter reflecting the nutritional evolution of man. This is very much true also for more recent periods like the first half of the 19th century which we intend to study in this paper.

Archaeologists and osteological specialists who have scrutinized skeletons from remote times have been able to show that there existed surprisingly tall individuals as far back as the hunting-gathering period. They have also argued that these people have lived in a comparatively sound surrounding, enjoying a diet of a satisfactory composition. The result was well-fed populations. Thus the scholars infer from the bodily height a whole pattern of life. The bone material from hunting cultures does not disclose much of severe illness or epidemics.

The implication will be that the transition from hunting to agriculture, from migratory mobility to stable settlements turned out to be more problematic. This fact has been revealed by the skeleton material. This means that mankind had to pay a rather high price for the improved security of the agricultural society. As a consequence of a higher density of population we can register a series of epidemical diseases which have tormented rural as well as urban populations ever since. Through history peasants have a height 15 centimetres less than hunters-gatherers. In Sweden height of man seems to have been rather stable from Neolitic age to the Medieval period.

However, there are exceptions to short height in the Middle Ages. Rural populations from this period may show quite impressive heights which has been proved by Vilhelm Hultcrantz who has studied an osteological material from a site just outside the walls of the city of Visby, where a battle took place in 1361 between the army of the Danish King and a band of badly armoured peasant soldiers living on the isle of Gotland. This massacre has left us with a huge bone material which discloses that the average height among the peasants was almost 169 centimeters. At the turn of the century 1900 the modern Swedish population just passed 170 centimeters!

Later on we will comment upon the fact that the height development from the early 19th century and onwards does not show a steady progression. On the contrary we can register several set-backs and a varied rate of growth. But we have still a rather scanty information about the period before 1840.

Hesitant historians

It is somewhat embarrassing to notice that our fellow historians in Sweden have devoted no interest what-so-ever to the health development of earlier populations as mirrored in Sweden's quite satisfactory height information about the young soldiers. This is even more astonishing if we consider the strong position medical and demographic history have reached lately. Therefore the attitudes may change pretty soon. Maybe this article can act as an inspiration for further studies in the field.

As a matter of fact Hultcrantz who was a medical doctor started his studies already in the 1890's. At that time Adolph Quetelet and others have been studying the height development of different populations in several countries like Belgium, France and Germany for half a century. This research was not that much removed from the new school of historical height studies inspired by Robert Fogel, Roderic Floud and others in the late 1970's. Also their forerunners tried to establish a correlation between health and standard of living on one side and the measures of bodily height and weight on the other in order to find a proxy for the changing welfare of preindustrial and industrial populations.

Begging the question

In the literature treating the standard of living we have found a tendency to pass over the crucial problem of correlating health and height to the general economic situation. We have a suspicion that this may be dangerous, that there are still reason to study if and how the bodily height reflects living conditions in general in a society. This means that we would like to question a simple and uncomplicated combination of stature and economic conditions in general.

In our opinion passing over this crucial problem means that we easily end up in a circular reasoning. By combining poor and inexact variables of an economic, social or cultural kind with our height measures we may find ourselves performing something very much like the well-known Indian rope trick. There are still some evidence that does not fit into the picture of a strong positive correlation between height and economic development. To our mind the demographic and medical information more easily lend itself to a correlation effort. That is why in this moment we have decided to use such an angle of approach. We may also add that the basic empirical evidence about the height development during the last 200 years needs to be reconstructed and specified for Sweden as well as for many other comparable countries.

Why measuring the recruits?

As historians we often have to be satisfied with source materials gathered for quite other reasons than to improve our knowledge about a society. Strangely enough this situation does not apply to the registration of different groups of military personnel. As a matter of fact the military organization as well as the government wanted to know already in the 18th century the "power" and "vigor" of the young men intended for military service. Therefore they paid attention to the bodily shape of the young recruits as well as to sickness and handicaps which could be revealed during the enrollment procedure. That is why most information from the muster rolls is quite adequate and relevant for our present purposes. Especially the possibility to treat not only aggregates but also individuals is of great value. We can only regret that we lack weight information for all the observed periods and that no information about women can be found. This of course creates an extrapolation problem when we try to reconstruct the situation for both sexes in a certain time period.

There are still good reasons to apply a very strict source criticism to our material. There are many pitfalls we must be aware of. Therefore we have to learn thoroughly the military organization of different countries especially when we intend to establish comparisons between nationalities.

Sweden's military organizations in former times

In the Swedish case we can notice that the defense organization was very complicated. There were remnants from different time periods. Thus we find at least three different categories of soldiers and military personnel. On one hand we have the enrolled who had been voluntary drafted as well as a special category of soldiers-crofters; on the other hand there were the conscripts. The soldiers-crofters were living in the midst of the rural population, a special solution for the Swedish defense, and their military training and obligations were performed during a short period in the summer time when they were gathered to certain meeting places in every military district. Voluntary drafted soldiers were living in garrisons, thereby being a more mobile force. The conscripts were only trained during a couple of summer weeks intermittently.

Earlier research has used either the information about the soldiers-crofters or the information about the conscripts. In our opinion this is not satisfactory. To have a richer empirical evidence we must eagerly combine the existing

416

sources since the different groups of soldiers have different characteristics. There are also a lot of other technical problems, some of them rather difficult to handle.

The material about the conscripts is however the best starting point for our analyses. This material covers more fully the main part of the actual population (age cohorts). It also helps automatically to control the age variable, which is of course of most crucial interest in this type of analyses. The material about the conscripts also has a much better social coverage which also turns out to be important. But there are also weaknesses: even if the main part of the growth spurt has taken place at the age of 21 there remain some millimeters up to the point where final height is reached. Since this spurt has a different timing and length in different socio-economic and cultural settings it is important to discuss the effects of different measuring points. In this respect the material gathered about the soldiers-crofters is better, since there was a consecutive measuring of this personnel even when it was quite old but still in service.

Another advantage of the soldier-crofter material is the early starting point of measuring. Height information has been gathered since 1776 which allows us to make reconstructions already from the 1740's. Aggregated statistics about the conscripts can be found from 1840 and onwards but we have been able to recover local material from certain areas from 1813. A draw-back in all materials is the truncation of the height information covering the smallest individuals. Different minimal height demands existed both for the conscripts and even more for the soldiers-crofters. To complicate things these demands varied over time and could also be lowered temporarily because of difficult recruitment situations during war times.

The ordinary military personnel was taller in average than the conscripts and they were not included among the conscripts in the muster rolls. They were measured in a special procedure. That is why as we mentioned earlier the distribution curve based on the muster rolls for the conscripts has to be combined with information about the ordinary personnel. Since the latter category was scattered over many age groups the corrections we have to make are, however, rather limited. In the 20th century the enlistment of conscripts took place already at the age of 20; therefore we have to make special arrangements to combine the older material with the modern one.

It must be added that during the period 1813-1860 persons who were rejected because of illness or mental or bodily handicaps are not included in the measurements. After 1860 we have the same information about them as about the accepted individuals.

From the very beginning there were not many draft dodgers but their number increased and reached the level of 6.000-8.000 persons out of about 40.000 every year in the middle of the 1870's. This complication has been neglected in earlier research. This substantial loss of people in every age cohort in the last part of our investigation period has probably introduced a bias. We know that a substantial part of these draft dodgers emigrated to North America and that this contingent tends to be taller than the average population.

Even if we consider all these problems and complications the height material must be characterized as an excellent source, especially compared with different measurements of the economic standard of living. As was intimated we are also able to correct most deficiencies in the material. Not even the possibility for well-to-do persons to hire someone else who could do their military service has been a real draw-back for us. For different reasons this possibility was not practised very often.

A reinterpretation of the late pre-industrial period is needed

Like in England there is in Sweden some confusion about what really happened in a social and economic dimension during the period 1810-1870. Technically more advanced and sophisticated research has not as yet been able to solve these problems. On the contrary widely different interpretations and suggestions based on huge amounts of data and statistics have added to the confusion. For Sweden we do not even know if the standard of living was rising or declining during the period. Thus there are good reasons to try to find new and more relevant information about individuals and households as Roderic Floud has pointed out for England.

During the period 1810-1870 we can notice a heavy proletarization of the Swedish countryside. Something like 900.000 people out of 3.5 million had lost their footing in the peasant society making up a group we sometimes call the potato-people. They had their dwellings on the outskirts of the peasant society literary speaking and their houses and shacks were in general in a deplorable condition. Before the onset of the industrialization, urbanization and transatlantic migration these people had to live a very unsecure life on the margin of peasant society. Their numbers were still growing in the 1870's. In the same time period the mortality rates decreased rather drastically and this does not apply only to the infant mortality.

Against this background some questions must be asked: was there an improved health standard and living conditions in Sweden 1810-1870? Can we notice and isolate the effects of the proletarization? Were there deepening cleavages between different social groups? Can we explain the mortality decline during the period? Were there geographic differences as regards the height development of the population? Can we imply that the pace of pauperisation was different from region to region dependent on different economic levels?

418

Study design

We have chosen to catch the main development by treating three age cohorts or generations. As was mentioned earlier we are able to start already in the year 1813. Thus our first cohort contains people who were enlisted in 1813 and 1814. Our investigation area consists of the main part of the region Uppland north of Stockholm. This region is in general a rather wealthy part of the country but contains also poor districts in the periphery of the central, fertile plain of Uppsala.

A second and a third cohort were constructed of those who enlisted in 1843-1844 and 1873-1874 respectively. It could have been possible to use shorter intervals between the cohorts for example 20 or 25 years, but we have preferred to get enough space between the cohorts to be able to register a substantial change. Normally the increase of the bodily height happens quite slowly as was mentioned earlier. The time span between generations is often approximated to thirty years.

Research material

Our empirical evidence is homogeneous and in principle it also covers all social strata and every corner of our geographical unit. Our data have been stored in the so called general muster rolls which comprised all youngsters of the actual recruiting age. A small contingent of older recruits, who had been rejected temporarily, is present as well. Some hired people, often much older than 21 years, are added to the registers. A bunch of doctor's certificates belongs to every muster roll containing information about the reasons why the actual person could not serve as a soldier. This material of course is highly relevant for our study but has not as yet been used systematically. The situation concerning the archival material for the conscripts is a little bit confused. The military archives in Stockholm *(Krigsarkivet)* do not cover more than small parts of the material. We have to consult the local county archives to find more information. Still we lack some important parts of the muster rolls even on the county level. That is why we were unable to construct a final age cohort for the late 19th century for Uppland, which was our original plan. For other regions such a cohort may very well be possible to build up though.

The height information is stated in feet and inches and not in centimeters. It is important to observe that the inch was measured a little bit differently during the investigation period. Not only the name of the enlisted appear in the muster rolls but also sometimes his father or employer. Information about the residence tells us in which village, parish and county they were staying. As was mentioned earlier we have height information about the rejected but only after 1860.

As we are interested in the health development of the population and the possible associative or causative relationships between the mortality decline and height increase, we have also collected aggregated statistics of mortality rates from the study districts where the conscripts came from. The health statistics include birth rates per thousand of the population, death rates per thousand of the population, still-born rates per hundred births, infant mortality rates per thousand live births, toddler (age 1-5) mortality per thousand population and maternal mortality per hundred thousand live births. We have chosen to collect these vital statistics from the districts during the periods 1793-1795, 1813-1815, 1833-1835, 1853-1854 and 1873-1875. Furthermore, specific death cause statistics regarding deaths below the age of 10 have been collected at an aggregated level in the Uppsala diocese for the period 1793-1794, and in the Uppsala county 1874.

Results

The total number registered in the muster rolls were 5.707. Of those 1.081 were rejected and 1.698 were registered but with missing height. That is, the total number studied was 3.077 individuals in the three age cohorts of conscripts during the study period (see Table 1). The mean height was 163.9 centimeters during the period 1813-1814 and increased with almost three centimeters to the next cohort during the years 1843-1844 and with almost two centimeters up to the next cohort of 1873-1874 (Table 1). The percentage of rejected by social background is shown in Figure 1. Evidently, students have been evading the enrollment procedure more than other categories, especially during the latter part of the study period. However the number of registered students is considerable in all cohorts.

The height increase at district level was found to be rather uneven. The general pattern was a definite increase from the first to the second cohort in all districts. But from the second to the third age cohort, that is from the years 1843-1844 to 1873-1874, a decrease of mean height was observed in some districts like the town of Enköping and the rural districts of Hagunda and Lagunda. Furthermore, a stable height was noticed in four of the twelve

Table 1. Three age cohorts of conscripts 1813—1874 of muster of Uppland.

Conscripts	1813—14	1843—44	1873—74
registered	2311	1637	1759
rejected	244	317	520
hired	197	0	0
with missing height	550	419	729
with height information	1639	1208	1030
mean height (cm)	163.9	166.6	168.4

Source: General Muster Rolls. Landsarkivet, Uppsala.

districts from the second to the third cohort. It was only in four of the twelve districts that a definite increase of height was registered from the years 1843-1844 up to 1873-1874. This concerns the districts of Bälinge, Habo, Oland and Ulleråker (see Figure 2). All of them situated in the more prosperous parts of Uppland.

Social differences in the same age cohort are more pronounced than geographical differences or differences between the age cohorts over time. Students had a mean height of 168.7 centimeters during the years 1913-1914, that is the mean height of the years 1873-1874 of the total cohort. This means that students as a matter of fact were two generations before the mean population as regards the bodily height development. The mean height of students during the years 1873-1874 was 173.2. Not until the 1930's this was the mean height of the population in general in Sweden. Peasants from the age cohort 1813-1814 were taller than crofters and farmhands; this difference was not that much pronounced in the age cohort of 1873-1874 (see Figure 3). It is, however, quite difficult to make clear-cut divisions between the subgroups of the rural population (like sons of peasants or farmhands).

Figure 1. The percentage number rejected of concripts by social background in the county of Uppsala 1813-1874.

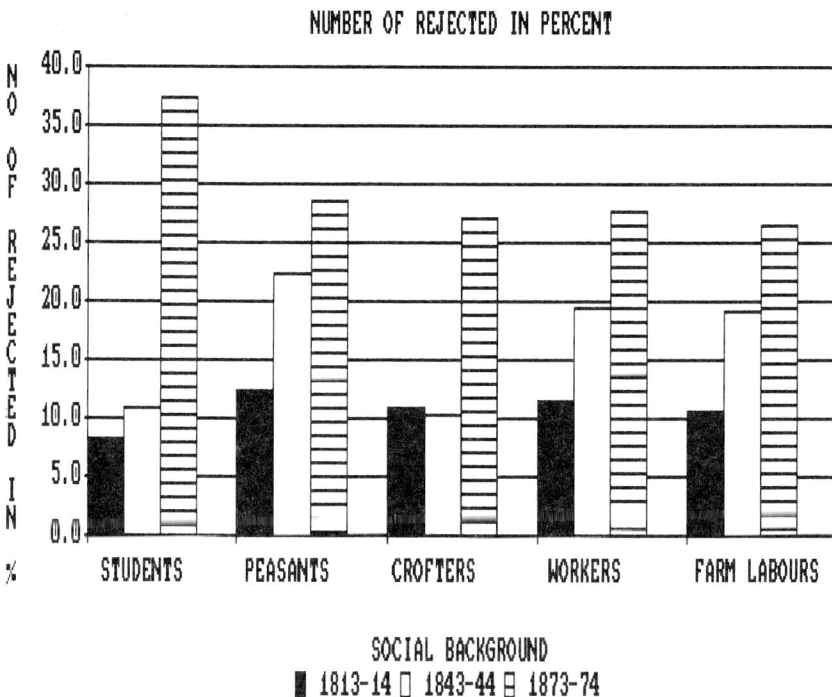

NUMBER OF REJECTED IN PERCENT

SOCIAL BACKGROUND
■ 1813-14 ☐ 1843-44 ⊟ 1873-74

Figure 2. 3-D display of height development among conscripts in twelve districts in Uppsala county in three cohorts during the years 1813-1874.

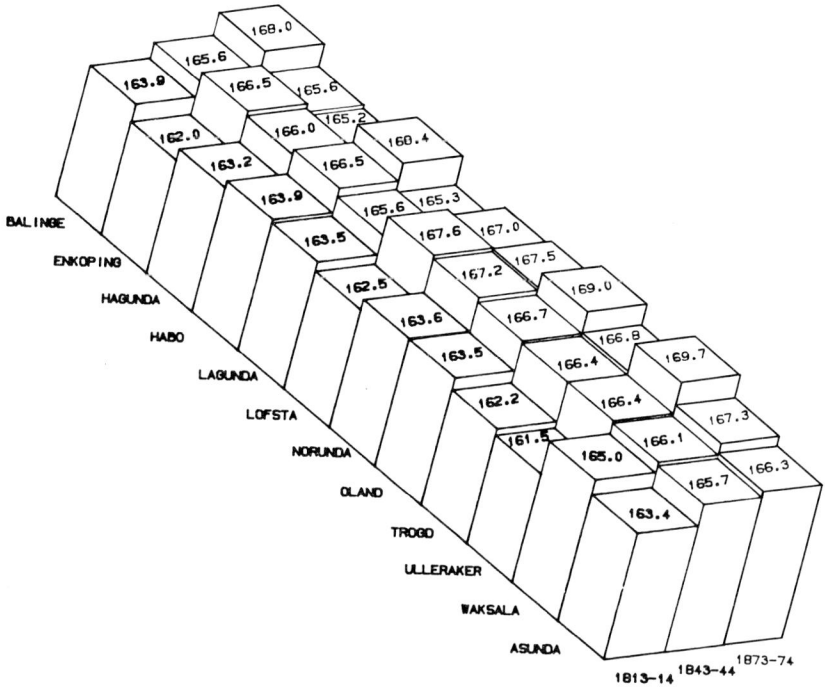

BALINGE
ENKOPING
HAGUNDA
HABO
LAGUNDA
LOFSTA
NORUNDA
OLAND
TROGD
ULLERAKER
WAKSALA
ASUNDA

168.0
165.6 163.9 166.5 165.6
162.0 166.0 165.2
163.2 166.5 168.4
163.9 165.6 165.3
163.5 167.6 167.0
162.5 167.2 167.5
163.6 166.7 169.0
163.5 166.4 166.8
162.2 166.4 169.7
161.5 165.0 166.1 167.3
165.7 166.3
163.4

1813-14   1843-44   1873-74

Well, what did happen with the mortality decline during the study period? Here we find a 60 % decline of infectious diseases among children below age of 10 from the years 1793-1794 up to 1874. Certainly there are problems connected with the interpretation of special death causes during such a long time period. However, the total mortality decline should be correct (see Table 2).

Our material has certain short-comings. It would have been desirable to gather more data on the conscripts, not only information on height, but also about the mortality of the individual conscript and his family. In the available material it has only been possible to get aggregated health statistics for the comparison with the height information; the health statistics are, however, comparable over time and as regards geographical situation, since our health statistics are based on the home districts of the conscripts.

422

Figure 3. 3-D display of height increase by social background in three cohorts of concripts of Uppsala county during the years 1813-1874. (Studenter = students, bönder = farmers, torpare = crofters, arbetare = workers, drängar = farm labourers.)

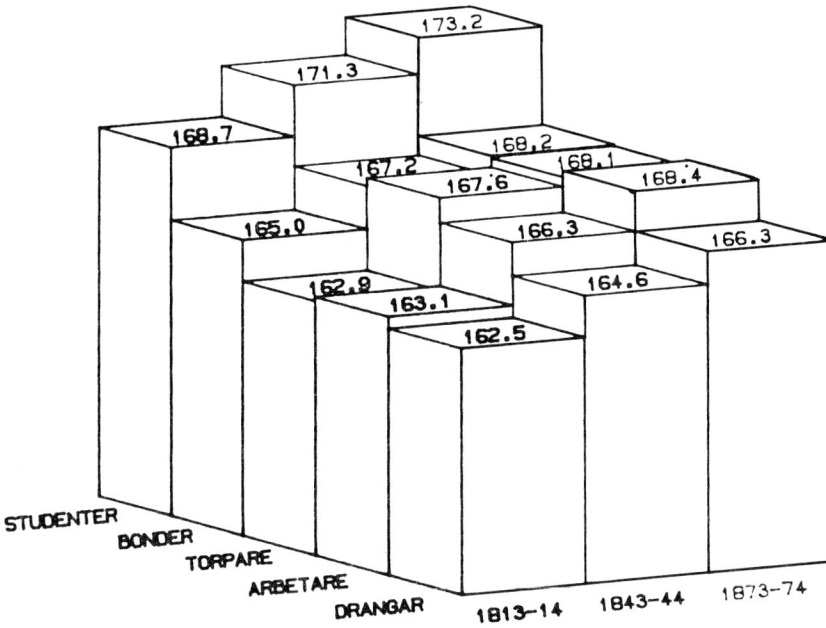

Table 2. Death causes in the diocese of Uppsala 1793—1794 (5.329 deaths) and the county of Uppsala 1874 (465 deaths) for children with age below ten years per thousand population.

Death Cause	Mortality		Percentage Mortality Decline
	1793—94	1874	
Variola	1.48	1.30	12
Malaria	0.11	0.08	27
Whooping-cough	0.31	0.44	—
Measles	0.97	0.02	98
Dysentery	0.38	0.02	95
Epiglottitis	0.48	0.45	6
Others	7.12	2.13	70
Grand total	10.85	4.43	60

Source: Central Bureau of Statistics in Sweden.

The observed health indicators are presented in Table 3. Graphically the relationships between the increase of height of the three cohorts and the decline of bad health in the population is shown in Figure 4. Evidently, there is a relationship between declining maternal mortality, declining infant mortality, declining toddler mortality on one hand and increasing height of the conscripts on the other (that is 20 years after the observed death rates). Our material does not permit regression analyses as the observation points are too few. However, the results give us an indication of an associative or causative relationship of health improvement during the 19th century in Sweden. The common denominator should be improved nutrition.

Figure 4. 3-D display of height development among three cohorts of concripts from twelve districts in Uppsala county and different death rates in the population from same districts 1813-1874.

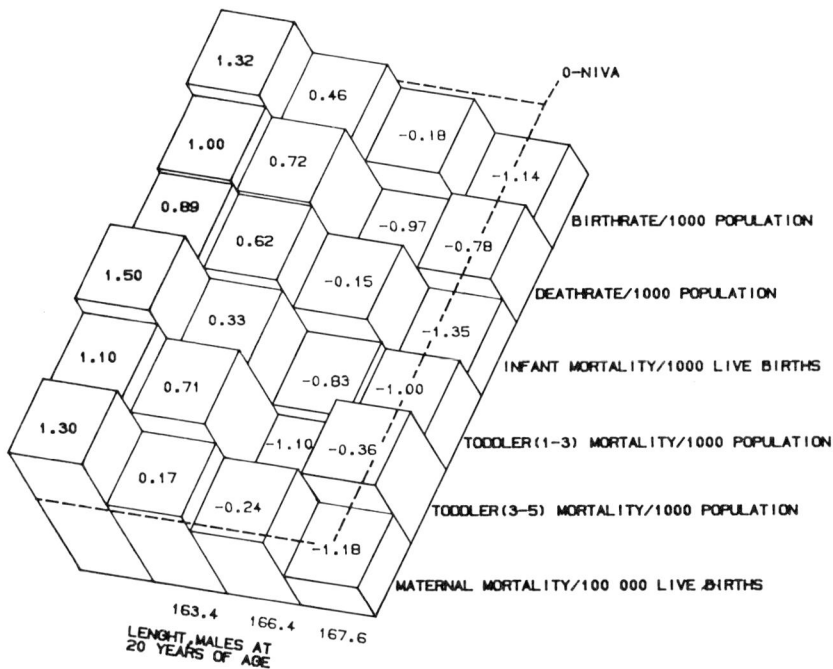

Table 3. Health indicators in twelve districts of Uppsala county during the years 1793—1855, and for Uppsala county as a whole for the years 1873—1875, means and 95% confidence limits.

	1793—95	1813—15	1833—35	1843—45	1853—55	1873—75
Birthrate per 1,000 population	32.0 (30.5-33.6)	29.1 (27.1-30.8)	28.7 (27.2-30.0)		26.6 (25.6-27.6)	29.1
Deathrate per 1,000 population	27.9 (23.9-31.9)	27.0 (23.6-30.5)	21.6 (18.8-24.4)		22.2 (20.2-24.3)	22.2
Stillborn rate per 100 births	3.8 (3.0-4.7)	2.1 (1.6-2.7)	3.2 (2.6-4.0)		2.9 (2.1-3.6)	3.5
Infant mortality rate per 1,000 live births	194.8 (139.5-250.1)	187.6 (139.3-236.0)	167.9 (129.1-206.7)		136.8 (104.2-169.3)	160.7
Toddler (1-3) mortality per 1,000 population	2.5 (1.7-3.3)	1.8 (1.4-2.1)	1.0 (0.8-1.3)		1.0 (0.8-1.3)	1.1
Toddler (3-5) mortality per 1,000 population	1.0 (0.7-1.3)	0.9 (0.5-1.2)	0.4 (0.3-0.6)		0.6 (0.5-0.8)	1.4
Maternal mortality per 100,000 live births	1084.5 (736.0-1432.9)	818.1 (601.7-1034.4)	718.3 (478.6-957.9)		486.7 (293.3-680.2)	780.0
Length, males at 20 years of age		163.4 (162.9-163.8)		166.4 (166.0-166.8)		167.6 (166.3-168.9)

Source: Central Bureau of Statistics in Sweden.

Discussion

The most important part of former research in the actual field was performed by Vilhelm Hultcrantz as was pointed out above. His studies comprised aggregated statistics covering the whole period 1840-1926. Hultcrantz also participated some years as a medical officer in the enlistment of conscripts, an ideal situation for a researcher. His scholarly work was based on more than 3 million observations. Already in the 1890's he made some basic findings, very similar to what has been observed in international research lately. Among other things he noticed the bell shaped distributions of the height of the conscripts in every cohort. He was also quite aware of the fact that the smallest individuals were never registered or only partly treated. He also dealt with many other source critical problems connected with changing administrative routines as well as different losses.

According to Hultcrantz there was an increase in the height of the recruits starting from about 1850 and accelerating in the late 19th century. Even for the 1840's he could register a slight increase. He was not aware of the contradictory development we have noticed above. In line with Robert Fogel we could talk about a proletarization paradox. As we mentioned above this paradox must be dissolved one way or another. Hultcrantz suggested that a decreased alcohol consumption may be the most important part in this development. As a matter of fact the alcohol consumption in Sweden culminated in the 1830's whereafter a secular but slow decline took place. Hultcrantz' interpretation may very well shed light on an important change but our results imply rather some sort of improvement of nutrition as regards volume and composition at least for major parts of the Swedish population.

Gunnar Sandberg and Herbert Steckel have used the more fragmentary information about the soldiers-crofters treating the whole period between 1750-1850. Their investigation area happens to be the same as ours, the region of Uppland. Their sample comprises only 2.000 observations which of course is too scanty to constitute a firm basis for interpretations. What they have done is a first tentative study on the available material. For the period 1840-1860, which overlaps Hultcrantz' study they have found the same tendencies. According to Sandberg-Steckel's findings the first cohort born in the early 1790's coincides with a trough in the height development of the whole Swedish population; this finding seems to be confirmed by our results.

To conclude: we have established a definite height increase in our consecutive age cohorts during the 19th century. But this height increase has been unevenly distributed by district and social strata over time. In some districts there were observed set-backs of height development, while in others the increase was more uniform. Differences in height by social background were even more pronounced in the latest cohort, which of course shed light on the proletarization process that was going on. Students were in fact more than two generations before the general population. Evidently, environmental influences during childhood are responsible for these differences among adults and between different sub-populations. This is also indicated by the close association between height increase on one hand and declining mortality on the other which has been revealed in our study. The hypothesis that there might be differences between the central fertile area of Uppland and the out-skirts of the county has also been confirmed.

References

J. Abbolins, 'Utvecklingsförändringar under sista seklet', *Socialmedicinsk Tidskrift,* 43 (1964).

T. Bengtsson and R. Ohlsson, 'Levnadsstandard och mortalitet i Sverige 1750-1860', *Meddelande från Ekonomisk-historiska institutionen, Lunds universitet,* 37 (1984).

M. Essemyr, 'Food Consumption and Standard of Living. Studies on Food Consumption among Different Strata of the Swedish Population 1686-1933', *Uppsala Papers in Economic History,* 2 (1983).

R.W. Fogel, 'Nutrition and the Decline in Mortality since 1700: Some Preliminary Refindings', *Working paper no 1402, National Bureau of Economic Research* (1985).

J.V. Hultcrantz, 'Über die Zunahme der Körpergrösse in Schweden in den Jahren 1840-1926', *Nova Acta Regiae Societatis Scientiarum Upsaliensis, Volumen extra ordinem editum 1927* (Uppsala 1927).

O. Krantz and O.L. Schön, 'Om den svenska konsumtionen under 1800- och 1900-talen', *Meddelande från Ekonomisk-historiska institutionen, Lunds universitet,* 35 (1984).

C. Lundh, 'Levnadsstandarden—indikatorer och mått. Engelsk och svensk debatt om lönearbetarnas villkor 1750-1850', *Meddelande från Ekonomisk-historiska institutionen, Lunds universitet,* 92 (1982).

'Maternal Health Care and Development Assistance', *report to SIDA, The Health Division* (Stockholm 1986).

L.G. Sandberg and R.H. Steckel, 'Soldier, Soldier What Made You Grow so Tall?', *Economy and History,* 23, 81 (1983).

The New England Journal of Medicine, 213, 283 (1985).

Comments on the Session Change and Patterns in Rural Mortality

John Rogers

Change and patterns in rural mortality is the theme of this last session of the conference. Change, of course, provides us with the historical dimension, the unifying theme of the conference. Patterns indicate, however, that we are dealing with observable differences in the structure and scope of mortality in rural areas. In other words, we are assuming that there is no general rural or agrarian pattern of mortality. In contrast we often assume that it is possible to analyze and discuss urban mortality, in spite of the fact that there were in the past as there are today significant demographic variations within the urban sector. Although we generally consider towns and cities during the preindustrial era and the period of early industrialization as being more unhealthy than rural villages, many of the explanatory variables attributable to an urban environment, such as overcrowding, inferior sanitary conditions, low quality foodstuffs or contaminated water supplies, were also applicable to many rural milieus. The significant variable was population density. The mere fact that large numbers of people lived together in close quarters increased the negative consequences of such factors. The result, as we know, was a higher rate of mortality in urban areas. In Sweden, for example, the crude death rate for the period 1816-1840 was 22 o/oo in rural areas and 34 o/oo in urban areas. Although the national crude death rate in Sweden decreased steadily during the nineteenth century, urban mortality declined more rapidly than rural mortality, diminishing the rural-urban differential. By the second decade of this century urban mortality dropped below rural mortality, reversing the preindustrial relationship.[1]

The distinction between rural and urban has had an unusual effect on research. Although the analysis of variation within the urban sphere is common, we tend to stress similarities rather than differences with regards to mortality and its causes. On the other hand, most studies of rural mortality emphasize the fact that there were marked variations or patterns. This may explain why, under a general theme of rural mortality, we find a paper on the 1868 famine in northern Sweden, a paper on the role of smallpox vaccination in the decline of mortality in Norway, and a study of the causes of death in a mining parish in Sweden during the eighteenth and nineteenth centuries. Stressing the differences!

During this conference a consensus has been reached on at least one point, that the analysis of mortality change, be it the study of dramatic rises or gradual declines, is indeed a complex and difficult undertaking. The pitfalls are many and unambiguous results few. All three papers presented to this session address this problem, each in a different manner. Tommy Bengtsson's analysis of the changing structure of mortality in Västanfors uses information on age at death and cause of death to determine long-term trends. Ståle Dyrvik, on the other hand, attempts to assess the role of one particular cause of death, smallpox, in a general decline of mortality in Norway. Marie Clark Nelson, through a detailed analysis of local patterns, tries to sort out the complexity of factors associated with epidemic and famine related mortality. All three studies clearly reveal the disadvantages and advantages of working with historical sources on the micro-level.

The disadvantages are well-known, small numbers leading to spurious results making valid comparisons and generalizations difficult. Dyrvik's study illustrates several of the problems involved in working with a small number of observations. For example, in Table 7 (annual births and deaths among children 0-14 years of age during the period 1801-1840) Dyrvik considers an increase of two to three deaths in the age group 1-9 as indicating a smallpox epidemic. The 1823 epidemic is based on five deaths in this age group. To say the very least, we are on shaky ground here.

While Bengtsson's work is not hampered by small numbers, it is difficult to draw any general conclusions from the analysis. Studying one parish with a specific socio-economic structure and a changing mortality pattern very similar to the country as a whole, does not increase our knowledge of the underlying causes of changes in mortality, regardless of the amount of detail in the analysis. As Bengtsson pointed out, this is only the first of several parishes to be studied. We can only hope that an expanded sample together with the inclusion of other demographic variables will lead to a better understanding of the mechanisms behind long-term changes in mortality.

Nelson's work includes an analysis of several parishes and as such generally avoids the small numbers problem. Since the province under observation was in the center of the famine area, the problem of generalization is also partially avoided. Although Nelson uses a detailed analysis for the comparison of the various local areas within a larger region, the results are not directly compared with other famine areas. Nelson has been able to show that there was a significant amount of variation in mortality experience within the larger region and has offered plausible explanations for this. Yet the answer to the question of whether or not an increase in famine associated mortality was actually avoided because of measures undertaken by the authorities and other help organizations still eludes her, mainly because she has not compared her results with famine areas in nearby Finland where death rates reached exceptionally high levels. Oiva Turpeinen's earlier presentation of infant mortality during the famine period in Finland provides comparable demographic information (see O. Turpeinen's contribution to this conference). Turpeinen, however, does not consider the role of relief organizations. Without comparison the results will remain inconclusive.

Tommy Bengtsson's paper, "Mortality and causes of death in Västanfors parish, Sweden, 1700-1925", illustrates one of the distinct advantages of working on the micro-level; a large variety of variables can be analyzed over long periods of time. In this way we are able to study long-term trends while keeping changes in the environment under control. Bengtsson's stated purpose is to describe the panorama of causes of death and discuss problems in the source material. Several others, for example Imhof and Lindskog, Fridlizius and Ohlsson, Larsen, and Puranen have considered the problems involved in using Swedish sources on causes of death (see bibliography in T. Bengtsson's contribution to this conference). Since several of these experts are in attendance, this topic can be treated more thoroughly in the following open discussion.

Although Bengtsson clearly states that it is not his intention to discuss the underlying causes of mortality change, he cannot completely avoid the issue. There are two interesting problems which arise in this connection. In his discussion of tuberculosis Bengtsson compares death rates in Västanfors with Sundbärg's estimates for the entire country and finds that, except for one period, the share of deaths attributable to tuberculosis was on the same level and changes followed the same pattern as for the country as a whole. Sundbärg assumed a fairly stable level tuberculosis during the 1750's, 1760's and 1770's, approximately seven per cent of all deaths. Bengtsson found that in Västanfors about four per cent of all deaths were due to tuberculosis. Very little information is provided given in the paper on conditions in Västanfors during this period, making it difficult to speculate on reasons for the lower death rate associated with tuberculosis. Was Sundbärg wrong in his estimates or was there some factor in the parish, such as a decline in the mining industry, which might account for the discrepancy? Or is the lower rate of tuberculosis in Västanfors simply due to changes in nomenclature? According to the table in the appendix, during the twenty-five year period 1751-1775 unknown childhood diseases increased while diseases of the breast decreased, indicating that a change in classification occurred.

Bengtsson also notes that during the second half of the eighteenth century life expectancy in Västanfors was two years lower than the national average. The difference was due mainly to a higher rate of infant mortality. According to the diagrams presenting the major cause of death in Västanfors for twenty-five year periods, one of the major causes of death among infants for the period 1751-1775 was either scarlatina or stroke. Approximately thirty per cent of all infant deaths were due to one of these causes. Neither assumption is reasonable since according to the table in the appendix no deaths were caused by scarlatina and only 4.4 % were due to stroke. The graphic presentation in this series of diagrams is not an improvement over a simple tabular presentation and, as such, makes it more difficult rather than less difficult (which, of course, is the major reason for providing a graphic presentation of statistical data) to analyze the results.

On the whole the emphasis on a source critical discussion of causes of death is far less interesting than the few glimpses of relevant problems which turn up in the paper. One may hope that a larger sample and the planned analysis of other demographic variables will be related to important historical questions. Otherwise there is a risk that a vast amount of information will be processed and analyzed to no real purpose.

In Ståle Dyrvik's paper, ''The effects of smallpox vaccination on mortality'', the advantages of working with a small population in a spatially limited area when testing new methodological approaches are clearly revealed. Compared to the wealth of information Bengtsson has on causes of death in Västanfors, Dyrvik has none at all for Etne, the parish he has chosen to study. How then does one analyze the role of one particular cause of death, smallpox, in a general decline of mortality? Dyrvik, through an analysis of annual series of births and deaths, has attempted to locate outbreaks of smallpox in Etne. Combining this information with information on smallpox immunity (both natural and through vaccination), Dyrvik has tried to determine the relative role of smallpox in the general decline in mortality observed in Norway after 1815. He comes to the conclusion that, in spite of a government decree in 1810 making smallpox vaccination compulsory and a first mass vaccination in the parish in 1813, it was not until after 1840 that smallpox was brought under control. According to Dyrvik this delay was due in part to the uneven nature of the vaccination campaign and in part to the fact that a new virulent variety of smallpox appeared in the 1830's. Thus the influence of vaccination in reducing mortality during the early stages of a general decline has been overstated, raising new questions in Norway's demographic history.

Dyrvik's study is hampered not only by a small number of observations but also by the need to make numerous assumptions, as data on cause of death are lacking. Although experience has shown that methodologically sound approaches generally yield valid results even when small numbers are involved, caution nonetheless is advisable in judging the correctness of Dyrvik's interpretation of the historical situation.

In attempting to locate smallpox epidemics, Dyrvik relies largely on observable increases in deaths among children aged one to nine, using increases in infant mortality to support the findings. According to Bengtsson, one of the three major reasons for a decline in infant mortality in Sweden during the nineteenth century was the elimination of smallpox. If a similar development occurred in Norway, then prior to a general vaccination of infants a significant number of infants should have died during an epidemic. In Etne infant mortality rates during smallpox epidemics were higher than the average for the entire period. In epidemic years prior to the vaccination campaign, Etne experienced an infant mortality rate of 296 o/oo compared to an overall average of 196. During the vaccination period the rates were 238 and 168, respectively.

According to Dyrvik, during normal years about one fifth of all infant deaths occurred above the age of six months. During epidemic years one third to one half of all infant deaths occurred above the age of six months. The excess is attributed to smallpox. Assuming an increase of one half, we find that approximately six per cent of all infant deaths could be attributed to smallpox during the period prior to the vaccination campaign and 11 % during the campaign. We know that at least some of the infants were vaccinated during the campaign and yet the relative number of infant deaths increased. This would suggest 1) that not all of the epidemics during the pre-campaign period were identified, or 2) that because of a concentration on older children during the vaccination campaign, infants were more susceptible to smallpox during epidemics, or 3) a new and more virulent strain of smallpox, as Dyrvik suggests, appeared at this time. The fact that 35 % of all infant deaths during the period of vaccination compared to 22 % during the pre-campaign period occurred during epidemic years supports the above assumptions. Infant mortality, however, declined generally indicating, as Bengtsson suggests, that vaccination did play a role in reducing mortality. The problem, of course, is that far too many assumptions must be made in order to analyze Dyrvik's results. This is one of the major shortcomings of an otherwise stringent methodological approach.

Considering the pandemic nature of smallpox and the more reliable information on the disease available in the other Nordic countries, Dyrvik has probably localized most, if not all, of the major outbreaks of smallpox in Etne. Yet, because of the widespread nature of the disease and the irregular nature of the vaccination campaign coupled with the fact that the early vaccines did not provide life-long immunity, it appears highly improbable that valid inferences can be made on the basis of the Etne study for conditions on a national level. If other parishes experienced the same uneven pattern of vaccination observed in Etne, for whatever reasons, then a general outbreak would affect parishes differently. Should the methods introduced here be applied to a larger study, for example a stratified sample of all parishes in Norway or a larger sub-region? Very probably one could, with a larger sample population, more convincingly argue the dating of various epidemics but it is doubtful whether the extra effort, without better information on causes of death, would lead to a better understanding of the role of smallpox in the general decline of mortality in Norway.

Marie Clark Nelson's paper on mortality during the 1860's in Sweden's northernmost province actually does consider rural mortality patterns and although a period of one decade is short, certain changes are apparent. The starting point of the entire exercise is the significance attributed to the year 1868 in Swedish history. It is considered the year of Sweden's last famine.

There were distinct variations within the province of Norrbotten with a lower mortality in the inland regions and a higher mortality along the coast, a pattern observed in several earlier studies. This distinction remain during the famine, although mortality generally attained a higher level. Nelson avoids drawing definite conclusions on the major issues: why was there no significant increase in mortality in the famine struck areas in Sweden as there was in neighboring Finland? Was the Swedish relief program effective in combating famine? Was an increase in famine related mortality averted because of relief measures? As mentioned earlier, the only way of conclusively establishing that the help programs in Sweden actually did prevent a mortality crisis is to compare the effectiveness of the programs with measure taken in Finland. However, on the available evidence, it appears that the Swedish relief action, no matter how badly run (relief was unevenly distributed and often unreasonable demands were made on those receiving relief) was able to help alleviate the extreme consequences of famine.

An interesting relationship appears within the region with regards to the three main cultural groups, the Lapps, the Finnish speaking population and the Swedish speaking population. The distinction between the Lapps and the others is well-documented and, as Nelson points out, is the major reason why famine did not affect the inland regions to the same extent as the coastal regions. The herding of reindeer, hunting and fishing meant less dependency on grain crops and a healthier non-flour based diet. Thus the two inland parishes of Arjeplog and Arvidsjaur had crude death rates of 20.1 o/oo and 19.6 o/oo in 1868, compared to averages for the decade of 18.0 and 15.9. A point which Nelson does not consider is that in both parishes a number of new settlers had recently arrived. Considering the precarious positions of these settlers and the fact that they were at least partially dependent on grain growing, it might be of interest to determine who actually died during the famine in these parishes. The slight increases in mortality in 1868 may have been due to the deaths of newly established settlers.

The distinction between the Finnish speaking parish of Karl Gustaf and the Swedish speaking parish of Råneå is even more intriguing. Råneå experienced a diphtheria epidemic in 1864 resulting in a crude death rate of 57.7 o/oo. Although this increased the average for the decade, the death rate in 1868 was not extremely high, 30.7 o/oo (decade average 30.7 o/oo). Karl Gustaf, on the other hand, experienced a crude death rate of 55.5 o/oo in 1867 and 36.8 in 1868. The average for the decade was 34.6 o/oo. Nelson touches on some of the differences between the areas, noting that Råneå was becoming integrated into a market economy. The argumentation on this point tends to support a claim that Råneå was more susceptible to a famine crisis because an economic crisis occurred at about the same time with the bankruptcy of a major company in the area. There is no evidence indicating significant differences in

434

relief efforts in the two parishes. Under the assumption that the standard of living among the two population groups was on a similar level, the higher rate of mortality in the Finnish speaking area would suggest a cultural explanation, possibly with regards to choice or preparation of foods. This factor may, in turn, have eliminated part of the positive effects of the relief program in Karl Gustaf. That infant mortality was substantially higher in Karl Gustaf both in normal years and during the famine supports this supposition. On the other hand, smallpox was present in the parish during the famine and may account for the entire difference. The issue is certainly worth further study.

The papers presented here represent three ways of approaching the study of society, health and population in the past. Ståle Dyrvik begins by asking a specific question: what role did smallpox vaccination play in a general decline in mortality in Norway? Marie Clark Nelson is interested in a more general issue: why did the last great famine in Swedish history not lead to substantial increases in mortality? Both begin with important historical questions and attempt to answer them through an analysis of historical sources on a micro-level. Tommy Bengtsson, on the other hand, begins with a micro-level analysis in order to generate questions of general interest. The validity and usefulness of the results will vary, not only because the questions asked differ, but also because the emphasis is on small rural communities. As pointed out earlier, it is extremely difficult, if not impossible, to produce valid generalizations concerning rural mortality. As an analytical tool rural mortality only appears useful in relation to urban mortality. Now may be the time to discard the concept and discuss instead ecological regions, for example forest areas, coastal regions, mountainous regions or the mortality of the plains. Or why not urban and non-urban mortality?

Notes

1. *Historical Statistics of Sweden,* Part 1, Population. Second ed. 1750-1967 (Stockholm 1969).

Patterns of Mortality in Sweden's Northernmost County in the 1860's

Marie C. Nelson

The year 1868 has achieved notoriety in Swedish history as the great year of deprivation *(det stora svagåret)*.[1] A series of poor harvests in the 1860's culminated with the harvest failure in northern Sweden in 1867, while parts of southern Sweden were hardest hit in the autumn of 1868. In southern Sweden 1867, 1868, and 1869 were designated as *det våta året, det torra året, det svåra året* (the wet year, the dry year, the hard year).[2]

Weather conditions were extraordinary throughout the country in 1867, but had their most dire consequences in the north. The average monthly temperatures in Haparanda during the spring of 1867 were low, 3-4 °C below the average for the decade in April, May, and June. The following November and December were also unusually cold (Nov.: -10.7 °C compared with -6.1 °C, 1861-1870; Dec.: -17.4 °C compared with -9.8 °C, 1861-1870).[3] In May 1867 the snow lay deep in Råneå, and coastal steamboat passengers celebrated mid-summer on the ice off the coast when the vessel was unable to land in the city of Sundsvall.[4] Although low-lying areas were normally plagued by early frosts[5], the especially early frosts of 1867 spelled disaster for many.[6] The *Landsting* (county government) in Norrbotten, Sweden's northernmost county, placed the question of crop failure on the agenda for September 17 and 18, 1867. The emergency relief committee was activated, and a delegation sent to Stockholm to seek aid.[7] The machinery was put into operation to stem a crisis.

The question remains as to the traces which this famine left in the demographic picture of Norrbotten. Was there increased mortality due to the famine? Were there regional differences in mortality patterns within the county? If so, what caused these differences?

Famines were a common feature of the historical landscape up until the end of the eighteenth century.[8] Investigations of harvest failures and mortality have furthermore shown greater correlation in the eighteenth than in the nineteenth centuries.[9] In Sweden, as in other parts of Europe, the relationships become far less clear when one looks at the 19th century.[10] Nor are the reasons for this development evident. The decline of the importance of epidemic disease for increased mortality, the improvements of science and technology both in medicine and in other fields, the introduction and spread of new food crops, such as the potato and corn (maize), the general rise in the level of nutrition among the masses, and the greater effectiveness of government measures and organization have all been suggested as decisive factors in the declining mortality of the 19th century and with it the decline of the ancient plague of famine.[11]

Trends in mortality in Sweden

Mortality was on the whole decreasing in Sweden during the nineteenth century with the exception of the century's first decade and the second half of the 1820's.[12] Thus the question remains as to whether there were any marked short-term fluctuations which could in some way be related to the success or failure of the harvests.

Studies of nineteenth century Sweden have revealed a complex picture. D.S. Thomas has pointed out the correlation between a low harvest index, poor harvests on the aggregate level, and demographic changes. Marriage rates, the crude birth rate, and the fertility rates for both married and unmarried persons increased following ample harvests and fell in the wake of poor harvests, while the opposite was generally true of death rates. This pattern persisted until the late eighteenth century, after which it was only during the period 1863-1892 that there was a negative correlation between the death rate and the state of the harvests.[13] Lundsjö investigated the relationship between harvest results and poverty and concluded that in the areas where the crops were most likely to fail in the 1860's, poverty grew the most and that the growth of poverty was greatest in the north.[14] In a study of southeastern Sweden during the crisis of the late 1860's, J. Söderberg found that poverty increases were greatest in areas with a higher proportion of landless, but that there was a weak connection between poverty and the death rate.[15] In an analysis of mortality patterns in Sweden 1751-1802 on an aggregate level Fridlizius and Ohlsson could not establish a *direct* relationship between harvests and mortality, and found that certain diseases operated independent of harvest results.[16] On the other hand T. Bengtsson's investigation of harvest fluctuations and demographic response in southern Sweden on the county level, 1751-1859, showed that the impact of nutrition on mortality increased in the nineteenth century.[17]

The picture becomes even more complex when the question of "famine mortality" is superimposed upon the already existing regional variations. G. Sundbärg recognized three major demographic areas in Sweden: the eastern, the western and the northern. According to him the northern region, of which Norrbotten forms a part, had extremely high fertility, low mortality, little emigration, and few illegitimate children.[18] That the entire northern Scandinavian region was characterized by an inland-coastland pattern with high

438

mortality in the coastal areas and low rates inland was first noted by E. Sundt in Norway.[19] A study of regional variations of mortality patterns in Sweden concluded that, contrary to the generally declining death rates in the country, the death rate was increasing in the northern counties.[20] The mortality in the county might perhaps be better described as maintaining a level around 20 deaths per thousand with increased rates in the 1830's and to a greater extent the 1860's (see Figure 1).

When compared with the mortality rates of all counties Norrbotten's crude death rate exceeded that of all other Swedish counties for the decade 1861-1870 (24.9 per thousand) in spite of the high death rates experienced in individual parishes in Västerbotten in 1868 (see Table 1).[21]

Why then were Norrbotten's death rates higher than in other counties? The annual average crude birth and death rates were calculated for all the parishes in the county. What emerged was the pattern seen in figure 2. The Torne Valley region in the northeast on Finland's border generally had the highest death rate, a result similar to the pattern found in Finland for the period 1816-1865.[22] The mortality rates exceeded 25 deaths per thousand and, in some cases, 30 deaths per thousand. A low mortality rate dominated in the south-western part of the county well as Jukkasjärvi in the north. As the map indicates, this parish, Arjeplog, Arvidsjaur, and Malå all had death rates below 20 per thousand.

Figure 1. Crude death rate per thousand. Ten year averages.

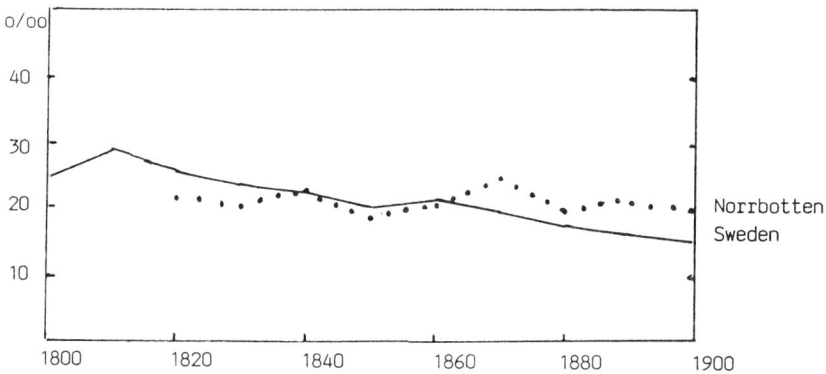

Norrbotten
Sweden

Source: Historisk statistik för Sverige. Stockholm 1969.

439

Table 1. The crude birth and death rates in the counties of Sweden 1861—1870 per thousand of the mean population.

County	Birth rate	Death rate
Stockholm	30.9	23.3
Uppsala	29.6	21.7
Södermanland	31.0	21.4
Östergötland	31.8	20.4
Jönköping	32.9	18.6
Kronoberg	32.9	19.9
Kalmar	33.2	19.9
Gotland	25.4	16.1
Blekinge	34.3	22.5
Kristianstad	30.8	18.6
Malmöhus	31.3	22.1
Halland	30.9	20.8
Göteborgs och Bohus	31.3	22.1
Älvsborg	30.9	19.8
Skaraborg	33.1	18.6
Värmland	32.0	19.0
Örebro	33.3	18.8
Västmanland	30.6	21.6
Kopparberg	30.9	20.2
Gävleborg	29.5	20.5
Västernorrland	33.2	21.0
Jämtland	29.0	15.3
Västerbotten	34.9	20.9
Norrbotten	37.5	24.9
Sweden	31.9	20.5

Source: BiSOS. Befolkningsstatistik.

The variations were thus great, the parish of Arvidsjaur noted an average crude death rate of 15.9 per thousand for the decade, while the parish of Karl Gustav, at the other end of the scale, experienced a rate of 34.8 per thousand. The towns generally followed closely the pattern of the surrounding parishes. Thus, the rate of Haparanda (25.6 per thousand) exceeded those of Piteå (22.9 per thousand) and Luleå (24.3 per thousand) (see Table 2). However, Haparanda had proportionately fewer deaths than the surrounding countryside, while Piteå and Luleå had more.[23] A number of observations may be made concerning the chronological distribution of the death rates during the 1860's (see Figure 3). First of all, the

Table 2. The mean crude birth rates and death rates for the parishes of the province of Norrbotten during the decade, 1861—70. Rates per thousand.

Parish	Death rate Mean	Range	Birth rate Mean	Range
Piteå rural	21.5	14.4—29.6	34.6	27.4—39.3
Älvsbyn	20.3	13.8—29.2	42.8	32.3—51.7
Neder-Luleå	22.5	16.8—32.3	33.7	25.4—39.0
Över-Luleå	21.7	12.8—32.7	41.0	34.8—46.0
Arvidsjaur	15.9	8.8—25.6	38.3	28.7—45.9
Malå	16.6	7.0—24.6[a]	35.4	23.2—41.9[a]
Arjeplog	18.0	9.3—28.8	30.4	24.7—36.5
Råneå	30.7	16.8—57.7	41.2	36.0—48.0
Över-Kalix	22.7	11.6—29.2	40.5	35.2—46.7
Neder-Kalix	28.6	20.7—44.4	39.0	30.2—43.2
Jokkmokk	23.3	11.7—33.3	28.7	22.3—37.6
Kvikkjokk	22.3	11.5—46.7	17.2	7.4—26.2
Gällivare	24.6	12.0—37.3	35.9	24.8—43.2
Pajala	25.2	15.4—37.6	37.2	32.0—46.5
Över-Torneå	26.6	15.9—34.3	37.7	30.7—45.7
Hietaniemi	27.2	18.7—34.2	37.5	27.2—44.8
Korpilombolo	34.6	15.2—57.4[b]	45.2	35.1—53.7[b]
Neder-Torneå	31.7	21.2—52.0	37.3	26.6—45.6
Karl Gustaf	34.8	24.3—55.5	38.9	31.2—46.6
Jukkasjärvi	18.4	12.3—29.0	35.1	22.6—40.4
Karesuando	21.8	16.5—31.2	27.4	20.8—35.2
Luleå city	24.3	15.6—35.6	32.1	25.4—37.3
Piteå city	22.9	16.2—33.0	31.2	27.1—35.7
Haparanda city	25.6	11.8—34.5	36.7	28.3—46.1

[a] The statistics for Malå are for the years 1862—68.
[b] The statistics for Korpilombolo are for the years 1862—70.

Sources: SCB. Summarisk redogörelse för folkmängden; Arbetstabeller. Sammandrag över döda; Utdrag ur dödböckerna.

general variations in the level of the crude death rate have already been mentioned. Most parishes experienced two periods with high mortality, the first generally falling between 1862 and 1865, and the second between 1867 and the end of the decade. In the inland parishes of Arvidsjaur, Jokkmokk, and Kvikkjokk 1865 represented the top year. Although it is the years 1867-1868 that have received the most attention, the earlier years of the decade represented an extreme period as well. Furthermore, in some of the parishes, for example Råneå, the crude death rate of the earlier part of the period exceeded that of the later.[24]

Figure 2. The crude death rate in the parishes of Norrbotten 1861-1870.

1. Karesuando	20. Arjeplog
2. Jukkasjärvi	21. Malå
3. Pajala	
4. Gällivara	
5. Kvikkjokk	
6. Korpilombolo	
7. Jokkmokk	
8. Över Kalix	
9. Over Torneå	
10. Hietaniemi	
11. Karl Gustaf	
12. Neder Torneå	
13. Neder Kalix	
14. Råneå	
15. Över Luleå	
16. Neder-Luleå	
17. Älvsbyn	
18. Piteå (rural)	
19. Arvidsjaur	

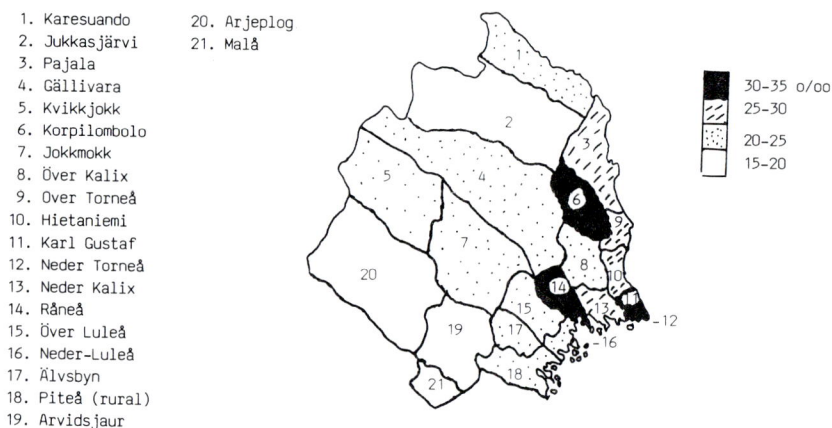

Legend:
- 30-35 o/oo
- 25-30
- 20-25
- 15-20

Suorces: SCB. Summarisk redogörelse för folkmängden, Norrbottens län 1861-1870; Arbetstabeller, Sammandrag över döda.

It is necessary to examine the death rates of the 1860's more closely in comparison with those of the preceding and following decades. A comparison shows that in 17 of 23 parishes the death rates of both the preceding and the following decades were less than those of 1860's. In the case of Råneå and Korpilombolo this difference exceeded 10 per thousand. A number of parishes in the inland suffered higher mortality rates during certain years in the 1850's and 1870's (see Figure 3). The death rates of these parishes differed little during the three decades.[25]

Clearly defined areas of Norrbotten were subject to increased mortality rates during the 1860's, and this increase was not exclusively confined to the later part of the decade. However, the problems of this ten-year period did not leave significant tracks in the death rates of the remainder of the county.[26] Several problems must then be considered: the sharp increase in the death rate in the early 1860's; the overall difference in death rates in the various parts of the county during the entire decade: and the relationship of the "famine" to mortality in the last years of the 1860's.

442

Figure 3. The crude birth and death rates in the parishes of Norrbotten 1851-1880.

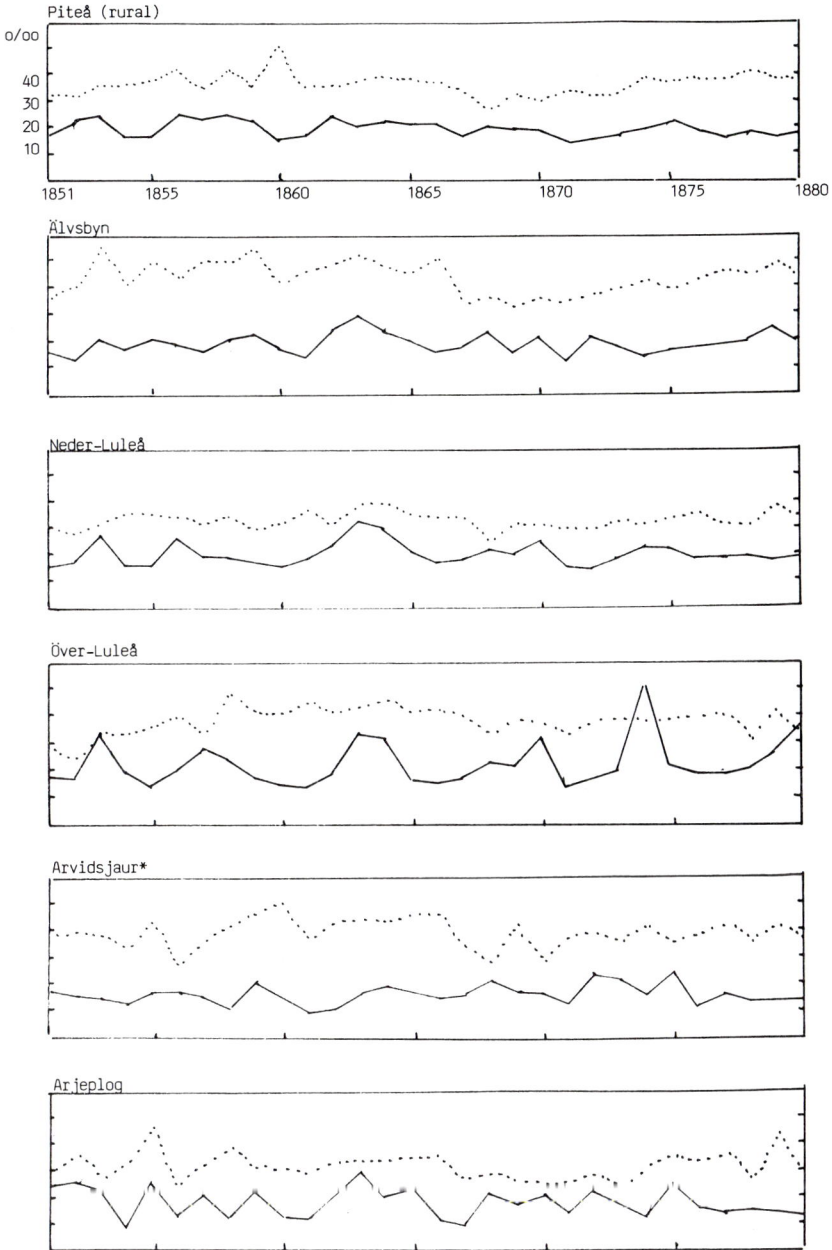

*Arvidsjaur included during the 1850's Malå and the villages of Nordenås and Fjellnäs. The latter are not included in the statistics for the two following decades.

cont.

Råneå

o/oo

Över-Kalix

Neder-Kalix

Jokkmokk*

Kvikkjokk

Gällivare

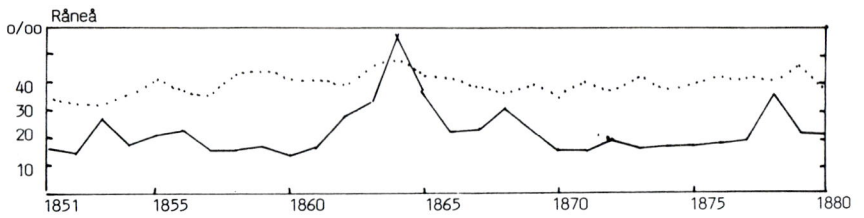

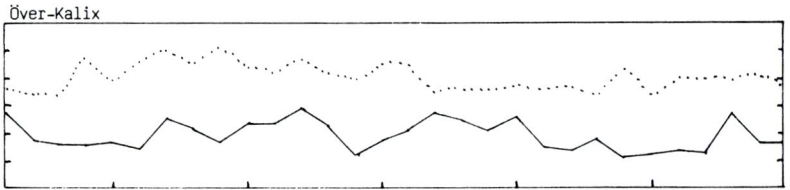

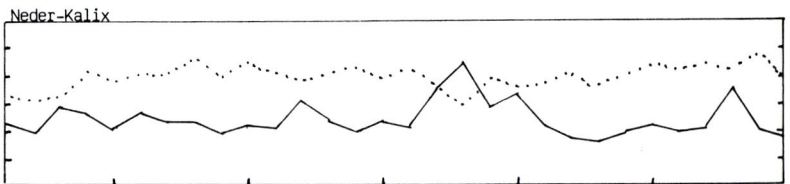

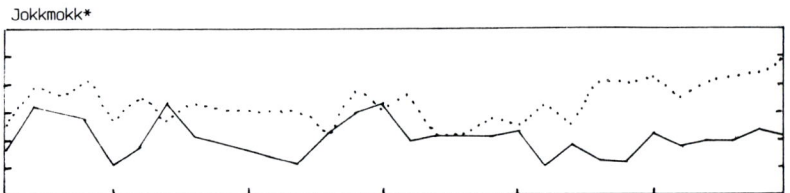

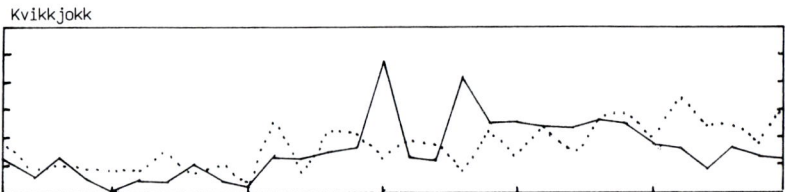

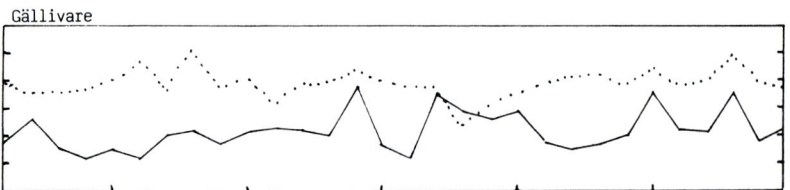

*There is reason to believe that the statistics for the period 1851-1860 may have been incomplete. The small size of the sample caused large fluctuations.

cont.

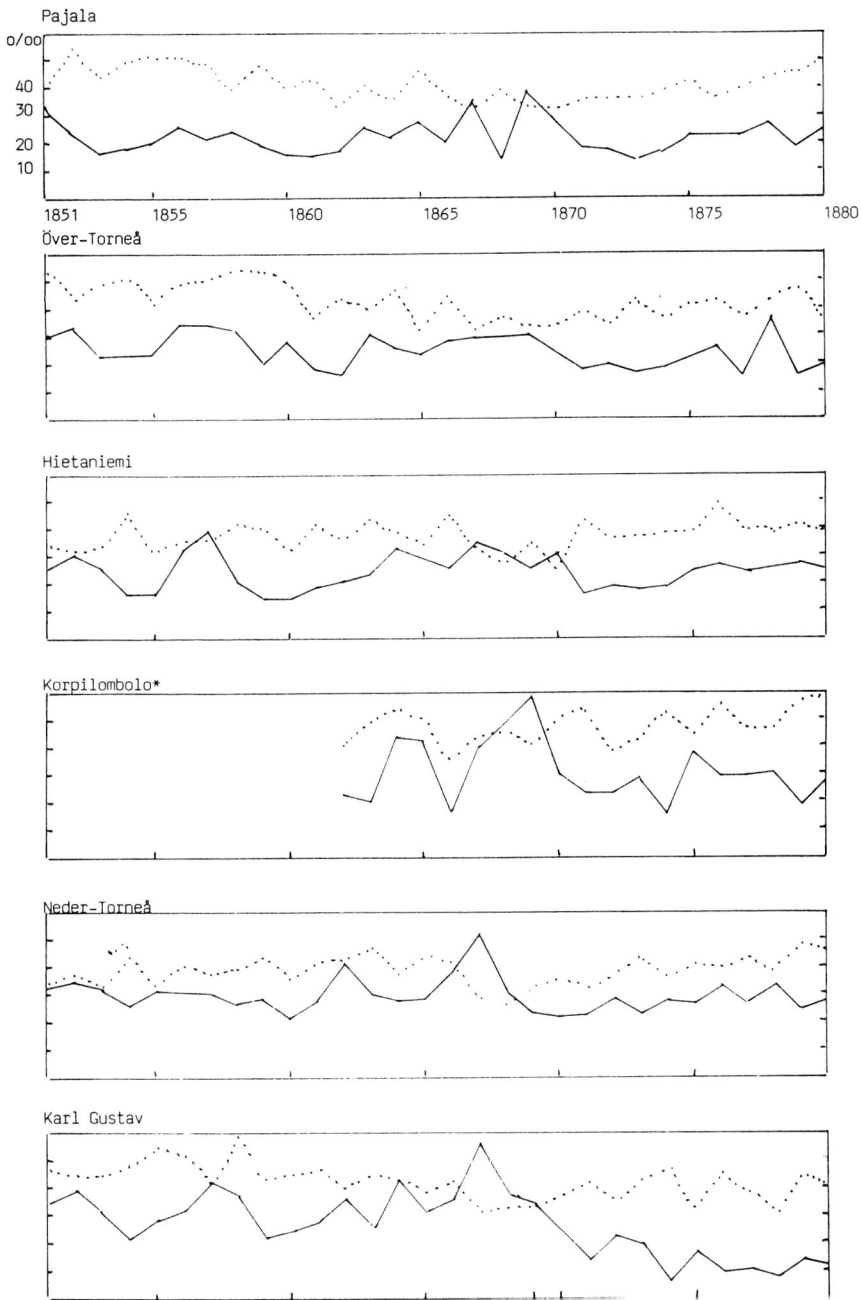

Pajala

Över-Torneå

Hietaniemi

Korpilombolo*

Neder-Torneå

Karl Gustav

* Korpilombolo was formed in 1856, prior to which it was part of Över Torneå, Över-
Kalix, and Pajala.

cont.

445

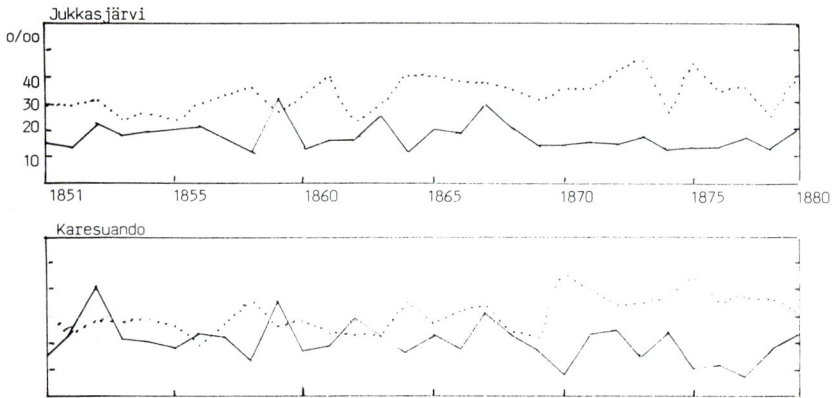

Sources: SCB: Nativiteten, Mortaliteten och Ingångne Äktenskap i Rikets församlingar 1851-1860; Summariska redogörelser för folkmängden, Norrbottens län, 1861-1870; 1870-års folkräkning, Tioårssammandrag av befolkningsrörelsen, Arbetstabeller; BiSOS A 1880.

Local studies

In order to attempt to look more closely at this pattern and to determine whether or not poor harvests played a significant role, some parishes were selected for study: Råneå on the coast, Arjeplog and Arvidsjaur in Lapland, and Karl Gustav in the Torne Valley Region.[27]

Råneå, a parish whose history also dates back to the fourteenth century, was in the nineteenth century occupied by a Swedish-speaking population. Agriculture was combined with animal husbandry and hunting and fishing and other sources may have provided some subsidiary income. The number of units of cultivation increased rapidly during the nineteenth century. There were three sawmills in 1850 as well as the iron works, Avafors, Melderstein, and Vitåfors. Tar was also produced, although its production began to decline early in the century.[28] Råneå was also affected by the foundation and the bankruptcy of The Gellivaara Company Limited (1864-1868), whose aim was to purchase all the iron works and their property and to develop iron mining and manufacturing. Improvement of transportation was undertaken in the form of the construction of a canal to bypass falls in the Lule River. The company also owned sawmills and a number of the farms in the parish.[29] While having a crude death rate of the middle range (30.7 per thousand) among the county's parishes for the decade as a whole, Råneå experienced the highest death rate of the decade in Norrbotten (57.7 per thousand) in 1864.

446

This parish served as a representative for the extreme increase in deaths in the beginning of the decade. It soon became apparent that diphtheria raged in Råneå beginning in 1863, culminating in 1864, and lingering on in 1865 (see Table 3 and Figure 3).[30] This epidemic reaped its greatest number of victims in the third quarter of 1864, especially during August and September. The deaths in that quarter were nearly three times as great as other peak periods. A comparison of age-specific mortality in 1861 and 1864 shows that, as might be expected, these deaths occurred among children. (See figure 4). Infant mortality had risen, but most striking was the dramatic increase of the deaths among children above one year of age up to age 15.[31] Nor was this epidemic confined to Råneå. During the years 1861-1863 several fatal cases were reported in Lappland. The disease made its appearance in the Kalix medical district in 1860, reaching epidemic proportions in 1862. Haparanda district reported cases in the beginning of 1862, whereas the Luleå district was stricken in 1864 and 1865.[32] Some areas in Lappland were hard hit in the mid-1860's (see, e.g., Table 3).

This epidemic, part of a diphtheria pandemic which was not under control until the beginning of this century, not only accounts for the high death rates in the early part of the 1860's in Norrbotten. The extreme mortality due to the diphtheria epidemic may also help explain the higher death rates earlier observed for this period, but not explained.[33]

Arvidsjaur and Arjeplog in Lapland contained market and church centers located in the interior. The land area of each of these vast parishes exceeded that of entire counties in southern Sweden. A large proportion of the population consisted of Lapps dependent on reindeer husbandry.[34] The majority was listed as being occupied in agriculture and/or its subsidiary occupations in 1870, the latter being lumbering, animal husbandry or fishing, although agriculture was less important than in the other parishes. There were also numerous new settlers *(nybyggare)*.[35] Arvidsjaur had the lowest crude death rate in Norrbotten for the entire decade (15.9 per thousand).

It is evident that the inland parishes in general had lower birth and death rates than the coastal region. This pattern has long been in evidence, as noted above. There was little change in the crude death rate over three decades, and it constantly remained at a lower level than in the remainder of the county. The rise in mortality in the mid-1860's in Arjeplog appears to have been caused by measles in 1863 and "old age" in 1865 (see Table 4). The infant mortality rate was slightly higher than in Råneå, but far lower than in Karl Gustav.[36]

Karl Gustav, originally part of Torneå parish, was formed in 1782. The area, first named in documents as early as 1345, had a predominantly Finnish-speaking population. Fishing, hunting, animal husbandry, and agriculture were the main sources of livelihood. Lumbering was insignificant.

Table 3. The causes of death in six parishes in the province of Norrbotten, 1861—1870. (When more than 25 % of the causes were reported.)

Parish	Year	% reported	(No.)	Disease	% of reported	% of total	Age	Range
Piteå rural	1863	29.8	(68)	diphtheria	42.7	12.7	>10m	≦8
				measles	36.8	11.0	5d	7
	1866	27.4	(66)	diphtheria	22.7	6.2	77m	14
				throat dis.	16.7	4.6	7m	14
Karl Gustav	1862	42.0	(34)	scarlet fever	88.2	37.0	6m	14
	1864	36.1	(35)	"nerffeber"	77.1	27.9	19	68
	1865	25.0	(18)	"nerffeber"	83.3	20.8	5	74
	1866	29.3	(13)	"nerffeber"	54.2	15.9	13	70
	1867	38.8	(47)	small pox	46.8	18.2	1m	39
				"nerffeber"	27.7	10.8	5	57
Råneå	1861	28.4	(27)	chest dis.	22.2	6.3	38	57
				tuberculosis	18.5	5.3	30	75
	1862	71.4	(110)	measles	20.0	14.3	1m	8
	1863	62.9	(122)	diphtheria	21.3	13.4	3m	8
				throat dis.	13.9	8.8	1	68
				whooping c.	18.9	11.9	1m	9
	1864	86.4	(280)	throat dis.	82.5	71.3	23d	25
				diphtheria	4.3	3.7	4m	13
	1865	67.7	(138)	throat dis.	66.7	45.1	7m	31
				diphtheria	3.6	2.5	2	10
	1866	40.3	(52)	throat dis.	34.6	14.9	2m	12
	1867	40.0	(55)	throat dis.	23.6	9.4	10m	24
	1868	49.4	(89)	pox	14.6	7.2	4m	60
				"nerffeber"	13.5	6.7	14	67
	1869	51.8	(74)	small pox	33.8	17.5	13d	78
	1870	60.4	(125)	scarlet fever	60.0	36.2	4m	15
Kvikkjokk	1861	85.7	(6)	child birth	33.3	28.6	31	36
	1862	48.9	(3)	child birth	66.7	28.6	24	27
	1863	50.0	(4)	child birth	75.0	37.5	19	25
	1864	100.0	(9)	diphtheria	33.3	33.3	8	19
	1865	100.0	(25)	diphtheria	88.0	88.0	6m	23
	1866	37.5	(3)	child birth	66.7	25.0	24	37
	1867	40.0	(2)					
	1868	54.5	(12)	"nerffeber"	50.0	27.3	21	70
	1869	72.7	(8)	old age	62.5	45.5	64	74
	1870	50.0	(6)	old age	50.0	25.0	69	79
Korpilombolo	1861	54.2	(13)	tb	38.5	20.8	2	27
	1862	63.6	(14)	tb	35.7	22.7	16	51
	1863	35.0	(7)	influenza	28.6	10.0	2m	1
	1864	33.3	(15)	diphtheria	80.0	26.7	9m	3
	1868	48.6	(35)	"nerffeber"	74.3	36.1	1	68
	1869	40.7	(24)	whooping c.	50.0	20.3	7d	5

(cont.)

Arjeplog	1861	92.3	(12)	old age	33.3	30.8	69	82
	1862	100.0	(23)					
	1863	100.0	(36)	measles	27.8	27.8	13d	38
	1864	100.0	(26)					
	1865	100.0	(27)	old age	18.5	18.5	62	93
	1866	100.0	(15)	old age	26.7	26.7	75	86
	1867	100.0	(12)	old age	50.0	50.0	70	101
	1869	95.5	(21)	old age	33.3	31.8	60	95
	1870	100.0	(26)	old age	26.9	26.9	67	86

Sources: SCB. Utdrag ur dödböcker, Norrbottens län, 1861—1870.

With time fishing and hunting had become of relatively less importance, partly because various fishing rights had been curtailed. Barley was the major agricultural crop. The parish, in general, reached no great heights except in the southeast corner, and its many low-lying bogs was subject to frosts.[37] This parish exhibited the highest crude death rate for the decade as a whole (34.8 per thousand).

A comparison of the age-specific mortality during a "normal year" (1861) and an extreme year (1867) reveals a strikingly high rate of infant mortality in 1867. The rate of death for children in the age group 1-4 was also excessive, nearly seven times as great as the year used for comparison. Furthermore, there are relatively more deaths among nearly all groups, but especially among women over 35.

Although the causes of death were not reported as frequently as in other parishes, it can be assumed that smallpox was a probable cause of much of the increased mortality among children in 1867. Less clear is the case with *nerffeber* ("nerve fever", a type of typhus). Smallpox struck children, whereas *nerffeber* more often afflicted adults. The high infant mortality accounted for much of this high rate.[38]

It is also interesting to compare the birth and death rates in Karl Gustav (see figure 4). It has often been pointed out that malnutrition and food shortages affect the fecundity of women.[39] S. Sogner has demonstrated the usefulness of using birth rates as an indicator of poor nutrition. In her study of the Norwegian crisis of 1783 she has found that, while sharply increased mortality was conspicuous with its absence, a decrease in the birth rate occurred.[40] The other parishes studied showed little or no decline in the birth rate in the late 1860's. In Karl Gustav, however, there was a marked decline in births, although the sharpest decline occurred in 1867, not 1868. Similar results may be seen when comparison is made with the neighboring parish of Neder-Torneå (including Haparanda) (see Figure 3). Thus the question of the relationship of mortality to hunger in the Torne Valley has not been clearly resolved.

Further comparisons may be made with both neighboring Västerbotten County and with Finland. The highest death rates of the 1860's in Norrbotten are compared in Table 4.

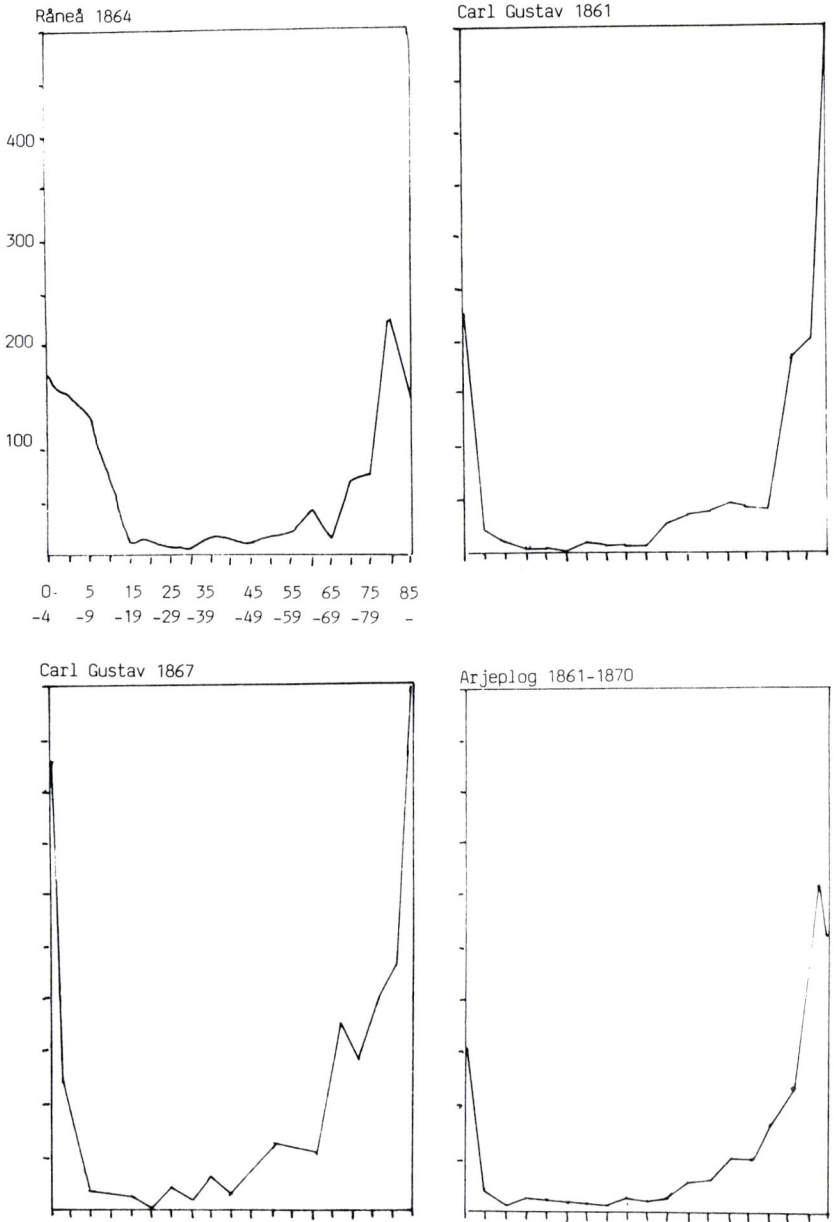

Figure 4. The age-specific mortality in selected parishes.

Table 4. Comparison of crude death rates in years of high mortality during the 1860's.

Area	Year	Crude death rate per thousand
Norrbotten		
Råneå	1864	57.7
Korpilombolo	1868	44.8
	1869	57.4
Neder-Torneå	1867	52.0
Neder-Kalix	1868	44.4
Kvikkjokk	1868	42.3
Västerbotten		
Robertsfors	1868	84.0
Bygdeå	1868	65.1
Burträsk	1868	59.6
Säfwar	1868	54.8
Finland		
Parkano (Åbo län)	1868	231.8
Reisjärvi (Uleåborgs län)	1868	219.2

Sources: Jensen (1978), pp. 13, 21, 28, 34; Bidrag till Finlands Officiella statistik. VI. Befolkningsstatistik, Andra häftet. Födde, Vigde och Döde åren 1865—1868 jemte en öfversigt af folkmängdens förändringar sedan 1812.

The differences speak emphatically for themselves. There were sixteen additional parishes named in Finland in which the crude death rates in the same year were between 10 and 20 *percent* of the population.[41] The total number of deaths in Finland in 1868 (137, 720) was nearly a doubling of the 1867 figure and more than twice as great as the total for 1866. Births in 1868 decreased by more than one-third when compared with 1864. Typhus was rampart, and 2,349 persons were recorded as having died of hunger or "hunger diarrhea", a figure assumed to be an underregistration of the actual starvation deaths.[42] The death rates in modern famines in non-European countries or during the Irish Potato Famine could provide further contrast. People did not die in such comparatively great numbers in Norrbotten. Thus the situation might best be compared with the aversion of a potential demographic crisis as was the case in Norway in 1783.[43]

Conclusion

The demographic evidence shows us that much of the increased mortality of Norrbotten in the 1860's may be explained by the presence of epidemics, particularly the diphtheria epidemic which struck early in the decade and began to wane in the second half. The pattern of low mortality in the interior and higher mortality on the coast was preserved. The role played by the crop failures and subsequent destitution and hunger are far less clear. An important point, however, should be born in mind. Death is only the *final step* in a long process of malnutrition and starvation.[44] The fact that mortality did not always increase does not deny the suffering and wretched deprivation of which there is more than ample evidence, but on the whole the populace managed to keep itself above the final threshold in most parts of Norrbotten.[45]

However, the difficult question of the relationship of nutrition and disease must be considered. Many volumes have been written in this question and the debate rages. T. McKeown has been a spokesman for the interpretation that decreasing mortality rates were the result of improvements in nutrition rather than because of the advances of medical science and health care.[46] The implications of his arguments are far-reaching. Others have completely refuted McKeown and maintained that disease, or at least specific diseases, are not affected by malnutrition.[47] Attempts have been made to categorize the relationship between nutrition and disease. One such characterization summarizes the situation thus: some diseases are definitely encouraged and exacerbated by malnutrition; other diseases are not affected by nutrition at all and cause epidemics which readily cross all social boundaries; still other diseases remain very much debatable or the picture may be blurred by a number of circumstances.[48]

If malnutrition does foster illness and mortality for certain diseases, then it is necessary to determine whether or not the people were malnourished in the areas that suffered most. That is not an easy task, but there is some evidence to support this notion. It has often been pointed out that a cereal and milk based diet which was gradually supplemented by potatoes during the nineteenth century long persisted in central and northern Sweden's agricultural areas. Little meat or fish was consumed.[49] A government-sponsored investigation of nutrition in the area of Norrland in the early 1930's revealed that this diet favored the existence of certain types of anemia and gastric disorders.[50] While one may argue that changes in diet probably occurred in fifty years, contemporary reports of the district doctor in the Pajala district described the food in the Torneå Valley in 1867 as follows:

> their food consists nearly exclusively of sour milk *(pimä)*, sour fish, and unleavened barley bread *(rieska)*, their drink of soured (rotten?) buttermilk *(kirnopimä)*, and their nearly only warm drink of coffee. Meat is seldom eaten and boiled food an exceptional Sunday. On the other hand the foodstuffs in the parishes of Lapland are on the whole more substantial.[51]

The greater dependency of the coastal regions and the Torne Valley on a flour-based diet is supported by the fact that the estimated yearly grain requirement per person for the Swedish-speaking and Finnish-speaking population was 12.85 ft.³ while the Lapps were estimated to need only about half that amount.[52] If more people in the Torne Valley lived closer to the subsistence margin, and if the people in the interior had a better diet, then this might at least partially explain some of the regional differences.

There is evidence that much of the population lived at or near the subsistence level. The common use of bark breads and other surrogates both in Norrbotten and elsewhere is well documented.[53] Efforts were also made by the authorities to convince people to use more nourishing food substitutes, such as lichens, in their bread.[54] The margin between survival and severe malnutrition may have been very small.

Yet, there are other factors which must be considered. In the 1860's the county was on the edge of integration into the market economy of the nineteenth century. The lumber industry was growing, although its real breakthrough came after 1870.[55] In spite of a certain amount of homogeneity in the economic system, there were some regional differences which cannot be entirely ignored on the local level.[56] While reindeer husbandry was important in the inland, agriculture dominated elsewhere with animal husbandry gaining ground. Furthermore, the economic recession of the 1860's, accompanied by repeated crop failures, brought about unemployment, rising prices for grain (but not for meat), and a lack of both readily available cash and credit.[57] The situation was further exacerbated by the failure of The Gellivaara Company Limited and the subsequent loss of production and jobs in the county. There were also complaints of that company's failure to observe its patriarchal obligations in regard to obtaining grain for "its people".[58]

The character and the success or failure of the aid given must also be considered. Early in the fall of 1867 the Emergency Relief Committee was activated on both the county and the local levels. Aid was requested from Stockholm and guidelines were established for the distribution of all aid which was to be channelled through the committees.[59] There were great variations in the distribution of the aid locally. For example, in Överluleå the committee decided that each homeowner who could post bond would receive 4 ft.[3] of grain for each person in his household, while others received 1 ft.[3] per person. The remaining 700 ft.3 were to be reserved for seed grain for the spring. These terms greatly displeased the county governor and aroused public opinion. In Jokkmokk, held up as an example of fairness by Luleå's newspaper, one-tenth of the grain was reserved for seed. Grain was allotted by a committee. Provisions for repayment were made for those who could not pay cash; if a bondsman could not be provided, then a contract for a payment in kind could be made. In many parishes flour was dealt out in return for work.[60]

It is difficult to determine the actual results. This point needs further investigation. However, there are a number of questions which may be pondered. Crucial in the distribution of aid often seems to have been the question of the repayment of these "loans" of grain, the extension of credit, and the ability to find bondsmen. There were numerous complaints of the lack of cash and of the failures to obtain extensions of credit; bankruptcies were frequent.[61] It is evident that many Finnish peasants found themselves in a similar predicament during the same year. Loans that had been made during earlier crop failures, especially 1862, were due to be paid when the even more severe failure of 1867 took place. A further extension of credit was impossible.[62] If one is to believe the contemporary reports, the harvest failure of 1867 was the final blow to an already hard-pressed peasantry. Government responded, but perhaps did not fully understand the problem nor the implications of some of its actions.

Another dimension should also be considered. Adherence to certain "moral" considerations made it impossible for the leaders of that day to respond otherwise: the morality of the peasantry should not be undermined by giving food; the repayment of debts for credit extended during the poor years of the 1860's should be made promptly regardless of the circumstances; and collateral or bondsmen were often deemed essential for a household to be considered for the distribution of food.[63] While such regulations were designed to prevent both the economic ruin of the local governments and leading merchants (the largest taxpayers) in the short run and the moral decline of the peasantry, they spelled poverty, destitution, and beggary for the many.

The increased mortality in Norrbotten County in the 1860's was mainly the result of epidemics, particularly diphtheria, during the first part of that decade. The questions of the reason for this pattern and of the relationship of the hardships that followed the 1867 harvest failure to mortality are far from clear. It is probable that malnutrition contributed to the higher death rates in the Torne Valley in the late 1860's, but the differentiated pattern of mortality within the county appears to follow cultural boundaries and the differences in the most important sources of livelihood. No single explanation emerges. Rather, some factors have been suggested which may have played a role in the creation of these patterns.

454

Notes

1. O. Häger, C. Torsell and H. Villius, *Ett satans år* (Stockholm 1978).

2. E.G. Holm and E. Lönnberg, 'Nödåren i Norra Småland 1867-1869', *Medd. från Norra Smålands Fornminnesförening och Jönköpings Läns Hembygdsförbund* (1944), p. 3; G. Sundbärg, *Betänkande i utvandringsfrågan och därmed sammanhängande spörsmål* (Stockholm 1913), p. 157.

3. M.C. Nelson, 'Through a Looking Glass. Report on the Famine in Norrbotten as Seen through the Eyes of Norrbottens-Kuriren, 1867-1869', *Historisk Tidskrift,* 2 (1984), p. 184. (hereinafter referred to as Nelson 1984a); *BiSOS. Helso- och sjukvården.* I. Sundhets-Collegii Underdåniga Berättelse. Ny följd. 1-10: (1861), p. XVIII; (1862), p. II; (1863), p. I; (1864), p. I; (1865), p. I; (1866), p. II; (1867), p. II; (1868), p. II; (1869), p. II; (1870), p. II.

4. *Norrbottens-Posten* (Piteå) N:o 18, May 4 (1867); *BiSOS. Helso- och sjukvården.* I. Sundhets-Collegii Underdåniga Berättelse. Ny följd. 7 (1867), p. 15.

5. See, for example, E. Bylund and Å. Sundborg, 'Lokalklimatets inverkan på bebyggelsens läge i Arvidsjaurs socken', *Meddelanden från Uppsala universitets geografiska institution,* 77 (Uppsala 1952), passim.

6. *BiSOS Helso- och sjukvården.* I. Sundhets-Collegii Underdåniga Berättelse. Ny följd. 7 (1867), p. 15; *Norrbottens-Kuriren* (Luleå), September 12 (1867), September 26 (1867); *Norrbottens-Posten,* August 24 (1867), August 31 (1867).

7. *Norrbottens-Kuriren,* September 19 (1867), October 3 (1867), December 12 (1867).

8. See, for example, F. Braudel, *Capitalism and Material Life 1400-1800* (London 1977), pp. 38-42.

9. J.D. Post, 'Famine, Mortality, and Epidemic Disease in the Process of Modernization', *The Economic History Review,* Second series, XXIX, 1 (1976), pp. 22-26.

10. D.S. Thomas, *Social and Economic Aspects of Swedish Population Movements 1750-1933* (New York 1941), pp. 83-84.

11. Post (1976), pp. 22-26.

12. A. Norberg, H. Norman and S. Åkerman, 'Regional and Local Variations of Mortality in Sweden 1750-1900', *Scandinavian Population Studies,* 5 (Oslo 1979), pp. 55-73.

13. Thomas (1941), pp. 131-132.

14. O. Lundsjö, *Fattigdomen på den svenska landsbygden under 1800-talet* (Stockholm 1975), pp. 131-132.

15. J. Söderberg, 'Interrelationships between Short-Term Economic and Demographic Fluctuations in a Period of Crisis: South Eastern Sweden 1866-1872', T. Bengtsson, G. Fridlizius, and R. Ohlsson (Eds.), *Pre-Industrial Population Change* (Stockholm 1984), pp. 264-267.

16. G. Fridlizius and R. Ohlsson, 'Mortality Patterns in Sweden 1751-1802: A Regional Analysis', T. Bengtsson, G. Fridlizius and R. Ohlsson (1984), pp. 306-324.

17. T. Bengtsson, 'Harvest Fluctuations and Demographic Response: Southern Sweden 1751-1859', T. Bengtsson, G. Fridlizius and R. Ohlsson (1984), pp. 352-353, 339-343.

18. G. Sundbärg, *Emigrationsutredningen,* Bilaga V (Stockholm 1910), pp. 4-9.

19. E. Sundt, *Om dødeligheten i Norge* (Christiania 1855), pp. 111-124; In a study of infant mortality in Västernorrland and Jämtland during the nineteenth century J. Hellstenius noted a similar pattern. J. Hellstenius, 'Barnadödligheten i Vesternorrlands och Jemtlands län', *Statistisk Tidskrift, 73* (1884), pp. 153-168; S. Wahlund observed a low mortality rate among the Lappish population. See S. Wahlund, *Demographic Studies in the Nomadic and the Settled Population of Northern Lapland* (Uppsala 1932); Norberg, Norman and Åkerman (1979) have pointed out the existence of such a pattern for the northern regions of Sweden; Brändström reconfirmed the existence of such variations in his recent study of infant mortality in A. Brändström, *"De Kärlekslösa Mödrarna". Spädbarnsdödligheten i Sverige under 1800-talet med särskild hänsyn till Nedertorneå* (Umeå 1984); O. Turpeinen has found a similar pattern in Finland. See O. Turpeinen, 'Regional Differences in Finnish Mortality Rates 1816-1865', *The Scandinavian Economic History Review,* XXI, 2 (1973), pp. 145-163.

20. Norberg, Norman and Åkerman (1979), pp. 58-59. The following crude death rates were cited for Norrbotten county: 23.0 o/oo, 1816-40; 21.5 o/oo, 1851-55; 24.2 o/oo, 1861-65; and 20.00 o/oo, 1891-95.

21. T. Jensen, 'Dödligheten i fyra Västerbottenförsamlingar år 1868', *Historiska institutionen, Uppsala universitet* (Unpublished paper 1978), pp. 13, 21, 28, 34. In 1868 the following crude death rates were recorded: Robertsfors, 84.0 o/oo; Bygdeå, 65.1 o/oo; Burträsk, 59.6 o/oo; and Säfwar, 54.8 o/oo.

22. Turpeinen (1973), pp. 146-151.

23. On December 31, 1860, Luleå had 1516 inhabitants, Piteå 1554, while Haparanda recorded 737 citizens; M.C. Nelson, 'Some Baked their Bread from Bark, Lichen, and Straw. Mortality in Norrbottens län 1861-1870', *Historiska institutionen, Uppsala universitet* (Unpublished paper 1984), appendix. (hereinafter referred to as Nelson 1984b).

24. Nelson (1984b), appendix.

25. In the case of Korpilombolo the comparison could only be made with the 1870's. Nelson (1984b), appendix.

26. Cf. Söderberg (1984), pp. 265-267.

27. Sundbärg's description of these parishes in 1900 indicates that their production of grain for bread was by then insignificant (1-2 kg. per person; 0 kg. per person in Arjeplog) compared with a calculated need per inhabitant of 210 kg. per person and an average national production of 144 kg. per person. Although the validity of agricultural statistics may be questioned and changes has occurred between the 1860's and the period covered by the statistics, the small amount of grain for bread produced is striking. Sundbärg (1910), EU, Bilaga V, pp. 262-266. More investigation is necessary on this point.

28. E. Byström, 'Råneå socken', E. Byström (Ed.), *Råneå socken 1654-1954* (Luleå 1955), pp.9-20; E. DeGeer, 'Finländska och svenska språkgrupper/minoriteter i Sverige och Finland'. *Historiska Institutionens Tidskrift,* Nr 26 (1981), pp. 5-21; M. Öhlund, 'Socknens näringsliv: Översiktlig framställning', Byström (1955), pp.328-338; Å. Edlund, 'Socknens näringsliv: Socknens jordbruk', Byström (1955), pp.350-358.

456

29. A.W. Axelsson, *Gällivare-verken, investerings- och spekulationsobjekt 1855-1882. En lokalhistorisk studie kring kampen om naturtillgångarna i Norrbotten* (Luleå 1964), pp. 103-182, 198 and map in the appendix.

30. Diphtheria was generally acknowledged to be the major killer in the reports of the district doctor, even if throat disease was often listed in the causes of death in the church records. RA. Medicinalstyrelsens arkiv. Provinsialläkare rapporter. Råneå; A virulent form of diphtheria made its appearance in England in 1858 and spread over the world. B. Macfarlane, *Natural History of Infectious Disease,* 2nd ed. (Cambridge 1953), pp. 262-263; See also, M. Bergmark, *Från pest til polio* (Stockholm 1960), pp. 224-225.

31. M.C. Nelson, 'The Year the Children Died: The Diphtheria Epidemic in Råneå Parish, Sweden 1863-1865', *Meddelande från Familjehistoriska projektet,* 6 (Uppsala forthcoming).

32. J. Waern, *Om Difterins och Strypsjukans uppträdande i Sverige* (Stockholm 1885), pp. 26-29.

33. Cf. Norberg, Norman and Åkerman (1979); Usually high mortality rates for the ages 1-15 in the period 1850-1870 have been noted by E. Hofsten and H. Lundström. If the death rates due to diphtheria, which swept the county in a new, more virulent form during this period, were as high as in other afflicted areas as they were in Råneå, then this disease might partially account for their observation. Cf. E. Hofsten and H. Lundström, *Swedish Population History: Main Trends 1750-1970* (Stockholm 1976), p. 47.

34. In 1860 ca 29 % of the population in Arvidsjaur and 44 % in Arjeplog were classified as Lapps. SCB. Folkräkningen 1860. HIb:3 arbetstabeller.

35. SCB. Folkräkningen 1870. HIb:1. arbetstabeller.

36. Cf. Wahlund (1932).

37. See G.W. Lindfors, *Karl Gustavs sockens historia. 1543-1934* (Haparanda 1941), pp. 15, 19, 96-98 for information on Karl Gustav parish; DeGeer (1981), pp. 15-16, 18; SCB, Folkräkningen 1860: HIb:3, arbetstabeller. Folkräkningen 1870: HIb:1, arbetstabeller. In DeGeer and the material from SCB the distribution of the Finnish- and Swedish-speaking and Lapp populations may be seen. However, marginal notations in the working papers from SCB indicate that the categorizations were far from clear even for contemporaries because of intermarriage and the adaptation to different life styles.

38. For a discussion of infant mortality, see U-B. Lithell, *Breast-feeding and Reproduction. Studies in Marital Fertility and Infant Mortality in 19th Century Finland and Sweden* (Uppsala 1981), pp. 15-17; Brändström (1984).

39. Lithell (1981), pp. 15-17.

40. S. Sogner, 'A Demographic Crisis Averted?', *The Scandinavian Economic History Review,* XXIV, 2 (1976), p. 117-.

41. *Bidrag till Finlands Officiella Statistik* VI. Befolkningsstatistik. Andra häftet. 'Födde, Vigde och Döde åren 1865-1868 jemte en öfversigt af folkmängdens förändringar sedan 1812', p. 35.

42. A. Meurman, *Hungeråren på 1860-talet* (Helsingfors 1892), pp. 55-58.

43. Sogner (1976), pp. 116.

44. W.R. Aykroyd, 'Definition of Different Degrees of Starvation', in G. Blix, Y. Hofvander and B. Wahlquist (Eds.) *Famine. A Symposium dealing with Nutrition and Relief Operations in Times of Disaster, Symposia of the Swedish Nutrition Foundation,* IX (Uppsala 1971), pp. 17-21.

45. R.E.F. Smith and D. Christian, *Bread and Salt* (Cambridge 1984), pp. 327-360. This book presents the following scale (p. 332), briefly summarized below, which might prove helpful for categorizing the nutritional level of the peasants. Note that the individual peasant families could move between the various levels according to the seasons and the levels of prosperity.

(1) *affluence* — abundance of all foods, regular livestock products, some luxuary — reduced grain and potatoes an improvement.

(2) *adequacy* — most staples available, meat a luxuary, with a little meat and fresh vegetables — probably adequate.

(3) *mild difficulty* — animal foods and fresh vegetables luxuries, some staples not available — probably not adequate and "hard on the very young".

(4) *inadequacy* — animal foods insignificant, quantity and quality of staple food, bread declines — approaching the nutritional minimum.

(5) *begging* — area still capable of protecting from death by starvation, if not from disease.

(6) *starvation* —

46. T. McKeown, *The Modern Rise of Population* (London 1976), pp. 128-142 and T. McKeown, *The Role of Medicine* (Oxford 1979), pp. 59-63.

47. G.V. Mann, 'Food Intake and Resistance to Disease', *The Lancet* (1980), pp. 1238-1239.

48. See the 'The Relationship of Nutrition, Disease, and Social Conditions: A Graphical Presentation', *Journal of Interdisciplinary History,* XIV, 2 (1983), pp. 503-506, where the following categorization is presented:

Nutritional Influence on Outcomes of Infections

Definite	Equivocal	Mimimal	
Measles	Typhus	Smallpox	
Diarrheas	Diphtheria	Malaria	
Tuberculosis	Staphylococcus	Plague	
Most	Streptococcus	Typhoid	Respiratory
Infections	Influensa	Tetanus	
Pertussis	Syphilis	Yellow Fever	
Most	Systematic Worm	Encephalitis	Intestinal
Parasites	Infections	Poliomyelitis	
Cholera			
Leprosy			
Herpes			

49. G. Blix, 'Kostförhållanden i Sverige sedan äldsta tider', *Kungl. Vetenskapssocietetens Årsbok* (1954), pp. 60-61.

50. M. Odin, 'Sjukdomar och sjukdomsfrekvens i övre Norrland särskilt med hänsyn till födans sammansättning', N. Hellström (Ed.), *En socialhygienisk undersökning i Västerbottens och Norrbottens län,* (Lund 1934), II, p. 78 ff.

51. RA. Medicinalstyrelsens arkiv. Provinsialläkare rapporter: Pajala 1867.

52. HLA. Länsstyrelsens handlingar 1866-1870: DV. Norrbottens län.

53. N. Keyland, *Svensk Allmogekost. I. Vegetabilisk Allmogekost* (Stockholm 1919), pp. 111-114; L. Levander, *Livet i en Älvdals-by före 1870-talet* (Stockholm 1914), pp. 34-35.

54. M. C. Nelson and I. Svanberg, 'The Use of Lichens as Food: Historical Perspectives on Food Propaganda', *Linnésällskapets årsbok* (forthcoming).

55. See, for example, E. Heckscher, *Svenskt arbete och liv*, 8. uppl. (Stockholm 1976), pp. 262-271; H. Wik, *Norrlands Export 1871-1937* (Uppsala 1941), pp. 45-46; H. Östman, *Norrlands ekonomiska utveckling sedan mitten av 1800-talet* (Stockholm 1911), passim.

56. M. Nyström, *Norrlands ekonomi i stöpsleven* (Stockholm 1982), pp. 158, 162-163.

57. S-O. Bergström, 'Nödåren i Övre Norrland under 1860- talet', *Ekonomisk-historiska institutionen, Uppsala universitet* (Unpublished paper 1963), pp. 16-24; Lennart Jörberg, *A History of Prices in Sweden 1732-1914*, 1 (Lund 1972), pp. 145, 161, 309; *Kongl. Maj:ts. Befallningshafvandes Femårs-berättelser*, (1866-1870), p. 3; RA. Medicinalstyrelsens arkiv. Provinsialläkare rapporter (Piteå 1867); Nelson (1984a), p. 183.

58. *Norrbottens-Kuriren*, October 5 (1867).

59. Nelson (1984a), pp. 191-192; *Norrbottens-Kuriren*, December 5 (1867).

60. Nelson (1984a), pp. 193-194; *Norrbottens-Kuriren*, November 21 (1867). November 28 (1867).

61. See, for example, *Norrbottens-Kuriren*, September 19 (1867).

62. Th. Rein, *Johan Wilhelm Snellman, Senare delen*, (Helsingfors 1901), p. 577 ff.

63. Nelson (1984a), passim.

Mortality and Causes of Death in Västanfors Parish, Sweden, 1700-1925

Tommy Bengtsson

The present examination of mortality and causes of death in the parish of Västanfors is a pilot study of a larger study of Central and Southern Sweden. The entire investigation, which will comprise some fifteen parishes, is not only confined to mortality; fertility, nuptiality and migration will also be analysed. In this paper we shall limit ourselves to a description of long term changes in the death panorama and discuss problems in interpreting the causes of death in the parish registers. The determinants of these changes will be analyzed in a forthcoming study.

Västanfors is a mining parish in Bergslagen, i.e. in the central part of Sweden. The number of inhabitants was around 1,300 by the mid-18th century and approximately 2,200 one hundred years later. The parish is located in a hilly district with many water courses and with ample resources of high-quality iron ore. The iron industry has existed in this area since the 12th century. Surrounding parishes are dominated either by mining, like Västanfors, or by ironworks. Agricultural production existed, but was of minor importance in these parishes.

The population development of the district is similar to that of the country as a whole. During the second half of the 18th century the life expectancy was slightly higher than the national average, 36.8 years compared to 35.2 years.

As demonstrated in Figure 1, showing age-specific death risk and survivalship in five Bergslagen parishes, the increase in life expectancy during the 19th century was due to a decline in infant mortality as well as a decline in mortality in older ages. On the other hand, the death risk in ages 10-60 years was almost unaltered. From this figure one can also observe that the decline in infant mortality commenced after 1815 whereas the death risk in older groups declined somewhat later.[1]

The development in Västanfors was largely the same as in Bergslagen. However, some particularities could be discerned in the development of mortality. During the period 1770-1810 the level of mortality in the age group 25-50 was higher than the district average. Life expectancy too was somewhat lower in Västanfors, 35.8 years, and thereby closer to the national average. In a broad sense Västanfors is typical for its region, for which the development of mortality largely resembles that of other parts of Sweden. This does not mean that the development in Västanfors can be generalized to the whole of Sweden.

The data

As in the studies of Southern Sweden and in the case study of Central Sweden the source material consists of parish registers. However, on one point there are divergences in the data. While for the southern part of the country we have built our own family reconstitutions our analysis of the central part is based on reconstitutions done by Karl Arvid Edin.

In the early 20th century Edin made family reconstitutions for a number of parishes, mainly from Central Sweden. Edin's reconstitutions include not only data on births, deaths, and marriages but on migration as well. For these reconstitutions he used the regular parish registers, records from catechetical meetings, census registers, migration certificates and tax records.

Edin's investigations were aimed at filling the major lacunae in the official population statistics, namely the lack of data on age specific marital fertility. His study covers thirteen parishes, most of them neighbouring parishes in Bergslagen, the mining area in the middle of the country. He was then, at least to some extent, able to follow migrants from one parish to another. Thus, the family reconstitution data set for Västanfors used in this study includes events that have taken place outside the parish.

Figure 1. Age-specific death risk and survival in five parishes in Bergslagen 1751-1850.

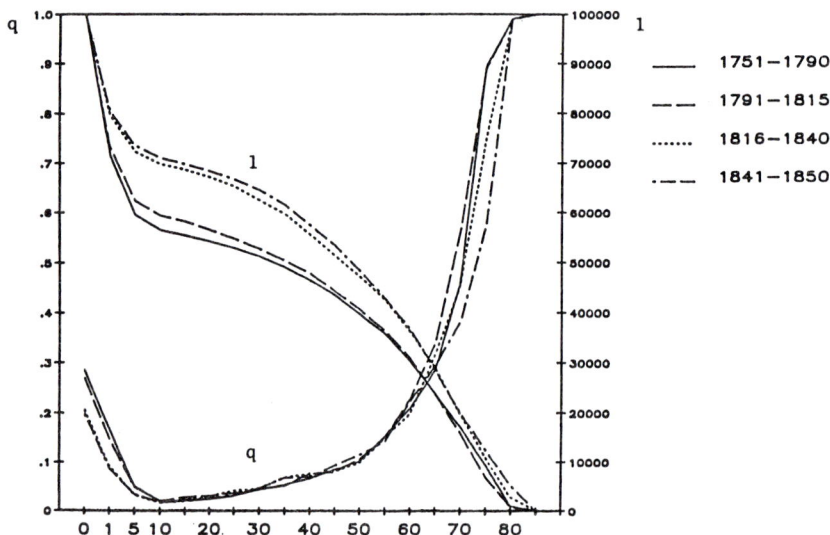

Table A.

	18th century	19th century
Number of deaths	3 993	3 860
with age	92%	98%
with cause	85%	75%
with age and cause	77%	73%

Edin was unable to complete his revisions of all thirteen parishes. Västanfors is one of the parishes for which the revisions appear to have been completed. An interesting point is that Edin used the same technique and form system that was used in the French studies half a century later.

One problem when studying a single parish is the tiny size of the population. When the number of events are few, random variation will dominate the series.[2] This is one of the reasons why our final study is to comprise around fifteen parishes. Thus, the aim of the present study is not, and cannot be, to trace general patterns and causes but to describe the panorama of causes of death and to discuss the problems in the source material.

In Edin's reconstructed material for Västanfors there are 3 993 deaths during the 18th century and 3 860 in the 19th century. In some cases, data concerning age of death is missing, whereas in other cases data for the cause of death is missing. In a few hundred cases more than one cause of death is stated. The following table gives an overview of the range of the data.

Thus, the data for causes of death, which is our prime concern is less frequent during the 19th century, specially during the second half of the century.

In addition to data on time of birth, time of death and cause of death, Edin's reconstitution comprises data on sex, date of marriage, date of migration, place of residence, profession and data referring to other members of the family.

In this study, the different causes of death will not be added together in various classes such as epidemic-endemic or diseases diffused by water or air. Instead, we confine ourselves to discussing them separately with emphasis on the most frequent causes. In Table 1 we list the total number of causes given in the death registers of Västanfors after standardization of the spelling of the names of the causes. Thus, we have made no aggregation or coding of any kind. If several causes are given, which is so in about 3 percent of the cases, we have chosen the first cause stated.

The validity and reliability of the death cause data

The Swedish data on causes of death from the 18th century are almost unique in an international perspective but for a number of reasons they are difficult to interpret. These difficulties have been discussed by a number of researchers including Sundbärg, Fridlizius, Imhof, Lindskog, Widén, Brändström,

Puranen, Ståhl et al, Lindahl, Nordenfelt, Nyström and others.[3] Some have a pessimistic view of the value of these data while others are optimistic.

In general, Ståhl et al, Lindskog and others with medical training are the pessimistic ones. From their own experience, they are aware of the difficulties in determining the cause of death even after an autopsy.

Lindahl and Nordenfelt discuss the problem from a philosophical point of view, distinguishing between direct and indirect causes in the chain of causality. For example, what is the cause of death if an old person breaks his leg slipping on an icy pavement and catches pneumonia at the hospital? In this paper we shall limit ourselves to a discussion of the direct causes of death, that is the medical, or rather biological, cause of death leaving a discussion of indirect causes for a forthcoming study.

Discussing the reliability and validity of the data on causes of death there are three major problems: (1) What are the effects of the development of medical science, (2) How do changes in the nomenclature and instructions affect the registration of the cause of death, and (3) How much did the diagnoses depend upon who made them, i.e. what are the effects of the individual priests or medical practitioners.

The medical knowledge of the time is the ultimate limitation of how correctly the cause of death could be diagnosed. At the time when the priests started to record causes of death in the 17th century there was no uniform nomenclature or classification.[4] Different medical systems existed side by side in Europe, and during the 18th century the nosological system was developed.[5] In this system, diseases were classified according to symptoms and not according to biological causes. The nomenclature used in *Tabellverket*, the Swedish population statistics that started in 1749, was a nosological system. From that time the causes of death were reported in a similar way all over the country. Printed forms were distributed and the priests made annual summaries of the causes of death according to age and sex.

Table 1. Causes of death in Västanfors 1700—1899. Percentage of the total number of deaths with cause specified.

Causes of death	Percent	Cumulative percent
1. Stitch and sting (håll och styng)	14.0	14.0
2. Chest disease (bröstsjuka)	12.5	26.5
3. Infirmities of old age (ålderdomssvaghet)	9.4	35.9
4. Consumption in the lungs (lungsot)	7.5	43.4
5. Smallpox (koppor)	7.1	50.5
6. Stroke (slag)	5.5	56.0
7. Unknown child disease (okänd barnsjukdom)	3.9	59.9
8. Dysentery (rödsot)	2.7	62.6
9. Stomach disease (magsjuka)	2.5	65.1
10. Dropsy (vattusot)	2.4	67.5
11. Whooping-cough (kikhosta)	1.8	69.3
		cont.

12. Putrid fever (rötfeber)	1.5	70.8
13. Fever fits (hetsig feber)	1.5	72.3
14. Childbirth (barnsbörd)	1.4	73.7
15. Drowning (drunkning)	1.4	75.1
16. Stillborn (dödfödd)	1.4	76.5
17. Hysteria (moderspassion)	1.4	77.9
18. Measles (mässling)	1.4	79.3
19. Accident (olycka)	1.4	80.7
20. Swelling (svullnad)	1.3	82.0
21. Thrush (torsk)	1.3	83.3
22. Cancer (kräfta)	1.2	84.5
23. Nerve disease (nervsjuka)	1.1	85.6
24. Heart disease (hjärtsjuka)	1.0	86.6
25. Inflammation of the lungs (lunginflammation)	1.0	87.6
26. Ague (frossa)	0.9	88.5
27. Shortness of breath (andtäppa)	0.8	89.3
28. Cold (förkylning)	0.8	90.1
29. Headache (huvudvärk)	0.8	90.9
30. Scarlatina (scharlakansfeber)	0.7	91.6
31. Weakness (svaghet)	0.7	92.3
32. Pain (värk)	0.7	93.0
33. Burning disease (brännsjuka)	0.6	93.6
34. Gout (gikt)	0.6	94.2
35. Coughing (hosta)	0.6	94.8
36. Kolera (cholera)	0.5	95.3
37. Fever (feber)	0.5	95.8
38. Colic (kolik)	0.4	96.2
39. Blood disease (blodsot)	0.3	96.5
40. Haemorrhage (blodstörtning)	0.3	96.8
41. Diarrhoes (diarré)	0.3	97.1
42. Falling sickness (fallandesot)	0.3	97.4
43. Sick from birth (sjuk från födseln)	0.3	97.7
44. Suicide (självmord)	0.3	98.0
45. Brock	0.2	98.2
46. Difteria (difteri)	0.2	98.4
47. Jaundice (gulsot)	0.2	98.6
48. Throat disease (halssjuka)	0.2	98.8
49. Brain disease (hjärnsjuka)	0.2	99.0
50. Gangrene (kallbrand)	0.2	99.2
51. Weak from birth (svag från födseln)	0.2	99.4
52. Boil (böld)	0.1	99.5
53. Rickets (engelska sjukan)	0.1	99.6
54. Piles (hemmorojder)	0.1	99.7
55. Head disease (huvudsjuka)	0.1	99.8
56. Influenza (influensa)	0.1	99.9
57. Sick (sjuk)	0.1	100.0
58. Itch (skabb)	0.1	100.0
59. Executed (avrättad)	less than 0.05	
60. Drunkenness (fylleri)	less than 0.05	
61. Convulsion (konvulsion)	less than 0.05	
62. Murder (mord)	less than 0.05	

The total number of deaths with cause specified are 5 051.

Population statistics were collected from the middle of the 1730s but were not made on a nationwide basis until 1749. At the beginning they were built up by special commissioners. From 1756 to 1858 this work was done by the Tabular Commission. From then onwards the population tables and other statistics were prepared by the Statistical Tabular Commission, a new government office. Its executive arm was later to become the Central Bureau of Statistics.

In many parishes causes of death were registered even before 1749. We do not know how far these registrations go back and how frequent they were. They were probably started on a more regular basis in 1686 when a new Church Law was passed. From then on the church was obliged to register births, deaths and marriages continuously as well as class, age and some other things.[6] Although they did not have to record the cause of death they often did so.

How common was it that the priests recorded causes of death prior to 1749? Puranen states that in most parishes causes of death were not properly registered until after the mid-18th century. However, she does not say on what grounds this conclusion is arrived at.[7] In the case of Västanfors, causes of death were first registered at the end of the 18th century when some deaths in smallpox, consumption in the lungs, and drowning were recorded.

The question is then which system was used prior to 1749, when a nosological nomenclature came into practice? Nyström argues that several systems were used as in the rest of Europe.[8] On the other hand it is obvious that Abraham Bäck, who designed the first two nomenclatures for population statistics must have been well-aware of the medical knowledge of those who were going to fill in the statistical tables. Therefore, it is likely that he started from what was common knowledge in Sweden at the time. Thus, the cause of death statistics shortly prior to 1749 must be similar to the statistics after 1749. Without making any attempt to generalize, this is what we have found for Västanfors, with a single exception discussed in the following.

By studying medical handbooks and textbooks we can get an idea of the medical knowledge of the time. Such a study has been made by Puranen for tuberculosis and other chest diseases.[9] The medical training for priests is also discussed in this context. An interesting comparison of the medical books with the population statistics has been performed by Imhof and Lindskog.[10] However, an analysis in which the medical books are compared with the recordings in the church books and the population tables has not yet been undertaken.

The instructions to the priest changed over time, reflecting changes in the needs of the society, medical advances and other things. As discussed above some priests interpreted the 1686 Church Law in such a way that they made diagnoses and recorded the cause of death in the parish register. From 1749 they received more precise instructions. Among other things, they were to report the number of deaths by 33 different diseases specified in a printed form.

In Västanfors, the priest continued to register the causes of death in the parish registers very much as before. This information was the base for the yearly population tables he made. The number of causes of death was about the same after 1749 as before. Thus, the priests in Västanfors had to add different causes together when reporting to the Tabular Commission. For example, while smallpox and measles were always registered separately in the parish registers in Västanfors, they were accumulated in the population tables.

Thus, the nomenclatures did not have any direct impact on what was registered in the parish registers. However, in one case there is a strong indirect effect. In the 1749 nomenclature one cause of death was called "unknown child disease". It had never been used before in Västanfors but from this year onwards the priests started to use it. It is clear that the cause was not introduced by a new priest as the same priest, Eric Todenius, was in service from 1731 to 1770 (see Appendix).[11]

Eight children died of "unknown child disease" in Västanfors in 1750. Earlier the diagnosis "unknown disease" had been used a couple of times for children. For the next fifty year period deaths from "unknown child disease" were registered in the parish registers almost every year. After 1796 it appears very sparsely, and in the early 19th century it is used only a couple of times.

In analyzing the changes in the death panorama for children below one year of age we find that the number of deaths from stitch and sting decreases rapidly as unknown child disease increases, but deaths from other, less frequent diseases, like chest disease, stomach disease and smallpox, diminish as well (see the following table).

Thus, it is very likely that unknown child disease to a large extent is the same as stitch and sting.

The nomenclature then changed in 1774, 1802, 1811, 1821, 1831, 1860, 1873, and 1891. The changes in 1774, 1802, 1811 and 1821 do not seem to have had any effect on what the priests in Västanfors registered in the parish registers. Thus, the problems with changes in the nomenclature when constructing continuous time series based on the population statistics does not exist when analyzing the parish registers.

Table B.

	1740—1749	1750—1759	difference
Chest disease	23	19	- 4
Stitch and sting	53	13	-40
Smallpox	9	3	- 6
Unknown child disease	0	25	+25
Other diseases	17	5	-12
No cause specified	18	27	+ 9
Totally	120	92	-28

The statistical tables of death causes almost come to an end in 1831 as a result of pressure from the priests who argued that they were not competent to make the diagnoses. From then on they only had to register deaths from smallpox and other epidemic diseases, deaths in child birth, accidents, crime and suicide.[12]

The new instruction had no immediate effect on Västanfors. Eric Eggertz, who came to the parish in 1806, continued to register causes of death in almost the same way as long as he was in service. In fact, he rather improved the registration during the 1830's. Only 11 percent of deaths were left without a registered cause.

His successor, Georg Fredric Seseman, who started his duties in 1843 and died in 1861, adopted the new instruction. About one quarter of the deaths were left without any notice of the causes. According to the instructions, only deaths from epidemic diseases, childbirth, accidents, crime and suicide were to be reported. However, the number of causes reported in the 1840s are almost as many as before, 30 as compared to 32 in the 1830s, when the cause of death was very frequently registered.

The diseases still reported, although less frequently than before, are, in particular, chest disease, stitch and sting, consumption in the lungs and stroke. Some causes of death became more frequent, such as cholera, cold, nerve disease, and weakness. Concerning cholera and nerve disease, the change is probably real but the increase in cold and some other diseases may very well be a result of a change in the diagnoses of chest disease, stitch and sting, and consumption in the lungs. However, the increase in these causes of death is not as large as the decline of the other causes. Thus, it is likely that an increasing number of deaths from chest disease, stitch and sting and consumption in the lungs were not registered. This change in registration and reporting is then a result of the new instructions in 1831, although these did not come into practice until a new priest came to Västanfors in 1843.

The obligation to register causes of death changes again in 1859. Now, the causes of death should be based on the doctor's diagnoses. If no medical practitioner was available, and this was the case in most of the parishes in the countryside, the priest had to report deaths from suicide, crime, accidents, epidemic diseases and so-called endemic disease. A year later, the list was extended to include deaths from alcoholic-poisoning as well. Thus, the instruction for the countryside from 1831 is more or less confirmed.[13] The only difference is that endemic diseases are mentioned.

This time the new instruction came only a couple of years before a new priest, Harald Vedholm, came to Västanfors. During his period the proportion of unspecified deaths increased considerably, as shown in Figure 2. The number of different causes used in the 1870s is slightly lower than before. In many cases it is a question of real changes. There are, for example, no deaths from cholera in the 1870s. Vague diagnoses, like shortness of breath, are not used any longer. Deaths from chest disease declined while deaths from con-

468

sumption in the lungs and inflammation in the lungs increased considerably. In the 1880s the number of different causes of deaths decreases further.

Figure 2. Deaths in chest disease, stitch and sting, consumption in the lungs and deaths with no cause specified in Västanfors. Average of first and last ten years of the service of each priest (bars) and ten year averages from 1700-1709 and onwards (dotted line). Dark blocks in the time axis show the length of the service of each priest. See also text.

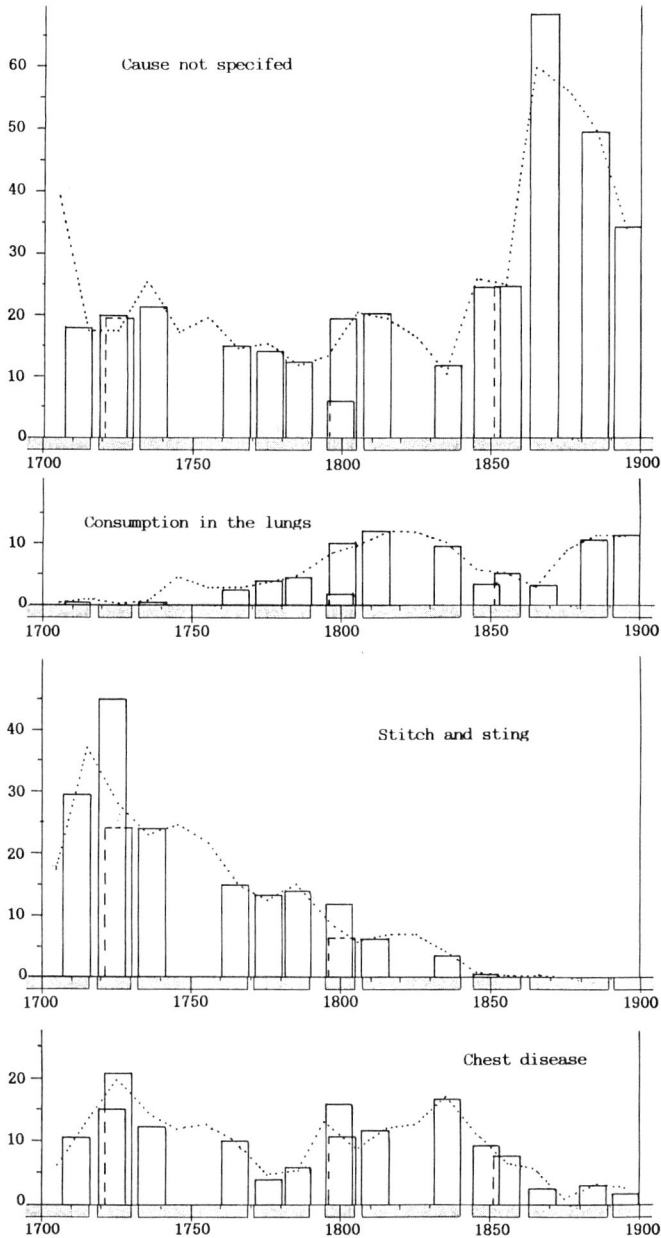

Our impression is that the effects of changes in the nomenclature in 1859 are small. The general view from society, put forward in the instructions, that all deaths did not have to be specified, had the effect that almost the same diseases were diagnosed as before, although in different proportions, but that the number of unspecified deaths increased.

Some changes took place in the nomenclature in 1874 and 1891. The latter change was more radical as the number of causes was substantially reduced and as some causes are etiological while others are still nosological. In addition, the 1891 nomenclature was a change from primary and secondary causes of death (introduced in 1860) to main cause and contributory causes of death.[14]

In the 1890s only 13 causes are registered in Västanfors. These thirteen causes account for 66 percent of the total number of deaths. Again, a new priest came to the parish at the same time as the nomenclature was changed.

We shall now turn to the question of the effects of the persons making the diagnoses and the registration of the death causes. It is obvious that even today persons with the same medical training will make different diagnoses. It is equally evident that this problem was greater during the 18th and 19th centuries. All priests had some medical training but it differed considerably. Some were very well educated although they did not have the same practice as a doctor, even if they discharged his duties, which was particularly the case in the countryside. It may also very well be that they interpreted their instructions in different ways, particularly prior to 1749.

On the other hand, during the 18th and 19th centuries, many died at early ages from acute diseases which, in many cases, were fairly easy to diagnose in comparison with our day, when most people die at an advanced age. Furthermore, epidemics appeared abundantly for short periods of time so that there was not only one but a number of deaths with the same disease to diagnose. Besides, the priest had good knowledge of the persons in his parish and saw them while they were alive, which made the diagnoses easier.

How shall the effects of the individual priests on the causes of death registration be detected and measured? It would have been much easier to analyze a number of similar parishes located close to each other. In this case we could compare the diagnoses of the different priests. Comparing parishes from different parts of the country or the same parish during different time periods is more problematic, the reason being the difficulties in separating the effects of the priests from real differences. In some cases the difference is of a magnitude that makes it obvious that the individual priest had a strong influence. But this is by no means always the case.

Puranen has come to the conclusion that the effect of the priests is large during the 19th century.[15] However, her study is not fully convincing. Puranen compares parishes in different parts of the country, but does not ask the question whether the differences found could be due to real differences in the death panorama.

Nor is Puranen's comparison of different priests within a parish conclusive. She calculates the percentage of deaths from different diseases during the entire period for which each priest was in service. Comparing these periods, which in some cases are more than thirty years long while others are less than ten years, she finds considerable differences. From the way the result is presented, one has the impression that the entire change occurred when a new priest arrives to the parish. No attempts have been made to differentiate between real development and the effects of individual priests. If a certain disease gradually declines during the entire period the picture is changed to a step by step decline, according to the way Puranen presents it.

It is evident that we cannot compare the death panorama for the entire period during which each priest was in service regardless of how long it was. On the other hand it is impossible to compare the records of the last one or two years for one priest with those of the first years of a new priest. The reason is that the death panorama could change very rapidly due to epidemics. We have to compare longer periods at the ends of each priest's period so that extreme situations are evened out. For this purpose, we have tried to take both five and ten year periods.

We found that a five year period is too short, i.e. that the influence of extreme situations is still strong. Even ten year periods are almost too short and must therefore be used with caution. Figure 2 shows averages for the first and last ten years of the service of each priest as vertical bars. The period each priest had served is shown as shaded blocks on the time axis. The gaps between the shaded blocks are the time it took to install a new priest. A so called "year of grace preacher" served during this time. Deaths that occurred during these years are excluded. The dotted line shows ten year averages from 1700-1709 onwards irrespective of changes of priests. The diseases shown in Figure 2 are consumption in the lungs, stitch and sting, and chest disease, i.e. diseases that change fairly slowly. The percentage of deaths for which no cause was registered is also shown. All other diseases have been analyzed as well.

As shown in Figure 2, the differences between the first and last ten years of a priest's period could be greater than the difference when a new priest came into office. This is not surprising since the periods served by most priests were rather long. Often the difference is very small between the last ten years of one priest and the first ten years of his successor.

What would the effect be if one priest had over-diagnosed one cause of death at the expense of another? One consequence would be that the number of deaths from that disease would be high during his period as compared to the periods of his predecessor and successor. Parallel to this, it would be lower for some other disease. A shift between two diseases *during* the working period of a priest may be due to wrong diagnoses but may just as well reflect a real change.

There is no obvious sign of over-diagnosing in Figure 2. Deaths from stitch and sting fall almost constantly over the entire period. It is probably under-registered during the first decade of the 18th century, when the number of deaths for which no cause is specified was twice as high as in the following decade.

Deaths from consumption in the lungs increase gradually in time with a peak around 1820. From 1840 they go down at the same time as a number of unspecified deaths go up. Finally, they increase at the end of the 19th century when diagnosing again becomes more frequent. Generally speaking, the percentage of deaths not specified is too high after 1860 and before 1710 to make it possible to study effects of individual priests. The high proportion of unspecified deaths is no effect of the individual priests, but of changes in the Church Law and the instructions.

The curve of chest disease is fairly parallel to the one for stitch and sting in the 18th century, and of consumption in the lungs in the 19th century. The disease became less common when Eric Fermelin was in service in 1771-1790. This may be a result of under-diagnosing, but other explanations are possible. It may as well be a result of competition from other diseases. In 1773, more than twice as many died as in a normal year. The following three years, the number of deaths was below average. After two years of extremely bad harvests, numbers of people died, particularly from dysentery and smallpox, in Västanfors and all over the country. In this and the following couple of years, the number of deaths from several diseases, including chest disease, went down. In 1779 there is another outbreak of smallpox and in 1783 dysentery hits hard again. In some of the years between the epidemic years, the number of deaths from chest disease goes back to a normal level. However, on average, chest disease became more uncommon.

This is an example of how real changes in the death panorama could, incorrectly, be interpreted as the effects of individual priests. How individual years with peaks of deaths from different diseases could influence the average of a period as long as ten years is also illustrated in Figure 2. Comparing the first and last ten years of Hellenius' service, i.e. 1719-1728 and 1721-1730 (with eight years overlapping) we get very different averages for deaths from chest disease and stitch and sting. The effect of an extreme year can also be seen when Dillman was in service 1795-1805.

An example of a priest who made diagnoses which differed from those of his predecessor is Georg Seseman, who was in service from 1843 to 1861. Cold, as a cause of death, was almost non-existent before 1843, but in the years of Sesemans' service it became rather frequent with peaks in 1845, 1850, 1851, 1854 and 1858. His successor never made this diagnosis. Similarly, weakness as a cause of death was only used by Seseman. His over-diagnosing of cold seems to have an effect on the number of deaths from consumption in the lungs, chest disease and stitch and sting which are all particularly low during his period. This will be discussed further below. This is the only clear example in Västanfors of how an individual priest influenced the diagnoses.

To summarize the discussion of the quality of the data: First of all, one of the major problems of an analysis based on aggregated data in the population statistics, from parish to national level, is the changes in the nomenclature. Causes of death are aggregated into classes in different ways in the different nomenclatures, which makes it very difficult to analyze long term changes in the death panorama. This is no problem at all when analyzing the registration of causes of deaths in the parish registers of Västanfors since no aggregation of different diseases is needed.

The influences of the nomenclature is of a different kind. The fact that new diseases are introduced to the priests by the nomenclature affected the diagnoses. This is certainly the case with "unknown child disease", a cause of death almost never used in Västanfors prior to the first nomenclature from *Tabellverket* in 1749. From 1750 to the beginning of the 19th century, this cause of death was frequently diagnosed in the parish.

Secondly, the instructions to the priests related to changes in the nomenclature had a strong effect on the registration of the causes of death in Västanfors. This was the case in 1831 when the priests no longer had to report all causes of death. The proportion of deaths with no cause specified increased rapidly in Västanfors. This did not happen immediately since the cleric in service between 1806 and 1841 continued to register the causes of deaths as he had always done, irrespective of the changes in the Church Law. When a new priest came to the parish in 1843 he adopted the new instructions and the proportion of deaths with no cause specified increased. Puranen comes to the same conclusion for the parishes she analyzed.[16]

Thirdly, the ideal situation when discussing effects of the individual priests is to have a number of similar parishes located close together. This will be the case in a forthcoming study, but in this case we are analyzing only one parish. The problem is to separate the effects of the priests from real changes in the death panorama in time. Analyzing consumption in the lungs, stitch and sting and chest disease during the first and last ten years of the service of each priest and comparing with the development of competing diseases gives the conclusion that the effects of individual training etc of different priests have no strong influence on the cause of death registration in Västanfors.

Age profiles and seasonality of the most frequent causes of death

Of the sixty-two causes of deaths registered in Västanfors, only ten causes account for more than two percent of the deaths with cause specified. Together these ten diseases account for 67.5 percent of all specified deaths in the parish. The two most common causes of death are *stitch* and *sting* and *chest diseases*, both lung diseases. They account for a quarter of all specified deaths during the 200-year period but for more than 50 percent in the beginning of the 18th century. *Consumption in the lungs* adds another 7.5 percent to the deaths from lung disease. As shown earlier, some deaths from *unknown child disease* are stitch and sting which adds a few percent to deaths from lung diseases. We also had to add a number of less common causes of death to the lung disease group namely *inflammation of the lungs, shortness of breath, cold, coughing, haemorrhoea*, and *blood disease (blodsot)*. Together they account for 3-4 percent of the total number of deaths with cause specified. This means that about 40 percent of the specified deaths were due to lung diseases. In addition, some deaths in *infirmities of old age*, yet another frequent cause of death, may be due to lung diseases as discussed below. The figure is still probably a bit low as these exact diseases did not need to be reported after 1831. As shown earlier, they are also under-registered in the first decade of the 18th century. We believe it is fair to say that approximately half of the deaths in the 18th and 19th centuries were due to chest and lung diseases.

Other frequent diseases are *smallpox, stroke, dysentery, stomach disease and dropsy*. Smallpox and dysentery are well defined compared to the others. The age distribution and seasonality of the most frequent diseases will be studied below. Age-distributions have been calculated for men and women separately. The profiles are very similar except in the fertile ages, for which deaths in childbirth account for 8-15 percent of the specified deaths for women. Therefore, we limit ourselves to a presentation of the age-distributions for men and women together.

This section is a description of Västanfors with few references to works of other scholars. This is due to one fact. We would like to present some basic results from Västanfors that will be used when we discuss the changes in the death panorama in time in the next section, in which we will relate our results to other studies.

Mortality from *stitch* and *sting* was most frequent among infants, but people in active ages were hit hard as well. As can be seen from Figure 3, a shift in the age-distribution occurred during the 19th century towards a larger share of adult mortality.

It must be kept in mind that Figure 3 gives the percentage distribution of the disease in different age groups only. Therefore, the share of deaths in old age groups tends to be low simply because these age groups are small. The age-specific mortality for different diseases and its causes will be analyzed in a forthcoming study.

The seasonality of *stitch* and *sting* is the same for both centuries. Like the crude death rate, it has the shape of a sinus curve with a pronounced peak in March, April, and May and a trough in September. Adjustments have been made for differences in the lengths of months.

Chest disease has characteristics very similar to *stitch* and *sting* with two minor differences. The age distribution is more stable and there are two peaks in the seasonality during the 19th century: one in January and one in April and May.

Figure 3. Age-distribution (left), and seasonality (right) of deaths in frequent diseases in Västanfors.

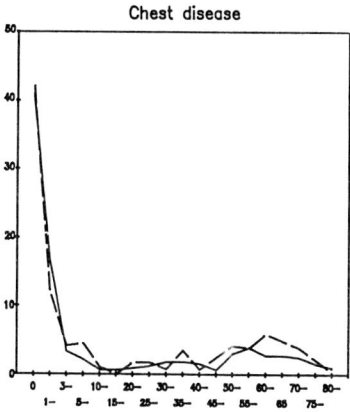

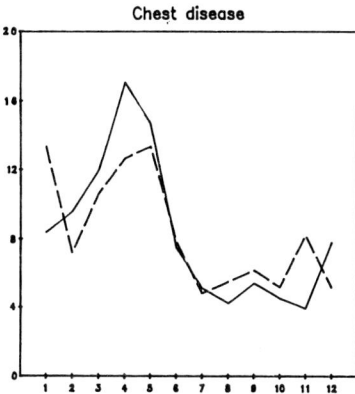

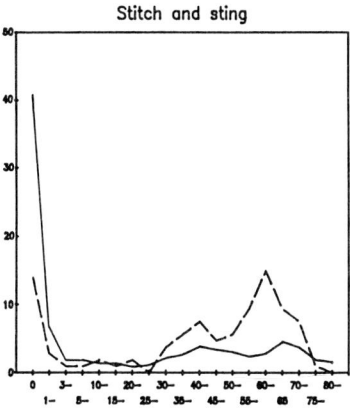

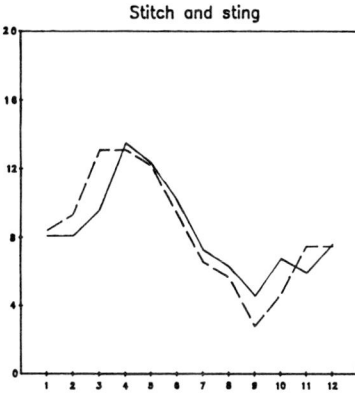

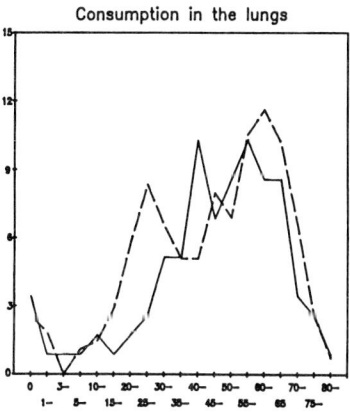

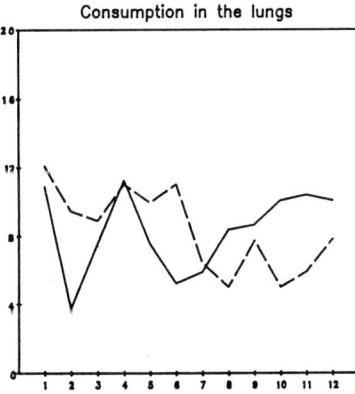

Figure 3. continued

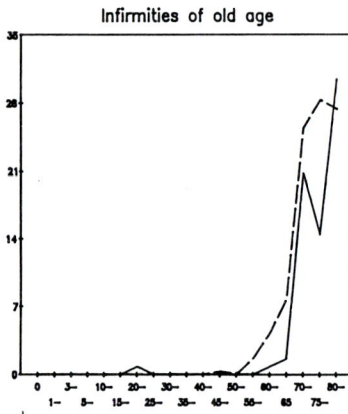

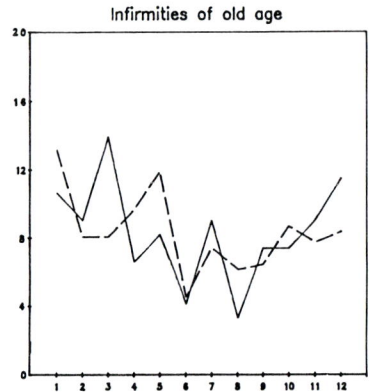

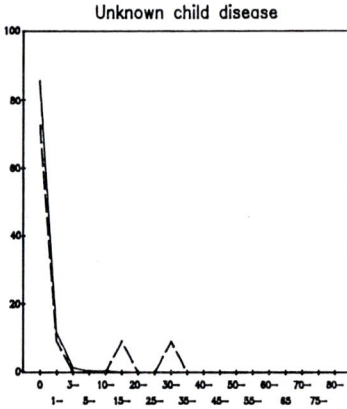

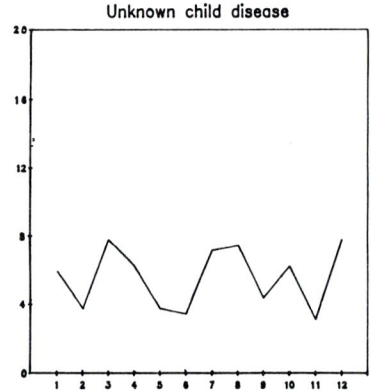

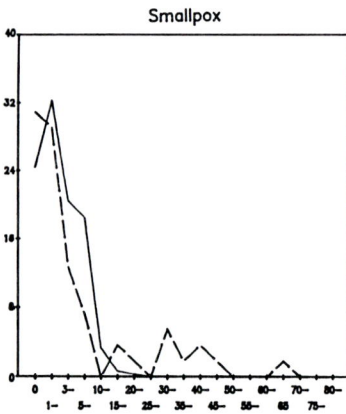

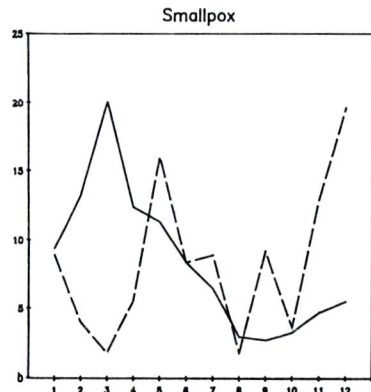

476

Figure 3. continued

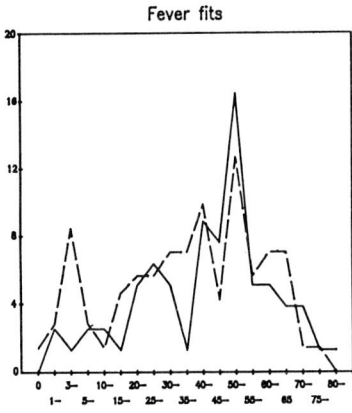

Fever fits

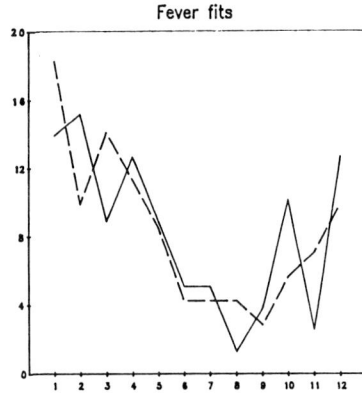

Fever fits

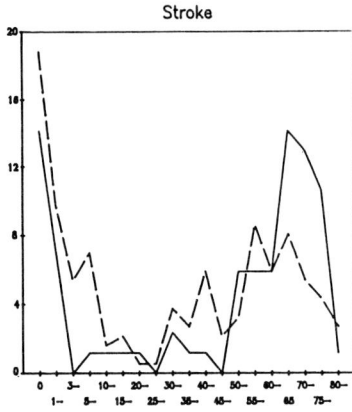

Stroke

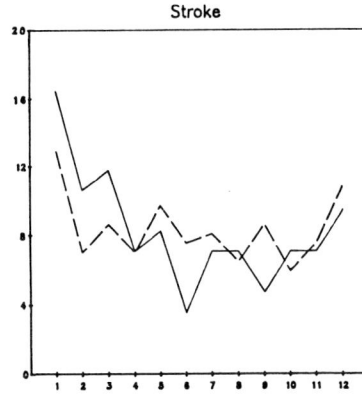

Stroke

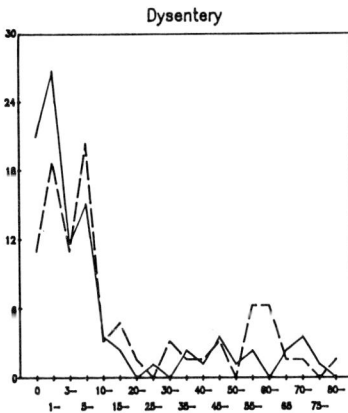

Dysentery

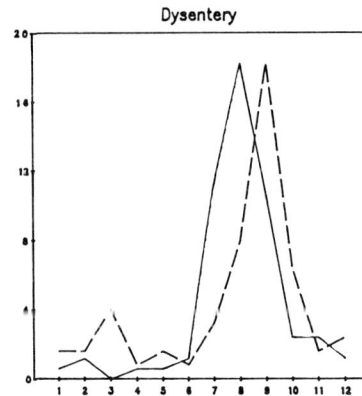

Dysentery

Figure 3. continued

Other diseases

Other diseases

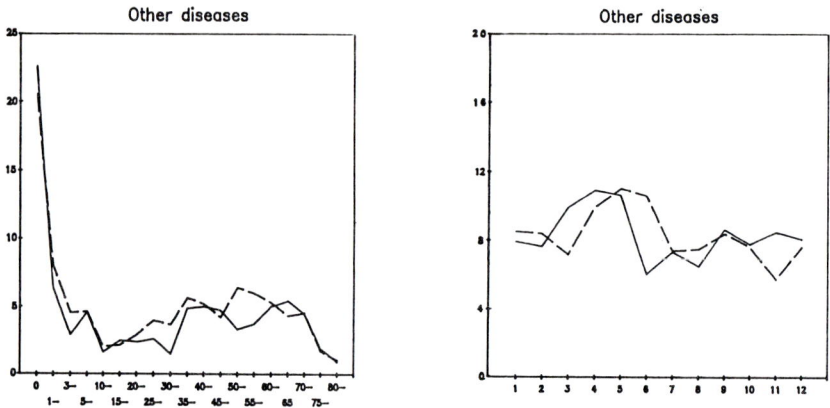

Between the 18th and 19th centuries the age profiles for *consumption in the lungs* differ somewhat with a minor shift towards older ages during the 19th century. The main difference in comparison with *stitch* and *sting* and chest disease is that the mortality for consumption in the lungs is much lower for infants. The seasonality is very weak. The mortality is somewhat higher in the first half of the year as compared to the rest of the year, at least during the 19th century. The irregularities during the 18th century are probably a result of the few deaths from *consumption in the lungs* during this period. Thus, it resembles *stitch* and *sting* and chest disease with higher mortality for adults compared to children aged 3 to 10, and a somewhat higher mortality in the first half of the year.

Infirmities of old age is a very vague cause of death. It may comprise anything, but is probably dominated by *pleurisy, pneumonia, edema, heart failure* and *cerebral hemorrhage.* As can be seen from Figure 3, the classification applies almost exclusively to very old people. Furthermore, the classification is not frequently used before the 19th century.

The graph of the seasonal pattern is u-shaped with high values in the winter and low in the summer. It differs considerably from *chest disease* and *stitch* and *sting* although during the 19th century it has a second peak in May during the 19th century.

An example of a disease with a more precise definition is *smallpox,* which was rather easy to diagnose. An interesting finding is that during the entire 18th century smallpox almost exclusively affected children. When it was becoming less frequent - it disappeared almost completely at the beginning of the 19th century—it affected people in active ages as well. Thus, it seems as if the entire population was exposed to the disease during the 18th century, and that those who survived received a life-long immunity. Later, when it was

478

becoming less common, people could have their first contacts with the disease as adults.

During the 18th century, when it was very frequent, it had a very regular seasonal pattern with a peak in March. It starts increasing slowly in the autumn, increases rapidly in the first months of the year and then falls again. The seasonal pattern during the 19th century is very irregular due to the few deaths from this disease.

Stroke is another common cause of death during the period 1700-1899. Also in this case it is rather a question of symptoms. The classification conceals diseases leading to sudden death, such as *infarct of the heart, cerebral hemorrhage* and other internal hemorrhages. These were diseases primarily affecting children and old people. The age-distributions differ between the two centuries. During the 19th century it did not affect people in ages above 65 as much as it had done during the previous century. Today, stroke is one of the most common causes of death for old people.

Stroke has a u-shaped seasonal pattern similar to the one for infirmities of old age. The seasonality is less pronounced during the 19th century.

The age profiles of *unknown child disease* differ very little between the two periods. The classification which was primarily used during the second half of the 18th century indicates that the disease almost exclusively affected children below the age of one year. This is the same as for the country as a whole.

Unknown child disease was common in Västanfors during the second half of the 18th century only. By the beginning of the 19th century the classification had disappeared almost completely.

The seasonal pattern is only shown for the 18th century, as it became very irregular during the 19th century due to few events. The pattern is flat with several small peaks of equal amplitude.

Dysentery is a stomach disease primarily affecting children. It has an epidemic character but was very common during the years of severe crop failures in the early 1770s. As on the Continent, it is spread in the summer. During the 18th century, the peaks are in August during the 18th century, and in the following century they are in September.

Other prevalent diseases are *dropsy* and *fever fits*. The latter primarily hits adults. It has a pronounced u-shaped seasonal pattern. Dropsy is another disease with a diffuse pathological picture. The classification covers diseases leading to an accumulation of body fluid in the stomach, lungs, brain or other parts of the body, the underlying reason being some kind of heart disease. The age-profile is similar for the two centuries. It affects primarily middle-aged men and women.

At the end of the 19th century, the diagnoses were becoming more differentiated. *Cancer* and *heart disease* are frequent causes of death in the parish registers. It is somewhat surprising to note that heart disease to a very large extent affected infants. Other prevalent diseases were *scarlatina*, affecting children, and *cholera* which primarily hit people in active ages.

As is demonstrated by the discussion above, several of the most frequent causes of death are rather vague. Unfortunately, many of the more unusual diseases, such as *measles, whooping-cough, malaria, typhus* and *thrush* were easier to diagnose. From the point of view of medical history, these diseases are of course as interesting as the more common diseases, but from a social and economic historical point of view they are less important. This does not mean that they are not interesting at all since they may, for example, be used as indicators of living conditions etc or of medical and hygienic development. But as a first step, we will focus on the most common diseases.

Changes in the panorama of death causes

The long-term development in mortality from different diseases has primarily been studied by Sundbärg and Fridlizius. The development of *tuberculosis* has been studied by Puranen. A number of other authors, such as Lind-skog/Imhof and Widén, have analyzed shorter time periods.[17]

A major problem when analyzing long-term changes in the death panorama on the basis of the population tables is the changes in the nomenclature. Since this problem is very limited when the analysis is based on the parish registers, our references to works discussing this topic are few.

A main problem in analyzing the parish registers is how to interpret the cause of death, as a nosological system was used. To what extent can we identify different biological causes of death from the parish registers in the 18th and 19th centuries?

Most researchers working with data for causes of death are of the opinion that certain features of the development could be pictured in spite of the deficiencies in the material. Fridlizius and Fridlizius/Ohlsson argue that it is possible to arrive at a reasonable understanding of the development of *smallpox, measles, whooping-cough and dysentery* for the period 1749-1830. These diseases are rather easy to diagnose. Furthermore, they argue that for *tuberculosis, chest disease, typhus* and possibly also *fever fits* the statistics are fairly good.[18]

With respect to *whooping-cough* and *dysentery*, we are in full agreement with this argument and would even suggest that *cholera* and *scarlatina* could be added, diseases which are becoming common after the period analysed by Fridlizius/Ohlsson. With respect to smallpox and measles there could be some under-estimations since, according to Fridlizius and other authors, they are not always combined with rash.[19]

It is correct that *tuberculosis pulmonum* could be traced or estimated on the basis of the population tables, but Fridlizius/Ohlsson as well as Sundbärg are aware of the possibility that the groups "chest disease" and "stitch and sting" comprise cases of tuberculosis also during the periods when they were reported separately.

For the same reason we must question the correctness of the long-term development of *chest disease* and *stitch* and *sting*. Another problem concerning these diseases is the two unspecified causes *unknown child disease* and *infirmities of old age*. These groups could include cases of different lung diseases. In the case of unknown child disease we have already shown that *stitch* and *sting* is included.

Stroke, another frequent cause of death, is rather well defined today, but was more vague in the period we are studying. It probably included all different death causes that gave a sudden death, as discussed above, and not only attacks of cerebral hemorrhage and thrombosis in the brain. The fact that it breaks out in different years in the 1830s and 1840s suggests a wider interpretation.

Cancer and *heart disease*, the latter is likely to be heart attack, both became more frequent compared to other diseases at the end of the 19th century. They are also quite well-defined, at least in the case of cancer.

Figure 4 shows a transition from a society dominated by different lung diseases and smallpox to a society with more differentiated causes of death. This is not mainly a result of a better specification and improvements in diagnosing as shown above. Our problem is that almost all of the different lung diseases are vague. Because of their dominance, we shall primarily discuss these diseases when analyzing the long-term changes in the death panorama.

Figure 4. Causes of deaths in different age-groups in Västanfors. Cumulated percentage in the most frequent diseases.

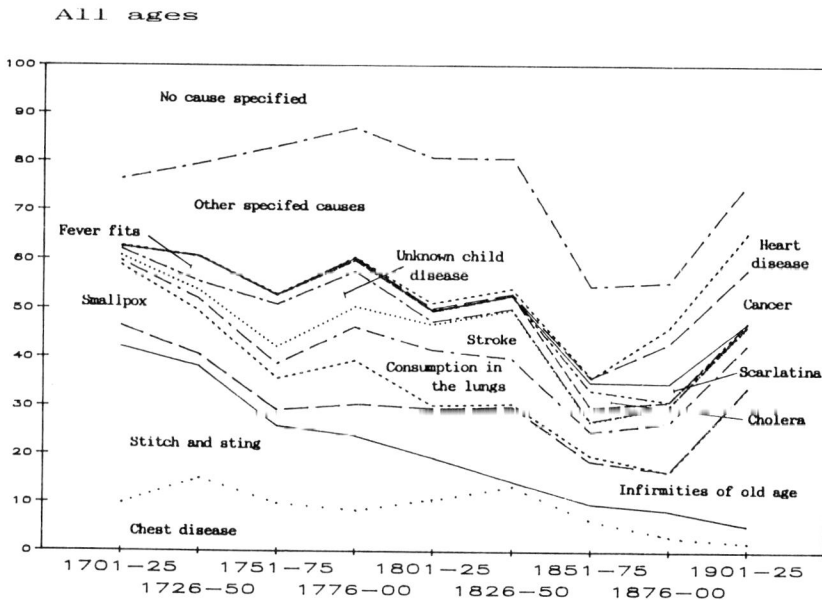

481

Figure 4. continued

Infants

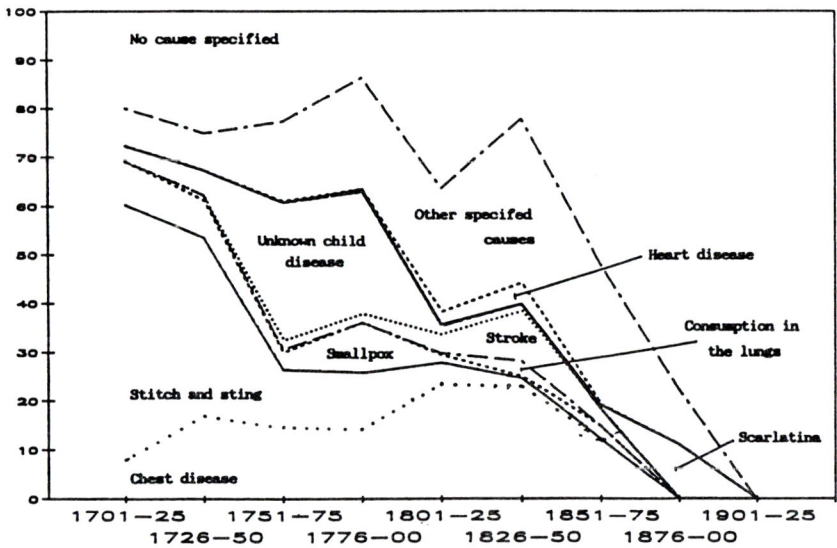

Ages 1 - 2 years

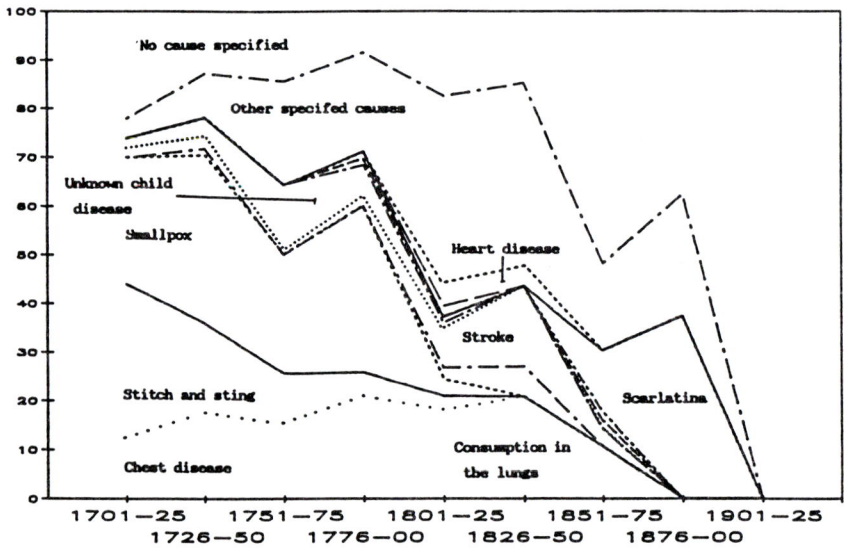

482

Figure 4. continued

Ages 3 – 4 years

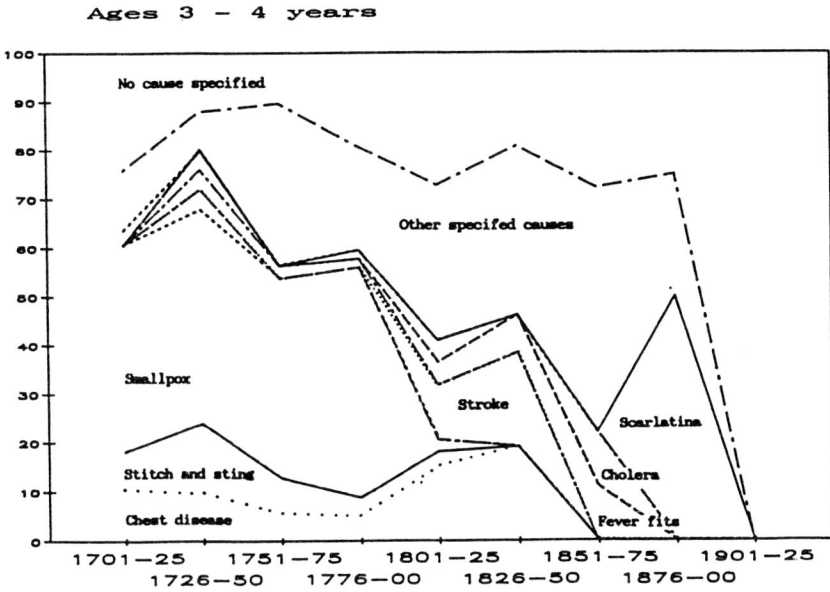

Ages 5 – 9 years

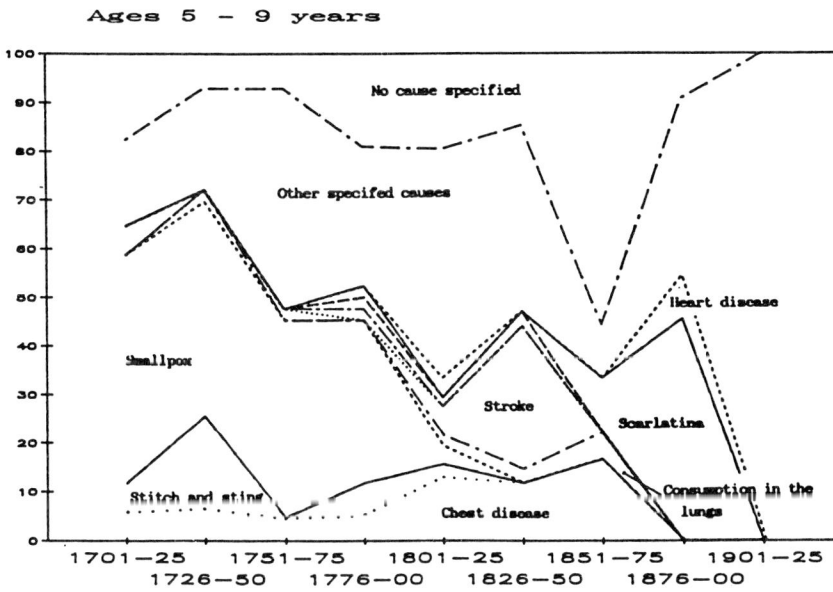

Figure 4. continued

Ages 10 - 19 years

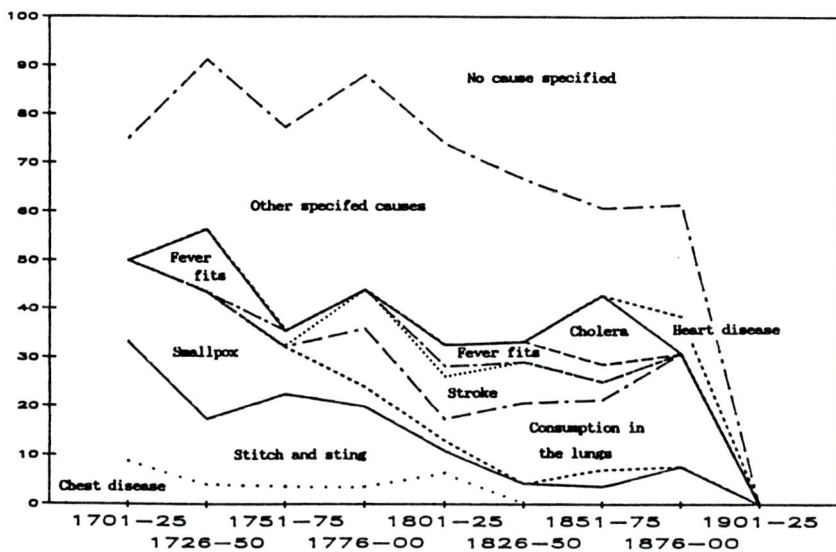

Ages 20 - 49 years

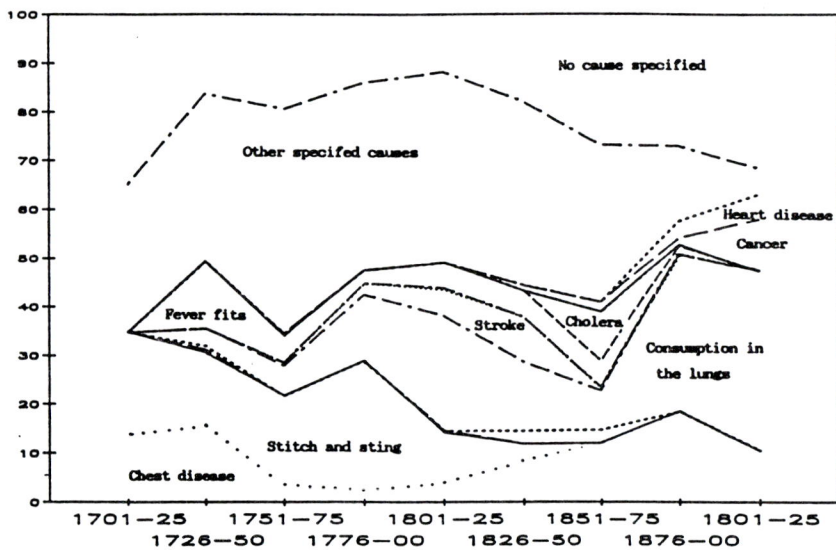

484

Figure 4. continued

Ages 50 – 69 years

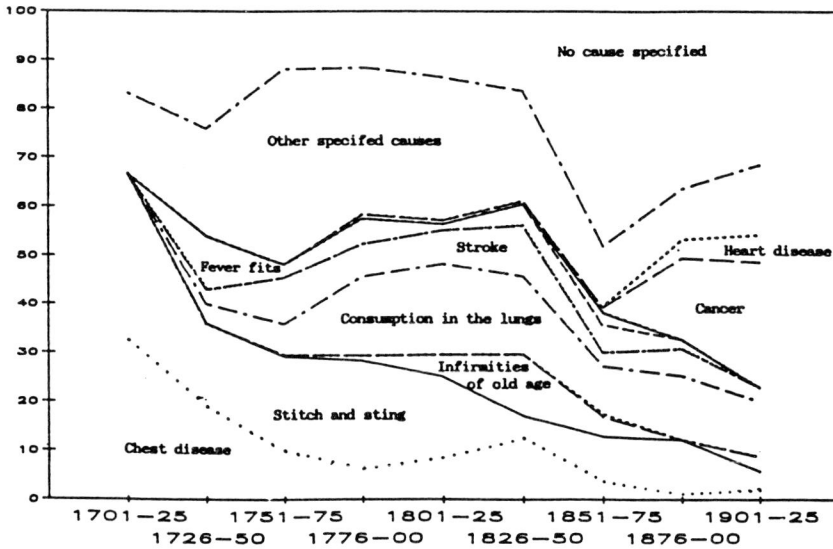

Ages 70 and over

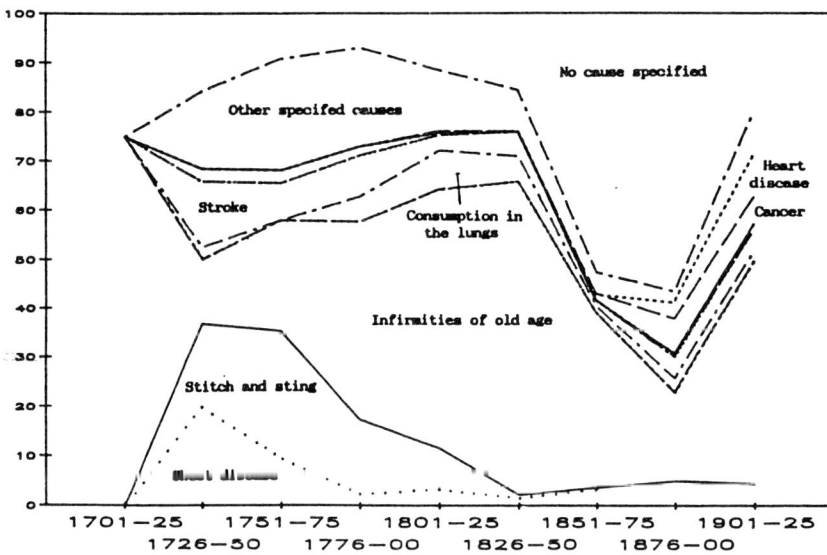

When analyzing the long-term development of mortality from lung and chest diseases, we have to consider the following diseases (percent of total number of specified deaths in parentheses): stitch and sting (14.9), chest disease (26.5), infirmities of old age (9.4), consumption in the lungs (7.5), unknown child disease (7.1), fever fits (1.5), burning disease (*brännsjuka*) (0.6), inflammation in the lungs (1.0), shortness of breath (0.8), cold (0.8), coughing (0.6), hemorrhage (0.3), throat disease (0.2) and influenza (0.1).

We have already shown that *unknown child disease* includes *stitch* and *sting* (indirect nomenclature effect), that cold includes *consumption in the lungs* (priest effect), *infirmities of old age* may include different lung and chest diseases, and that *stitch* and *sting* and *chest disease* have very similar age-distributions and seasonality.

Fever fits is an inflammation in the blood without any specific part of the body being affected. According to Bäck, it is synonymous with burning disease (*brännsjuka*). Possibly it is influenza.[20] Both fever fits and *brännsjuka* mainly hit adults in Västanfors. They also have similar seasonal patterns with a peak during the winter. Imhof and Lindskog find in their analyses of southern Sweden that fever fits is prevalent every year but that it breaks out as an epidemic disease in certain intervals.[21] The pattern in Västanfors is similar, but the disease completely disappears some years. The difference in this respect is explained by the fact that we are analyzing a much smaller population than Imhof and Lindskog. Thus, both fever fits and burning disease appear more epidemical than endemic in Västanfors. Neither of them is related to changes in the nomenclature or to a change of priests. Our conclusion is that in our analysis of Västanfors there is no reason to relate them, or influenza, to consumption in the lungs, stitch and sting or chest disease as Puranen has done in her study.[22]

Coughing has almost exactly the same age-distribution as *whooping-cough*. The seasonal pattern, too, is very similar, with a high abundance in autumn and spring. Both causes of death disappear in some years and appear in others. Almost no deaths from coughing occur in the 19th century, major outbreaks are in 1771-1772, 1777, 1781 and 1785-1788. Whooping-cough was very rare until the end of the 18th century. Years with high frequencies are 1796, 1846-1847 and 1852. The two diseases overlap in time, but it seems as if they are the same disease. The fact that they had an epidemic pattern gives us reason to distinguish them from stitch and sting, chest disease and consumption in the lungs.

Hemorrhage and *throat disease* are diagnosed as causes of deaths for adults only. A number of different diseases have these symptoms, for example consumption in the lungs. As they are very rare, there is no reason to discuss them in the context of the long-term development of lung and chest diseases.

Shortness of breath is a cause of death in old people. It has no pronounced seasonal pattern. Several diseases have this kind of symptom, and as this cause is rare, we have left it out of the further analysis. Altogether 1.3 % of the specified diseases have been left out of this part of the analysis.

To sum up:

1. Cold is aggregated with consumption in the lungs.
2. Inflammation in the lungs is aggregated with stitch and sting.
3. Unknown child disease and infirmities of old age have to be considered when analyzing the long-term development of lung and chest diseases.
4. Fever fits, *brännsjuka*, influenza and coughing are not connected with stitch and sting, chest disease or consumption in the lungs.
5. Hemorrhage, throat disease and shortness of breath may be connected with these diseases but their vagueness and low abundance are strong arguments for leaving them out.

The abundance of cold and inflammation in the lungs is so small and similar as compared to consumption in the lungs and stitch and sting that it will not alter the seasonality and age-distribution of the latter two.

The next question is how many deaths from *unknown child disease* were actually deaths from *stitch* and *sting*. If we make the assumption that deaths from *smallpox* and other easily- diagnosed diseases were always specified, the increase in deaths in *unknown child disease* should mainly be distributed among *stitch* and *sting* and *chest disease*. The ratio of chest disease to *stitch and sting* is one to ten during the 1740's. Approximately 90 percent of the deaths from *unknown child disease* should then be transferred to deaths from *stitch* and *sting*.

As is shown in Figure 4 "Infants" there is another problem in the early 19th century when deaths from *unknown child disease* vanished. The number of unspecified deaths increases almost as much as the former decreases. These unspecified deaths may very well be due to *stitch* and *sting*. This is also the case after 1850, but from then on the number of unspecified deaths is so large that it is meaningless to try to obtain a picture of the long-term development in lung and chest disease for this age group. If we only adjust *stitch* and *sting* for deaths from *unknown child disease*, it is very likely to be under-estimated for the period 1801-1825.

Imhof and Lindskog make no suggestion of how to interpret deaths from infirmities of old age. There is no such discussion in the medical books of the 18th and 19th centuries.[23] Its seasonality looks like that of stroke and fever fits, but like chest disease and stitch and sting it has a peak in the spring. Furthermore, it is much more like the latter two diseases in terms of year-to-year changes. There are no outbreaks in specific years which was the case for fever fits and stroke.

Figure 4, "Ages 70 and over", shows very clearly that what was diagnosed as stitch and sting and chest disease in the middle of the 18th century was called infirmities of old age in the 19th century. Looking at the long-term changes, there is reason to believe that at least one-third of the deaths from infirmities of old age were due to chest disease and stitch and sting. It is probably the case that the death panorama for old people is more stable than for any other age group.

Figure 5 shows how the adjustment discussed above affects the long term change in consumption in the lungs, stitch and sting and chest disease.

Referring to 18th and 19th century medical literature, Imhof and Lindskog come to the conclusion that the group "chest disease and consumption of the lungs" in the first nomenclature is probably *pulmonary tuberculosis*.[24] According to the same sources, stitch and sting is difficult to distinguish from chest disease but it is more likely to be *pleurisy,* possibly in connection with *pneumonia.* Imhof and Lindskog analyzed the period of the first nomenclature when chest disease and consumption in the lungs was reported as one group and stitch and sting as another. In the second nomenclature, consumption in the lungs was reported as a cause of its own, while stitch and sting and chest fever were reported together.

The age-distributions and seasonal patterns of stitch and sting and chest disease are almost identical in Västanfors, as shown above (Figure 3). Consumption in the lungs has a quite similar age-distribution but a lower abundance for infants than stitch and sting and chest disease. Furthermore, its seasonality is somewhat different from the latter two.

Chest disease is present almost every year until the end of the 1860s. The variation from year to year is not very strong. Stitch and sting has a very similar pattern although it vanishes around 1850.

Consumption in the lungs is less abundant, and it is not until the 1770s that it becomes present almost every year. Unlike the two other diseases, it is present during the entire period, but like them there were no outbreaks of the disease.

Our conclusion is that chest disease and stitch and sting are, if not the same, very similar diseases. Given their patterns and abundance in the middle of the 18th century, when consumption in the lungs was diagnosed, it is unlikely that it is pulmonary tuberculosis. However, with its vague symptoms, parts of the deaths from stitch and sting and chest disease may very well be the same as pulmonary tuberculosis.

The result of the adjustments is that our picture of the long-term development in the death panorama based on the original series (Figure 4) must be modified. The transition from a society dominated by smallpox and chest and lung diseases to a society with more differentiated causes of death is not entirely true. The elimination of smallpox for children is still an important feature for the 19th century, but deaths in chest and lung diseases do not change the way we first thought.

Figure 5. Adjustments of chest and lung diseases.

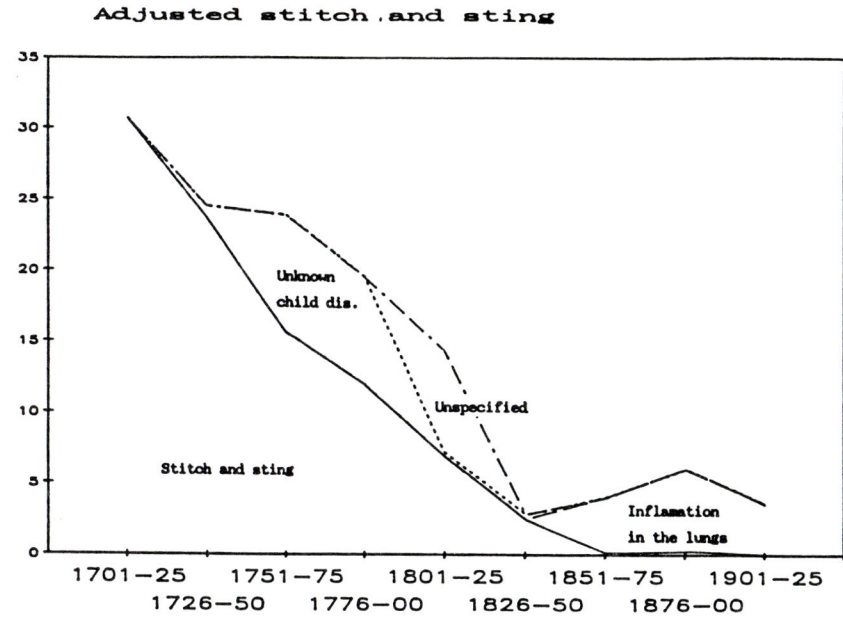

Adjusted stitch and sting

Unknown
child dis.

Unspecified

Stitch and sting

Inflamation
in the lungs

1701—25   1751—75   1801—25   1851—75   1901—25
   1726—50   1776—00   1826—50   1876—00

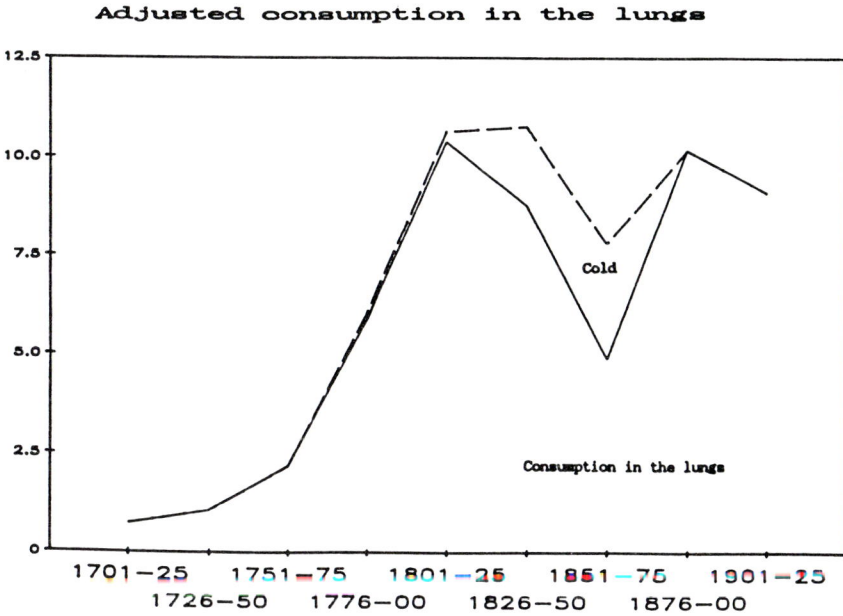

Adjusted consumption in the lungs

Cold

Consumption in the lungs

1701—25   1751—75   1801—25   1851—75   1901—25
   1726—50   1776—00   1826—50   1876—00

Figure 5: Continued

Adjusted chest disease

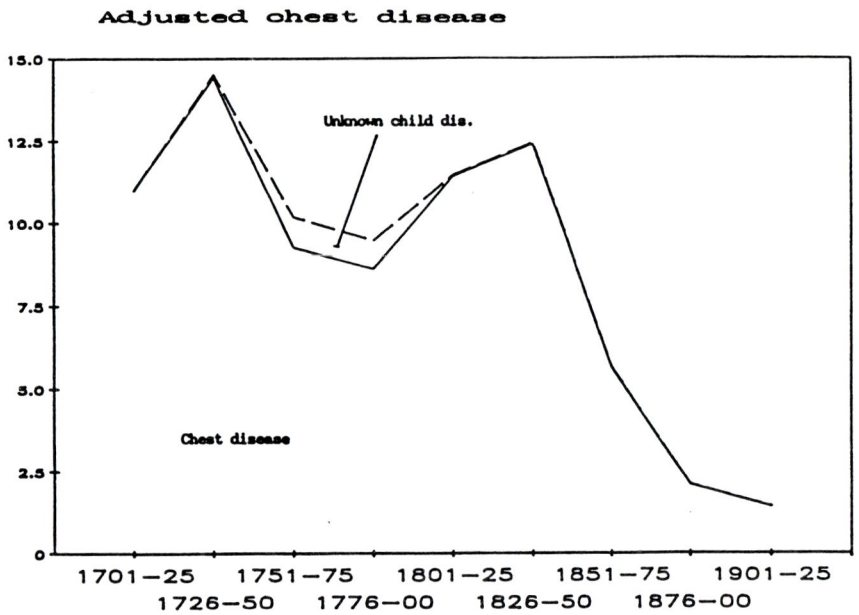

Adjusted chest and lung diseases

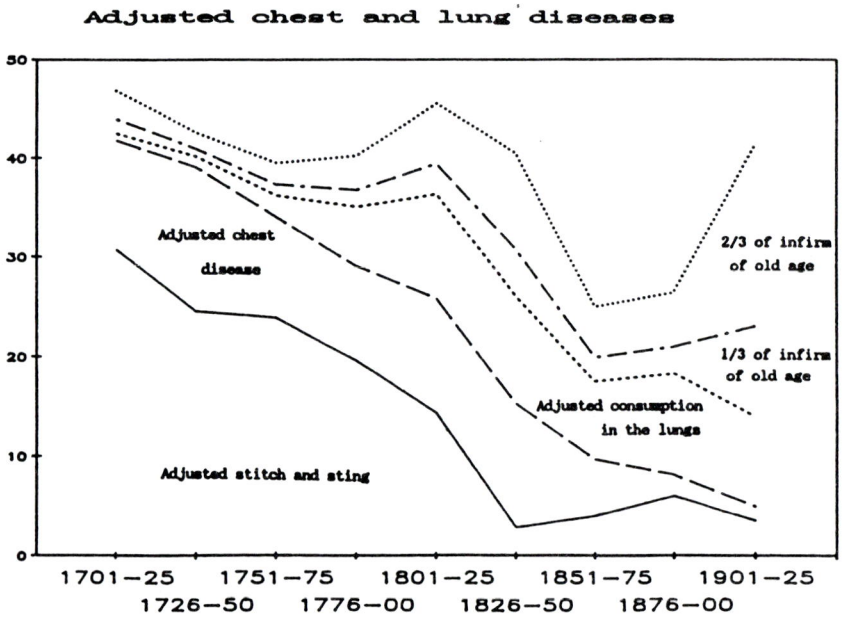

For the period for which we have the best data, i.e. where the number of deaths is high and the proportions specified also high, which is the case for the period 1725-1850, the percentage who died from chest and lung diseases is almost stable. The decline prior to 1825 is so small that may it as well be zero, given the fact that the cause of death is not specified for about one fifth of the deaths. From 1801-1825 to 1826-1850 there is a substantial drop in chest and lung diseases. At the same time, deaths from infirmities of old age and stroke increase. As we do not know for sure how many of the deaths from infirmities of old age were actually a result of chest and lung diseases, we cannot say how large this decline was.

Our conclusion is that the transition in the death panorama is totally dominated by the elimination of smallpox. But another transition takes place within the group chest and lung diseases. Stitch and sting, the most common cause of death in the early 18th century, when about one third died from it, gradually diminishes and has almost vanished by 1826-1850. Chest disease, another common disease with characteristics very similar to stitch and sting is much more stable. The disease that becomes more prevalent when stitch and sting decreases is consumption in the lungs. As stitch and sting and chest disease are very similar, and as they both include cases of consumption in the lungs, i.e. of pulmonary tuberculosis, it is very hard to know to what extent the changes between the three diseases are real or imaginary. We have, however, found no evidence that changes in the nomenclature had any influence or that the individual priests played any important role concerning these diseases. Thus, this part of the puzzle still remains.

Appendix. Clergymen in Västanfors.

	Started	Ended
Jacobus Gussarvius	1694	1717.06.04
Olof Hellenius	1719	1731
Eric Todenius	1731	1770.05.08
Eric Fermelin	1770.10.15	1791
Died 1794.05.08		
Carl Petter Dillman	1794.12	1806.01.13
Hit by stroke in 1802,		
yet usually able to do his service		
Eric Eggertz	1806.11.12	1841.06.29
Georg Seseman	1843.05.29	1860.06.06
Harald Emanuel Vedholm	1862.07.17	1890.01.17
Per Södergren	1890.10.31	1924.04.30

Västanfors was a Chapel of Ease until 1811 when it became a parish in its own right. The priests listed above were the ones who lived and served in Västanfors. There is reason to assume that they are the ones making the diagnoses of the cause of death.

Source: See footnote 11.

Notes

1. The data on age-specific mortality and life expectancy are from a forthcoming study by Rolf Alexandersson based on the statistical tables from 1749 to 1859. I am grateful to Rolf Alexandersson for helping me in preparing the data used in this study.

2. T. Bengtsson, *Notes on the Effects of the Choice of Time Period and the Level of Aggregation*. Paper for the SSHA Conference in Toronto 1984 (Lund 1984).

3. G. Sundbärg, 'Dödligheten af lungtuberkulos i Sverige åren 1751/1830', *Statistisk Tidskrift* (1905); C. Runborg and G. Sundbärg, 'Dödligheten i lungsot i Sveriges städer 1861/1900', *Statistisk Tidskrift* (1905); G. Fridlizius, 'The Mortality Decline in the First Phase of the Demographic Transition: Swedish Experiences', T. Bengtsson, G. Fridlizius, and R. Ohlsson (Eds.), *Pre-Industrial Population Change—The Mortality Decline and Short-Term Population Movements* (Stockholm 1984); G. Fridlizius and R. Ohlsson, 'Mortality Patterns in Sweden 1749-1914', T. Bengtsson, G. Fridlizius and R. Ohlsson (1984); A.E. Imhof and B. Lindskog, 'Dödsorsakerna i Sydsverige 1749-1773', *Sydsvenska medicinhistoriska sällskapets årsskrift* (1973); L. Widén, 'Mortality and Causes of Death in Sweden During the 18th Century', *Statistisk Tidskrift*, 2 (1975); A. Brändström, *"De kärlekslösa mödrarna". Spädbarnsdödligheten i Sverige under 1800-talet med särskild hänsyn till Nedertorneå* (Umeå 1984); B-I. Puranen, *Tuberkulos. En sjukdoms förekomst och dess orsaker. Sverige 1750-1980* (Umeå 1984); R. Ståhl, et al, *Synpunkter på dödsbevisens validitet* (undated); B.I.B. Lindahl, *On Weighting Causes of Death* (in this volume, Umeå 1988); L. Nordenfelt, 'Causes of Death—a Philosophical Essay', *Forskningsrådsnämnden, Rapport 83:2* (Uppsala 1983); L. Nordenfelt, and B.I.B. Lindahl, *Om grunden för svensk dödsorsaksstatistik. Reflektioner kring grundbegrepp, regler och praxis* (Linköping 1984); E. Nyström, *The Development of Cause of Death Statistics in Sweden 1749-1911. A Survey of Problems, Sources, Possibilities* (in this volume, Umeå 1988).

4. G. Lext, 'Studier i svensk kyrkobokföring 1600-1946', *Meddelande från Ekonomisk-historiska institutionen vid Göteborgs universitet,* no 54 (Göteborg 1984), pp. 57-122.

5. Nyström (1988).

6. Lext (1984), p. 85. Lext also describes the development prior to the new church law, pp. 57-84.

7. Puranen (1984), p. 53.

8. Nyström (1988).

9. Puranen (1984), pp. 54 onwards.

10. Imhof and Lindskog (1973).

11. *Vid hundraårsminnet av Västanfors kyrkas grundläggning 1824-1924. Fästskrift utgiven av Västanfors kyrkoråd till biskopsvisitationen den 9-12 oktober 1924* (Köping 1924), pp. 5-6.

12. SOS: *Folkmängden och dess förändringar. Dödsorsaker 1911* (Stockholm 1915), p. 2.

13. SOS (1915), pp. 3-4.

14. Puranen (1984), p. 38.

15. Puranen (1984), pp. 64-72.

16. Puranen (1984), p. 64.

17. Imhof and Lindskog (1973); Widén (1975).

18. Fridlizius and Ohlsson (1984), p. 327.

19. Fridlizius (1984), p. 104.

20. Imhof and Lindskog (1973), p. 130.

21. Imhof and Lindskog (1973), pp. 129-130.

22. Puranen (1984), pp. 383-385. In one context is fever fits aggregated with chest disease, in another with stitch and sting and yet another with all kinds of fevers depending on which data is analyzed.

23. Imhof and Lindskog (1973).

24. Imhof and Lindskog (1973), p. 128.

The Effects of Smallpox Vaccination on Mortality. A Norwegian Case Study 1770-1840

Ståle Dyrvik

Introductory remarks

Norwegian historians have not dedicated much work to the demographic transition of their country. Instead, they have recently been quite occupied by a particular phase of it, namely the great mortality decline that Norway experienced just after the Napoleonic Wars.

Until 1815, the Norwegian crude death rate remained at an average level of approximately 25 per 1000, but with strong annual fluctuations, especially during the war years 1807-1814. From 1815 the rate, on a five year basis, declined to well below 20 and the fluctuations were much reduced. During the period 1800-1814 annual rates from 20.7 to 35.9 were observed. They were contained between 17.5 and 20.5 during the following 15 years.

This sudden change was soon registered by contemporary Norwegian economists, but the sociologist Eilert Sundt was the first one to submit it to scientific investigation, mainly in his book "On Marriage in Norway" (1855). Sundt summarized the debate by stressing two main causes for the mortality decline: *Smallpox vaccination*, made compulsory by a Royal Decree in 1810, and *potato cultivation*, known from the late 18th century and greatly promoted during the Napoleonic Wars.

After Sundt more than a century should pass until a new push was given to the scientific discussions. In his book "Population and Society in Norway 1735-1865" (1969), the English demographer and historian Michael Drake presented an enlarged documentation on vaccination and potato cultivation, and tried to evaluate the possible effects of each. In his opinion, the amelioration of nutrition was by far the most important factor behind the fall in mortality.

An even stronger turn in the direction of agrarian history took place in 1975 when Kåre Lunden gave the lecture "The Cultivation of Potatoes and the Acceleration of Population Growth in Norway after 1815" as part of the defence of his doctoral dissertation. Lunden did not dispute that the country was gradually better fed after 1815, but claimed that the contribution of the potato had been small (less than one fifth of the increase in the food supply measured in calories). Several scholars joined in the discussion opened up by Lunden. As a whole, the debate since 1969 has provided valuable new knowledge on Norwegian agriculture and nutrition in the early 19th century. But I personally doubt if we have got any closer to a solution of the original question, the causes of the mortality decline.

The few scholars maintaining a more strict demographic perspective have taken quite extreme stands. Kjell Haarstad (1980) claims to have demonstrated a close connection between official appraisements of grain and the crude death rate, which should indicate the important role plaid by nutrition. Rolf Engelsen (1983) argues that the social differences in mortality about 1800 were small, and thereby shifts the emphasis from food and economy to epidemics and disease.

What seems quite evident, however, is that the recent agrarian and demographic discussions both have forgotten *smallpox vaccination.*

The aim of the investigation

In this paper, we intend to explore source material and approaches with a view to renew the study of smallpox vaccination and its demographic effects.

Let us start by making a few summary observations and deductions: We do not have statistics on causes of death from the period concerned. Consequently, it is impossible to ascertain how many died from smallpox before and after the decree of 1810. If we are to believe results from smaller areas where causes were registered, or observations from abroad, between 5 and 15 percent of all deaths may be attributed to smallpox. These numbers are extremely uncertain. However, if we tentatively say that 10 percent is valid for our country, a complete disappearance of smallpox will represent a decline of about 2.5 per 1000 in the Norwegian crude death rate. This is less than half the actual decline about 1815. It is still sufficient to confirm the importance of vaccination.

But the 10 percent is a mere guess. In addition, we need to know whether vaccination became effective immediately or only gradually. Thus, we have to consider the *practice of vaccination.* We are lucky to possess sources which allow that. In the Norwegian parish registers of the 1820 model (adopted somewhat later in most parishes) there is a separate section for vaccinations. In the registers of the 1812 model a column was reserved for information on vaccination in the section of confirmed, and from 1820 the same information was collected from people who married. The decree of 1810 stated that no one could present himself to any of these ceremonies without a certificate of vaccination. Not only do these sources tell how protection against smallpox was built in the population. They also name those persons who were naturally immune through having suffered the disease. This particular information offers clues to the actual outbreaks of smallpox, replacing in some way the causes of death in the registers.

In the present paper advances will be made into some of these fields. We are conducting a micro study, which imposes severe restrictions both on statistical significance and the possibilities of generalisation. The effort might nonetheless be of some methodological interest.

The practice of vaccination

The vaccination lists proper for the parish of Etne start as late as 1832. Earlier, the number of vaccinated can only be reconstructed retrospectively, by information given for all those who pass confirmation (from 1816) and marriage (from 1831). This means that the number of vaccinated may be somewhat greater than can be traced. Some of those confirmed before 1816 must have been vaccinated, and some vaccinated children presumably died before reaching registration at confirmation from 1816 onwards. In a table presented later we shall see that the number of deceased children between the ages of infancy and confirmation is quite low in the actual period, so the loss is probably small.

How is the date of vaccination to be understood? The standard certificate contained no less than three different dates: That of the vaccination, that of the vaccinator's control of the result and issue of the certificate, and that of the parish priest's verification of person and certificate. When vaccination is declared in connection with confirmation or marriage, we have reason to believe that the date is that of the issue of certificate. But when the vaccination lists proper begin in 1832, registration is normally done only twice a year, and the date refers to the day when the vicar convened children and parents, checked scars and put his signature of final approval on the certificates. For reasons of convenience we have used these dates and not taken the bother of correcting them when certificates are mentioned later at the moment of confirmation or marriage. From 1832 onwards registration thus lags the factual vaccination, but probably never by more than half a year.

The vicar Jørgen Brochmand was the first to practice Jenner's invention in Etne. In 1806 and 1807 he vaccinated five children from adjacent farms — he had no children of his own. Two persons vaccinated in 1811 and 1812 have been found, and then comes the tremendous break-through: 227 vaccinations during a mass operation in 1813. A gentleman called Wisbech was in charge most of the time. A certain Mr. Knudsen also signed a few certificates that year, as well as one called Niels Svendsen, who continued to vaccinate until 1820.

Who were they? Christian Wisbech (1740-1822) was from 1789 county surgeon in Søndre Bergenhus (now Hordaland). Fredrik Tobias Knudsen (1785-) was a dyer and a merchant living in Bergen except for the years 1809-1811, when he stayed first in Etne and later in the neighbouring parish Fjelberg where he owned a farm. He had started to experiment with vaccination on his own, but in 1813 he was probably engaged in public service. Niels Svendsen was a school teacher and deacon residing at Tungesvik in Skånevik, the parish north of Etne. He was appointed vaccinator for the three parishes Skånevik, Fjelberg and Etne.

Not until 1821 do people from Etne itself take over. That year the farmer's son Velom Torsson Ekrheim started vaccinating, and he was replaced in 1825 by the farmer and shopkeeper Jan Berntsson Børretzen. In the late 1830s the farmer Lars Bjørnsson Hordland was working alongside Børretzen.

Figure 1 shows the annual number of vaccinated persons to 1840, the terminus of this study. Until the end of 1840, a total of 1591 persons had got artificial protection against smallpox in the parish of Etne. No dissimilarities appear according to sex. The two main social groups (farmers and cottagers) are represented in the vaccination material as they were in the actual population. Since no bias is observed according to sex or social status, these characteristics will be left out of the following analysis.

The striking feature of Figure 1 is the violent annual fluctuations in the number of vaccinated persons, going on till the late 1830s. The early vaccinations had the character of big razzias. This is understandable before 1820, when outside agents were in charge of the work. It becomes more intriguing after 1820, when Etne had its own vaccinators. Did for instance the supply of vaccine constitute a bottle-neck?

Figure 1. Vaccination in the parish of Etne 1806-1840

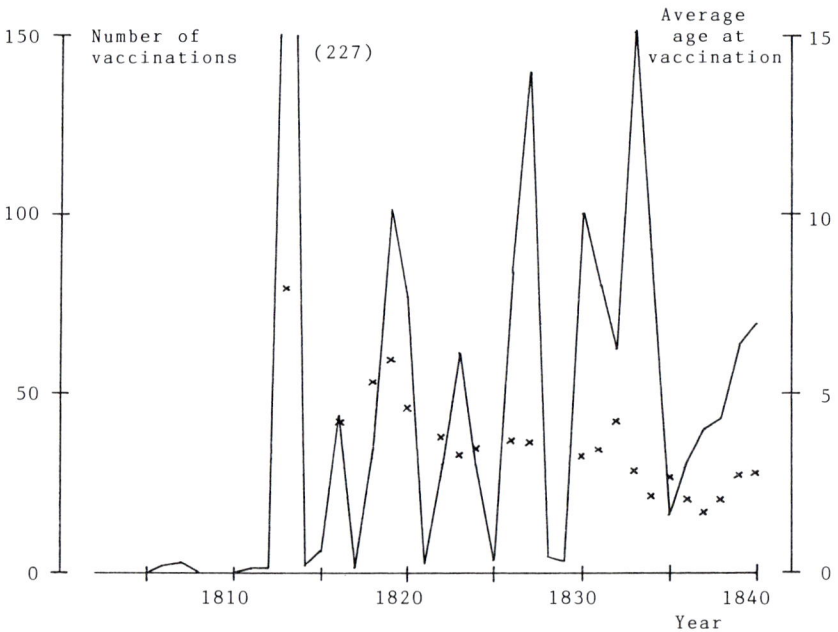

Another interesting aspect of the vaccination practice is the age distribution. To prevent strange effects, we will exclude persons over 15 years of age — they were very few in any case. The average age of the remaining persons is plotted into Figure 1 (leaving out years with less than 10 vaccinations). As had to be expected, average age is quite high in the opening year of 1813, almost 8 years. The distribution is smooth and large, with modal values a little over the average, in ages 9-11. Only six infants (aged less than one year) are to be found. After this start the average age centers on 4-5 years up to the 1830s, when it suddenly declines to 2-3 years. The main reason for that is that the vaccination of infants became much more extensive from 1833 onwards.

What conclusions should be drawn from these observations? It took a long time to establish a regular practice of vaccination. Not until the 1830s was a routine vaccination practice established. Both the unstable frequency and the high average age at vaccination made the number of unprotected children in the population before 1830 dangerously high. Then we have not even checked that *all* were vaccinated sooner or later.

This is an important point. The population of Etne was 1412 in 1801 and rose to 2416 in 1845. A total of approximately 1600 vaccinations before 1840 suggests that one was far from the goal of reaching all the inhabitants. But a comparison of this kind in fact makes no sense. Earlier, when the smallpox epidemics were ravaging, natural immunity was conferred to those who got the disease and survived. At the start in 1813 a considerable part of the children and certainly a majority of the youths and adults were already protected. The aim of the vaccinators was to protect the arriving cohorts of children, preferably at the lowest age possible. The 1600 vaccinated persons should not be compared to the total population, but to the number of births during the same period. From 1813 to 1840 about 2500 children were born in the parish. Even if many of these died early in life, we now realize that the coverage *may* have been dubious. To investigate this question further, we shall proceed to a cohort analysis.

Vaccination in the birth cohorts

The present study comprises all inhabitants of Etne born from 1771 to 1840 inclusive, both natives and in-migrants. According to the type of vaccination information, they are divided into three categories:

1. Data on vaccination is lacking.
2. "Natural smallpox" (having had the disease).
3. The date of vaccination is known.

In Table 1 the persons are arranged in five-year birth cohorts, with natives and immigrants in separate columns. As was to be expected, a gradual transfer from type 1 to type 3 takes place as one moves forward in time, but even in the

Table 1. Birth cohorts of natives and immigrants according to the type of vaccination information.

Birth cohort	Natives			Immigrants		
	Unkn.	Nat.	Vacc.	Unkn.	Nat.	Vacc.
1771—1775	192	6	0	47	4	0
1776—1780	196	9	0	68	3	0
1781—1785	176	10	0	57	5	0
1786—1790	190	15	0	56	6	0
1791—1795	213	30	3	67	11	0
1796—1800	208	27	25	46	11	2
1801—1805	106	15	134	61	14	24
1806—1810	100	16	117	61	6	30
1811—1815	66	10	145	33	2	34
1816—1820	58	9	217	52	5	35
1821—1825	69	46	217	48	5	37
1826—1830	81	14	265	27	0	39
1831—1835	80	26	262	40	4	45
1836—1840	69	1	299	44	0	69

youngest cohorts there remains a considerable number without information. As already mentioned this does not immediately signify that a lot of children escaped vaccination. In this category are included all those who died shortly after birth, at an age when the question of vaccination had not yet arisen. Immigrants pose a more serious problem. Since we have not checked vaccination lists in their places of origin, only confirmation or marriage inside Etne can inform us about them. There is no reason to believe that the immigrants generally were in a different situation according to vaccination than the natives. In the following tables we shall therefore concentrate on the native inhabitants of Etne.

In order to obtain a more correct impression of how vaccination was extended into the birth cohorts, we shall in the next step limit the group under scrutiny to native born residents of the parish who survived to their 15th birthday. What was their ultimate status according to vaccination? Did people and vicar obey the order that no one should be allowed to confirmation or marriage without having had "natural smallpox" or being vaccinated? For once, this table will also separate according to sex.

We have now obtained a picture that is more revealing. From the birth cohort 1811-1815 onwards vaccination becomes practically general. What surprises us, and this will be discussed later in the paper, is that a significant number still receive "vaccination" in the natural way, by having real smallpox.

Table 2. Birth cohorts of boys and girls attaining 15 years of age, according to type of vaccination information. Native born only.

Birth cohort	Boys Unkn.	Nat.	Vacc.	Girls Unkn.	Nat.	Vacc.
1771—1775	50	4	0	51	2	0
1776—1780	47	4	0	52	4	0
1781—1785	40	3	0	54	7	0
1786—1790	41	10	0	49	5	0
1791—1795	62	9	2	60	20	1
1796—1800	53	8	14	60	19	11
1801—1805	9	9	69	12	6	65
1806—1810	10	8	55	14	8	59
1811—1815	3	4	66	1	6	78
1816—1820	0	6	94	0	3	98
1821—1830	0	15	110	0	30	79
1826—1835	2	10	126	1	4	106
1836—1845	0	8	111	0	15	114
1846—1850	1	1	125	0	0	120

Table 3. Age at vaccination for children attaining their 15th anniversary, in selected birth cohorts. Native born only.

Age	1801—05	1806—10	1816—20	1826—30	1831—35	1836—40
0	0	0	14	12	41	29
1	0	0	30	61	101	61
2	1	8	29	64	31	48
3	2	14	26	41	7	23
4	0	17	11	30	9	17
5	0	17	23	9	9	9
6	0	14	15	3	4	9
7	9	6	14	2	5	5
8	13	3	5	2	1	2
9	22	6	6	0	2	1
10	31	10	3	0	2	6
11	26	7	5	1	0	8
12	13	0	1	0	1	2
13	2	4	1	0	3	3
14	6	0	8	5	6	17
15	0	8	1	2	3	5
Total	134	114	192	232	225	245
Average	10.4	6.6	4.8	3.1	2.8	4.3

(The average age is calculated on the basis of vaccinations done before the 15th birthday.)

Table 4. Percentages of vaccinated children in different age groups at the end of the years 1820, 1830 and 1840. Native born only.

Age	1820	1830	1840
0	6	2	4
1	31	16	47
2	40	39	71
3—4	63	53	78
5—6	72	73	74
7—9	78	71	87
10—14	68	89	92
Sum			
0—14	58	62	74

But even if it is now evident that all were finally vaccinated or immunized, the moment, that is to say the age at which vaccination took place, remains to be investigated in the new cohort perspective. Table 3 starts with the first five-year cohort that underwent massive vaccination, that of 1801-1805. At this early stage, mainly children between 10 and 15 years were vaccinated, but then the modal age embarks upon a long decline, to about 10, then to 5, then to 2 and finally down to 1 year of age. But the good clustering obtained during this process does not last: In the cohort born 1836-1840 we can observe an increasing leak by persons who avoid vaccination and are not caught until the eve of confirmation.

Now let us try to capture the native-born population at three points in time, to see what proportions of children in the different age groups were protected against smallpox (Table 4).

In 1820 close to 60 percent of the children were protected through vaccination. The proportion hardly changed up to 1830. Among the youngest under 5 years of age it even declined, but this was counterbalanced through a better coverage among those over 10 years. However, considerable progress was done in the course of the following decade. In 1840 three quarters of the children under 15 were vaccinated, and protection of the very youngest was strikingly ameliorated.

The preceding discussion of the practice of vaccination may be summarized in the following way: In spite of the massive effort from the start in 1813, at least two decades passed until vaccinations assured a satisfactory protection against smallpox in the population. Measured as the percentage vaccinated before the age of confirmation, coverage was quite good already in the early phase. But it was not until the 1830s that a majority of children were vaccinated in the first years of their life. In fact, it might be argued that the population in the period 1813-1830 was left gradually *less* protected against smallpox if new cohorts of children escaped the earlier natural immunization without having it fully replaced by the artificial one. This particular subject will be discussed later. To summarize, defence against smallpox was not set up at the moment the Royal Decree was issued in 1810. Neither was it established after the mass vaccination of 227 children in 1813. It was only slowly becoming a reality in the 1830s.

Smallpox in the pre-vaccination period

We shall now turn our attention from the medical action against smallpox to the disease itself. The first objective is to find out how smallpox acted in the period before vaccination, for practical reasons limited to the 25 years from 1776 to 1800. In later sections we shall try to shed some light upon the question of when and how smallpox was eradicated.

The task may seem difficult. No source will tell us who were ill or what diseases prevailed. The parish registers show who died, but causes of death are only incidentally declared before the middle of the 19th century. The historian is therefore forced to trace epidemics by means of the mere *number* of deceased children.

Table 5 contains information on annual births and deaths under 15 years of age from 1776 to 1800. Please note that only children born from 1771 onwards are counted in the latter category: Due to this, there is a certain under-registration of deaths in some age groups until 1785.

The age groups under 10 are the most interesting ones, particularly the 1-4 years group. Four major years of mortality can be pointed out: 1779, 1786, 1791 and 1798. In 1779 and 1791 mortality also spills over into the following year. We have no guarantee that epidemics caused these concentrations of deaths, even if this is likely. The local sources do not mention diseases in the actual period. Consequently, the four peaks should be investigated more closely.

Epidemics are usually conceived as being short and intense. Unfortunately, the chronological pattern can only be studied in 1798, as the vicars earlier had the bad habit of leaving out dates. In 1798 deaths are concentrated between April and August. This confirms our suspicion of an epidemic. In spite of the uncertainties of dating, we will include deaths in 1780 and 1792 in those of the preceding years, presuming them to belong to the same eruption of disease.

Table 5 indicates the number of deaths in different ages. It may also be useful to relate deaths to the groups at risk. But who were exposed? If we are in presence of smallpox, those who get the disease and survive will be out of danger later. For this reason it may be useful also to make a calculation which only puts children born after the latest epidemic in the group at risk. This has been done in Table 6.

It appeared from Table 5 that the age group 1-4 was most seriously afflicted during these years of death. The first calculation in Table 6 confirms this, but age differences are somewhat smoothened when one takes into account that some of the older children might have been immunized by earlier epidemics.

Table 5. Annual births and deaths in the age groups 0—14 years in the period 1776—1800. Deaths only counted in the birth cohorts from 1771 onwards. The whole population.

Year	Births	Deaths				Total deaths
		0	1—4	5—9	10—14	1—9
1776	44	11	0	(0)	—	0
1777	40	9	1	(0)	—	1
1778	42	9	2	(0)	—	2
1779	28	14	8	(2)	—	+ 10
1780	51	12	5	(2)	—	+ 7
1781	43	10	1	0	(0)	1
1782	33	9	0	1	(0)	1
1783	35	11	2	1	(1)	3
1784	41	8	3	1	(0)	4
1785	34	7	1	0	(1)	1
1786	31	7	5	4	4	+ 9
1787	45	10	1	0	0	1
1788	41	17	0	0	0	0
1789	38	11	1	0	0	1
1790	50	13	2	1	0	3
1791	43	18	16	3	3	+ 19
1792	58	10	4	2	0	+ 6
1793	51	7	0	0	0	0
1794	49	11	3	0	0	3
1795	45	9	0	0	0	0
1796	57	9	2	0	2	2
1797	46	14	3	0	0	3
1798	57	20	11	7	2	+ 18
1799	65	16	2	1	0	3
1800	35	5	2	2	1	4

— = no observations
( ) = partial coverage of the age group

Most commonly about 5 percent of the unprotected children seem to have died in the course of these outbreaks. Even if numbers are small, they suggest a majority of boys among the dead, as if their resistance to the disease was weaker.

Did this mortality also penetrate down into infant age? Answering that is difficult because many children less than one year old die also in normal years. Still peaks of infant deaths are traceable in all of the years except 1786. Counting shows that what sets the years 1779-1780, 1791-1792 and 1798 apart is an unusually high proportion of deaths over approximately 5 months' age. Between one third and one half of the infant deaths are in this age span, compared to less than one fifth in normal years. Our suspected epidemics

Table 6. Mortality during the four probable epidemics before 1800, according to age and type of exposed group.

Year		All in the age group			Born since the last ep.		
		1—4	5—9	10—14	1—4	5—9	10—14
1779	Deaths	8	2	0	8	2	0
—80	At risk	166	114	0	166	114	0
	Quotient	0.05	0.02	—	0.05	0.02	—
1786	Deaths	5	4	4	5	4	4
	At risk	151	194	165	151	76	0
	Quotient	0.03	0.02	0.02	0.03	0.05	—
1791	Deaths	20	5	3	16	3	3
—92	At risk	151	179	179	151	0	0
	Quotient	0.13	0.03	0.02	0.13	—	—
1798	Deaths	11	7	2	11	7	2
	At risk	204	218	180	204	135	0
	Quotient	0.05	0.03	0.01	0.05	0.05	—

therefore seem to hit the older half of the babies. In fact mortality is extremely high: Out of approximately 20-25 exposed infants each year, 7 die in 1779-1780, 10 in 1791-1792 and 7 in 1798.

As far as infants were concerned, we got a deviant mortality pattern in 1786. This year also exhibits a different geographical spread of the disease. Most of the deaths this year are confined to only two farms or hamlets. Not so in 1779-1780, 1791-1792 and 1798 when the fatal cases are quite evenly dispersed throughout the parish, in good accordance with the number of children living in each locality.

On the basis of this analysis we will put forward the hypothesis that the parish was in fact visited by epidemics during the four occasions of accumulated deaths among children. We suggest that the disease was smallpox in 1779-1780, 1791-1792 and 1798, but leave the question open as regards 1786, due to its particular age pattern and geographic extension. It might have been another child epidemic, for instance measles.

Was smallpox eradicated through vaccination?

We now turn to the 19th century and continue Table 5 in the new Table 7.

The main impression is that after 1800 children did not experience years of death comparable to those in 1798 and earlier, although the population was growing and the exposed groups likewise. We nonetheless find years with a noticeable number of fatalities in the younger age groups. Were they caused by smallpox, or should they be imputed to other diseases?

In the search for an answer, four ways are open to us. Firstly, we can look for common characteristics between these years of death and those of the previous century. Small absolute numbers and spurious variations make this procedure less recommendable. The second solution consists in searching the parish register for some mention of cause of death. We may have luck in one or the other of the actual years. Thirdly, we can utilize the information we possess on "natural smallpox", that is, immunity conferred by the disease itself. Fourthly, we may try to collect information on smallpox epidemics outside of our parish.

Searching the parish registers gives a meager harvest, but it might turn up a valuable one:

1830: Two deaths from measles
1831: Two deaths from measles
1834: One death from smallpox
1835: Three deaths from smallpox
1840: One death from smallpox

All of a sudden, we have documented the presence of smallpox in three different years. The cases from 1834 and 1835 happened in rapid succession during the winter and probably belong to the same epidemic. Both in 1834-1835 and in 1840 our findings correspond to the peaks signalled in Table 7. The peak of 1831 might have been caused by the measles observed during the previous winter 1830-1831.

There is a lacuna of no less than 36 years from what we believed was a smallpox epidemic in 1798 until the next solid proof of smallpox in 1834. Did the disease really stay away from the parish during this considerable period? If we study the prevalence of "natural smallpox" (refer to Tables 1 and 2), the answer must be no.

The information on natural immunity is picked up in the lists of confirmation and of marriage. It tells us that the person has suffered the disease at some moment between his birth and the religious ceremony in case. To identify this moment may appear impossible. Still, let us try to arrange the occurrences of natural immunity according to the person's year of birth (Table 8).

The persons carrying natural immunity do not distribute randomly according to year of birth. By rule of the thumb, four concentrations may be delimited: 1799-1800, 1804-1806, 1821-1823 and 1832-1835. For those born after the introduction of mass vaccination in 1813, a kind of race will take place between attracting smallpox and being vaccinated. If we presume roughly (see Table 3) that vaccination happened at an average age of 3 years for those born in the 1820s and 2 years for those born in the 1830s, we are tuning in smallpox epidemics about 1822-1826 and 1833-1837.

506

Table 7. Annual births and deaths among children 0—14 years of age during the period 1801—1840.

Year	Births	Deaths				Total deaths 1—9
		0	1—4	5—9	10—14	
1801	56	7	2	1	0	3
1802	59	14	2	1	1	3
1803	40	9	3	1	0	4
1804	58	15	3	0	0	3
1805	42	7	0	0	0	0
1806	56	15	0	0	0	0
1807	38	9	2	0	0	2
1808	58	10	0	0	0	0
1809	46	12	2	0	0	2
1810	35	8	6	1	0	+ 7
1811	45	10	0	1	1	1
1812	45	8	4	0	0	4
1813	41	4	0	0	0	0
1814	36	8	2	1	1	3
1815	54	11	0	0	0	0
1816	53	12	0	1	0	1
1817	50	11	0	0	0	0
1818	52	7	1	0	0	1
1819	65	8	0	0	1	0
1820	64	11	3	0	1	3
1821	63	9	2	1	0	3
1822	73	9	2	0	0	2
1823	68	16	4	1	0	+ 5
1824	69	11	2	0	1	2
1825	59	7	0	0	0	0
1826	85	12	2	0	1	2
1827	69	14	4	2	0	+ 6
1828	68	10	9	0	0	+ 9
1829	73	8	2	0	1	2
1830	65	17	3	2	3	+ 5
1831	70	20	7	1	1	+ 8
1832	72	13	0	0	0	0
1833	75	9	1	1	0	2
1834	74	12	10	0	1	+ 10
1835	77	14	8	1	2	+ 9
1836	85	21	1	0	2	1
1837	65	10	1	0	1	1
1838	71	12	0	0	3	0
1839	75	7	3	1	0	4
1840	73	8	5	1	2	+ 6

Table 8. Persons with natural smallpox according to year of birth 1799—1840. Native born only.

Year of birth	Persons	Year of birth	Persons	Year of birth	Persons
1799	+ 8	1813	1	1827	4
1800	+ 7	1814	2	1828	4
1801	1	1815	3	1829	2
1802	3	1816	4	1830	1
1803	0	1817	1	1831	3
1804	+ 9	1818	1	1832	+ 7
1805	2	1819	3	1833	+ 5
1806	+ 7	1820	0	1834	+ 6
1807	1	1821	+ 16	1835	+ 5
1808	3	1822	+ 9	1836	0
1809	3	1823	+ 12	1837	1
1810	2	1824	4	1838	0
1811	1	1825	5	1839	0
1812	3	1826	3	1840	0

A glance at Table 7 shows an upsurge in childrens' deaths in 1823, 1823-1828 and 1834-1835. We already know that smallpox visited the parish in 1834-1835 and 1840. The deaths in 1827-1828 have to be considered outside the actual area of search, while 1823 is inside and therefore will be retained as a possible smallpox epidemic. For the period immediately after 1800, the delimitation of the disease is more intricate. We are inclined to believe that outbreaks must have occurred before the start of vaccination in 1813. Using Table 7 once more, we find that 1810 stands out as a possible epidemic year.

By combining observations of years of unusual child mortality, years of birth of persons having natural smallpox, and random information on causes of death, we have arrived at the following list of epidemics:

Illustration A

Year	Disease	Degree of certainty
1810	Smallpox	Possible
1823	Smallpox	Possible
1827—1828	Measles	Uncertain
1830—1831	Measles	Certain
1834—1835	Smallpox	Certain
1840	Smallpox	Certain

It may be of interest to compare these findings with information available on smallpox epidemics in other parts of Norway and the Nordic countries:

Illustration B

Etne	Northern Norway	Eastern Norway	Sweden	Åland Islands	Finland
1798	1798—1803	1801—1802	1799—1801	1799—1801	1798—1899
					1803—1804
1810	1810—1811	1808—1810	1807—1809		1808—1809
				1814—1815	1813—1814
					1820
1823			1824—1827	1823—1824	1822—1824
1834—1835 (no data available)			1831—1834	1833	1832—1833
1840			1838—1844	1840—1841	1839—1840

Sources: Brockmann (1936), Sogner (1979), Mielke et al. (1984).

Even if Norwegian material after 1815 is lacking in this Tableau, the number and timing of smallpox outbreaks are surprisingly similar throughout the Nordic countries. Smallpox appears in great pandemics, and we are tempted to interpret these findings as a confirmation of our assumption concerning the disease in the parish of Etne.

The four certain or probable smallpox epidemics will now be studied from three points of view: Calendar time pattern, level of mortality (in age groups over one year and among infants) and geographical diffusion.

In 1840 deaths are accumulated from January to May, in a pattern that might be called epidemic. 1834-1835 is different: Deaths are quite evenly spread from January 1834 through October 1835. In 1823 and 1810 deaths are fewer, but quite concentrated again: October-December in 1823 and April-September in 1810. These observations do not bring us far, perhaps: We possess evidence of both short and long outbreaks in the two certain years of smallpox, but only find short durations in the two probable years. In this respect, they remind us of 1798.

During the examination of the 18th century epidemics, we tried to delimit realistic risk groups in order to have a good estimate of the mortality. The task is difficult because one never knows who has had the disease previously and obtained immunity. This point loses importance after the start of vaccination. At the four possible outbreaks of smallpox after 1800 we will consider all no-vaccinated persons as belonging to the risk group. The classification of children later declared as naturally immune creates a problem, as we do not know the date of their immunization. But if there were no more epidemics than the four traced by us, it should be quite safe to include all children born after an epidemic in the risk group at the outbreak of the following. We shall

509

also consider all the deaths in a year of disease as deaths from smallpox. Now even a third dimension can be reconstructed: The number of those who got the disease. If smallpox had only two outcomes, dying or surviving with natural immunity, the sick can be found by adding these two groups (from Tables 7 and 8). This is done in Table 9 for the age group 1-9 years. The possible years of smallpox can then be compared according to two measures: The proportion of the risk group attracting the disease, and the proportion of the sick dying.

One would expect the disease to be hampered in attaining its possible victims as the risk group was reduced in the wake of vaccination. The opposite seems to happen, however: Smallpox attacks increasing percentages of the unprotected. Lethality (deaths among the sick) reaches its lowest point in 1823 by 11 percent and subsequently rises tremendously. An extremely dangerous variant haunts the parish in 1834-1835, and only the small risk group keeps the number of deaths down. But in 1840, something new is intervening and disrupts one of the longtime trends: Lethality has sky-rocketed (because of the small numbers, it should not be dramatized), but in spite of an increased risk group, the disease gets through to only 5 percent of the exposed persons.

The small number of deaths during the outbreaks prevents a thorough analysis of possible geographical patterns. However, it looks as if all the epidemics spread evenly or randomly in the parish. This observation is corroborated by the distribution of children having obtained natural immunity. The pattern appears quite reasonable in case of a disease that is extremely contagious and difficult to constrain in an early phase of outbreak. Exactly in this respect, a very interesting change may have taken place between the two certain smallpox epidemics in 1834-1835 and 1840. Because of extensive vaccination of children of low age in 1833, the exposed group was much reduced when smallpox erupted early in 1834 (see Table 9). It should have been feasible to round up and suffocate the disease. Instead, it lingered on in the population for one year and a half. This is not only an indication that the epidemic was dangerous, but also that preventive measures were lacking.

Table 9. Cases of sickness and death during smallpox epidemics 1810—1840. The age group 1—9 years.

Epidemic	Risk group	Sick = dead + immune	Deaths	Percentage of sickness lethality	
1810	336	36	7	11	19
1823	206	44	5	21	11
1834—35	81	53	19	65	36
1840	138	7	6	5	86

When smallpox reappeared in 1840, the initial situation was much more un-favorable. Vaccinating in the previous years was below standard and the risk group had expanded considerably since 1834. Still the outbreak was brief, causing a few deaths but only one single immunization. The possible inter-pretation could be that the parish was visited by the same aggressive variant of smallpox as in 1834-1835, but that it was arrested this time by measures taken against the mechanisms of contagion. If this is true, we have met the first case of an "administrative" campaign against the disease.

We now turn to the subject of how the epidemics hit infants. 1834-1835 shows no particular effect on the total of infant deaths (Table 7). Out of 26 dead under one year of age, 6 have passed 6 months of age, a proportion that differs so little from the average that it is very doubtful if smallpox reached in-fants at all. In 1840 data are more scarce, but the results even more clear-cut: At most one out of 8 infant deaths takes place in an age span where smallpox can be suspected. During the epidemics of 1810 and 1823 all infants die less than 6 months old, and only one is over 3 months age. Consequently, smallpox should be left out as a cause of death.

Concluding this discussion of mortality and lethality, one common characteristic of the 18th century epidemics has to be mentioned: There is a pronounced surplus of boys among the dead. We suggested earlier that this might be due to a lower resistance in boys. The latest epidemics allow us to develop that point. Table 2 showed that in birth cohorts after 1820 a greater number of girls than boys got natural immunization. We conclude from this that girls were at least as vulnerable as boys in getting the disease. The majori-ty of boys among the dead therefore demonstrates that the difference resided in lethality.

Conclusions

In the previous section we have seen that smallpox did not vanish when vac-cination began in 1813, but continued to visit the parish till 1840 and even later. Still it is obvious that the disease counts less in the total pattern of mor-tality than before 1800. How then can this change be explained?

Vaccination may have had a positive effect in two ways. It reduced the size of the exposed part of the population. It may even have facilitated the discovery and arrest of the disease when the chains of contagion became weaker and diffusion slower. But our investigation indicates that these favorable effects did not have any real break-through until the 1830s, and not even then in a manner that offered full security against smallpox epidemics. In fact, we can observe a relapse after a good effort of vaccination around 1833. During the last outbreak in 1840, the lucky outcome should probably be ascribed as much to administrative action as to vaccination.

For events between the 1798 epidemic and the outbreaks of the 1830s, vac-cination probably is of minor importance. It is surprising that only two possi-ble epidemics, both of them mild, can be pin-pointed during this period. We know little about the development in neighbouring parishes and districts, but it does not seem likely that the practice of vaccination or the measures of quarantine differed much from those of our parish. The immediate explanation of the mild interregnum should apparently be sought in the disease itself: Smallpox had changed, not the inhabitants of Etne or their environment. The society we are investigating did not experience great changes between the late 18th century and 1840. Nevertheless, there are two striking alterations in the way smallpox manifests itself. Firstly, it ceases to claim victims among infants after 1798, at the same time as the spacing of epidemics increases. Secondly, evidence is quite convincing that the variant of smallpox which visited the parish in 1834-1835 and 1840 was more virulent than any observed from 1779-1780 till 1823. This change is quite impossible to explain by any reference to living conditions in the 1830s compared to earlier. The same has to be said about the mild epidemics of the preceding 35 years.

We therefore end by drawing the conclusion that smallpox got less virulent after 1798 due to a mutation of the disease itself. A new and much more serious type of smallpox appeared in the 1830s. Only from that decade did vaccination have any impact upon the mortality of the parish.

If the case of Etne is representative of the whole country, as it may well be, our results will force us to give up vaccination as a factor in the mortality decline of Norway at the end of the Napoleonic Wars. Instead, a notable role must have been played by smallpox itself, which for some decades turned less dangerous. Long-term fluctuations of this kind were nothing new — they can be traced back into the early 18th century. Human action through vaccination did not become of any importance until a quarter of a century after the spectacular fall of mortality about 1815.

References

Brochmann, S.W, 'Bidrag til epidemienes historie i Norge i eldre tider', *Tidsskrift for Den Norske Laegeforening* (saertrykk), 7-24 (1936).

Drake, Michael, *Population and Society in Norway 1735-1865* (Cambridge 1969).

Engelsen, Rolf, 'Mortalitetsdebatten og sosiale skilnader i mortalitet', *Historisk tidsskrift*, 2 (1983).

Haarstad, Kjell, 'Sult, sykdom, død. Et teoretisk problem belyst med empirisk materiale', *Historisk tidsskrift*, 1 (1980).

Lunden, Kåre, 'Potetdyrkinga og den raskare folketalsvoksteren i Noreg frå 1815', *Historisk tidsskrift*, 4 (1975).

Malm, Ole, *Kopper og vaccination i Norge* (Oslo 1915).

Mielke, James H., et al, 'Historical Epidemiology of Smallpox in Åland, Finland: 1751-1890', *Demography*, 21, 3 (1984).

Sogner, Sølvi, *Folkevekst og flytting. En historisk demografisk studie i 1700-årenes Ost-Norge* (Oslo 1979).

Contributors

Tommy Bengtsson, Dept. of Economic History, University of Lund, Sweden

Anders Brändström, Dept. of Historical Demography, Umeå University, Sweden

Gösta Carlsson, Dept. of Sociology, University of Stockholm, Sweden

Reinhold Castensson, Graduate School of Water in Environment and Society, University of Linköping, Sweden

Mats Danielsson, Demographic Data Base, Umeå University, Sweden

Ståle Dyrvik, Dept. of History, University of Bergen, Norway

Robert W. Fogel, Graduate School of Business, Center for Population Studies, University of Chicago, USA

Gunnar Fridlizius, Dept. of Economic History, University of Lund, Sweden

Jean-Pierre Goubert, École des Hautes Études en Sciences Sociales, Centre de Recherces Historiques, Paris, France

Fritz Hodne, Dept. of Economic History, School of Economics and Business Administration, Bergen, Norway

Ulf Högberg, Dept. of Obstetrics and Gynecology, Umeå University, Sweden

Karin Johannisson, Dept. of History of Science and Ideas, Uppsala University, Sweden

Gerry Kearns, Dept. of Geography, University of Liverpool, England

John Knodel, Population Studies Center, University of Michigan, USA

Øivind Larsen, Dept. of Medical History, University of Oslo, Norway

Margareta Larsson, Dept. of Sociology, University of Stockholm, Sweden

Robert Lee, Institute for European Population Studies, University of Liverpool, England

D. Ingemar D. Lindahl, Dept. of Social Medicine, Huddinge University Hospital, Sweden

Ulla-Britt Lithell, International Health Unit, Dept. of Paediatrics, Uppsala University, Sweden

Marianne Löwgren, Graduate School of Water in Environment and Society, University of Linköping, Sweden

Dan Mellström, Dept. of Geriatric and Long-Term Care Medicine, University of Göteborg, Sweden

Marie C. Nelson, Dept. of History, Uppsala University, Sweden

Hans Norman, Dept. of History, Uppsala University, Sweden

Eva Nyström, Dept. of History of Ideas, University of Stockholm, Sweden

Per-Gunnar Ottosson, Graduate School of Health and Society, University of Linköping, Sweden

John Rogers, Dept. of History, Uppsala University, Sweden

Margit Rosenberg, Dept. of Informatics, University of Oslo, Norway

Walter Rödel, Historisches Seminar, Johannes Gutenberg-Universität, Mainz, Federal Republic of Germany

Sølvi Sogner, Dept. of History, University of Oslo, Norway

Jan Sundin, Graduate School of Health and Society, University of Linköping, Sweden

Oiva Turpeinen, Dept. of History, University of Helsinki, Finland

Peter Ward, Dept. of History, University of British Columbia, Canada

Sune Åkerman, Dept. of History, Umeå University, Sweden